Common Medical Problems in the Tropics

Third Edition

A reference manual for health workers in health centres and small hospitals

Christopher R. Schull

MB BS (Hons) (Qld), DPH (Eng), FRACP

Senior Lecturer,
School of Medicine,
The University of Queensland,
Australia

Consultant Physician,
Thoracic and Sleep Medicine,
Greenslopes Private Hospital,
Brisbane, Australia

Formerly Specialist Medical Officer (Physician),
Madang; and Honorary Senior Lecturer and
Clinical Tutor (Internal Medicine) College of Allied Health
Sciences, Madang, Papua New Guinea

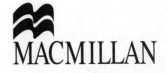
MACMILLAN

Macmillan Education

Between Towns Road, Oxford OX4 3PP

A division of Macmillan Publishers Limited

Companies and representatives throughout the world

www.macmillan-africa.com

ISBN: 978-0-230-03104-3

First edition 1987

Second edition 1999

Third edition 2010

Designed by Macmillan Publishers Limited

Illustrated by Tech Type

Cover design by Macmillan Publishers Limited

Cover illustrations by Tim Kahane

Macmillan Education received assistance in the production of this third edition from the members of the Queensland Branch of the Australian Medical Association in Australia.

Printed and bound in Malaysia

2014 2013 2012 2011 2010
10 9 8 7 6 5 4 3 2 1

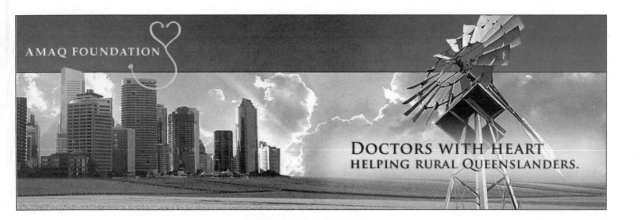

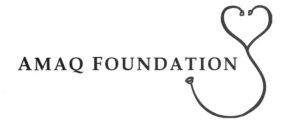

Judith,
who made this possible
and also
Rebecca, Susan, Marcus and Daniel

Contents

Foreword   vii
Preface to the First Edition   viii
Preface to the Second Edition   xi
Preface to the Third Edition   xii
Acknowledgements   xiii

1   On Being an Effective Health Worker   1
2   Some Clinical Definitions   7
3   Pathology   14
4   A Classification of Disease – the causes of diseases   16
5   Epidemiology   19
6   Diagnosis of Disease   21
7   Treatment, Drugs and Pain Relief   30
8   Notification of Disease and Death   36
9   Control and Prevention of Disease. Summary of patient management   37
10   Infection, Immunity, Immunisation and Allergy   40
11   Infectious Diseases, Chemotherapy and Universal Precautions   52
12   Septicaemia and other Acute Severe Bacterial Infections; and HIV Infection   64
13   Malaria   68
14   Tuberculosis   101
15   Leprosy   127
16   Some Common Infectious Diseases   151
17   Some Serious Acute Infectious Diseases with Limited Distribution   158
18   Some Serious Subacute and Chronic Infectious Diseases with Limited Distribution   173
19   Sexually Transmitted Diseases Including HIV Infection and AIDS   192
20   Disorders of the Respiratory System   262
21   Disorders of the Blood and the Blood Forming Organs   312
22   Disorders of the Lymphatic System and Spleen   330
23   Disorders of the Gastrointestinal System and Nutrition   346
24   Disorders of the Liver, Bile Ducts and Pancreas   390
25   Disorders of the Nervous System   403
26   Disorders of the Urinary System   437
27   Disorders of the Heart and Blood Vessels   456
28   Disorders of the Bones and Muscles   476
29   Disorders of Joints (Arthritis)   480
30   Disorders of the Endocrine Glands   495
31   Disorders of the Eye   505
32   Disorders of the Skin   521
33   Bites and Stings   554
34   Poisoning and Drug Abuse   561
35   Psychiatric Conditions   567
36   Some Common Symptoms and Signs   585
37   Emergency Resuscitation   606

Appendix: Incubation Periods   615
Useful Publications   616
Index   617

Important notes about drugs and drug doses

1. *Manufacturer's recommendations*. Always check the drugs you use with the manufacturer's recommendations (these are usually on a leaflet with the drugs) and with your country's treatment guidelines. The author has made every effort to ensure that the drugs and doses recommended in this book are the most appropriate for 'tropical countries' at the time of writing. However, errors and omissions may have occurred, or time and tests may have shown that other drugs or doses are better.

2. *Doses*. Use the doses of drugs given in weight, e.g. mcg or μg, mg or g. Where only one size of tablet or one strength of a solution is commonly used, the dose may also be given in brackets as number of tablets or volume of solution. Always use the dose of drug given by weight (and not the number of tablets or volume of solution) until you have checked that the strength of tablets or solution in the book is the same as that in use in your country.

3. *Drug doses and children*.

   All drug doses in this book are for adults.

   Some of the doses of drugs given to adults would be dangerous or even fatal for children.

   For details about children with diseases and especially for the correct doses of drugs for children, you MUST look in a book on child health and children's diseases.

4. *Drug doses and drug choices in all patients*. If your country has a national essential drugs list and/or standard treatment guidelines for drug doses, you MUST use those drugs and the doses listed in them. The drugs and doses recommended in these lists and guidelines will be the most safe and effective for people in your country.

Foreword

TALC is delighted that a further edition of this most useful book has been developed. At the present time, many standard books on tropical health are going out of print and *Common Medical Problems in the Tropics* is now perhaps the only low-cost widely available book for doctors and other health workers working in developing countries on adult tropical diseases. All those who practise medicine and the patients who receive better treatment thanks to this book owe Dr Chris Schull a very deep sense of gratitude. On their behalf I would like to express my sincere thanks. Dr Schull has not only undertaken a massive re-write, but also has been in touch with many experts around the world to make this book up to date. If this was not enough, he is accepting no royalties for all his months of work. He and his family have found the financial resources to bring this book to you at a phenomenally low price. His fellow Australians should be proud that he has made such a wealth of knowledge and experience available to some of the most needy populations worldwide.

David C. Morley
Emeritus Professor of Tropical Child Health
Institute of Child Health
University of London

Preface to the First Edition

If you are a health worker in a rural health centre in a tropical or developing country, this book was written specifically for you. If you are a health worker in a small provincial hospital, an urban health centre, or the outpatients' department of a large hospital, this book was written especially for you also. If you are a health worker of any other sort interested in the promotion of good health, prevention of disease and treatment of medical problems of adults in tropical and developing countries, this book was written for you too.

Most of you will be paramedical workers such as Health Extension Officers, Medical Assistants, Nurses and similar workers. Some of you will be Medical Officers working outside a large well-equipped hospital. Most of you will be doing most of the work which most medical 'general practitioners' in the industrialised western countries do. This book was written in the way it is as you usually (1) work without direct or easy contact with a Medical Officer in a well-equipped hospital; (2) cannot easily and quickly get pathology tests done in a reliable laboratory; but you (3) can refer or transfer patients to a Medical Officer in a hospital – if this is needed. An important feature of this book is helping you to make decisions based on clinical findings without waiting for laboratory help. It is very important for you to be able to do this, as experience in a number of countries has taught that even when laboratory services are supposed to be available, they are in fact not available or give very unreliable results which are misleading or even dangerous. Another important feature of this book is helping you to decide if and when a patient of yours should be referred or transferred to a Medical Officer in a hospital.

If you are a Medical Officer and especially if you are a consultant physician (in internal medicine), this book was written in the hope you also could use it – summarise it, expand it, or alter it, to make it specific and more useful for the health workers in the area in which you live and practise medicine. It is hoped you can do this without your having to first do all the groundwork to get basic information together and then make it relevant to the above health workers and the people in tropical and developing countries.

When you read this book, especially if you are a Medical Officer, please remember that some things stated as facts and some explanations given are so stated and so given for the Health Extension Officers, Medi-

cal Assistants and Nurses who have only a very short training in the basic medical sciences and pathology. Discussion of controversial subjects and pathophysiological explanations can be found in standard texts and journals.

This book grew out of work and teaching done with Health Extension Officers and Nurses in Papua New Guinea in the 10 years up to 1982, and also time previously spent in Nigeria and other places. The author worked for a year in a rural health centre without hospital facilities in post-war Nigeria and for another year in a rural health centre in Papua New Guinea. After these years, from a new position as consultant physician for an area as well as a hospital, the author regularly visited health centres and their staffs of paramedical workers and discussed with the staff all their patients and also any of their other problems. Also, all the adults with medical problems transferred by the health workers from health centres were received into the author's hospital ward. Also, about half the author's time each day was spent teaching paramedical workers in the half of the hospital ward which was run (with the aid of the trainee paramedical workers and their tutors) as a health centre and not a hospital ward. (All new urban patients were admitted to and managed in the health centre ward, and were transferred to the Medical Officer section of the ward only if transfer to Medical Officer and hospital care became necessary.) (Patients transferred from rural health centres were admitted directly to the Medical Officer section of the ward.) Half of most nights and the majority of most weekends were spent by not only the author but also his wife, devising the management regimes, the indications for transfer or referral of patients and all the other things which went into the preparation of books such as this. These regimens and books were then tried out by the health workers locally and later in all of Papua New Guinea; and then in the light of the usefulness or otherwise of parts of them, modifications were made and new editions of books produced. Many parts of these books, which some Medical Officers said should be removed, were left in because Health Extension Officers and Nurses repeatedly asked for that information and were certain it should not be removed.

This present book is a modification of the final reference book produced for Papua New Guinea *Adult*

Internal Medicine in Papua New Guinea – A Reference Book for Health Workers in Health Centres and Hospital Outpatients Departments, 1984, C.R. Schull, published by the Government Printer, Port Moresby, Papua New Guinea. The author was asked to try to make the Papua New Guinea book useful to paramedical workers in other parts of the world. The author realised that he was not knowledgeable enough or experienced enough to do this adequately. It was clear, however, after searching in vain for a similar book for the rest of the world through all available libraries, that no one else had felt qualified or experienced enough to write it; or if they had, they had not been motivated enough to do it. Although there were books for paramedical workers in Child Health, Surgery and Obstetrics and Gynaecology, there were none along these lines in Adult Internal Medicine for senior paramedical workers. Hence this book.

This book is a reference book. It is not meant to be all learned. It is meant to be read during the years of student life when training to be a health worker; and then to be referred to during working life to help when problems arise. The book is therefore large and has many words to try to explain things as clearly as could be done.

It is hoped that supervising or teaching Medical Officers in each country, who do not have time to prepare all the books needed by paramedical workers, may be able to take the parts from this book which apply to their country, simplify and summarise those parts (and alter or amplify or add to other parts if needed), and produce perhaps two other more useful books.

One book probably needed would be a 'summary', i.e. a book with just those things which the student and health worker must know, i.e. be able to recite orally or write, interpret on patients and use in practice to solve the problems of patients and the common health problems of the area. Such a book for Papua New Guinea is *Common Medical Problems of Adults in Papua New Guinea – A Summary*, 1979, C.R. Schull, Kristen Press Inc., Madang, Papua New Guinea.

The other book which is probably needed is a small book that can be carried in the health worker's pocket all the time and which has the details of the management of the common health problems in that area including drug doses (and it is much safer to look these up than to try to remember them and perhaps make a fatal mistake). Of course, the health worker must be actually taught to look up the book when he is seeing the patient. Such a book is *Diagnosis and Treat-*

ment of Common Health Problems of Adults in Papua New Guinea, 1980, C.R. Schull, Kristen Press Inc., Madang, Papua New Guinea.

Experience with Health Extension Officers and Nurses has taught that only one part of the book is likely to be consulted at any one time. Experience has also taught that repetition is a good teacher. The above will also partly explain some of the repetition in the book.

After the introductory chapters, most chapters are set out using the following plan (modified as needed). At first, there is a short description of the anatomy and physiology of the system. Then there is a list of the symptoms and signs which can be caused by abnormal structure or function of that system. This section includes details of how to examine the patient to find these signs. Next, there is a section which includes the common conditions and diseases of the system. Finally, there is a section which summarises the cause of and management of the common symptoms and signs caused by disorders and diseases of the system.

Although this is a reference book, the health worker student should become familiar with it before graduating. During student life you should read the following.

1. All of the first *eleven* chapters including diagnosis of disease, management of a patient and control and prevention of disease.
2. All sections on Anatomy, Physiology, Pathology, Symptoms and Signs in chapters which have these discussed.
3. The sections on all the common important diseases in the country in which he is working.

These will include the following in almost all countries:

1. Severe bacterial infections including septicaemia (Chapter 12).
2. Malaria (Chapter 13).
3. Tuberculosis (Chapter 14).
4. Leprosy (Chapter 15).
5. The common infectious diseases which occur almost everywhere (Chapter 16).
6. Any of the other infectious diseases which occur in your area (Chapters 17 and 18).
7. Syphilis, gonorrhoea, and HIV infection and AIDS (Chapter 19).
8. Otitis of various types, the common cold, influenza, acute bronchitis, pneumonia, asthma and chronic bronchitis; and causes of cough, sputum, haemoptysis, shortness of breath and pain in chest (Chapter 20).

9. Anaemia, hyperreactive malarious splenomegaly and, if it occurs in your area, sickle cell anaemia (Chapter 21).
10. Filariasis (Chapter 22).
11. Gastroenteritis, intestinal parasites and peptic ulcer; and causes of vomiting, haematemesis, diarrhoea and dysentery (Chapter 23).
12. Jaundice, hepatitis, liver abscess, hepatoma and cirrhosis (Chapter 24).
13. Meningitis of all types, cerebral malaria and other types of 'encephalitis', convulsions, epilepsy, paralysis, unconsciousness and headache (Chapter 25).
14. Urinary tract infections, causes of urinary frequency and pain, nephrotic syndrome, chronic kidney failure and causes of proteinuria (Chapter 26).
15. Osteomyelitis and pyomyositis (Chapter 28), acute bacterial arthritis, 'tropical arthritis', tuberculous arthritis and osteoarthrosis (Chapter 29).
16. Foreign bodies in the eye, conjunctivitis, corneal ulcer and iritis (Chapter 31).
17. Tinea, impetigo and scabies and the principles of treatment of all skin conditions (Chapter 32).
18. Snakebite (Chapter 33).
19. Swallowed poisons (Chapter 34).
20. Acute and chronic organic psychoses, schizophrenia, manic-depressive psychoses, acute psychotic reactions, anxiety states and 'acting out' states (Chapter 35).
21. Some important symptoms and signs including fever, generalised oedema, generalised wasting, dehydration, abdominal pain, abdominal tenderness – guarding – rigidity, abdominal masses and abdominal distension.
22. Resuscitation including artificial ventilation (Chapter 37) and treatment of shock (Chapter 27).

Any other diseases which are common in the area where the health worker is, must be added to this list.

Malnutrition is not only a cause of disease, but it also interacts with infection in a number of ways. Malnutrition decreases immunity or resistance to infection. Malnutrition makes any infection present more serious, and makes it less likely for the body to overcome that infection, even when correct treatment of the infection is given. Infection in a person who already has malnutrition makes that malnutrition even worse. As these conditions are even more important for children than adults, and as they are dealt with at length in the books on child health and children's diseases, malnutrition has not been discussed in a separate chapter in this book and the interaction of malnutrition and infection has not been emphasised. This is not meant to indicate that malnutrition and its relation to infection and its prevention and its treatment are not important for adults – they are. For detailed discussions of these, however, see books on child health and children's diseases; but remember that these things apply to adults also.

If the health worker does decide to purchase some other books on adult internal medicine, the first three to consider are:

Edwards, C.R.W. *et al.* (latest edition) *Davidson's Principles and Practice of Medicine*. Edinburgh, Churchill Livingstone.

Lawrence, D.R. (latest edition) *Clinical Pharmacology*. Edinburgh, Churchill Livingstone.

Munro, J. and Edwards, C. (latest edition). *MacLeod's Clinical Examination*. Edinburgh, Churchill Livingstone.

All of these books are available in low-priced editions. The latest edition should, of course, be obtained.

The author is only too well aware of the many imperfections in this book. If the book is to be improved, advice on how to do this is needed from those who use it. If Health Extension Officers, Medical Assistants, Nurses, Tutors and Medical Officers who use this book in any way for any purpose would be kind enough to write to the author and tell him of errors or omissions noted or things which are hard to understand, etc. and also make specific suggestions for improvements, this would greatly help. PLEASE WRITE.

It is hoped that the content of this book will show how health workers using only simple and cheap items (available in most health centres and hospital outpatients departments) are able to manage almost all of the medical health problems of adults safely and effectively.

C.R. Schull
1987

Preface to the Second Edition

I was asked by Professor Morley from TALC, some staff from The Australian College of Tropical Medicine at the James Cook University, Townsville and others, to update the first edition of this book, as apparently no other similar book has recently been published. As I now live and work in Australia, I no longer have constant contact with paramedical workers to make sure what I write is truly relevant to them and what they want. However, the first edition of this book has been used by an even greater range of health workers and teaching institutions than I expected. As well as this, situations in one country do still differ very greatly from situations in another country. No book could possibly cover all of the practical aspects needed for all users of this book for all countries. No book could do this for many of the users without including many details not important to them.

I have therefore done my best to retain in the book what paramedical workers have told me they want and I have added what appears to be new and important. Great changes in health have been caused by the epidemic of HIV infection; increasing numbers of people living in cities but still without access to good health services; increase in diseases associated with urban living, such as vascular disease; some diseases, such as leprosy, becoming less of a problem; some diseases, such as tuberculosis, becoming more of a problem; and exciting changes for possible control of some of the helminthic and other diseases which previously could not be controlled. I have tried to alter the text to take account of these developments.

It is still essential that a specialist in internal medicine in each country indicates to paramedical health workers in that country, what they do and do not need to know. They can then delete from this book what is not important in their country and add anything missed out that is important. I am of course happy for such Medical Officers to use this book as a basis for any local literature produced, if an explanation of what has been done is included.

It is also still essential that such a Medical Officer produces a summary of what the paramedical health worker needs to learn and to know. If a photocopy of such booklets as *Diagnosis and Treatment of Common Health Problems in Papua New Guinea* and *Standard Management of Common Medical Problems of Adults in Papua New Guinea*, which I previously wrote, would help as a basis for the production of such local booklets, I would be happy to send these copies on request, although they now are out of date.

This book is a reference book to be used throughout training. It is then to be used as a source of information by the health worker when he is working independently and he comes across a problem not covered by his existing knowledge.

In many places I have added explanations of treatment carried out and names of drugs used by Medical Officers in hospitals but not available at health centres. This is so that when patients, who have been referred to hospital, return to the health centre, the paramedical workers will understand about the treatment and drugs the patients has been given. Paramedical workers should not try to learn those sections where such things as 'Drugs used by Medical Officers in hospitals will include …' are written.

To try to save space and time the words 'he, him, his' stand also for 'she, her, hers' where the text could refer either to a man, boy or woman, girl.

Publications of particular value to paramedical workers and Medical Officers include those listed on page 616 at the back of this book.

I would like to thank those few people who did write with suggestions for improvement of the first edition. Most of these suggestions have been included in this second edition. If you have any suggestions for improvement of this second edition, please write.

Sheila Jones, Freelance Editor, has done the difficult and thankless task of editing the whole manuscript – not only for the first edition but also for this second edition. I am grateful for her help and acknowledge how much she has contributed.

Shirley Hamber, Freelance Publisher, who has overseen all the work, could not have been more helpful.

My wife, Judith, has not only helped more than anyone else in the re-writing of this second edition but has in fact been the one who has made it possible.

C.R. Schull
Greenslopes Private Hospital
Newdegate Street
Greenslopes, 4120
Queensland
Australia

Preface to the Third Edition

All of the book has been updated. The sections on HIV/AIDS, malaria and some others have had to be greatly expanded. World Health Organization (WHO) policies and the drugs in the WHO essential medicines model list form the basis for the recommendations in the book. All errors, however, are the author's, who is no longer working in a developing country and who is getting older.

This book is not a book to be learned. This is a reference book for paramedical health workers (but often used also by Medical Officers new to this sort of medical work). Important parts to learn and remember can be marked; however, these are usually indicated or put in 'boxes'. The health worker as a student will hopefully understand what he (or she) is trying to learn by reading the explanations in the book. The health worker after graduation, and often working alone and not able to discuss with a Medical Officer unusual or difficult problems in patients or unusual treatments a patient has been given, hopefully will find an answer or explanation in the book and be helped to make a plan to cope with the patient's problems.

The health worker in every country also needs the following:

1. A printed guide on what conditions occur and are important in that country; and what he needs to know about these things.
2. A Standard Management (or Treatment) Book which fits into the pocket and which sets out for that country what drugs and other treatments are available and how these should be used.

These things will be different in every country. The Health Department on the advice of the Medical Officers and specialists in internal medicine in each country should supply this. This textbook or other similar textbooks cannot be specific for every country. Always follow the policies of the country in which you are working.

As many health workers have so few books, the Medical Officers in Queensland, Australia, who are members of the Australian Medical Association Queensland Branch (AMAQ), have generously contributed money to the publishers to help keep the selling price of the book far below the cost to produce it. The Australian doctors did this in the hope that this will help their paramedical colleagues in far away and less privileged circumstances. They did it to express their gratitude to those of you who work so hard in difficult circumstances to also look after our fellow human beings in the family of man.

Again, the staff of TALC and the publishers, Macmillan, have been very helpful.

Again, the ability to produce this edition has been achieved solely due to the understanding and the enormous amount of typing and other work done by my wife Judith, and the acceptance of our doing this work by our four children (three born in and all of whom enjoyed growing up in developing countries).

C.R. Schull
702 Musgrave Road
Robertson 4109
Queensland
Australia

Acknowledgements

This book was prepared with the help of many of my friends and colleagues. So many helped in so many ways over so many years, it is now no longer possible to record all the people who helped – even in major ways.

Foremost among those who made this book possible were my wife and children. They not only went without many things so that this and the other books for Papua New Guinea could appear; they also gave encouragement and help and my wife did all the typing for the numerous Papua New Guinean drafts and editions.

Many of my colleagues in Papua New Guinea gave encouragement and help. In particular, Doctors John and Narelle Stace helped in very many ways and in every way they could. Dr Brother Andrew SSF contributed significantly to the chapter on mental illnesses. Professor George Wyatt made valuable suggestions and Dr Greg Lawrence read the whole of the Papua New Guinean edition and made numerous suggestions for improvement. Papua New Guinean health workers, and in particular Dr Puka Temu and HEO Tutor Mr Mika Kenas, gave invaluable guidance. Of course, many of the ideas in the book came from observation of what happened to patients and other situations that arose during health centre work and then discussion of these with the staff involved.

For the International edition, Dr F.J. Wright of Edinburgh kindly and helpfully checked the various chapters dealing with diseases with which the author had not had significant practical experience. Dr C.J. Ellis of Birmingham then read through the text and made many valuable suggestions. Both of these doctors have had vast experience in tropical and developing countries and are internationally recognised authorities in tropical diseases. The author is very grateful to them for their invaluable advice.

Two editors, at first Mrs Jennifer Gamel and later (for the bulk of the work) Mrs Sheila Jones, did a large amount of important work in preparing and improving the text for publication.

As the author did not plan to publish any works for distribution outside Papua New Guinea until he was requested to do so just before he had to leave Papua New Guinea to return to Australia, and as there was no copyright law in Papua New Guinea, no particular record of the origin of diagrams and descriptions of laboratory procedures, etc. collected for use of health workers was kept. Most of those which the author did not produce in Madang were obtained from slides or photographs in the Medical Learning Resources Unit of the University of Papua New Guinea in Port Moresby, and most of these were not documented as to origin. If, therefore, there are any parts of the book, and especially any diagrams, which have been inadvertently reproduced without appropriate acknowledgement made, the author apologises for this and would make such acknowledgement if permission for the use of these were granted for any future edition, and the publishers would make the necessary arrangements.

Money to assist in travel for library research and typing of the International text was kindly supplied by the Damian Foundation, Belgium, Boehringer Ingelheim Australia and the World Health Organization, Geneva. Large grants were then given by both the Swedish International Development Agency and the Australian Government's Australian Development Assistance Bureau to Teaching Aids at Low Cost, London, to provide money for the printing and sale of the first edition by Macmillan at a price well below the normal price for a book of this size. The author has and will accept no payment of any kind in a further attempt to keep the price as low as possible. It is only through the generous assistance of the above charitable, company and government bodies, however, that it has been possible to produce and distribute this book.

Despite all the above help, however, the production of this and the other books has been an 'after hours' effort by a clinician who considers himself in no way an academic or an author. Responsibility for errors and omissions, therefore, rests with the author, and not those who helped in so many ways.

To all the people, as well as the above, who helped the author, he gives his thanks. The author knows these people well enough to be certain that if this book helps to improve the health of people in tropical and developing countries, then those who contributed to the production of this book will be thanked enough.

C.R.S

Acknowledgements

The publisher and author wish to thank the following rights holders for the use of copyright material:

The World Health Organization for the following items: Table 10. 1 from DIP 755 Immunization in practice: module 2: the vaccines www.who.int/vaccines-documents/iip/word/manu755-2.doc; Table 10.3 reproduced from www.who.int/vaccines-documents WHO Global Immunization vision and strategy 2006–2015; Fig 13.1 reproduced from http://rbm.who.int/wmr2005/html/map5.htm; Table 14.3 reproduced from Treatment of Tuberculosis: guidelines for national programmes, 3rd ed, Geneva 2003; Table 14.4 from Tuberculosis Care with HIV Co-management (IMAI), 2007; Fig 14.5 reproduced from Tuberculosis infection control in the era of expanding HIV care and treatment 2006 – Appendix B Information on ventilation and fans www.who.int/tb/publications/2006/tbhiv_infectioncontrol_addendum.pdf; Table 14.6 Symptom-based approach to management of drug side-effects adapted from Harries A D & Maher D TB/HIV: a clinical manual 1996 Geneva WHO 2nd ed table 10.6; Fig 15.1 reproduced from WHO Technical Report Series no 874; Fig 17.6 reproduced from http://www.who.int/csr/resources/publications/WHO_HSE_EPR_2008_3w.pdf;
Fig 17.11 reproduced from www.who.int/csr/disease/yellowfev/impact1/en; Fig 18.2a & b reproduced from Where does leishmaniasis occur in the world? www.who.int/leishmaniasis/leishmaniasis_maps/en/index2.html; Fig 18.10 reproduced from Control of Human African Trypanosomiasis: a strategy for the African Region – Regional Committee for Africa AFR/RC55/11 17 June 2005 fig 1; Fig 18.11 The distribution of Chagas vectors in Latin America reproduced by kind permission of Pan-American Health Organization (PAHO/WHO), Program of Communicable Diseases, January 2003; Figs 18.13a & b reproduced from WHO Technical Report Series no 830; Fig 19.3 reproduced from AIDS Epidemic Updates December 2007 UNAIDS/WHO http://whqlibdoc.who.int/unaids/2007/9789291736218_en.pdf; Text and Appendix 21.1 & 21.2 reproduced from WHO Haemoglobin Colour Scale information leaflet; Fig 22.6 reproduced from Lymphatic Filariasis http://whqlibdoc.who.int/hq/2001/WHO_CDS_CPE_SMT_2001.7.pdf; Fig 32.23 reproduced from WHO Technical Report Series no 852; Table 35.2 adapted and reproduced from WHO ICD-10 International Classification of Diseases 10th ed; Tables 10.2 and 14.6 from *Guidelines to rational drug use* by Fr von Massow & R Korte, © 1997, reprinted by permission of Macmillan Education; Fig 19.19 from *AIDS epidemic update* December 2009 reproduced by permission of UNAIDS/WHO, November 2009; Appendix 3 reproduced from Mini-Wright's Peak Flow Meter leaflet by permission of Clement Clarke International Ltd; Table 23.5 reproduced by permission of vertex42.com; Table 27.1 from Manson's Tropical Diseases ed G G Cook and A Zumla 21st ed. reproduced by permission of Elsevier © 2003.

The author and publishers wish to acknowledge, with thanks, the following photographic sources:
Dr M.M. Minter (from A Colour Atlas of Tropical Medicine and Parasitology by W. Peters and H.M Giles, Wolfe Medical Publications Ltd) pp180, 537(t), 538;
St Bartholomew's Hospital, Department of Medicine Photography pp214, 215, 275;
TALC pp117, 213, 333, 418, 549;
Tropix pp178, 179;
WHO pp181 (b), 608, 609, 610, 611, 612;
C. James Webb pp181 (t), 398, 410.

All other photographs are courtesy of the author.

The publishers have made every effort to trace the copyright holders, but if they have inadvertently overlooked any, they will be pleased to make the necessary arrangements at the first opportunity.

1 On Being an Effective Health Worker

If you are a new student, you should probably read and try to understand only the first two sections in this chapter. Come back to read and understand the other sections when you:
1. have learned more about diseases, sick people in the community and being a health worker;
2. have seen, during your work with people with diseases and with the many other people of the community, the situations, problems and possibilities for good written about in the rest of this chapter;
3. can talk with your teachers about how these things really are, in the place where *you* actually live and work.

Evidence-based medicine

Our present scientific, evidence-based system of health care has developed only in the last 100 years. For thousands of years, health care has been just caring for (looking after) people with diseases. Few cures existed. Health care has now, however, come to be much more – curing disease, preventing (or stopping) people getting disease and promoting (or encouraging) good health; as well, of course, and still very importantly, caring more effectively for the people with disease.

There are a number of reasons why the art of caring for people with disease has now been joined by science with the ability to cure disease, prevent disease and promote good health.

Knowledge about anatomy and physiology and disease has been collected for centuries. A large amount was known, but many things, now known to be untrue, were also believed. The invention of the microscope allowed people to see how the body was made up of cells. Then the development of modern chemistry and physics allowed people to find out how the body really worked. The microscope showed micro-organisms and explained how infectious organisms could cause disease. Simple epidemiological experiments showed how these organisms and diseases could pass from one person to another and how these could be stopped. Chemicals were then discovered that killed some micro-organisms which caused disease without hurting the patient as much. These chemicals have gradually been made safer, until today many are very safe for people, while many have been made very effective in killing harmful micro-organisms. Knowledge about causes and treatments of other types of diseases followed. Clinical trials were begun, which showed which treatments were more effective than other treatments. The results formed the basis of what we now call 'evidence-based medicine'. Almost unbelievable cures can now at times be possible. Most infections and many other diseases can be prevented or cured until our bodies get old.

Good health is now a possibility for almost all people if the social environment (the way families and communities live together), the government, and the absence of famine and war, allow it.

The purpose of the health worker

It is this sort of modern scientific evidence-based health care that we want to give to the people in our community. There are many things that need to be done by ourselves as health workers and by others, however, before people in our community actually get this kind of health care. None of us can do all the things needed by ourselves. Only a very few of us get the chance to do any great thing. All of us, however, can play our small but very important part in our own community to try to get this kind of health care to our people.

For this kind of health care to be delivered, this will involve not only health workers, but parents, teachers, agricultural workers, council and government persons, law enforcement officers, religious workers, business development officers, cultural performers and many others, all working together.

You (and all of us who are really effective health workers) must have three aims (as well as giving care to sick people):
1. to promote good health;
2. to prevent disease;
3. to treat disease.

These three aims must be for both
1. individuals and
2. the whole community.

When you treat disease, again you have three aims:
1. to cure the patient (this is not always possible);
2. to relieve the patient's symptoms (this is almost always possible);

3. to comfort and encourage the patient and his relatives (this is always possible).

By what you say and do, you need to reassure the patient and his relatives that you are also a real person and that you do understand his health problems and the worries these cause him. The patient should understand that you will not leave him without all the medical and personal help that you are able to give him. You need to be optimistic (hopeful and cheerful) and continue to be optimistic about your being able to give good relief of his symptoms, to cure him if possible, and if this is not possible, to help him die without distress and in dignity.

It is very easy to spend all your time treating disease and so have no time to prevent disease and promote health. This is not the best way to spend your time. Of course you must treat patients with disease. This helps the patient and his relatives. It also shows the community that you know how to help them and that you do want to help them. It is only when the community discovers these things that they will take any notice of your work to prevent disease and promote health. Unless, however, you really do prevent disease and promote good health, your work in treating the sick will not help the community very much. It is no good curing a patient if you do not prevent the patient getting the same disease again when he goes home. His family and friends may also get the disease. So:

1. You must use some of your time to treat patients with disease.
2. You must use some of your time to prevent disease.
3. You must use some of your time to promote good health.

You can do a lot to control and prevent disease and promote good health in the health centre. When a person comes to you in the health centre and you diagnose his disease, you can give the patient and his family and friends education about how to control and prevent disease, and about other things which would improve their health. Remember the following two things.

1. When people are well they usually take little notice of health education as they feel they will not get a disease. But when they are sick, the patient and his family and friends will often take notice of health education, as they then know they can get the disease.
2. Most cases of undiagnosed infectious diseases such as leprosy, tuberculosis (TB) and human immunodeficiency virus (HIV) are in the family and friends of patients with these diseases. Therefore, before you

go out of the health centre to look for these sorts of diseases in the whole community, first make sure you educate and examine all the family and friends who have come (with the patient) to you in the health centre.

This does not mean you should stay in the health centre all the time. It means you should never miss the chance to control and prevent disease and promote health anywhere, including when a sick person comes to the health centre.

You will often find it difficult to leave your work in the health centre and go out into the community to prevent disease and promote health. But you must also do this. Unless you and other workers are successful in getting people in the community to drink only safe water, use only safe toilets, eat a healthy diet, wash their hands after going to the toilet and before preparing food, exercise, keep their body and houses clean, be immunised against common diseases, have only safe sexual intercourse, etc. disease and unnecessary death will continue to spoil the lives of many people.

You, the Health Worker, must also remember that what you *do* to treat and prevent disease and promote good health will have much more effect than what you *say* about these things. (Your actions will speak louder than your words.) Your life (and that of your family) should be a living example of how to have a healthy body and mind, and how to contribute all that is possible from the position you hold in life to the good of all in the community. Your effectiveness as a Health Worker will depend on what sort of person you really are and the way you live and work.

Traditional healers

Health workers know (mostly from personal experience) that there is a traditional system of health care or healing that exists parallel to (or alongside) the system of health care we give. In fact, most patients have used it before they come to our system of health care. In the traditional system, some illnesses may now be recognised as being due to causes which respond to modern medical treatment and surgery, because this has become so obvious to everyone. However, many illnesses and many conditions are still thought to be due to spirits, bewitchment, curses, breaking taboos or at times behaving badly towards other people. Some illnesses are no doubt due to worry, anxiety and fear about these things. Although some traditional healers now send people to the health centre for treatment of certain conditions (e.g. malaria, TB, injuries), they often still keep many patients to themselves. If these patients cannot be cured by modern scientific health care (e.g. incurable cases of cancer, etc.), and as long as they are not in a great deal of pain that could be relieved and do not have an infectious disease which can spread to others, this is not necessarily a bad thing. At times, however, patients with treatable and even curable conditions are not sent by traditional healers for diagnosis and treatment, and this directly hurts the patient and others to whom the disease spreads. At times, drug treatments are given in the form of 'bush teas', leaves, bark and other mixtures. At times, operations are done where soil or leaves are put into cuts made in the skin. At times, treatment involves prayers, rituals, diets, sacrifices, etc. Occasionally, this treatment can be successful because it relieves anxiety and there is no doubt that a few of the drugs used do have helpful effects. Much more often, however, the treatment can cause harm, e.g. liver failure as a result of drinking 'bush teas' (we now know the dangerous chemicals they contain) and infections as a result of unsterile cuts and other 'surgical' procedures.

Most people all over the world continue with some customs and traditions even though they know they are no longer of any particular value. For this reason, it is unlikely that just opposing traditional healers will help sick people. This may only make it more likely that patients will stick to their customs and their traditional healers and not come to the health centre.

Some health workers ignore the traditional system of health care and behave as if it did not exist. It does, however, exist, and probably most patients have used it before coming to the modern health care worker. Unless a worker knows what diagnosis and treatment has already been given, he is at a great disadvantage in helping the patient (especially if traditional treatment has caused a further condition in the patient, who then has two conditions which need diagnosis and treatment).

Other health workers try to cooperate with traditional healers. Some traditional healers refuse, but a surprising number are happy to cooperate. If they can be helped to recognise infections, especially TB, leprosy, pneumonia, meningitis, gastroenteritis, malaria, etc. which are easily treated and cured by modern drugs, and if they agree to send such patients to the health centre, this will prevent the patient having disease or dying and will control or stop the spread of the infection. The traditional healer can sometimes even be taught to give basic treatment for some diseases such as malaria and then to refer the patient if necessary. Some traditional healers have been supplied with 'first-aid boxes' with simple treatments not only for malaria, but also for dehydration, sores, etc. and have become quite skilled in their use. They can also be taught to recognise other conditions needing medical treatment such as anaemia, and refer such patients. It may not matter if the traditional healer uses his methods first, before sending the patient to the health centre, as long as there is only a little delay and the patient does not have traditional treatment which causes harm or much expense. The traditional healer may be in a much better position to help patients with mental disorders caused by anxiety about things they have or have not done in the past, than a health worker in the health centre, who may not know the patient's family history or social circumstances. The traditional healer could be encouraged to keep and help these patients, but send them if his treatment does not help.

There are some things that are unacceptable, however, when working with traditional healers. Some ideas may not only be medically wrong, they may be also morally wrong, e.g. the belief in some areas that having sexual intercourse with a virgin (person, usually young, who has never had sex before) will cure sexually transmitted diseases, especially HIV infection/AIDS. This does not help the patient with the disease and spoils the other person's life. Of course, simply opposing this sort of belief will not work. Ways have to be found to show that it does not work and it is wrong. In addition, ways also have to be found for the traditional healer to come to this conclusion himself and to think that it is his own idea. Then he is likely to advise patients correctly.

These are all very difficult things to do. The help of other people, especially health educators and other people in your health department, will be needed to make these big changes.

The situation with traditional healers will obviously be different from one place to another place. It is important to recognise this parallel system of traditional medicine and, together with your other health workers, try to get that system to do the following;

1. look after the patients it can (especially those with incurable disease we cannot greatly help);
2. try to get that system to give only treatment which will do no harm;
3. if possible supply 'first aid' (or immediate correct basic health care);
4. recognise those symptoms which are important (as they suggest a condition which can cause disease or death or may spread to other people, but can easily

be cured or prevented by modern medical methods) and send those patients to the health centre.

How to manage diseases and conditions we do not understand

There are some diseases which

1. we do not yet recognise as a disease; or
2. the cause is not yet known; or
3. even if we do recognise and know the cause of the disease we have no treatment which helps, apart from relieving its symptoms; or
4. may go away themselves even if the diseases are not recognised and not treated, as the body often can and does 'cure' itself.

If you do not know what disease a patient has, or if the disease has no known treatment,

1. tell the patient you do not recognise the disease and/or you do not know a cure for it;
2. do not give drugs (except to relieve symptoms and treat any other severe disease which could possibly be present);
3. tell the patient you will, if the condition is serious, transfer him to see a Medical Officer, or if the condition is not serious, refer him to the next visiting Medical Officer for further diagnosis and possible treatment;
4. tell the patient the body may 'cure' itself without any treatment;
5. tell the patient that if he has any worries or fears about things he has done in the past which he thinks may be a cause of the condition, then he should do the correct things to put these right and this may help him; tell the patient to try a non-specific but worthwhile thing you think would be helpful for its 'placebo' effect (see below), even if it may not help with the patient's specific problem.
6. as long as any traditional healer does not
   (a) give treatment which could be harmful, or
   (b) take a lot of the patient's money or goods for treatment,
   there is no reason to try to stop the patient from seeing a traditional healer. First, however, make sure that you have explained the above five things to the patient.

Remember that if a person's disease runs its course, or the body 'cures' itself, the person giving treatment at the time this 'cure' takes place, will be the one thought to have 'cured' the patient. The treatment, however, may have nothing to do with the 'cure'. It is only when epidemiological and controlled clinical studies show a close association between a certain treatment and a likely chance of 'cure' that we know whether a particular treatment is effective or not.

The placebo effect

It is also important to know that by just taking an interest in patients and giving them any treatment (even if the treatment has no effect on their illness), many patients 'feel' improved. This is often called a 'placebo' effect.

If a health worker is willing to listen to the patient, is understanding, is kind and is helpful (even if it is only in non-medical ways), many sick people feel much better just for these things.

If the health worker can get people to remember feeling well and to have positive or good thoughts about improving their health, some patients may actually improve, i.e. what the person thinks may influence what their body does. (The opposite is also true – if a person thinks about getting worse or dying, it may be more likely that the patient will actually get worse.)

It is probably through the placebo effect and by being interested and helpful, and also by using the power of positive thinking and remembered wellness, that popular traditional healers do seem to be able to help some people.

We can and we should do all of these things. If no specific treatment is known to you, always try something sensible or give the patient something sensible to try, to help the illness. (It need not be a drug or medicine; adding something good to the diet or using only safe water or starting exercise if the patient exercises little, are safe and may be effective.) However, do not tell the patient it will heal or cure him. Tell him only that it may help, but is worth trying. Be interested in your patient, his family, his work and how his illness affects all these things. Talk to him and try to help him solve any problems the illness causes. Find some positive things in the patient's illness and situation that you can use to start him thinking hopeful and positive thoughts. These may be just that you will not 'give up' trying to help him no matter what happens, as well as the fact that the body's defences and healing powers sometimes unexpectedly overcome what seem to be even fatal diseases. Get the patient to remember what he felt like when he was really well, and to do all he can to follow these paths to wellness again. These things will help many people. Our scientific evidence-based medicine helps only the patients it has been shown to help. Do not, however, neglect or forget to use all other possible means to help the patient – scientific medicine alone is not enough. Medicine is an 'art' as well as a 'science'.

It is most important you do not tell a patient that you know what the disease is and how to treat it, if this is not true. If you try to scientifically treat something you do not recognise, the treatment is not likely to be effective, and people will soon believe that you are not reliable and not be trusted to treat even the things which you do know and can treat effectively. Always tell (the patients and the relatives) the truth.

How to work together with other community leaders

There are two further important things you can do to promote good health, prevent disease and treat those suffering from disease in the area where you work.

The first is to identify (i.e. find out) who are the leaders in the community. These will include the traditional leaders, the religious leaders, young people's leaders, the opinion (i.e. the things people believe in and act on) leaders as well as those who are the government leaders. The second is to find out if you can make these key (i.e. very important or needed for success) people key parts of your health programmes.

An example of this was the identification and use of a key traditional and religious leader from a place where the author worked for some time. This person was a traditional leader. He was given some basic medical training and did this medical work in his village. He then did some religious training and became a full-time religious leader. He then decided it would be better for him to do ordinary work together with other people of the community during the week and carry out his religious duties at the weekend. He took a low paid job as an orderly in the hospital. He was of outstanding character and highly respected by everyone in the community. Other health workers helped to identify him to the author. After thinking about it and further training, he agreed to be the psychiatric orderly and became the key worker for thousands of people with mental disorders and diseases. He came from the area and knew the local language and the beliefs and customs. He really knew what local people thought and felt and why they acted as they did. If a person was reported as having a mental problem, this key worker was able to quickly find out the two important things about mental problems and act on them.

1. Did the patient have a psychotic problem (i.e. the person did not think or feel or act in ways the rest of the community did or could understand) and did the patient have an underlying organic condition (i.e. an actual disease of the brain or abnormality of the blood going to the brain of which there were only a few important treatable ones in the area)? If either of these were the case, this worker would immediately bring the patient to the author and tell him he should quickly do tests and give treatment for organic causes of psychosis or give drugs for a non-organic psychosis.

2. Did the patient have a non-psychotic condition and a non-organic condition? If both of these were the case, this key worker and other health workers could find out the causes for the stress, anxiety or worry which caused the mental condition and help the patient solve the causes of the illness and so get well. This key health worker could do this work much better than the author who came from a different country, race, language and culture.

The above is only an example. You may be able to identify a number of such persons where you work, most of whom will probably not be health workers. They do need to understand and be respected by the community and are usually people who come from the area. As well as being able to communicate health messages, they must be a genuine (or real) example of what the health message is. Such people may be teachers or educators who can give health education but who also live in healthy ways. Such people may be opinion leaders. These people should not only make public statements (give talks, write, etc.) about eating a good diet, drinking safe water, always using a proper toilet, washing hands after going to the toilet and before preparing food, having only safe sex, not smoking tobacco and not drinking enough alcohol to cause drunkenness or disease, etc.; they themselves should be an example of such a lifestyle.

If you can identify such key people in the community and get them to help you in your main health programmes, this will make the programmes far more effective.

You yourself must have a good idea of the programmes actually needed in your area. This will depend on the epidemiology of the diseases where you are (see Chapter 5).

You also need to be humble enough (not too proud) to get advice and help from others in organising these programmes. You need to be so dedicated to your work of treating people with disease and preventing disease and promoting good health that you yourself are respected. You need also to be a person who does not try to keep the success of any programme to yourself, but shares it with the others. It is only if you do all these things that these key community leaders will be willing to work with you.

Rewards for health workers

If you can do all of these things and successfully treat those with disease, prevent disease and promote good health, just seeing the help you have been to the community (as long as you get your proper pay) will be its own reward – you will need no other. You will, however, reap other rewards. The most important will be the respect in which the community will hold you and to occasionally hear others saying how much good you do for the community and how much they like, respect and value you.

You will, however, have one great problem. If the Health Department wants to promote you or send you to another area, the people where you are will do all they can to try to keep you there, as you are so valued. If you can study, work and live to make this your problem, it is a good problem to have.

A good soldier thinks that it is worth his while to give up his life (and never again be able to experience and enjoy life) to serve his country. A good health worker will think that it is worth his or her while to live his life (probably with less money and possessions and status than he would otherwise have had) to save the lives of and make more healthy and happy the people of his country.

2 Some Clinical Definitions

Do not try to learn these definitions until you have:
1. read more about them in later chapters,
2. talked about them with your teachers, and
3. used the things they are about in your practical work.

Anatomy

Anatomy is the science (or study of and knowledge of the facts) of the *structure* of the body; or *how the body is made*.

Physiology

Physiology is the science of the normal *function* of the body; or *how the living body works*.

Definition of a disease

In this book the definition of a disease is a short statement about the nature of the disease; or what kind of disease it is. Other important facts may be added.

Frequency

The frequency is how often the disease occurs. There are more accurate terms. These include the following:

Prevalence: This is the *total* number of persons with the disease at a *stated* time in a *stated* population.

Incidence: This is the number of *new* persons developing the disease during a *stated* time in a *stated* population.

A classification of the causes of disease (aetiology or etiology)

There are ten common kinds or classifications of disease (congenital, traumatic, inflammatory (four types), neoplastic, degenerative, chemical-induced, malnutrition, psychological, body system failure (especially vascular) and others including unknown). The causes of many of these classifications of diseases are known (see Chapter 4). In fact, some of the classifications are based on the cause of disease. However, there are also causes that are not yet known about. For example, it is said that a patient's disease may be degenerative (or due to the body wearing out); but it is not completely known why the body, which can repair itself, eventually wears out. The most common causes of disease in tropical and developing countries are infections with organisms, trauma and malnutrition. (See Chapter 4.)

Pathology

The cause of the disease can make changes in the normal anatomy and physiology of the body. These changes are called pathology. (See Chapter 3.)

Epidemiology

Epidemiology is the name of the science that gives the known answers to the questions:

1. *Who* gets a particular disease and *how many* people get it?
2. *When* and *where* do these persons get the disease? and
3. *How* and *why* do they get the disease? (See Chapter 5.)

Symptoms

Symptoms are *what the patient feels*.

The patient *tells* you his symptoms when he talks to you about what he *feels*.

You can usually discover symptoms when you take a *medical history* from the patient. When you take a medical history you must ask about:

1. General information (name, age, where he lives, etc.).
2. The patient's symptoms and how long he has had each one. (Record these in the patient's own words.)
3. The history of the present illness (or the story of how the patient went from being well to sick).
4. The specific questions (or specific interrogation) that you must ask to discover if there are also symptoms of a disease of any other system of the body (as well as those the patient has already talked about).
5. The past history – you ask the patient about the drugs he has taken, treatment he has been given by traditional healers, previous attacks of this illness and their treatment, other illnesses and their treatment, operations, accidents and previous and present pregnancies, etc.
6. The family and contact history – you check if an illness in the family or in one of his contacts could be affecting the patient.

There are three other things you must do when you take a medical history.

1. If the patient may have a mental condition, take the history again from a relative or another witness.

2. Check the patient's outpatient card and any inpatient notes for any history in them.
3. Tell the patient a summary of the history as you have understood it and ask him to correct anything wrong.

See Chapter 6 page 21.

Signs

Signs are *what you find (see, feel, percuss, hear, etc.) when you examine the patient.*

You do the *clinical* or *medical* or *physical* examination to discover all the patient's signs. You must do it systematically (or in a special order), usually in nine sections, so that you never forget anything.

1. Basic observations. These help you decide if the patient is 'sick' or not. They also help you to look for common diseases (even if the patient does not complain of their symptoms). If you find these diseases while they are still not serious you can treat them and prevent them from getting worse. These observations include: level of consciousness and signs of meningeal irritation; temperature; pulse rate; breathing rate and type of breathing; blood pressure, weight with observations about dehydration, oedema, malnutrition or chronic wasting illness; and colour, especially anaemia.
2. Head and neck including ear, nose, throat, lymph glands and thyroid.
3. Chest, including spine.
4. Abdomen.
5. Skin.
6. Muscles, bones, joints.
7. Ear, nose and throat (if not done before).
8. Any special examinations, if needed.
9. Examination of mental state (psychiatric examination), if needed.

See Chapter 6 page 23.

Course and complications

The *course* is what usually happens to a person who has the disease. *Complications* are other things which do not usually happen in the course of the disease. Complications are other clinical conditions which can happen on top of the original clinical condition.

Tests or investigations

You do tests for one or more of three reasons:

1. to help you decide between different possible diagnoses,
2. to confirm a diagnosis, and
3. to provide a baseline by which you can judge if the patient is getting better or worse.

There are three groups of tests:

1. Those you can do at the health centre, e.g. haemoglobin, urine tests, lumbar puncture, etc.
2. Those you cannot do, but you take a sample at the health centre and send it to the hospital laboratory to be examined there, e.g. 'serum tests', malaria smear, sputum smears, etc. (In some large health centres there is a medical laboratory assistant who can do some of these tests at the health centre.)
3. Those where you cannot do the test or take a sample at the health centre, and must send the patient to the hospital for the test, e.g. X-rays, etc.

Differential diagnosis

The differential diagnosis (DD) is the list of all the diseases *which could* be causing the patient's main symptoms and signs. See Chapter 6 page 25.

Diagnostic features

In this book diagnostic features are the most typical things about the disease (in a short list). These features are nearly always present if that disease is present.

Provisional diagnosis

The provisional diagnosis (PD) is the disease (or diseases) you think the patient really has. You decide this after eliminating all the other diseases in the differential diagnoses because they do not fit the patient's symptoms and signs and tests as well as the provisional diagnosis does. When you have made a provisional diagnosis, you manage the patient for this disease. See Chapter 6 page 25.

Management

Management is not only the treatment of the patient. A patient who has a disease creates problems for many people. To manage these problems you must do at least these four things:

1. treat the patient;
2. notify or advise certain other people;
3. control the spread of the disease, if necessary;
4. prevent other members of the community from getting the disease and the patient from getting it again.

These things are considered separately below. See also Chapters 7, 8 and 9.

Treatment of the patient

Treatment includes the following nine things:

1. *Decision on outpatient treatment or admission for inpatient treatment.*

2. *Nursing care* of many types including at times, bed rest; special positions; special care of respiratory tract, eyes, bladder, pressure areas, etc.; isolation; observations; food; fluids, etc.
3. *Specific treatment* to attempt to *cure* the disease, e.g. drugs, fluids, food, surgery, dressings, plasters, physiotherapy and psychiatric counselling.
4. *Symptomatic treatment*, to attempt to relieve the patient's symptoms and make him *feel* better, e.g. drugs, etc. as in 3 above; nursing care as in 2 above.
5. *Giving an explanation, reassurance and comfort* to the patient and relatives.
6. *Giving health education* about control and prevention of the disease to the patient and to the relatives.
7. *Consultation if needed about the patient with the preventive medicine/administrative Health or Medical Officer or hospital Medical Officer* (sometimes). This can be for advice or about transfer of the patient to Medical Officer care or referral of the patient to the next visiting Medical Officer.
8. *Discharging the patient* and giving final health education.
9. *Following up the patient*, if needed.

See Chapter 7.

Indications for consultation, transfer or referral

Some symptoms and signs mean that you should do one of the following three things:

1. Describe the patient's condition to the Health Officer or hospital Medical Officer by telephone or radio, and ask for advice (that is 'consult').
2. Transfer.
   (a) Send the patient to the hospital as an emergency case for urgent treatment by a Medical Officer as soon as you can find a plane or car or boat to take him there, i.e. 'urgent transfer'.
   (b) Send the patient to the hospital as a non-emergency case using the next available usual transport, i.e. 'non–urgent transfer'.
3. Ask the next Medical Officer who visits the health centre to see the patient, i.e. 'referral'.

See Chapter 7 page 30.

Prognosis

The prognosis is what the likely result of a condition will be (e.g. cause the patient's death, get better quickly, last for a long time, etc.).

See Chapter 6 page 26.

Notification

1. You must notify certain diseases to the Health Officer or Health Department if they occur. Some have to be notified immediately if any new case occurs. Some have to be notified immediately if an epidemic occurs. This second group and another group usually have to be notified monthly if any cases occur.
2. You must notify certain cases to the police and coroner. These include all cases of 'sudden and unnatural death' and cases when you do not know the cause of death, including persons who are 'dead on arrival'. Notify all fights, accidents, alleged poisoning, etc. if the patient is ill.
3. You should notify relatives and friends (and sometimes other people) and advise them that the patient is not well. You must, however, get the patient's permission to inform them of things which are private, i.e. the patient's condition, treatment and probable future.

See Chapter 8.

Control

Control is what you must do to stop the disease spreading. You need to know the epidemiology of the disease so that you can choose the best means of control. You may need to use one or more or all of the following four ways:

1. inactivating the specific agent/cause in the reservoir (usually killing an organism in the body of the original host);
2. blocking the means of spread of the specific (or causative) agent from the reservoir to susceptible persons;
3. increasing the resistance of the susceptible persons; and
4. giving prophylactic treatment to susceptible persons who are probably infected.

See Chapter 9.

Prevention

Prevention is what you need to do to stop the disease occurring. You need to know the epidemiology of the disease so that you can choose the best means of prevention. The means used for prevention are the same as are used for control. (See above and Chapter 9.)

Acute

Any condition which comes suddenly and lasts a short time may be called 'acute'. This often means less than one month.

Chronic

Any condition which lasts a long time may be called 'chronic'. It usually starts slowly, but an acute condition may become a chronic condition. This usually means more than one month.

Subacute

A subacute condition is one which is somewhere between acute and chronic.

Lesion

Lesion is a general or non-specific term for a pathological change in a body tissue. It is often used to mean damage to the structure of part of an organ, especially damage caused by an injury or infection.

Syndrome

Syndrome is the name given to a *group of symptoms and/or signs*. When these symptoms and signs *all occur together* this usually means that a certain pathological process is present. There may be a number of possible causes of this syndrome.

Curative or clinical medicine

Curative medicine or clinical medicine are terms sometimes used for the processes of seeing a patient, taking a history, doing an examination, doing tests, making a diagnosis and treating the patient.

Note on prefixes and suffixes

Certain words or syllables may be added to the beginning of a word (prefix) or the ending of a word (suffix) to form a new word with a different meaning. Some of the prefixes and suffixes often used in medicine are listed below.

Common prefixes

hypo- less than normal or under.
> e.g. hypothermia: temperature less than normal; hypodermic: under the dermis or skin.

hyper- more than normal or above.
> e.g. hyperthyroidism: thyroid makes more hormone than normal.

an- without.
> e.g. anuric: without urine or no urine made.

exo- outside.
> e.g. exophthalmos: eye pushed out.

endo- within or inside (not to the outside).
> e.g. endocrine: gland which secretes into the blood.

macro- large.
> e.g. macroscopic: large enough to be seen by the naked eye.

micro- small.
> e.g. microscopic: so small can be seen only with the aid of a microscope.

Common suffixes

-aemia or -emia refers to the blood.
> e.g. anaemia: without normal amount of blood.

-uria refers to the urine.
> e.g. haematuria: blood in the urine.

-pathy disease.
> e.g. encephalopathy: disease of the brain.

-itis inflammation of.
> e.g. conjunctivitis: inflammation of conjunctivae.

-oma tumour of organ.
> e.g. meningioma: tumour of meninges.

Abbreviations (short terms for long words) and other words often used in medicine

+	and/with
>	more than
<	less than
%	per cent (or how many out of each one hundred)
↑	raised
↓	lowered
→	leading to
+ve	positive
−ve	negative
ACT	artemisinin-based combination therapy (for malaria)
AFB	acid fast bacilli
AIDS	acquired immunodeficiency syndrome
ARD	anti-retroviral drug
ART	anti-retroviral therapy
BCG	bacillus Calmette-Guérin (immunisation for tuberculosis)
bd	twice daily
bid	twice daily
BP	blood pressure
bubo	swollen pus-containing lymph nodes
CD4 cells	those T lymphocytes which are an important part of cellular immunity

chemotherapy	treatment with a chemical or drug	IM(I)	intramuscular (injection)
°C	temperature in Celsius or in Centigrade scales	IPT	intermittent prophylactic treatment (for pregnant women to prevent effects of malaria)
cm	centimetre		
CMV	cytomegalovirus	ITBN	insecticide-treated bed nets
CNS	central nervous system	IU	international unit
contacts	people, often family, close to patient, and at risk of getting the patient's infectious disease	IUD	intra-uterine contraceptive device
		IV	intravenous
co-amoxyclav	amoxicillin and clavulanic acid in one capsule, tablet or mixture	JVP	jugular venous pressure
		kg	kilogram
		l	litre
co-trimoxazole	trimethoprim and sulfamethoxazole in a single capsule, tablet or mixture	lesion	a damaged area of an organ or tissue
		LP	lumbar puncture
COLD	chronic obstructive lung disease	♂	male
COPD	chronic obstructive pulmonary disease	m	metre
		M	mile
CSF	cerebrospinal fluid	mcg (µg)	microgram or one-millionth of a gram
CVS	cardiovascular system		
CXR	chest X-ray	MDT	multidrug therapy (for leprosy)
dl	decilitre	mg	milligram (one-thousandth of a g)
DOT	directly observed treatment	mm	millimetre
DOTS	directly observed treatment short course	mmHg	millimetres of mercury
		mmol	millimol
dyspnoea	feeling of being short of breath (i.e. a symptom, not a sign)	MMR	measles, mumps and rubella vaccine
e.g.	for example	MO	Medical Officer
ENT	ear, nose and throat	mosmol	milliosmol
EPI	Expanded Programme for Immunization (WHO)	MR	measles rubella vaccine
		NIDDM	non-insulin-dependent diabetes mellitus (Type 2)
exudate	fluid containing much protein and many inflammatory cells (from an inflamed area)	NNRTI	non-nucleoside (and nucleotide) reverse transcriptase inhibitor
♀	female	NRTI	nucleoside (or nucleotide) reverse transcriptase inhibitor
FBC	full blood count		
ft	feet (measurement)	NSAID	non-steroidal anti-inflammatory drug
g	gram (also used for more than one, e.g. 2 g)	OPV	oral polio vaccine
GI	gastrointestinal	ORS	oral rehydration solution
GU	genito-urinary	PO	per os – by mouth
HAART	highly active anti-retroviral therapy	PR	pulse rate
		PR	per rectum – through the rectum
Hb	haemoglobin	PV	per vaginam – through the vagina
Hg	mercury	qid	four times in the day
HIV	human immunodeficiency virus	q2h	every 2 hours
HMS	hyperreactive malarious splenomegaly	q4h	every 4 hours
		regimen	a drug or several drugs given in certain doses for a stated condition
hrs	hours		
IDDM	insulin-dependent diabetes mellitus (Type 1)	relapse	disease starting again after the patient seems to be cured
i.e.	that is	RR	respiratory rate

SC(I)	subcutaneous (injection)
SMX/TMP	sulfamethoxazole/trimethoprim (co-trimoxazole)
STD	sexually transmitted disease
STI	sexually transmitted infection
TB	tuberculosis – usually used for disease and not just infection by *M. tuberculosis*
Td	tetanus toxoid and low-dose diphtheria vaccine
tid	three times in the day
TMP/SMX	trimethoprim/sulfamethoxazole (co-trimoxazole)
TT	tetanus toxoid vaccine
µg	microgram (one-millionth of a gram), often written 'mcg'
URT	upper respiratory tract
URTI	upper respiratory tract infection
WCC	white cell count
WHO	World Health Organization
ZN	Ziel–Neelson stain (for AFB)

SI units

The International System of Units (SI) is based on the units; metre, kilogram, second, ampere, kelvin, candela and mole. It is already used by many countries as their only legal system.

Names and symbols for basic SI units

Physical quantity	Name of SI unit	Symbol for SI unit
length	metre	m
mass	kilogram	kg
time	second	s
thermodynamic temperature	kelvin	K
amount of substance	mole	mol

Prefixes for SI units

Prefixes can be used to show decimal fractions or multiples of the basic (or derived) SI units.

Fraction	Prefix	Symbol
$\frac{1}{10}$ or 10^{-1}	deci	d
$\frac{1}{100}$ or 10^{-2}	centi	c
$\frac{1}{1000}$ or 10^{-3}	milli	m
$\frac{1}{1,000,000}$ or 10^{-6}	micro	µ *or* mc

Multiple	Prefix	Symbol
× 10 or 10^1	deca	da
× 100 or 10^2	hecto	h
× 1000 or 10^3	kilo	k
× 1,000,000 or 10^6	mega	M

Length

The SI unit of length is the metre (m).
  1 micron (µ) (obsolete) = 10^{-6} m = 1 µm.
  1 inch (in) = 2.54 cm = 0.0254 m.
  1 foot (ft) = 0.3048 m.
  1 yard (yd) = 0.9144 m.

Volume

The SI unit of volume is the cubic metre (m^3); but since this is inconveniently large for most measurements in medicine, the litre (l) has been kept as an alternative to the cubic decimetre (dm^3).
  1 m^3 = 1000 l.
  1 fluid ounce (oz) = 28.41 ml.
  1 pint = 20 fluid oz. = 568 ml.
  1 gallon = 4.55 l.

Mass

The SI unit of mass is the kilogram (kg).
  1 kg = 1000 grams (g).
  1 grain = 64.8 mg.
  1 ounce (oz) = 28.35 g.
  1 pound (lb) = 16 oz = 453.6 g.
  1 ton = 2240 lb = 1016 kg.
  1 tonne = 1000 kg = 0.984 ton.

Amount of substance

Where the molecular weight of a substance is known, its amount should usually be expressed in terms of the mole (mol). One mole of a substance is that amount of the substance which contains the same number of particles (whether atoms, molecules, ions or radicals) as 12 g of carbon 12. In short, 1 mole is the particle weight (such as atomic weight or molecular weight) expressed in grams.

The 'equivalent' is now not used. It was used to express the amount of an ionised substance; it is the number of moles multiplied by the valency.
Thus 10 mol Na^+ = 10 equiv.;
but 10 mol Ca^{++} = 20 equiv.

Concentration and osmotic pressure

Concentrations of substances in biological fluids should be expressed in molar terms if the molecular weight is known; and in terms of mass if not. Thus plasma glucose is expressed as mmol/l, while plasma albumin is expressed as g/l. In each case the reference unit of volume is the litre. A special exception is haemoglobin, whose concentration in blood is expressed as g/dl.

Osmotic pressure is expressed as osmolarity (moles per litre of solution) or osmolality (moles per kilogram of water).

Pressure

The SI unit of pressure is the pascal (Pa); this is the pressure exerted by 1 newton acting on an area of a square metre ($1\ Pa = 1\ N\ m^{-2}$).

1 cmH$_2$O = 98.1 Pa.
1 mmHg = 1 torr = 133.3 Pa = 0.1333 kPa.
1 kPa = 7.50 mmHg = 10.1 cmH$_2$O.
1 normal atmosphere = 760 mmHg = 101.3 kPa.

Temperature

The SI temperature scale is the kelvin scale (K), but this is inconvenient to use in medicine and the Celsius (formerly 'centigrade') scale (C°) has been retained.

Degree Celsius = K − 273.15.

Conversion from the Fahrenheit scale to the Celsius scale can be carried out with either of these formulae:

$$F = (9/5\ C) + 32$$
$$C = 5/9\ (F - 32)$$

where F is the temperature in degrees Fahrenheit and C is the temperature in degrees Celsius.

Time

1 hour (h) = 60 minutes (min) = 3600 seconds (s).

The use of hertz (Hz) for frequency to replace cycles per second is recommended provided it is not used for the timing of discontinuous events, i.e. not, for example, for the frequency of passing urine or the dispensing of doses of medicine. It should not be used for frequency of rotation.

3 Pathology

The normal human body is made in a certain way. This is called its structure or its *anatomy*. The normal human body works in a certain way. This is called its normal function or *physiology*. Many things can damage the normal anatomy of the body or upset the normal physiology of the body and cause changes in the anatomy and/or the physiology. These are called *pathological changes*.

Pathology (or pathological change) is the change in the normal anatomy and physiology made by the cause of disease.

The pathological changes (and sometimes the causes of them) show themselves as the symptoms, the signs and the abnormal tests of disease.

When a part of the body is attacked by things which may damage it (see Chapter 4 page 16), this can cause many different types of pathological change. Three very important pathological changes are:

1. death of part of the body (often called necrosis) or death of all of the body,
2. inflammatory reaction (or inflammation), and
3. neoplasm (or 'cancer' formation).

Inflammation

Inflammation is the change which happens in a tissue when it is injured, if the injury does not completely destroy the tissue.

Some causes of inflammation are:

1. trauma or physical injury,
2. infection,
3. chemicals,
4. allergy (see Chapter 4 page 16).

There are two main types of inflammation:

1. acute,
2. chronic.

The type and amount of inflammation depends on the cause. Acute serious injury or infection with some organisms cause acute inflammation. Chronic mild injury or infection with other organisms (especially those which cause leprosy and TB and HIV) cause chronic inflammation.

Acute inflammation

In acute inflammation more blood flows to the area. This is because the blood vessels become more widely open. Fluid (containing white blood cells, antibodies and other proteins from inside the blood vessels) goes through the capillary walls into the tissues of the area. Then some or all of the following processes happen, depending on the cause of the inflammation.

- Fluid dilutes the cause, e.g. a chemical.
- White blood cells try to digest and destroy the cause, e.g. dirt in a wound.
- Proteins make a wall around the area to limit the spread of bacteria, e.g. TB (see Chapter 14 page 102 and Chapter 10 page 42).
- Antibodies attach themselves to bacteria or viruses and destroy them or make it easier for white cells to digest them.
- Immune white cells attach themselves to bacteria or viruses and destroy them.
- Pus, made of dead cells and tissue, is formed in the area.

Some of the symptoms and signs of acute inflammation are:

1. swelling,
2. redness or shininess,
3. heat,
4. pain and tenderness,
5. loss of function,
6. sometimes, fluid or pus in the area.

Chronic inflammation

Chronic inflammation can happen because of a chronic mild injury or infection by some types of organisms or because an acute inflammation has been in the area for a long time and the body has not quite been able to destroy the cause.

In chronic inflammation the blood vessels become only a little wider and fluid, protein and cells escape only slowly into the area. However, the structural body cells normally present in the area are slowly killed and replaced by fibrous tissue. As the fibrous tissue gets older, it shrinks and causes scarring. The tissue in the area of the chronic inflammation is slowly destroyed. Pus may be made if many white cells are killed.

Symptoms and signs of chronic inflammation in an area include:

1. swelling, but not usually very much,
2. redness is not usual,
3. heat, but only slight,
4. pain and tenderness, but not usually very much,
5. loss of function is usual,
6. there can be fluid or pus.

Chronic inflammation will stop if the cause is removed. Healing will then happen. However, if the organ has been badly damaged or if the area of the body has been very scarred, it may never function properly again.

General (whole body) effects of inflammation

In both acute and chronic inflammation, *certain toxins and other chemicals are put into the blood.* Some of these chemicals are made by the body to help the defensive inflammatory reaction. Some of these chemicals cause more white blood cells to be made, fever, fast pulse rate, etc. Some of these chemicals may be from the cause of the inflammation, especially if it is an organism. Some of these chemicals may be toxins which cause high fever, damage to blood vessels with bleeding, wasting of the body (muscles get thin and weak), damage to the bone marrow and blood cells with anaemia, etc.

In acute inflammation, more acute changes are caused – high fever, shivering (rigors), fast pulse, bleeding, etc.

In chronic inflammation less acute changes are caused – low fever, wasting, anaemia, etc.

Neoplasm (also called newgrowth or tumour or cancer)

Normal body cells grow only where and when they are needed, e.g. during growth of a child, or to repair a wound, or to make new parts for the body to replace worn out parts. These normal cells stop growing after they have done their work.

A neoplasm is the growth of *abnormal body cells* which *keep on growing either where or when they are not needed.* The body cannot stop them growing.

The cause of some neoplasms is not known. Known causes of neoplasm include:

1. Chemicals, e.g. tobacco smoke causes lung cancer; betel nut and lime causes mouth cancer.
2. Some drugs, but not those used by most health workers.
3. Some viruses, e.g. hepatitis B virus causes hepatoma.

4. Too much sunlight in people with light coloured skins (or albinos) causes skin cancer.
5. Radiation from atomic bombs, etc. causes blood cancers.
6. Hereditary factors.

There are two types of neoplasm:

1. Benign (or simple) neoplasms. The cells of benign neoplasms stay in the place where they started to grow and do not spread to other organs.
2. Malignant neoplasms. The cells of malignant neoplasms do not grow only at the place where they started to grow. These cells also spread directly or in the blood or in the lymph to other parts of the body where they also start to grow. Malignant neoplasms can therefore be of two types:
   (a) Primary – the neoplasm at the place where it started,
   (b) Secondary – the neoplasm at the place it has spread to from the primary neoplasm.

Neoplasms damage the body in many ways:

1. Destruction of the tissue in which it is growing, e.g. neoplasm in the liver causes liver failure with jaundice.
2. Obstruction of the organ in which it is growing, e.g. neoplasm in the intestine causes intestinal obstruction with abdominal pain, constipation and vomiting.
3. Pressure on other important structures, e.g. Burkitt's tumour in the face pushes an eye out so that the eyelids cannot close.
4. Ulceration of the surface with bleeding or infection, e.g. stomach cancer causes vomiting of blood and anaemia.
5. Wasting and malaise (not feeling well).

The ten most common tumours in developing countries are of

1. the uterine cervix,
2. stomach,
3. oropharynx (of mouth and throat),
4. oesophagus,
5. breast,
6. lung,
7. liver,
8. colon and rectum,
9. lymphatic system (lymphomas),
10. bone marrow and blood (leukaemia).

4 A Classification of Disease – the causes of diseases

Diseases can be grouped or classified in many different ways. One good way to classify diseases in a health centre is by a *combination* of cause and pathology and clinical findings. Like this:

Congenital

These are diseases or abnormalities that were present when the patient was born. There are three sub-groups:

1. inherited or hereditary, i.e. passed on from the mother or the father – these diseases are in the family (e.g. thalassaemia);
2. damage done to the baby while it was in the mother's womb (e.g. blindness or congenital heart disease from an attack of rubella (German measles) in the mother);
3. unknown (e.g. talipes or club foot).

Traumatic

These are injuries. *Causes* include:

1. mechanical injuries (e.g. cuts, bruises, fractures),
2. heat (e.g. burns).

Inflammatory

Inflammation is a reaction of part of the body to things which can injure it but do not completely destroy it. The most important part of the inflammatory reaction is that the blood vessels become wider and bring much more blood to the area. The blood vessels then allow fluid, proteins and cells to go into the area to fight the thing that is attacking the body (see Inflammation, Chapter 3).

Causes include:

1. Infection with organisms including:
   viruses, bacteria, rickettsiae, protozoa, fungi, worms and insects (called 'infestations').
2. Trauma:
   mechanical, heat.
3. Chemicals, especially:
   toxins, bites, stings and venoms (e.g. insect stings, stonefish sting).
4. Allergic reactions.
   Allergy is an inflammatory reaction of part of the body caused by some foreign substance on or in the body. This substance does not cause inflammation in the body of normal people. But if a person develops allergy to this substance, he may develop abnormal antibodies or cellular immunity to this substance. When this substance comes in contact with the body again there is a reaction between the substance and the abnormal antibodies or immune cells which causes an inflammatory reaction. (See Chapter 10 page 44.)
   (a) Allergy can be caused by substances touching the skin, e.g. skin rash in some people due to 'hairy' caterpillars or some insects.
   (b) Allergy can be caused by substances being inhaled (i.e. breathed in), e.g. asthma and hayfever in some people from house dust.
   (c) Allergy can be caused by substances being injected, e.g. skin rash, asthma or shock in some people after penicillin injection or certain insect bites.
   (d) Allergy can be caused by substances being swallowed, e.g. skin rash in some people after swallowing aspirin tablets or cows' milk.

Neoplastic (also called tumours, cancers, new-growths, or growths)

Neoplasms are made of abnormal body cells. These cells grow both when and where they are not needed. They cause damage to the normal parts of the body where they are growing.

They may be:

1. simple or benign,
2. malignant, either
   (a) primary where the neoplasm started, or
   (b) secondary where the neoplasm has spread to.

(See Neoplasm, Chapter 3.)
Causes include:

1. viruses, e.g. EB virus together with malaria infection causes Burkitt's tumours;
2. chemicals, e.g. tobacco smoking causes lung cancer, lime and betel nut chewing causes mouth cancer;
3. some drugs, e.g. immunosuppressive drugs can cause lymphomas;
4. excess radiation, e.g. sun on skin of albino causes skin cancer;

5. inherited factors (e.g. certain genes);
6. other and as yet unknown causes.

Degenerative

These diseases are a wearing out of part of the body. *Causes* include:

1. Old age, e.g. cataracts cause blindness.
2. Habits or events during life can cause parts of the body to wear out more quickly than others, e.g. osteoarthritis when men play football and damage their knee joints many times.
3. Amyloid disease. This is an unusual condition in which an abnormal protein is put into the tissues and stops these tissues and organs working properly. It happens in old age and sometimes in chronic inflammatory diseases (e.g. leprosy) and some cancers and sometimes for no known cause.

Chemicals – drugs, poisons, toxins, venoms

These may have been given purposely or accidentally. They may have been given for good or bad reasons. They may have been given by the health worker, the employer, a traditional healer, an enemy or the patient himself.

1. Drugs should be given only by those who know the risks of their unwanted bad effects as well as their wanted good effects. These persons include health workers and patients who are instructed in the use of certain drugs, e.g. antimalarials. Drugs given by health workers and drugs patients themselves have taken to treat one disease, can be the cause of another disease.

   The patient may also give himself other drugs – alcohol, tobacco and lime with betel nut. These are very common causes of disease – accidents, chronic bronchitis and cancer of the mouth (respectively).
2. Poisons may be added to a person's food or drink by an enemy; but this in fact is very rare. Poisons may be taken by the patient himself to attempt suicide or attempt to treat a condition (e.g. unwanted pregnancy); but most commonly by accident (e.g. kerosene left in a soft-drink bottle).
3. Toxins may be formed by bacteria in food. When eaten, the toxins cause 'food poisoning'.
4. Venoms may be injected by insect stings or snake bites. They may cause various changes including pain, paralysis of muscles and abnormal bleeding.

Malnutrition

Not enough food, or not enough of some foods, or too much of some foods can cause disease, e.g.

• marasmus from not enough food,
• kwashiorkor from not enough protein,
• anaemia from not enough iron or folic acid,
• obesity from too much food.

Psychological

Situations causing worry, stress and anxiety often cause disease, e.g. tension headaches, anxiety states and acting out ('hysterical') paralysis.

Failure of an organ or system of the body (especially blood vessels)

Some conditions or diseases of parts of the body are caused by the failure of other parts of the body.

1. The most common of these conditions are those caused by the *failure of the blood vessels*. If an artery becomes narrowed or blocked, then little or no food and oxygen can go to the part of the body supplied by the artery. That part is then damaged and cannot function properly and may die. Death of just a part of the body, due to loss of blood, may be called gangrene. If veins become blocked, blood pumped into part of the body cannot go out of that part. That part then swells up, is damaged and cannot function properly. Such conditions have *vascular* causes.
2. *Blood volume failure* (not enough blood volume) may cause shock (shortness of breath, fainting, dizziness), etc.
3. *Heart failure* may cause oedema, enlarged liver, etc.
4. *Respiratory (lung) failure* may cause wasting, cyanosis, abnormal behaviour, heart failure, etc.
5. *Kidney failure* may cause oedema, high blood pressure, anaemia, weight loss, etc.
6. *Liver failure* may cause wasting, oedema, bleeding, abnormal behaviour, jaundice, etc.
7. *Endocrine gland failure* (e.g. pancreatic failure may cause wasting, passing a lot of urine, unconsciousness, etc., i.e. diabetes mellitus).

All body systems must be considered; but especially important are vascular, blood, heart, respiratory, kidney, liver and endocrine.

Others

Other groups do exist but are not as common as the nine groups discussed above. Some have known causes. Some have causes not yet discovered.

Summary

When a disease or disability is discovered in a patient and the diagnosis is not obvious, ask yourself and answer the following questions:

Is this condition:

1. Congenital?
2. Traumatic?
3. Inflammatory, caused by:
   (a) trauma?
   (b) infection?
   (c) toxins or bites or venoms?
   (d) allergy?
4. Neoplastic?
5. Degenerative?
6. Caused by chemicals – drugs, poisons, toxins, venoms?
7. Caused by malnutrition?
8. Caused by psychological causes?
9. Caused by the failure of an organ of the body – especially blood vessels?
10. Caused by other causes known or unknown?

5 Epidemiology

It is not enough to know only the causes of illnesses.

The presence of the cause of a disease (usually called the 'specific agent') does not mean that the disease will always develop. All people at times have the organisms that cause pneumonia (the specific agent of pneumonia) in their respiratory tracts. But few get pneumonia. Some, however, do. Why? Smoking tobacco causes lung cancer. But many people smoke all of their lives and do not get lung cancer. Some, however, do. Why? There are certain things about the specific agent, or about the person who has the specific agent acting on him, or in the environment, that determine if disease will or will not happen.

The study of the distribution of disease in the community (i.e. when it occurs, where it occurs and who gets it) and all the things that determine if disease will or will not happen, is called epidemiology.

> Epidemiology is the study of *who* gets a particular disease, *where* and *when* these persons get the disease, and *how* and *why* they get the disease. (See Figures 5.1 and 5.2.)

Epidemiology gives the known answers to these questions about a disease.

1. *Who* (including how many)
2. *When*
3. *Where*

are the people affected?

4. *How* does the whole process including the means of transfer of the specific agent (or 'cause') happen?
5. *Why* – or what are the factors (reasons) in:
   (a) the specific agent (i.e. the 'cause'); or
   (b) the means of transfer of the specific agent; or
   (c) man; or
   (d) the environment
   which determine if the disease happens or not.

Accurate terms to describe how often a disease occurs (or the *frequency* of a disease) include:

- *Prevalence* of a disease is the *total* number of persons with the disease at a certain time in a certain population.
- *Incidence* of a disease is the number of *new* persons getting the disease during a certain time in a certain population.

See Chapter 9 for other definitions and explanations.

Epidemiology has many uses. Many of these uses are not useful in your day-to-day work. Some, however, are.

If you know the epidemiology of a disease, it will help you in the differential diagnosis (see Chapter 6) of a patient who is sick. Some diseases do not affect some groups of people but may be common in other groups of people. By knowing which group of persons your patient is in and what diseases are common in his group, it is much easier to decide which disease your patient has.

If you know the epidemiology of a disease, it will help you to understand that there is often more than one 'cause' of a person getting sick. There may be more than one thing which you need to do, therefore, to make the patient well again.

If you know the epidemiology of types of disease, this may help you to find the reason for an outbreak of a disease in your community.

If you know the epidemiology of a disease, it will help you control and prevent a disease. You may have to try to kill or remove the specific agent which can cause the disease. You may have to change the environment to stop its means of spread. You may have to increase the resistance of the person who is susceptible to the specific agent. It is only if you know the epidemiology of the disease that you can decide which of these things is the best to do.

If you really want to improve the health of the people in your community, you need to use the methods of epidemiology to make a 'community diagnosis' of your own community. You need to find out who makes up your community and how many men, women and children there are. You need to know what illnesses really do affect these people. You need to know which members of the community have these illnesses. You need to know when and where and how and why these people get these illnesses. It is only when you have used epidemiological methods to make your own community diagnosis that you will be able:

1. to make the best use of epidemiological methods in diagnosing and treating individual patients, and
2. to give the best advice for disease prevention and health promotion to all the people of the community.

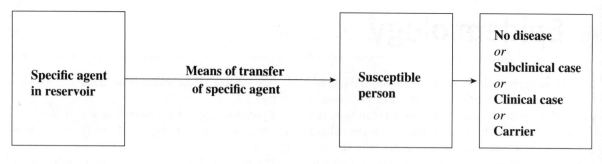

or, in more detail:

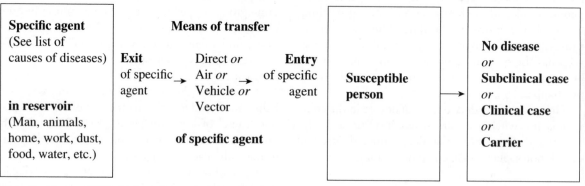

Figure 5.1 *Diagrams showing how disease may be caused.*

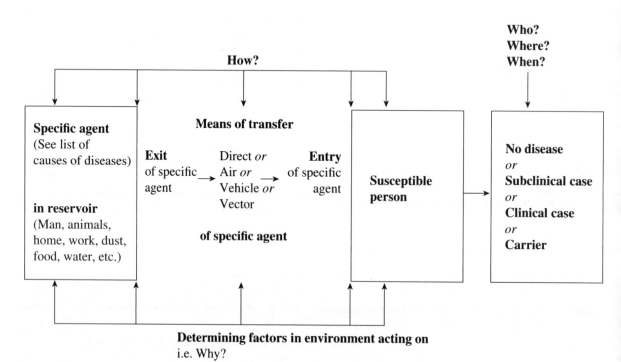

Figure 5.2 *A diagram showing the things that are studied in epidemiology.*

6 Diagnosis of Disease

Remember: you must diagnose before you can treat.

You must first diagnose what condition or disease a patient has before you can choose the proper treatment to help the patient. The only treatment which will help the patient is the proper treatment for the condition or disease which the patient really has. Treatment (even good treatment) for a condition which the patient does not have will not help the patient.

To make the correct diagnosis you must do all of the following six things:

1. Take a medical history.
2. Do a medical or physical examination.
3. Make a differential diagnosis (or make a list of the diseases that *could* be causing the patient's main symptoms and signs).
4. Do or order any tests that are needed:
   (a) to find out which of the diseases in the differential diagnosis the patient really has; *or*
   (b) to confirm a diagnosis; *or*
   (c) to give a 'baseline' to see if the patient gets better or worse.
5. Make a provisional diagnosis and decide:
   (a) which disease (or diseases) is most likely to be causing the patient's symptoms and signs;
   (b) how severe this disease is;
   (c) how quickly this disease is getting better or worse.
6. Decide on the prognosis of the patient.

Taking a medical history

If you know what questions to ask, you can take a full history in about 2–5 minutes in most ordinary cases.

If you make the patient give you a good history, you will often hear the patient tell you a story which you recognise. The story may be one you have heard before or it may be a story that you have read about in your medical books. In either case, you will recognise the patient's story as the story of a disease about which you know. Even if you do not recognise the story of a disease, you will hear about important symptoms which you can use in making the differential diagnosis.

Also the history will often tell you how you need to examine the patient.

The medical history is in nine parts (the medical examination is in nine parts too):

1. general information and admission notes;
2. complaints and their duration;
3. history of the present illness;
4. specific questioning (or specific interrogation);
5. past history;
6. family and contact history;
7. if the patient may have a mental condition, take the history again from a relative or another witness;
8. check the patient's outpatient card and inpatient notes for any history in it;
9. tell the patient a summary of the history – ask him to correct anything wrong.

1. *General information and admission notes*
   Write down:
   > Date.
   > Patient's name and address, etc.[1]
   > With whom patient lives and the address.[1]
   > Reason for the patient coming.
   > Who referred patient.

2. *Complaints and their duration*[2]
   Write down:
   > Only the main problems.[3]
   > Only short descriptions.
   > Only the patient's own way of describing them.

3. *History of present illness (HPI)*
   Ask questions like these and write down the answers:
   > How long ago was it that something first went wrong with you?
   > What was this first thing that went wrong?
   > What was the next thing that happened?
   > When did this happen?
   > What happened next?… When?…

   You should also:

   • Ask for a full description of pain or any other symptom.

---

1 The patient's exact present address and also a friend's or relative's name and address are most important. If you do not write this down it will not be possible to find the patient later if it is necessary. You may need to find the patient if he has an infectious disease (e.g. tuberculosis) and does not come for treatment.

2 When you have ordered treatment, look back at this list to make sure you have done something for the patient's complaints.

3 Make sure the patient tells you all of his complaints. He may leave the most important one till last.

- Ask about all the symptoms of all the body systems in which the patient has symptoms.
- Ask about the presence or absence of all the symptoms of any possible disease.
- Ask what treatment has already been given.

4. Specific interrogation (SI) or specific questioning

Ask the patient about (unless already talked about in the HPI):[4]

Fever.

Cough. Sputum. Haemoptysis.

Chronic cough.

Pain in the chest.

Shortness of breath.

Eating well. Vomiting. Diarrhoea.

Pain in the abdomen.

Urinary pain, urinary frequency, abnormal colour of urine, blood in the urine.

Date of last menstrual period.

Getting fatter or thinner or staying the same weight.

What the patient thinks is wrong.

What the patient thinks is the cause.

If the patient is *pregnant* also ask about:

Oedema? Treatment?

High blood pressure? Treatment?

Vaginal bleeding? Treatment?

Anaemia? Treatment?

Labour pains started? When?

Vaginal show or bleeding? When?

Membranes ruptured? When?

5. Past history (PH)

Ask about:

Drugs:

- given today,
- given for the treatment of this illness before today,
- given regularly,
- alcohol and tobacco – how much, how often.

Treatment given by traditional healers? What? Previous attacks of this illness? When? What treatment?

---

4 You must always get answers to all of these questions. If you already know the answers from the HPI, do not ask the questions again. You cannot think that the patient does not have these symptoms only because the patient has not told you about them. He may not think they are important. He may not want to talk about them. These questions are about the main symptoms caused by the main pathological processes in each of the major body systems. You must find out about each one of them. In some places where there are special diseases, other questions may have to be added to this list.

Previous other serious illnesses or operations or accidents? What? When?

HIV infection diagnosed or if there are risk factors for HIV infection (i.e. any unsafe sex ever)?

If the patient is *pregnant*, also ask about:

How many births? Dates?

How many miscarriages? Dates?

Any abortions? Dates?

How many stillbirths or neonatal deaths? When? Why?

Any difficult deliveries (Caesarian section, symphysiotomy, vacuum extraction, very long labour (> 24 hours)? Which births?

Any post-partum haemorrhage or retained placenta? Which births?

6. Family history and contact history (FH, CH)

This is especially important for those who live in the same house. Ask if there is:

anyone with this illness,

anyone with other serious illness,

anyone with tuberculosis (or cough for more than 4 weeks),

anyone with leprosy,

anyone with HIV infection.

7. If the patient may have a mental problem or condition, take all history again from a relative or other witness

8. Look at the patient's outpatient card (and also any inpatient notes) for any HPI, SI, PH, FH, etc. in it. (Return the patient's card to the patient.)

9. Tell the patient a summary of the history obtained. Then ask him to tell you if anything is wrong

If pain (or another symptom) is present, it will often help the health worker to ask about:

1. The site (or where it is).
2. The radiation (or if it spreads to any other place and where).
3. The character or type (e.g. constant [stays the same all the time] or colic [comes and goes again and again in minutes]).
4. The severity (or how bad it is).
5. The frequency (or how often it comes).
6. The duration (or how long it lasts).
7. Things that start it, make it worse or make it better.

Note: See Chapter 19 page 197 for further advice about taking the history.

Performing a medical or physical examination

The medical examination is in three parts.

1. Basic observations.
2. Examination of the part of the body that the symptoms suggest is diseased.
3. Examination of the whole body if needed.

The *first part or basic observations* should *always* be done on *all* patients for at least two reasons.

1. It will show you if the patient is 'sick' or not. This is not done by intuition (a feeling or an idea). This is done by observation during examination.
2. It is a simple test for the common and the serious or even fatal diseases. You may need to add some other observations to this list in places where there are special diseases. The following diseases are suggested by the 'basic observations':

   • Meningitis is suggested by the change in the level of consciousness and the stiff neck.
   • Malaria is suggested by a high temperature.
   • Penumonia is suggested by a fast and abnormal type of breathing.
   • Gastroenteritis is suggested by weight loss and signs of dehydration.
   • Malnutrition or wasting is suggested by the signs of malnutrition and wasting.
   • Anaemia is suggested by the colour.

Therefore, even if a patient has only a simple laceration, you should still do the 'basic observations' so that you can do any necessary preventive medicine. Diseases may be found while they are still mild. Treatment will stop these diseases becoming severe or causing death.

The *second part* is the examination of the part of the body which the symptoms suggest is diseased.

The *third part* of the examination is the examination of the whole body. You must examine the whole of the body if:

1. The patient is 'sick'.
2. The disease you think the patient may have could affect more than one part of the body.
3. You are not certain of the diagnosis.

In each part of a clinical examination you usually do these five things:

1. Inspection – look and see.
2. Palpation – feel and touch with hands.
3. Percussion – tap and listen (and feel).
4. Auscultation – listen (usually with stethoscope).

5. Measurement – apart from basic observations done every time any patient is seen, not often done in a health centre.

It is not always possible to do all these things. But you should do them all, in this order, if possible.

The full or complete medical examination, which includes all of the above three parts, will therefore include the following nine examinations.

1. Basic observations.
2. Head and neck including the ears, nose and throat, thyroid and lymph glands.
3. Chest and spine.
4. Abdomen.
5. Skin and hair.
6. Muscles, bones, joints.
7. Head and neck, etc. (if not done before).
8. Any special examinations suggested by previous history and examination.
9. Mental state.

1. Basic observations

Signs of meningeal irritation (drowsiness, or irritability or fitting, stiff neck, stiff back, Kernig's sign positive).

Does the patient have signs of meningitis or cerebral malaria?

Temperature (T°)
Pulse rate (PR)
Blood pressure (BP) (if needed)   } 5 vital signs
Breathing (respiration) rate (RR)
    and type of breathing (respiration)
Weight

Does the patient have signs of malaria or pneumonia or shock or weight change?

Dehydration – eyes sunken,
    mouth dry, inelastic skin,
    pulse fast, weight loss
Oedema (limbs, back, face)   } 5 general
Malnutrition   conditions
Wasting
Colour – anaemia, jaundice, cyanosis

Does the patient have any of these five signs?

Does the patient have HIV infection?

Is the patient 'sick'?

2. Head and neck including ears, nose and throat, thyroid and lymph glands in the neck and axilla

(See also Chapter 20 pages 265–268, Chapter 30 page 496, Chapter 22 pages 332–333.)
These may be left until 7.
Does the patient have a condition affecting these parts?

Does the patient have conditions affecting the lips, mouth, throat, lymph nodes, etc. suggesting HIV infection?

3. Chest
(See also Chapter 20 pages 269–275.)
Look for:

- rate of breathing (respiration),
- type of breathing (respiration),
- deformity of spine or chest.

Feel for decreased movement of:

- all of the chest,
- part or parts of the chest.

Percuss for:

- dullness or
- increased resonance

} in { all of the chest, or part or parts of the chest.

Listen for:

- amount of breath sounds
- breath sounds normal or bronchial
- crackles or crepitations
- wheezes or rhonchi

} in { all of the chest, or part or parts of the chest.

Ask the patient to cough – listen to the cough.
Look at the sputum (is there any pus or blood?).
Does the patient have pneumonia or tuberculosis or obstruction of bronchi?

4. Abdomen
(See Chapter 36 pages 593–605, Chapter 22 page 343, Chapter 23 page 348, Chapter 24 page 393.)
Look at:

- size (distension),
- shape (herniae, masses),
- surface (scars),
- movement when breathing.

Feel for:

- tenderness, rebound tenderness, guarding, rigidity,
- liver, spleen, uterus and bladder,
- lumps, including herniae and lymph glands.

Percuss, if needed, for:

- organs or masses,
- fluid (e.g. ascites).

Listen, if needed, for bowel sounds.

Pelvic examination through the rectum (PR), if needed, for:

- tenderness,
- enlarged organs,
- masses,
- faeces, blood or pus in rectum.

Pelvic examination through the vagina (PV), if needed, for:

- tenderness,
- enlarged organs,
- masses,
- blood or pus in vagina.

Does the patient have signs of 'peritonitis' or an enlarged organ, or an inflamed organ or an abnormal mass?

If the patient is *pregnant*, also:
Palpate for:

- size of uterus (height of fundus),
- lie of fetus, what is presenting part.

Auscultate for fetal heart rate.

If the patient is in *labour*, also:
Palpate for:

- size of uterus (height of fundus),
- lie of fetus, what is presenting part, engagement of head,
- frequency, duration and strength of contractions.

Auscultate for fetal heart rate.

Do pelvic examination PV for:

- state of cervix and start cervicograph,
- membranes ruptured or intact,
- level of head (above or below spines),
- caput.

5. Skin and hair
(See also Chapter 32.)
Look for:

- scabies,
- infections,
- other rashes,
- scars.

Does the patient have scabies or impetigo or leprosy or conditions suggesting HIV infection?

6. Muscles, bones and joints
(See also Chapter 28.)
Look and feel for:

- deformity,
- tenderness,
- swelling.

Does the patient have fracture, osteomyelitis, arthritis or abscess?

7. Head and neck, ENT, thyroid, lymph glands (if not done)

8. Any special examination indicated by previous history and examination

Five important examinations which you may need to do:

- If gynaecological disease is possible, do pelvic examination PV (see Chapter 19 page 200).
- If leprosy is suspected, do examinations for nerve enlargement and tenderness and for loss of sensation and for paralysis (see Chapter 15 pages 133–138).
- If there is pain in the eye or loss of sight, examine for iritis and corneal ulcer and corneal foreign body (see Chapter 31 pages 506–507).
- If there is a wound, check that nerves, tendons and blood vessels are all working.
- If there is oedema or if heart failure is suspected, examine for raised jugular venous pressure (see Chapter 27 pages 460–461).

9. *Mental state*

(See also Chapter 35 pages 571–572.)

- Ability to communicate (hear, see, move, talk, etc).
- Level of consciousness.
- Memory – recent past and distant past.
- Orientation: person, time, place.
- Intelligence.
- Thoughts by:

speech, appearance, behaviour } especially { logical or mixed up, hallucinations delusions, one particular idea

- Mood by:

speech, appearance, behaviour } especially { in keeping with thoughts, actions and circumstances; manic (too happy); depressed (too sad).

- Insight.

Does the patient have any evidence of confusion, delirium, dementia, non-organic psychosis or of a non-psychotic disturbance?

If you carry out a good examination, you will often see in the patient a 'picture' or 'pattern' which you recognise. The 'picture' or 'pattern' may be one you have seen before in another patient or it may be one you recognise from reading about it from your medical books. In either case, you will have recognised the 'picture' or 'pattern' as a disease which you know about. Even if you do not recognise a 'picture' or 'pattern' of a disease, you will have found important signs to use in making the differential diagnosis.

Making a differential diagnosis (DD)

The patient's symptoms and signs are caused by (1) an abnormality of the structure and/or function of a part of his or her body and (2) the cause of this abnormality.

A number of different conditions can cause the same symptom or sign. These different conditions, however, usually as well have other symptoms or signs or tests, which are not all the same. The different conditions which cause the same symptom or sign can be separated by using these other symptoms and signs and tests.

The differential diagnosis is a list of the conditions any one of which could be causing the patient's main symptoms and signs.

Write down the patient's main symptoms and signs in a row across the top of a page of paper. Then under each of these symptoms and signs, write down the list of conditions which could cause these symptoms and signs. The differential diagnosis is all the conditions in all the lists.

Next, look for a disease (or diseases) that is in each list (as a cause of each symptom and sign). This is the condition which is most likely to be the cause of the patient's condition. If there is more than one condition in all of the lists, tests will probably be needed to find out which of the conditions is the real cause of the patient's problems.

Doing or ordering tests (or investigations)

You may need a test:

1. to decide between the possible diagnoses in the DD;
2. to confirm a diagnosis;
3. to give a base line to be able to judge if a patient is getting better or worse.

See Appendix 1 (page 26) for how to take and send blood for tests in the hospital laboratory.

Making a provisional diagnosis (PD)

The provisional diagnosis (PD) is the condition you think the patient really has.

You decide the PD after considering all the conditions in the differential diagnosis that could cause the patient's main symptoms and signs. Reject the other conditions in the list if:

1. these conditions do not cause all of the patient's symptoms and signs; and
2. these conditions have other symptoms or signs or tests which do not fit the patient.

Choose the condition as the PD which:

1. is a cause of all the patient's symptoms and signs; and
2. has other symptoms and signs and tests, all of which do fit the patient.

In this book, the PD of most of the common symptoms and signs is set out.

The prognosis

The prognosis is what you think will happen to the patient because of the condition you have diagnosed, e.g.

• die or live,
• improve quickly or slowly,
• not improve at all.

The prognoses of the common diseases are set out in this book.

The signature of health worker and date should always be written after any of the above are written into the patient's notes.

Summary

> Diagnosis of disease includes:
>
> 1. Taking a medical history (nine parts).
> 2. Doing a clinical examination (nine parts).
> 3. Making a differential diagnosis.
> 4. Doing or ordering any tests needed.
> 5. Deciding the prognosis.

You must practise doing medical histories and examinations again and again until all of the things in this chapter can be done in 5–10 minutes.

Appendix 1   Method of taking blood for tests, making blood smears and sending pathology specimens to the hospital laboratory

> 1. Always use gloves when taking blood or handling blood. This is to protect you from HIV and hepatitis viruses and other infections which may be in the blood.

> 2. Always put lancets, disposable needles and other sharp pieces of equipment which may have blood on them into the special 'sharps' disposable container. This container should be itself disposable, strong enough that none of the 'sharps' can stick through the side of it and should never be overfilled. The filled container should be got rid of as has been decided by your health department, such as by burning it and then burying it or otherwise as you have been instructed.
> 3. All reusable equipment should first be washed well to remove all blood, etc. and then sterilised and not used again unless the sterilising is known to have been good enough to kill all the organisms which could be on the instrument.

Collection of blood

• Do not get the blood from the patient onto your skin and especially not into any cuts or sores or into the eyes, nose or mouth. This is to protect you from HIV and hepatitis viruses and other infections that may be in the blood.
• Always wear disposable (plastic) gloves or other gloves which can be and have been cleaned and sterilised.
• Always use needles, syringes, etc. which have no blood or body secretions from other people on them and have been sterilised. Use either disposable equipment or equipment which has been cleaned and sterilised.
• Do not try to put the cap back on the needle.
• Always put lancets, disposable needles and other sharp pieces of equipment which may have blood on them into the special 'sharps' disposal container. This container should be itself disposable, strong enough that none of the 'sharps' can stick through the side of it and should never be overfilled. The filled container should be got rid of as has been decided by your health department, such as by burning it and then burying it or otherwise as you have been instructed.
• All reusable equipment should first be washed well to remove all blood, etc. and then sterilised and not used again unless the sterilising is known to have been good enough to kill all the organisms which could be on the instrument.

Skin puncture (capillary blood)

1. In adults use the patient's finger or the lobe of the ear, choosing a site free from disease.
2. In infants use the heel.

3. Squeeze or flick the ear, finger or heel a few times. Clean it with spirit or antiseptic and allow to dry.
4. Make a good prick with a quick motion, using a sterile, dry, sharp lancet.
5. Try not to squeeze the finger or ear after you have pricked it because this spoils the specimen for some methods.
6. Make a blood film straight from the drop of blood or fill a blood pipette with it.
7. Label the specimen clearly.

Venepuncture (venous blood)

1. The syringe and needle *must* be clean, dry and *sterile*. Check that the syringe will suck. Fit a sharp sterile needle.
2. Place the tourniquet around the arm above the elbow; ask the patient to open and close his hand several times.
3. Clean the skin over the veins at the fold of the elbow with iodine or spirit.
4. Pull the skin tight over the vein with the thumb of the left hand. With a quick push, puncture the skin and vein with the needle which has the bevel upwards.
5. Do not move needle or syringe after the needle is in the vein.
6. Withdraw blood by pulling on the plunger of the syringe.
7. When ready to remove syringe, put a small piece of sterile, dry cotton wool over the needle. Remove tourniquet and withdraw needle from vein. Ask the patient to hold the cotton wool on the needle puncture for 2–3 minutes.
8. Remove needle from syringe and gently empty blood into a sterile test tube to clot; or into a bottle containing an anticoagulant (EDTA), mixing gently to prevent clotting.
9. Keep stopper in bottle to prevent evaporation.
10. Wash any non-disposable syringe and needle at once with cold water to remove blood before it clots.
11. The bottle containing the EDTA blood must be mixed for 3 minutes immediately before using the blood for a test.
12. Label the specimen clearly.

Anticoagulant used in haematology

1. It is necessary to have the correct proportion of blood to anticoagulant to prevent shrinkage of the blood cells which would give incorrect results.
2. *8% EDTA Solution*

(a) Pipette 0.1 ml of EDTA solution into small screwtop bottles. Allow the water to evaporate completely at room temperature. Fix the screwcaps and label them.
(b) This amount of EDTA prevents 4 ml of blood from clotting. It is important to try to add just 4 ml of blood to the bottle.

Preparation of thin blood films

To make a good thin blood film the slides must be perfectly clean; so first wash the slides in detergent and then clean water and store them in methylated spirit or 70% alcohol. Before use, wipe the slide dry with a clean cloth or paper (toilet paper will do). *Always hold the cleaned slide by the edges.*

Preparation of spreader (Figure 6.1)

Break off the corners of a glass slide, making sure that the edge of the slide is smooth. *It must not be chipped or rough* because this will spoil the blood film.

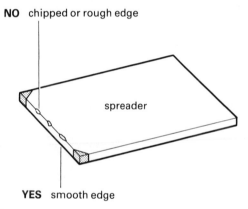

NO chipped or rough edge

spreader

YES smooth edge

Figure 6.1

Making the film (Figures 6.2 and 6.3)

1. Place a small drop of fresh blood, about 1 cm (½ inch) from the end of the clean slide.
2. Hold the spreader so that it slopes backwards.
3. Place the spreader just in front of the drop of blood, then move it back till it touches the blood. The blood will then spread along the edge of the spreader.
4. Push the spreader forward smoothly and quickly.
5. Immediately, hold the slide by the edges and wave it in the air quickly until the blood film dries.
6. Write the patient's name on the end of the slide with a marking pencil, or write the patient's name in pencil on the blood film.
7. Always wash the spreader with water after use, then dry it with soft paper, then sterilise it.

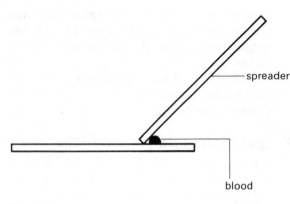

spreader

blood

Figure 6.2

Preparation of thick blood film

(Figure 6.4)

1. Place a drop or three small drops of fresh blood in the centre of a clean slide.

2. Spread the blood with the corner of a slide, making sure that it is spread evenly, until you can just see the print of a newspaper or book through it.

3. Leave the slide flat and allow to dry, protecting it from flies and insects.

Fixation of blood film

If the blood film is to be sent to another laboratory, it must be fixed immediately to preserve the blood cells.

Place the prepared film in a jar filled with *pure methyl alcohol* and leave it there for *10 minutes*. Then take it out and dry it in the air. Another method is to

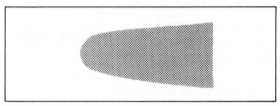

good film

Faults

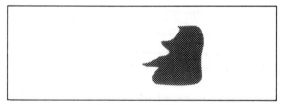

edge of spreader chipped

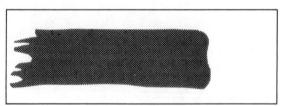

too much blood and film goes off the end

too short and thick

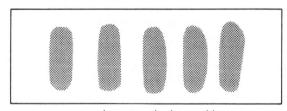

spreader not pushed smoothly

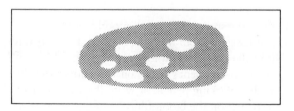

greasy slide making holes in the blood film

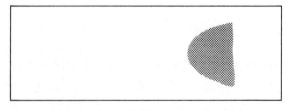

not enough blood film too small and thin

Figure 6.3

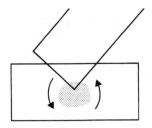

IF YOU CAN READ THE TYPE. THEN THE BLOOD FILM IS TOO THIN

IF YOU CA... THE TYPE. THE BLOO... O THICK

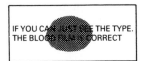

IF YOU CA... THE TYPE. THE BLO... CORRECT

Figure 6.4

pour a few drops of methyl alcohol over the film and allow 10 minutes for fixing before drying the film. Then wrap the fixed films in soft paper (e.g. toilet paper) and pack.

Make two films in case one is broken or damaged.

Details of how to take other tests are found in the appropriate chapters

Urethral smears for gonococci Chapter 19 page 206.
Smears for Donovan bodies Chapter 19 page 212.
Skin smears for AFB (leprosy) Chapter 15 page 141.
Skin biopsies Chapter 15 page 141.
Sputum smears for AFB (tuberculosis) Chapter 14 pages 108–109.
Etc.

Sending specimens to laboratory

1. Some specimens must be sent from a health centre to a laboratory. It is very important that specimens are packed and sent properly so that they do not spoil before they arrive.
2. *Histology specimens* are pieces of patient's tissues which are taken in the operating theatre. The speci-

mens are fixed in 10% formalin saline and sent to the laboratory. *Make sure that 10% formalin is used and that there is at least five times as much formalin as tissue.* The specimen must be kept in formalin for 24 hours to make sure that fixation is complete.
Packing
(a) Check that all specimens are labelled and see that the patient's name, age, sex, home village and census division, etc. are on the laboratory request forms, as well as details of his illness. Write these details into the record book and the date the specimens were sent to the laboratory.
(b) Small specimens such as liver biopsy, uterine scrapings and skin biopsy (in McCartney bottles) can be wrapped with cotton wool and packed with the request form in a small cardboard box.
(c) Big specimens can be sent in a polypot. Fix them first and pack them in a polypot with some cotton wool made wet with 10% formalin saline. Wrap them several times round in a polythene bag. Then seal this bag with sticking plaster. Pack the tissue wrapped in the polythene bag and laboratory request forms in a cardboard box.
3. *Bacteriology specimens.* Send specimen in a universal container packed in a cardboard box (see above). Swabs for culture should be sent in 'Stuart's transport medium' available from the hospital laboratory.
4. *Haematology, biochemistry and serology specimens*
(a) Blood specimens such as serum, EDTA blood and thin blood films may need to be sent. Fix the films by pouring a few drops of methyl alcohol over the films, allow 10 minutes for fixing, then dry them. Write on the laboratory request form that they are fixed with methyl alcohol. Wrap the slides separately with toilet paper and pack with the request forms in a small cardboard box.
(b) Wrap the serum and EDTA specimens carefully in cotton wool and put them inside a plastic bag. Seal the plastic bag with sticking plaster and pack with laboratory request forms in a cardboard box. Write '*BLOOD SAMPLES*' and '*Notify the department on arrival*' on top of the parcel.
(c) It is very important that all blood specimens should be sent by air freight or other quick delivery and not by ordinary post.
(d) *Specimens for biochemistry and serology.* Always send *serum*, if possible (if you have a centrifuge), not *whole blood*. The only time you send whole blood is for blood sugar that is collected into the special fluoride oxalate bottle. (These special bottles can be obtained from the hospital.)

7 Treatment, Drugs and Pain Relief

Treatment of the patient

Only when you have made a provisional diagnosis of the patient's problem can you decide how to treat the patient and manage the problem caused by the disease. Treatment of the patient only is not enough. You must do four things when you diagnose a disease:

1. Treat the patient (see this chapter).
2. Notify the necessary authorities and relatives (see Chapter 8).
3. Control the spread of the disease if necessary (see Chapter 9).
4. Prevent the disease occurring again in the patient and in the community if possible (see Chapter 9).

There are nine things you must do to treat a patient properly:

---

1. Decide on outpatient treatment or admit for inpatient treatment.
2. Order the proper nursing care.
3. Give specific treatment to cure the disease.
4. Give symptomatic treatment to relieve the symptoms.
5. Give explanation and comfort to the patient and to the relatives.
6. Give health education to the patient and to the relatives about control and prevention of the disease.
7. Consult with the Medical Officer *or* transfer the patient to Medical Officer care *or* refer the patient to the next visiting Medical Officer if necessary.
8. Discharge the patient and give final health education.
9. Follow up the patient if necessary.

Treatment of a patient may include any or all of these things.

---

1. Treat as outpatient or admit for inpatient care

2. Order proper nursing care (if necessary)

- Rest – in bed; in special position, etc.
- Special care of respiratory tract, mouth, eyes, ears, bowels, bladder, limbs, pressure areas, etc.
- Special fluids – orally or intravenously.
- Special diet.
- Special observations.
- Isolation. Barrier nursing (see page 35).
- Collection of specimens for tests.

3. Give specific treatment (to cure)

- Drugs. Which drugs; by what route; how much; how often; for how long?
- Surgery. What surgery; who will do it; when?
- Dressings, plasters, etc.
- Physiotherapy.
- Fluids – orally or intravenously. Food or diet.
- Psychiatric counselling.

4. Give symptomatic treatment (to relieve symptoms)

- To make the patient *feel* better (i.e. to relieve his symptoms, especially pain).
- 'Rule' treatment, e.g. 'Give antimalarials to every patient with a fever'. (There are different 'rule' treatments for different places and different countries.)

Symptomatic treatment may include any of the things in 2 and 3 above, especially:

- drugs,
- surgery,
- dressings,
- diet,
- psychiatric counselling,
- nursing in special positions,
- special nursing care of parts of the body.

5. Give explanation and comfort

Give explanation and comfort to the patient and to his relatives.

Many patients and relatives have very little knowledge about anatomy, physiology, pathology and what treatment means. One way of helping them understand is to get a book with good coloured anatomy pictures and explain to the patient and relatives using the pictures. There are also books and wall charts with the anatomy, physiology and pathology of each of the major body systems (e.g. lungs, gastrointestinal tract, etc.) on one page or one chart, which are even better if you can get them.

6. Give health education

Give health education about control and prevention of the disease to the patient and relatives.

7. Consult – Transfer – Refer (if necessary)

Consult with the Medical Officer (by phone or radio if necessary) if you are not sure of the diagnosis or what the management should be.

Transfer of patient to Medical Officer care in a hospital if necessary. Transfers are of two types: urgent (emergency); or non-urgent (routine).

Arranging transfer includes the following:

- Get permission from the Medical Officer if, when, where and how to transfer.
- Get written permission of patient or relative for any necessary treatment.
- Tell the hospital when the patient should arrive.
- Arrange for drugs, dressings, fluids, oxygen, splints, stretcher, pillow, blanket, etc.
- Arrange for a suitable person to accompany the patient.
- Arrange transport.
- Provide a letter.

Refer problem cases that are non-urgent to next visiting Medical Officer.

8. Discharge the patient

Arrange for patient to return for review on completion of treatment if necessary.

Write up patient's outpatient health record and give it to him.

Give final health education.

9. Follow up the patient (if necessary)

Management of the problem caused by the diagnosing of a case of a disease includes:

1. Treat the patient (nine things may be necessary) (see above).
2. Notify the necessary authorities and relatives.
3. Control the spread of the disease if necessary.
4. Prevent the disease occurring again in this patient and in the community if possible.

Drug treatment

A *drug* is any substance that can change the body or pathological states of the body.

Drugs act by changing the function or structure of parts of the body, or by changing the structure or function of organisms or substances which have entered the body.

Always use the '*approved*' generic or '*official*' name for a drug. Do not use the trade names given by companies to their brands of the drug, as the health department often changes the brands of the drug supplied from time to time.

Drugs may be given by a number of different ways (or routes) and are absorbed by the blood vessels there:

1. GI tract by mouth (orally or PO).
   Drugs are usually given by mouth. Drugs are not given by mouth if they would not be absorbed, because of any of the following reasons:
   (a) Their structure is such that they are not able to be absorbed from the gastrointestinal tract.
   (b) Vomiting and/or diarrhoea.
   (c) Shock (with little blood going to the gastrointestinal tract).
   (d) Swallowing not possible (e.g. unconscious).
   (e) The patient is not willing, or is not reliable enough, to swallow the drug.

2. By injection.
   Injections may be of different types:
   (a) intravenous injection (IVI),
   (b) intramuscular injection (IMI),
   (c) subcutaneous injection (SCI),
   (d) intradermal injection (IDI),
   (e) injection into special structures (e.g. intrapleural injection).

   Drugs are given by injection for any of the following reasons:
   (a) They may not be absorbed from the gastrointestinal tract (see above).
   (b) Oral administration is not possible – patient is not reliable enough, or is not conscious, etc.
   (c) Treatment needs to be effective quickly.
   (d) A high concentration in special structures in the body is needed.

3. GI tract, rectally (or PR), by suppository.

4. Lung (inhalation); skin (transdermal); under tongue (sublingual); nose (intranasal); or vaginally (PV) by pessary.

Drugs do not all go to all parts of the body. A drug has to be chosen which will go to the parts of the body where it is needed, but not go to parts of the body where it could cause damage.

Most drugs are destroyed ('inactivated' or 'metabolised') *and removed from the body ('excreted')* by either the liver or the kidneys. In liver or kidney diseases, therefore, drug doses may have to be lower than normal.

All drugs have unwanted side effects. These may include the following:

1. Effects that are normal actions of the drug other than the one action wanted for this patient.
2. Allergy (see Chapter 10 page 44) and other effects that do not normally occur, but do occur in a few special persons.

3. Damage to an unborn child in the uterus.

Give a drug only if its possible bad effects are less than the risk of the untreated disease.

Chemotherapy

Chemotherapy is the name given to the use of chemical substances as drugs for therapy or treatment.

The term chemotherapy is usually used only when the drug is used to treat either infections in the body or cancers in the body.

You will be using chemotherapy any time you treat any infection with a drug even though you do not often use the name chemotherapy when you do this; although you may, for such things as 'short term chemotherapy' for TB. You, yourself, will not be using chemotherapy for cancer, but you may send patients (with e.g. Burkitt's lymphoma or Kaposi's sarcoma) for chemotherapy for their cancer with drugs such as cyclophosphamide.

Drug treatment of pain – analgesia

The best treatment for pain is to remove the cause of the pain. While this is being done or if this is not possible, use one of the following groups of pain relieving drugs called analgesics.

1. General anaesthetics, e.g. ketamine.
2. Narcotic or opiate drugs, e.g. morphine, pethidine, codeine phosphate.
3. Acetylsalicylic acid (aspirin), and other non-steroidal anti-inflammatory drugs (NSAIDs), e.g. ibuprofen.
4. Paracetamol, also called acetaminophen.
5. Other systemic drugs with various actions, e.g. chlorpromazine, antidepressants and anti-convulsants.
6. Local anaesthetics, e.g. lignocaine, also called lidocaine; procaine; amethocaine; and local cooling agents.

Choice of analgesic

For mild pain, give paracetamol tablets or suppositories.

If paracetamol is not enough, add codeine phosphate.

If paracetamol and codeine together are not enough, add an NSAID as long as the patient has no problem with bleeding, peptic ulcer, BP, oedema, kidney or heart failure. (If the patient has these problems, do not add an NSAID.)

For bowel colic, use codeine phosphate.

For severe pain, use morphine tablets or injection. Do *not* use morphine drugs for chronic pain unless the patient is expected to die soon or you have discussed the matter with the Medical Officer. Pethidine is occasionally used instead of morphine, but for no longer than 3 days.

Use chlorpromazine in small doses together with the usual dose of morphine to make this drug more effective and last longer; but only in special cases such as cancer.

For very severe pain, give a general anaesthetic, usually a ketamine injection.

For some pains in only one part of the body (e.g. a sting from a 'stonefish') you can use an injection of a local anaesthetic around the painful area (although heating the area is usually more effective for some fish stings).

Morphine tablets and injection and codeine tablets

These are dangerous drugs. They are also called narcotic or opiate drugs. There are special rules for storing and using them. Effects and precautions include:

1. Pain is relieved. *Never use them in abdominal pain until the cause is definitely diagnosed and proper treatment started. Otherwise, when pain and tenderness are gone, diagnosis may not be possible.*
2. Breathing and coughing are less. *Never use in chronic obstructive lung disease or asthma or if the patient might have any difficulty in breathing. Otherwise the patient might completely stop breathing.*
3. Diarrhoea is stopped and constipation can be caused. They are a very effective treatment for severe diarrhoea.
4. Vomiting is caused sometimes.
5. Itch occurs sometimes.
6. Sleepiness and change in consciousness is caused. *Never use if the patient has a head injury as level of consciousness is then difficult to interpret.*
7. Happiness is often caused. Addiction occurs quickly. *Never use for chronic pain or for more than a few days unless the patient is soon to die or you have discussed this with the Medical Officer.* However, they are good treatment for pain in the dying patient.

Overdose is treated with artificial ventilation (see Chapter 36 page 607) and naloxone or nalorphine (see Chapter 34 page 564). If these are unavailable, try aminophylline (see Chapter 20 page 296).

Acetylsalicylic acid (aspirin)

Acetylsalicylic acid was the first non-steroidal anti-inflammatory drug (NSAID).

Effects include the following:

1. Pain is relieved (mild pain only).
2. Temperature is lowered. However, treatment of the cause of the raised temperature is much more important.
3. Anti-inflammatory effects occur if large doses are given regularly. This is done for arthritis and leprosy reactions.
4. Indigestion, peptic ulcer and gastrointestinal bleeding can occur. Do not give aspirin if the patient possibly has a peptic ulcer or any bleeding.
5. Platelets which help stop bleeding do not work well for 7–10 days. Do not give if the patient has a bleeding tendency or if surgery due in the next week.
6. Allergic reactions can occur.

Give acetylsalicylic acid when required for pain.

Give acetylsalicylic acid regularly for its anti-inflammatory effect.

If the dose of acetylsalicylic acid is too high, the patient may get:

1. 'ringing' or other noises in the ears; or deafness,
2. headache,
3. nausea, vomiting.

If these occur:
• stop the acetylsalicylic acid for 1 day,
• then give it in a lower dose.

A large overdose of acetylsalicylic acid is very dangerous. Immediately make the patient vomit if he is conscious. Treat immediately as described in Chapter 34 pages 562–563.

Do not use in children as it can cause liver and brain problems (Rye's syndrome).

Other non-steroidal anti-inflammatory drugs (NSAIDs), e.g. ibuprofen

Actions are similar to acetylsalicylic acid (aspirin) above. They are particularly useful for musculoskeletal pain.

Side effects also include decreased kidney function if given with diuretics and ACE inhibitors, raised blood pressure, fluid retention (and therefore in some patients heart failure).

Paracetamol (acetaminophen)

Paracetamol relieves pain and reduces fever. However, it is not usually as effective a drug as acetylsalicylic acid. It does not have the anti-inflammatory effects of acetylsalicylic acid. However, it does not cause gastrointestinal irritation and bleeding and other problems as acetylsalicylic acid does.

An overdose of paracetamol is very dangerous. Treat immediately as described in Chapter 34 page 564 and transfer the patient urgently to a Medical Officer for special treatment to try to stop severe liver damage.

Doses of analgesic drugs

Paracetamol (tablets, syrup and suppositories)

• 500–1000 mg each 4–6 hours if needed for pain in adults.
• No more than 4 grams in any 24-hour period.

Codeine phosphate (usually 30 mg tablets)

• 30 mg tablet each 4–6 hours if needed for pain (or diarrhoea).
• Give as well as paracetamol or acetylsalicylic acid for pain.
• This may cause constipation if more than 1 dose; if so, give also a laxative.
• No more than 180 mg in any 24-hour period.

Acetylsalicylic acid (aspirin) (tablets and suppositories)

• 300–1200 mg each 4–6 hours if required for pain.
• Use a small dose (300–450 mg) for a small adult or for mild pain in large adult. Use a large dose (900–1200 mg) only for a more severe pain in a large adult.
• No more than 4 grams in 24 hours.

Acetylsalicylic acid and codeine compound tablets (usually aspirin 300 mg and codeine 8 mg in each tablet) (codeine co; but other combinations of doses are possible).

• Before ordering, check the amount of each drug in the tablets being given.
• No more than 2 grams of acetylsalicylic acid or 180 mg of codeine in any 24-hour period.

Paracetamol and codeine compound tablets (usually paracetamol 500 mg and codeine 8 mg) (co-codamol tablets; but other combinations of doses are possible).

• Before ordering, check the amount of each drug in the tablets being given.
• No more than 2 grams of paracetamol or 180 mg codeine in any 24-hour period.

Ibuprofen tablet

• 400 mg each 6–12 hours.
• Add to paracetamol and codeine if more pain relief needed.

- Do not give if contraindicated (see page 33).
- Do not give as well as acetylsalicylic acid or any other NSAID.

Morphine (injection and tablets)
IMI or SCI

- 0.2 mg/kg each 4–6 hours if required.
- Small adult 7.5mg (7 ½ mg).
- Large adult 10 mg–15 mg.

Oral

- 20–30 mg each 4–6 hours if required.
- Thirty (30) mg of oral morphine gives about the same relief as 10 mg of injected morphine.

Pethidine (injection for IMI or SCI)
- 1–1.5 mg/kg each 4–6 hours if required for pain.
- Small adult, pain not very severe, 50 mg.
- Small adult, severe pain, 75 mg.
- Large adult, pain not very severe, 75 mg.
- Large adult, severe pain 100 mg.
- Do not use for more than 3 days.
- Morphine is usually preferred.

Lidocaine (or lignocaine) (plain 1% or 2% solution)
- Inject the smallest volume needed into or around the affected area to cause analgesia of the part of the body affected.
- Never inject more than 20 ml of 1% solution (or 40 ml of a 0.5% solution or 10 ml of a 2% solution) at any one time into a patient.

IVI ketamine, IMI ketamine for general anaesthetic.

IVI lytic cocktail for general analgesic effect.

IVI lignocaine (or lidocaine) for regional anaesthesia.

Do *not* use these last three drugs *unless*:

1. you have been trained in their use; *and*
2. you have all the necessary equipment for resuscitation and artificial ventilation available and ready.

Oxygen treatment

Oxygen is needed by all of the cells of the body to stay alive and do their work.

Normal air is made up of 20% oxygen. To get oxygen in the air to the body cells a person needs to:

1. have normal air to breathe,
2. breathe often and deeply enough,
3. not have a block to the air in the airways,
4. have lungs healthy enough to be able to take the oxygen out of the air and put it into the blood,
5. have a heart able to beat fast enough and strongly enough to pump around (circulate) the blood through the lungs and rest of the body,
6. have enough blood volume to circulate,
7. have enough haemoglobin in the blood to carry the oxygen,
8. have no block in the blood vessels which take the blood to the cells,
9. have no toxin or poison in the cells which stops them taking the oxygen out of the blood.

If there is any block in any of the above steps to get oxygen to the cells, called hypoxia, as long as the problem is not so bad that the oxygen cannot get through that block at all, one way of helping get more oxygen to the cells is to put more oxygen into the air that the patient is breathing. There is then a greater amount of oxygen at each step and a better chance of getting oxygen past wherever the block is. This is called 'oxygen therapy'.

Oxygen is often not available; and when it is, it is often scarce and expensive. It should be used only if the patient's body cells are short of oxygen and

1. it is possible to overcome the patient's problem,
2. the condition is acute (has come on quickly),
3. it is known oxygen will help (if so, this will be talked about in this book).

In a health centre, the usual dose is 2 litres by nasal prongs, which increases the amount of oxygen in the air the patient can breathe in from 20% to 28%. Occasionally, 4 litres are used, which increases the amount of oxygen to 32%.

Important notes for the health worker about drugs

There are other things we should keep in mind when administering drug treatment:

- *Counterfeit drugs.* In some countries, drugs are sold which have not been made properly and are therefore ineffective. Some tablets and injections on the market may have no effective ingredients at all. It is difficult or impossible to tell by looking at them which are effective and which are inactive or 'fake' (counterfeit) drugs. The World Health Organization

(WHO) states that up to 10% of drugs are counterfeit. Some counterfeit drugs contain harmful chemicals. In some regions of Africa and southeast Asia, over half of blood pressure or malaria treatment drugs are sometimes counterfeit. If the drugs supplied do not work as expected, discuss this with the Medical Officer. The WHO is trying to combat this problem and has a Rapid Alert System of communication which sends reports on the existence of counterfeit drugs and the places where they have been sent to national health authorities. People do not die from wearing a fake watch or clothes. People do die from taking fake drugs.

- *Traditional medicines.* As well as the drugs we give our patients, patients may also have been given other drugs by traditional healers or they may be actually buying and taking these drugs themselves. These other drugs may also cause illnesses or may stop the drugs we give from working. Always ask about other drugs the patient has taken.

- *Patient non-compliance.* The most common cause for drugs not working, however, is that the patient does not take them as prescribed. If a patient is not getting better as expected, not only should we ask if the patient is taking the medication, we need to check with staff, family and friends. If necessary, we may have to get the patient to actually take the drugs while the health worker is watching ('directly observed treatment').

- *Patients' lack of understanding.* It is often difficult for patients to know why they should take the drugs we give them as often or for as long as we say. It is very hard for those with little education or who are illiterate. Always give an explanation. If patients are not able to read, it is worth getting a special health worker or even a trained community member to not only tell but also show the patient when and how often to take his medication, and then ask the patient to repeat the information back. This may need doing several times before the patient really knows what to do.

- *Cost of medication.* There are many drugs available, especially new drugs, that are very expensive. It would be easy for a country to spend all its health budget on buying drugs and have none left for any other health work. Each country therefore has to set aside what it can for drugs and then buy the drugs which do the most good for that money. The WHO has helped governments to work out which drugs are the best value for money to provide treatment for the greatest number of diseases; these are contained in 'WHO Model List of Essential Medicines'. These are updated and published anew every 2 years. Although we would all like more drugs to be available to us, if we learn how to use those drugs that are available skilfully, we should be able to treat most of the illness we see better than those who have increasingly expensive drugs but do not use them skilfully.

Appendix 1 Barrier nursing

This is a way of nursing used to try to put a 'barrier' (or wall) around a patient with an infectious/contagious disease to try to stop the transfer (or spread) of the specific agent which causes the infection to staff, other patients and the outside world (see Chapters 5, 9 and 10).

Barrier nursing includes the following.

- Screens around the patient if the patient is in a ward with others; but this does not stop droplet, airborne and other spread well; it is much better if the patient is in his own room.

- Nurses and all who care for the patient must wear gowns, masks and gloves, etc.

- Strict hand washing rules by all who care for the patient in any way (including domestic and cleaning and other staff).

- All equipment used for the care of the patient is immediately treated by high level disinfection or sterilised.

- Special rules for handling clothes, sheets, etc.

- Special care with food and removal and disinfection of crockery, cutlery, etc.

- Visitors to the patients are kept to only a few and must use gowns, masks, gloves, etc. and wash hands, etc. as staff do.

Many of these rules are now carried out for all patients – see 'Universal precautions', Chapter 11 pages 61–63.

8 Notification of Disease and Death

There are three types of notification:

1. Notification of the Provincial or District or Regional Health or Medical Officer of:
   (a) the number of cases each month of the diseases which are under surveillance (being counted);
   (b) events of public health concern.
2. Notification of the police and the coroner of all cases of 'sudden and unnatural' death and cases where you do not know the cause of death – including persons who are 'dead on arrival'. Notify the police of all fights, accidents, alleged poisonings, etc. if the patient is ill.
3. Notification of the relatives and friends of a patient's illness. You must, however, have the patient's permission to tell details of the nature, treatment and prognosis of the patient's illness to anyone else.

Notification of the Health Officer

If certain diseases or conditions occur you must notify these to the Health Officer.

The Health Officer can then help you in your disease control and prevention work and can send you special advice or special help.

The Health Officer may have to report these things to Health Department Headquarters.

Headquarters need to know what diseases occur so that they can send the proper staff, drugs and equipment to help. Headquarters also have to report all 'events that may constitute a public health emergency of international concern' to the World Health Organization (WHO) under the 'International Health Regulations' (IHR).

At the time of writing four critical diseases are always to be notified to the WHO – smallpox, poliomyelitis (due to a wild type poliovirus), human influenza caused by a new subtype and severe acute respiratory syndrome (SARS). WHO will add to or change these diseases in the future as needed

There are two types of conditions which are notified to the Health Officer:

1. Diseases which are under surveillance and reported regularly at the end of each month.
   (a) Count and record every single case of these diseases (no matter whether an inpatient or an outpatient).
   (b) Send the number of cases of each disease to the Health Officer at the end of each month.

> Keep a copy of the list of diseases you must monitor and report in a safe handy place.

2. 'Events of Public Health Concern'. If any of these things happened, notify the Health Officer immediately, by the fastest possible method:
   (a) outbreaks or epidemics of known diseases;
   (b) outbreaks or epidemics of unknown diseases;
   (c) single cases of dangerous diseases not usual in the area, e.g. any case of cholera, plague, yellow fever, etc., and the (at present four) diseases to be notified to WHO;
   (d) natural disasters (floods, earthquakes, etc.) which may affect people's health;
   (e) unusual events such as diseases or deaths of animals (e.g. fish or rats or monkeys; or domestic animals kept for meat or milk) which may affect people's health.

9 Control and Prevention of Disease. Summary of patient management

Control and prevention of disease

To control and prevent disease, you need a knowledge of both:

1. the cause of the disease, and
2. the epidemiology of the disease.

You can then choose the most effective means (one or more) to control and/or prevent the disease. The four means for control and prevention of infectious diseases are:

1. Kill or inactivate the specific agent (an infecting organism) in the body of the original host (clinical case, subclinical case or carrier) or reservoir (man, animal, dust, etc.).
2. Block the means of spread from the reservoir to susceptible persons.
3. Increase the resistance of susceptible persons.
4. Prophylactic treatment. Give a drug to stop the infection in probably infected persons before the infection produces clinical disease.

Always give *health education to the patient and to his relatives* about those things which they can do to control and prevent the disease the patient has.

Always use a case of a disease as an opportunity to give *health education to all the community*.

Never forget to use each case of a disease to give *health education to your own health workers* about that disease including its prevention.

Figures 9.1 and 9.2 illustrate important points in control and prevention of infectious disease. *Use these five methods for the prevention and control of all (non-infective as well as infectious) diseases.*

See Chapter 11 for details of control and prevention of infectious diseases.

When giving health education to a patient or family or the community, all possible ways to prevent disease should be explained to them. The things which people can do to help themselves should be explained very clearly to them.

The most important health education to give about the prevention of infectious diseases is how people themselves can stop disease being passed on to others.

The most important ways of avoiding the transfer of disease include the following.

1. Drink only safe water, i.e.

   (a) water not contaminated by faeces, urine or bodily discharges from other people;

   (b) water not containing parasites which could infect people.

   If the water is not safe, it needs to be treated. Means of treatment might include the following.

   (a) Filtering the water if it is not clear (simple household sand filters as well as community sand filters can easily be made). Filtering the water is needed to remove ova, cysts and parasites that may not be later killed by chemicals such as chlorine. Also, higher levels of chlorine are needed if there is organic material in the water.

   (b) Adding chemicals to kill organisms. The cheap-

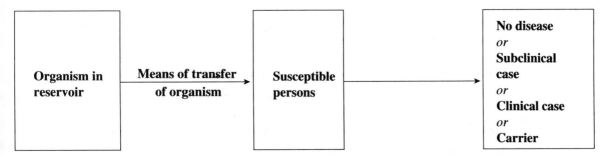

Figure 9.1 *Aetiology and epidemiology of disease.*

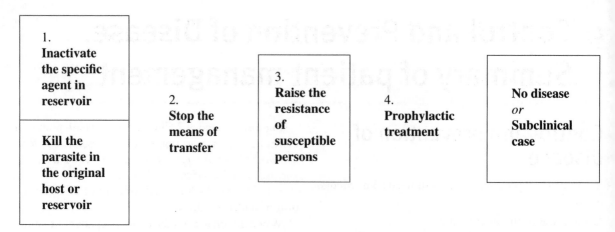

Figure 9.2 *Means of control and prevention of disease.*

est and most available is of course chlorine. Special preparations can be used, but even household bleach bought in the market is satisfactory as long as the right amount is used; this will depend on the strength of the bleach (see page 39).
(c) if the above two things are not possible, boil the water, preferably for 10 minutes (but even bringing it to the boil for 15 seconds helps).
2. Always use proper toilets and make sure all children always use the toilets. Each family can make a single compartment version of the Blair latrine (even if at first temporary walls, etc. made of sun-dried bricks, reeds or grass have to be used over the essential part, i.e. a concrete cover slab, brick collar and permanent pit lining).
3. Always wash hands after using the toilet.
4. Always wash hands before preparing food and eating.
5. Cover the nose and mouth when coughing or sneezing. Do not cough or sneeze onto other people or onto things other people may touch. Do not spit onto the floor or ground.
6. Wash hands before touching other people's food or drink or people with any respiratory infection.
7. Do not have sexual intercourse with anyone except one faithful, uninfected partner. If sexual intercourse is had with anyone else, always use a condom properly.

The above things are essential for everyone. The following things are essential but not as important as the above.
1. Cook food properly – long enough to kill any parasites or organisms it contains.
2. Wash food that is eaten raw (e.g. vegetables) only with safe clean water (see above).
3. Keep food covered so flies, etc. cannot get at it.
4. Do not drink milk or eat previously cooked meat if they are not kept in a refrigerator or a cold place unless it is cooked again.
5. Cover any wounds or sores so that flies and insects cannot get onto them.
6. Wash the whole of the body with soap and water regularly and dry properly afterwards.
7. Keep the environment clean and tidy and burn or bury rubbish so that flies, rats, etc. cannot eat it or live in it.
8. Do not have stagnant water near the dwelling in which mosquitoes can breed.
9. Do not have a lot of people sleeping in one room and keep all rooms well ventilated with open windows.

Simple things can have dramatic results. In a study reported in 'The Lancet' (Volume 366, July 16, 2005, pages 225–233), Dr Luby and colleagues reported on the effect of getting people in a low income population in part of Pakistan to wash their hands with soap and water regularly. No other change was made in the people's behaviour. In comparison to people not supplied with ordinary soap and not encouraged to wash their hands regularly,

- impetigo (skin infection) decreased by 34%;
- diarrhoea decreased by 53%;
- pneumonia decreased by 50%.

Washing the hands obviously helps to reduce the number of organisms transferred from one person in the family to another and to those outside the family. It is not easy to understand how it could be this effective, but it is.

Getting the authorities to provide plenty of safe water was essential to the success of the above study and this should be one of your major aims.

Once the safe water is available, getting people to wash their hands with soap and water should be one of the next aims.

Disease would be dramatically reduced if:

1. only safe water was drunk;
2. everyone always used proper toilets;
3. hand washing was always carried out after using the toilet, before handling or eating food, etc.;
4. sexual intercourse was always only by 'safe sex', as the means of transfer of the major sexually transmitted illnesses including HIV would be stopped.

Once these are achieved, other methods as above should be added.

Chemical treatment to make water suitable for drinking (potable water)

Water should first be filtered. This removes ova and cysts (e.g. *Giardia* and *Cryptosporidium*) which may not be killed by chemicals and it reduces the amount of chemical needed (the chemical would combine with the protein material in the cloudy water and not enough be left to combine with the organisms and kill them). If water cannot be filtered, at least twice the amount of chemical is needed.

Use sodium hypochloride 5%; or household bleach 4% available chlorine (but do not use one with perfumed cleaners (cleaning agents), sodium hydroxide or other additives. Read the labels of what you buy carefully). Add an average amount of chemical, e.g. 6.3 ml for 5 l of water or 125 ml for 1000 l of water. Mix well. Do not use the water for at least 30 minutes.

It is best to measure the amount of chlorine in the treated water. A swimming pool colour comparator is the cheapest way. Soon after treatment chlorine should be 5 mg/l and this will fall, but after 30 minutes should be at least 1 mg/l. The results will tell you if you need to add less or more chemical. If no measurement is possible, the water should have a slight smell of chlorine after 30 minutes. If it does not, treat the water with the same amount of chemical again.

If large amounts of water are being treated, use stronger chlorine solution 12.5% available chlorine (40 ml for 1000 l water or 'swimming pool' chlorine granules (5 g in 5 ml or 1 teaspoon) 65% available chlorine (8 g for 1000 ml water)).

The summary of the management of a person with a medical problem

When a patient comes to a health worker with a symptom, the management of this problem may well include some or all of these things:

1. taking a medical history;
2. doing a clinical examination;
3. making a differential diagnosis;
4. doing or ordering tests;
5. making a provisional diagnosis;
6. deciding on the prognosis;
7. deciding on inpatient or outpatient treatment*;
8. ordering proper nursing care*;
9. giving specific treatment to cure the disease*;
10. giving symptomatic treatment to relieve symptoms*;
11. giving proper explanations and comfort to the patient and to his relatives*;
12. giving health education about the control and prevention of the disease to the patient and to his relatives*;
13. consulting with a Medical Officer, transferring the patient to Medical Officer care or referring the patient to the next visiting Medical Officer*;
14. notifying the Health Officer, the Coroner, the police, the relatives, etc.;
15. controlling the spread of the disease;
16. preventing the disease occurring in the patient again and also in the community;
17. discharging the patient and giving final health education*;
18. following up the patient*.

(*These nine things were previously listed as 'treatment' of a patient.)

10 Infection, Immunity, Immunisation and Allergy

Infection

The specific agents (organisms) which cause infectious diseases are around people all the time. Why do these specific agents not cause disease in all people all the time?

There are many epidemiological answers. Here are some:

1. The specific agents – only some organisms cause disease.
2. The body – man's body has defences against the organisms that cause disease.
3. Transfer – the organism has ways of transferring to another person; sometimes it cannot use these ways of transferring.
4. The environment – changes in the environment can change the organism, man's body and the transfer of the organism.

This chapter considers:

1. the organisms which can cause disease, and
2. the body's defences against these organisms.

The specific agents which cause infections

The specific agents which cause infections are organisms such as:

- prions (very uncommonly at present),
- viruses,
- rickettsiae,
- bacteria,
- protozoa,
- fungi,
- worms,
- insects (called 'infestations').

Prions

We do not yet properly understand prions. Think of them as incomplete viruses (see below) which cause infection and destruction of the central nervous system but cause no inflammation and no immunity. Diseases caused include bovine spongiform encephalitis (BSE or 'mad cow disease') and when passed to people

'Creutzfeldt-Jakob Disease' (CJD). Other prions cause kuru. Diseases from prions as yet are very rare.

Viruses

Viruses are the smallest organisms. You cannot see them with an ordinary microscope. (You can see them only with a special 'electron microscope'.) They need to be inside body cells to multiply; but they can stay alive outside body cells and pass from one person to another. Most chemotherapeutic drugs and antibiotics at present available in health centres cannot kill them.

Examples of virus infections are the common cold in the respiratory system and the hepatitis viruses in the liver, and HIV in the immune system.

Rickettsiae

Rickettsiae are organisms that are bigger than viruses, but smaller than bacteria. You can see them, but not easily, with an ordinary microscope. Like viruses, they need to be inside body cells to multiply. Some antibiotics (tetracycline and chloramphenicol) can kill some of them. An example of rickettsiae is the typhus organism.

Bacteria

Bacteria are small organisms. You can see them only with a microscope. They can live in many places, inside and outside the body. Most bacteria are harmless – some are helpful to us. However, some bacteria can cause disease such as pneumonia in the lungs and leprosy in the skin and nerves. Chemotherapeutic drugs and antibiotics can kill most bacteria.

Protozoa

Protozoa are organisms of only one cell. They are much bigger than bacteria, but usually you can see them only with a microscope. Some protozoa cause diseases such as malaria in the blood and amoebic dysentery in the intestine. There are chemotherapeutic drugs that will kill most protozoa.

Fungi

Fungi are simple organisms usually with more than one cell, and are something like plants. Some cause disease such as tinea on the skin and thrush in the mouth. There are chemotherapeutic and antibiotic drugs that can kill most fungi, but some are very expensive.

Worms (helminths)

Worms are organisms with many cells. You can usually see them easily without a microscope. Worms are common parasites of man and animals. Many worms have complicated life cycles with different stages in man and other animals. Examples of worm infestations include filariasis in the lymph vessels and roundworm in the intestine. There are chemotherapeutic drugs that can kill most worms.

Insects

Insects are small animals that have three pairs of legs and a head, chest and abdomen. Many insects have wings. An example is the body louse, which can attach itself to hair or clothing and live by sucking blood. The bites often become infected with bacteria. Chemicals to kill insects are available.

> What determines if these organisms will cause infection and disease or not?

Pathogenicity

Some kinds of organisms *can cause disease* in *most* people they attack. These are called *highly pathogenic*.

Some organisms *can cause disease* in *only a few* of the people they attack. These are called *mildly pathogenic*.

Some organisms *cannot cause disease* in *any* of the people they attack. These are called *non-pathogenic*.

Virulence

The disease caused by organisms can be *mild* (e.g. common cold caused by the cold virus) or *severe* (e.g. meningitis caused by bacteria) or somewhere in between (e.g. influenza caused by influenza virus). Organisms that cause *severe disease* are called *virulent*. Organisms that cause *mild disease* are called *non-virulent*.

The number of organisms

The number of organisms that enter the body can determine if they will cause disease or not. A certain number of organisms must stay alive after entry to cause disease. This number is different for each specific agent. This fact is very important.

The body's defences against infection

The body's surfaces

The skin and the mucous membranes (or mucosa) act as a wall which can stop many organisms entering the body.

Secretions (or fluids made by the glands) on the body surfaces can contain antibodies which kill the organisms. Secretions can also wash away organisms. Damaged or diseased skin or mucosa makes it easier for many organisms to enter the body.

The body's defence cells

Some cells in the blood and in the tissues can surround and kill and digest many (but not all) organisms.

The body's immune system

When organisms enter the body, some lymphocytes in the blood and in the lymph glands start to grow and change. These lymphocytes can recognise protein parts of the attacking organism as not belonging to the body and being 'foreign' and therefore try to destroy them. Proteins which are recognised as not part of the body and are 'foreign' are called 'antigens'.

1. B lymphocytes change to plasma cells and then make proteins called antibodies. These antibodies go into the blood and then spread into the tissues. These antibodies then join to the antigens on the organisms. These antibodies may damage the organism or stop it growing or spreading. These antibodies may also help other body defence cells to digest the organisms or destroy them in a number of other ways. This immune response by B lymphocytes making antibodies is sometimes called 'humoral immunity' ('humoral' means 'travelling in the blood').

2. T lymphocytes are the most common lymphocytes in the blood and can cause 'cell mediated immunity'. T lymphocytes can change into at least four different kinds of cells. Cytotoxic T lymphocytes destroy body cells which have organisms in them before the organisms inside them have time to grow and reproduce. (Natural killer cells, which are not T lymphocytes and do not need to be activated by antigen, can also recognise and kill such infected cells.) Helper T lymphocytes help B lymphocytes to make enough antibody. Suppressor T lymphocytes stop B cells making too much antibody and also stop the body becoming immune to itself. Other T lymphocytes are responsible for the delayed hypersensitivity reaction. All of these are part of the 'cell mediated immunity' system. CD4 helper T lymphocytes are the lymphocytes most easily measured to be low in HIV infection, but all lymphocytes are affected.

Antibodies protect the body against bacteria, bacterial toxins and viruses that are floating free in the body fluids. Cellular immunity protects the body against bacteria and viruses and protozoa that are growing inside cells and therefore cannot be reached by antibodies. Cellular immunity also protects against other protozoa, fungi and some worms.

If organisms have previously entered the body and caused an infection and immunity, antibodies and the cells of cellular immunity may stay in the body after the organisms have gone. These antibodies and immune cells can then immediately attack any organisms of the same type that enter the body. If organisms have not entered the body and caused an infection before, there will be no antibodies and immune cells ready to attack them. It will take a week or more for the needed antibodies and immune cells to be made and start to attack the organisms.

Examples of infections

Acute infection with bacteria and the inflammatory reaction

This is what *can* happen:

1. The pathogenic organisms must first get onto the surface of the body (skin or mucous membrane).
2. The organisms must overcome the body's surface defences. Usually the organisms must find a break in the skin or mucous membrane. However, some organisms can break through unbroken skin or mucous membranes.
3. The organisms must then grow and multiply in the tissues more quickly than the body defence cells, antibodies and cellular immunity can kill them.
4. If the organisms are not immediately killed, the body usually establishes an inflammatory reaction. The blood vessels in the area dilate (open up more widely) and bring more blood to the area. Defence cells and antibodies then go through the dilated blood vessel walls into the affected area and attack the organisms.
5. A protein from the blood called fibrin sometimes makes a wall around the area so that the organisms cannot easily spread to other tissues.
6. The whole body prepares to fight the infection. The body cells in the area release chemicals. These chemicals cause more white blood cells to be made, raise the temperature and make many other changes.
7. If the body defences do not kill the organisms quickly, the organisms can release poisons called toxins. The blood then carries the toxins around

the body and they can poison the body in a number of ways. This is called 'toxaemia'. These toxins can cause malaise (feeling sick), raised temperature, fast pulse rate, nausea, vomiting and diarrhoea. Certain toxins can cause clinical disease, e.g. tetanus (see Chapter 25 page 419).

8. If the body defences do not kill the organisms quickly, the organisms can also destroy tissues in the area of the infection. The dead tissues and damaged blood cells and organisms are called pus.
9. The organisms can spread through the lymph vessels to the lymph nodes and cause inflammation in these places too – lymphangitis in the lymph vessels and lymphadenitis in the lymph nodes.
10. The organisms can be carried around in the blood stream. This is called bacteraemia. The infection can spread to other organs.
11. The organisms can grow and multiply in the blood. This is a very serious and often fatal disease. It is called septicaemia.

Acute infection with viruses and the inflammatory reaction

1. There can be all the symptoms and signs of acute inflammation.
2. There is no pus (e.g. there is only a watery nasal discharge in a viral common cold).
3. There can be a loss of function of the organ that is infected (e.g. viral hepatitis).
4. There can be the general symptoms and signs of toxaemia (e.g. influenza).

Chronic infection and inflammation produced by tuberculosis

1. There are the usual symptoms and signs of chronic inflammation.
2. There is slow destruction of the body tissues.
3. Thick pus (like cheese) (sometimes called 'caseation') is formed.
4. Fibrous tissue tries to make a wall around that area of the body so that the infection cannot spread.
5. Healing is by the contraction and shrinking of the fibrous tissue. This causes scarring.

There are many other types of reaction to infection.

Immunity and immunisation

Immunity is when a person has a resistance to a disease. Sometimes immunity is complete – the immune person can never get the disease again.

More often, the immunity is relative – the body has defences against infection; but, if the body is weakened or if the infecting agent is very strong or present in large numbers, the immunity can fail and disease can happen.

There are different types of immunity as shown in Figure 10.1.

1. *Inherent (inborn) immunity* is the immunity a person has without being infected or immunised, etc. It varies with race, gender (sex), family, etc.

2. *Acquired immunity* is due to specific antibodies or immune cells which develop in the body after an infection or immunisation. These antibodies or immune cells join onto the attacking organism or toxin and destroy it.

3. *Natural active immunity* follows a natural infection. After the infection some antibodies or immune cells can stay in the blood or another part of the body all the time. Also, the body 'remembers' how to make the antibodies immediately the organism tries to attack again.

4. *Natural passive immunity* is only in infants for the first few months of life. The infant gets the antibodies through the placenta or in its mother's milk if the mother has these antibodies. The antibodies do not last in the infant after 3–9 months.

5. *Artificial active immunity* is produced by immunisation (or 'vaccination') with any of the following three things:
   (a) Dead infectious organisms.
   (b) Living infectious organisms that are exactly like the organisms which cause disease, but cannot cause disease themselves (because they are avirulent or non-virulent organisms).

(c) A substance like the poison or toxin of an organism but not poisonous itself (called 'toxoid'). The body makes antibodies or immune cells against all of these three things. These antibodies or immune cells are also effective against the real live organisms or toxins that cause disease. Some of these antibodies and immune cells stay in the blood or other parts of the body after the immunisation. The body also 'remembers' how to make them immediately the disease-producing organism or toxin attacks.

6. *Artificial passive immunity* is produced by giving serum from another person or animal who has antibodies against the disease. This kind of immunity lasts for weeks or months, but after this time there are no antibodies left and there is no immunity.

However, if the antibodies come from a horse or other animal, the human body can have a severe or even fatal reaction to the other proteins in the serum when it is injected. This is even more likely if the serum is used more than once.

Active immunity is always better than passive immunity.

The WHO Expanded Programme on Immunization (EPI)

Immunisation should be given to produce artificial active immunity against all infectious diseases important to a population. This should be done for all infectious diseases that are common and for all infectious diseases that may not be common but which are usually serious. This will save those in the population who would otherwise have been infected from suffering the disease; from having permanent damage to their bodies

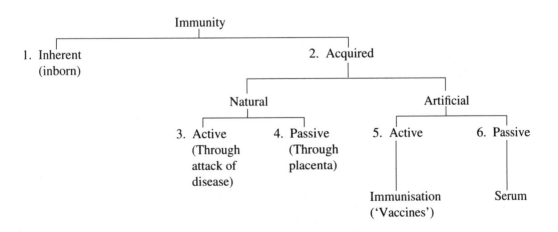

Figure 10.1 *Diagram to illustrate the classification of the different types of immunity.*

caused by the infection; or sometimes from death. It may also allow some diseases to be totally destroyed if there is no reservoir for the infection (as everyone is immunised and immune). This is becoming more important as some diseases such as tuberculosis and malaria are becoming resistant to drugs which used to kill the organisms causing them; and some diseases, such as poliomyelitis and HIV infection cannot be cured by any drugs that exist at present. Immunisation should be given to produce artificial passive immunity for patients exposed to or with infections to which they do not already have immunity, where the infection could have serious or fatal results.

The WHO has therefore recommended the programme given in Table 10.1 aimed at children. Your national government may have changed this programme a little or added other things to it to make it more effective for the diseases and the people affected by these diseases in your community. Adolescent and adult immunisation may be added. See Table 10.2 page 46. You must find out what your national

Table 10.1 The present WHO Expanded Programme on Immunization. Change this programme as your national government tells you. Add new immunisations as soon as they become available. Make sure everyone in your population gets all these immunisations.

Age	Vaccine	Hepatitis B vaccine* (two alternative schemes)	
		Alternative A	Alternative B
Birth	BCG, OPV-0	HB-1	
6 weeks	DPT-1, OPV-1, Hib-1	HB-2	HB-1
10 weeks	DPT-2, OPV-2, Hib		HB-2
14 weeks	DPT-3, OPV-3, Hib	HB-3	HB-3
9 months	Measles, yellow fever†		

BCG, used to prevent tuberculosis
OPV, oral polio vaccine; OPV-0 dose is given at birth only in polio endemic countries
DPT, diphtheria–pertussis–tetanus vaccine
HB, hepatitis B vaccine
* Hib is given in countries with carriage rates of HBsAg of 2% or more; scheme A is recommended in countries where perinatal transmission of HBV is important (e.g. SE Asia), and scheme B in countries where perinatal transmission is less important (e.g. sub-Saharan Africa).
† In countries where yellow fever poses a risk.
Hib-1 is used to prevent *Haemophilus influenzae* type b infection.

programme is and do all you can to make sure that all people in your community get all immunisations possible. As new immunisations become available, add these to your list. See Table 10.3 page 49.

See Appendix page 49 on 'The cold chain'.

For a very helpful guide for immunisation, read or do the training course by WHO 'Immunization in practice'.

Allergy or hypersensitivity

Allergy or hypersensitivity is an inflammatory reaction of part of the body caused by some foreign substance in or on the body. This substance does not normally cause inflammation in normal people. However, some people (who are called 'allergic' or 'hypersensitive') develop an abnormal immune reaction to these substances. If these people contact the substance again there is an immune reaction between the abnormal antibodies or immune cells and the substance. In this reaction, the body may release histamine and other substances. These substances cause an 'immediate' allergic reaction. Cellular immune reaction causes a 'delayed' hypersensitivity reaction.

Immunity is a helpful reaction of the immune system of the body to a foreign substance. Allergy or hypersensitivity is a harmful reaction of the immune system of the body to a foreign substance.

There are many types of allergy including:
• asthma,
• allergic rhinitis ('hay fever'),
• allergic or atopic eczema or dermatitis,
• urticaria ('hives'),
• oedema (angio-oedema), and
• shock.

Allergic reactions can be caused by things which:
• touch the skin,
• are inhaled (breathed in),
• are swallowed, or
• are injected.

Treatment includes:

1. Epinephrine (also called adrenaline), usually supplied as 1 mg/ml (1:1000 solution) 1 ml ampoule/ for injection is the most important treatment. For acute severe reactions; 0.5 ml (½ ml) is given by SCI or IMI; or if near death, 0.1 ml/minute IVI (dilute 0.5 ml with 4.5 ml 0.9% saline or dextrose saline and give 1 ml/minute) (see Chapter 27 page 469).
2. Antihistamine drugs IV or IMI if life-threatening; or orally if not severe reaction; and repeat the dose if needed, e.g.

- chlorphenamine (also called chlorpheniramine) is short acting (e.g. 4 hours) (4 mg tablets and 10 mg/ml injection for IVI diluted with saline to 5 ml and injected slowly over 1 minute); give 4–10 mg stat and repeat soon and each 4 hours if needed, but maximum dose in 24 hours is 24 mg by mouth and 40 mg by injection; *or*
- promethazine is long acting (e.g. 24 hours) (10 and 25 mg tablets; 1 mg/ml elixir; and 25 mg/ml injection); give 25 mg stat; and repeat once if needed; but maximum dose in 24 hours is 50 mg; *or*
- many other antihistamines exist but have different lengths of action and doses.

3. Other special drugs are sometimes used by Medical Officers, including adrenocorticosteroids, e.g. hydrocortisone, prednisolone, cortisone, dexamethasone, etc. For an acute allergic reaction threatening life hydrocortisone 100–300 mg or dexamethasone 4–10 mg IVI would be given immediately and 100 mg hydrocortisone or 4 mg of dexamethasone each 4–8 hours until the patient could swallow prednisolone/prednisone 1 mg/kg (e.g. 50–60 mg daily). However, this takes some hours to work and is not the most important treatment – epinephrine (followed by antihistamine) is the most important treatment.
4. The usual treatment of any complication.
5. Avoiding any further contact with the cause.

Autoimmune diseases

Very occasionally, the body's immune system attacks part of the normal body and can damage this part or destroy it.

It is thought that some types of diabetes mellitus (Type I), some types of overactive thyroid glands (hyperthyroidism or thyrotoxicosis) and underactive thyroid glands (hypothyroidism or myxoedema), perhaps rheumatoid arthritis and other conditions are brought about in this way.

Immunodeficiency disorders

Immunodeficiency occurs when either the antibody response or cellular immune response, or both, do not work properly to produce the immunity that would be expected in healthy people.

Causes of this include:

- congenital or inherited abnormalities;
- malnutrition (where not enough protein, etc. is available for the cells and antibodies to work properly);
- old age (where immune system starts to wear out);
- use of drugs which suppress immunity, especially adrenocorticosteroids (cortisone, prednisone, etc.) and some anti-cancer drugs;
- certain diseases, especially diabetes and kidney (renal) failure;
- the human immunodeficiency virus (HIV), which slowly destroys some of the T lymphocytes (CD4) but also affects all T lymphocytes and therefore the cellular immunity.

Sera and vaccines for prevention and treatment of infectious diseases

Table 10.2 is reproduced (with alterations and additions) with thanks from the book by Drs Fr. von Massow, J.K. Ndele and R. Korte *Guidelines to rational drug use* (1997, London, Macmillan) to try to help you remember when to give immunisations.

This section is intended to be a reminder of the importance of the WHO Expanded Programme on Immunization (EPI) and other immunisations possible for adults also. If you can immunise a person to prevent a disease, this is far more helpful to the patient and much cheaper for the Health Department than the patient getting the disease, having a lot of suffering, needing a lot of expensive treatment and then being left disabled or dying. Immunisation activities should be included in your daily routine.

Many vaccines already do exist. New vaccines are being developed all the time. If epidemiology shows diseases preventable by a vaccine are common in your country, your Health Department will try to provide them to prevent disease and death.

Table 10.2 Sera and vaccines for prevention and treatment of infectious diseases. (Source: Tables from *Guidelines to rational drug use* by Fr von Massow & R Korte, © 1997, reprinted by permission of Macmillan Education)

Sera and vaccines	Indication	Use			Notes
		In children	*In pregnant women*	*In non-immunised people*	
BCG vaccine (dried) injection	To build up immunity against: tuberculosis	*Age:* at or after birth	Avoid	Do not use in children with HIV with symptoms; or severe eczema	Tuberculin test may not be used for 3 months after injection
diphtheria–pertussis–tetanus vaccine (DPT) injection *	To build up immunity against: diphtheria, pertussis, tetanus	*Age:* 6 weeks, 10 weeks, 14 weeks, 18 months to 6 years		Full course of 3 doses: • 1st at the day of visit, • 2nd 4 weeks later; • 3rd another 4 weeks later	*In children* give polio **vaccine** at the same time (days) Give booster dose. After age 6–10 years use Td
diphtheria–tetanus vaccine (DT) * injection (different strengths for adults and children)	To build up immunity against: diphtheria, tetanus	*Age:* 6 weeks, 10 weeks, 14 weeks, 18 months to 6 years		**DPT** is contraindicated in patients with progressive neurological disorders or cramps; use **DT** instead	**DT** may be used instead of DPT Give booster at 6 years of age. After 6 years of age use Td
poliomyelitis vaccine (live attenuated) oral solution	To build up immunity against: poliomyelitis	*Age:* after birth 6 weeks in endemic countries 10 weeks 14 weeks	Avoid unless significant risk of exposure		*In children* give **DPT** at the same time (days) Give first booster dose after 5 years; then every 10 years. Extra doses in epidemic or eradication programme.
hepatitis B vaccine	To build up immunity against: hepatitis B	*Age:* 6 weeks, 10 weeks, 14 weeks or *Age:* after birth, 6 weeks, 14 weeks			Start at 6 weeks if not much infection near birth (e.g. Africa) Start at birth if a lot of infection then (e.g. Asia).

Table 10.2 (continued)

Sera and vaccines	Indication	Use			Notes
		In children	In pregnant women	In non-immunised people	
Haemophilus influenzae type b (Hib)	To build up immunity against: meningitis, pneumonia, epiglottitis	Age: 6 weeks 10 weeks 14 weeks			Does not prevent other bacterial infections
measles vaccine injection	To build up immunity against: measles	Age: > 9 months (never before 6 months) One booster	Avoid during especially first 3 months	Can have if HIV but well	If child is vaccinated before 9 months of age must give a 2nd dose after age of 9 months
measles–rubella OR **measles–mumps–rubella**	To build up immunity against: measles, mumps, rubella	9 months One booster	Absolute contraindication	If not had diseases All especially before puberty Can have if HIV	
tetanus vaccine injection	To build up immunity against: tetanus	See previous page	Give refresher at first visit If not already immunised see pages 48, 420	Give in case of accidents	Give booster dose every 10 years
	Prophylactic treatment after accident	*Application*			If a booster is needed use **DT** when available. Give in case of accidents or large burns; also give **antitetanus serum** or **antitetanus immunoglobulin**
		If person is not immunised or not fully immunised give a full course of 3 doses: • 1st at the day of visit; • 2nd 4 weeks later; • 3rd another 4 weeks later.			
antitetanus serum injection **antitetanus immuno-globulin (human)** injection	Prophylactic treatment after accident	Apply if person is not immunised or not fully immunised			Give in case of accidents or large burns; also give **tetanus vaccine**

Table 10.2 (continued)

Sera and vaccines	Indication	Use			Notes
		In children	In pregnant women	In non-immunised people	
rabies vaccine injection (prefer vaccine made from cell or tissue culture rather than duck embryo and especially brain culture)	To build up immunity against: rabies	*Pre-exposure* give a full course of 4 doses: • at day 0, 7 + 28, and 1 year later usually. Read manufacturer's leaflet as schedule may differ. *Post-exposure* Intradermal and intramuscular courses exist. Follow the manufacturer's recommendations carefully			Very expensive. Use only in groups at high risk exposure: wildlife services; veterinary services, animal handlers. Post-exposure prophylaxis is less expensive than pre-exposure vaccination. Give booster dose after 3 years
rabies immunoglobulin injection	Prophylactic treatment after bites				Extremely expensive. Follow dosage guidelines on the drug information insert
diphtheria antitoxin injection	Prophylactic treatment	Suspected cases only; sensitivity reactions are common			Also give prophylactic antibiotic treatment
meningococcal vaccine injection	Prophylaxis if significant risk of exposure	Give as *mass treatment* only after decision of national (or other relevant) health authority			
cholera vaccine injection		Has become *obsolete*			Concentrate on environmental hygiene and effective treatment
cholera vaccine oral	To build up immunity against: cholera	Effective. Two doses 1–6 weeks apart with a third for children under 6 years. Use possibly for staff caring for cholera patients			Expensive

* If pregnant woman not immunised against tetanus give TT (or Td)
1. when first seen in pregnancy,
2. at least 4 weeks after TT 1,
3. at least 6 months after TT 2 or during next pregnancy,
4. at least 1 year after TT 3 or during next pregnancy,
5. at least 1 year after TT 4 or during next pregnancy and continue for further pregnancies.
This protects not only the mother but the child by passive immunisation through the placenta.

Table 10.3 Vaccines and technologies available now. (Source: WHO Global Immunization vision and strategy 2006–2015)

Current vaccines

BCG [a]
Cholera (inactivated and live) [b]
DTP and DTP-based combinations [a]
Haemophilus influenzae type b [a]
Hepatitis A [a]
Hepatitis B [a]
Human papilloma virus [a]
Influenza [a]
Japanese encephalitis (inactivated and live) [b]
Measles [a]
Meningococcus (polysaccharide and conjugate) [a]
Mumps [a]
Pneumococcus (polysaccharide and conjugate) [a]
Polio (OPV and IPV) [a]
Pseudomonas [b]
Rabies [b]
Rift Valley fever [b]
Rotavirus [a]
Rubella [a]
Tetanus toxoid [a]
Tick-borne encephalitis [b]
Typhoid [b]
Varicella [a]
Yellow fever [b]

Available but underused immunisation supportive technologies

Pre-filled injection devices
Vaccine vial monitors on all vaccines

New or improved vaccines anticipated by 2015

Dengue [d]
DTaP (with two P antigens) [d]
Enterotoxigenic *Escherichia coli* (ETEC) [d]
Group A streptococcus [d]
Influenza for pandemic response [c]
Japanese encephalitis (improved) [c]
Malaria [d]
Measles (aerosol) [c]
Meningococcus A (multi-serotype conjugate) [c]
New combinations of existing vaccines [d]
Pneumococcus (improved conjugate or protein-based) [c]
Polio (monovalent OPV type 1) [d]
Respiratory syncytial virus [d]
Severe acute respiratory syndrome (SARS) [d]
Shigella [d]
Typhoid (conjugate) [d]
West Nile fever [d]

New immunisation supportive technologies anticipated by 2015

Jet injectors
Thermostable vaccines
Vaccine aerosols
Vaccine nasal sprays
Vaccine patches

[a] Available for immediate use in routine immunisation
[b] Available for specific regions or circumstances
[c] In a late stage of development
[d] Licensing expected 2010–2015
Source: www.who.int/vaccines-documents WHO Global Immunization vision and strategy 2006–2015

Appendix   The cold chain

Vaccines are damaged and no longer work if they are allowed to get hot or are frozen. They must be kept at the correct temperature from the time they are manufactured until they are used. The system used for keeping and sending vaccines in good condition to where they are used is called 'the cold chain'. The cold chain consists of a series of storage and transport links, all with the aim of keeping vaccines at a safe temperature of between 2°C and 8°C until they are injected.

The cold chain has to have vaccines and diluents:

• collected from the manufacturer or an airport as soon as they are available;
• carried between 2°C and 8°C from the airport and from one store to another;
• stored at the correct temperature in all vaccine stores and in health facilities;
• carried between 2°C and 8°C to wherever they are given;
• kept between 2°C and 8°C range during immunisation sessions; and
• kept between 2°C and 8°C during return to health facilities from where immunisation was given.

After vaccines reach the health facility you must:

• keep them between 2°C and 8°C in your health facility refrigerator;
• carry them to the immunisation session in a vaccine carrier with frozen ice packs or ice;
• keep the vaccines cool using a foam pad in the vaccine carrier while you immunise the children.

The following figure illustrates the cold chain.

Cold chain equipment used in health centres will include:

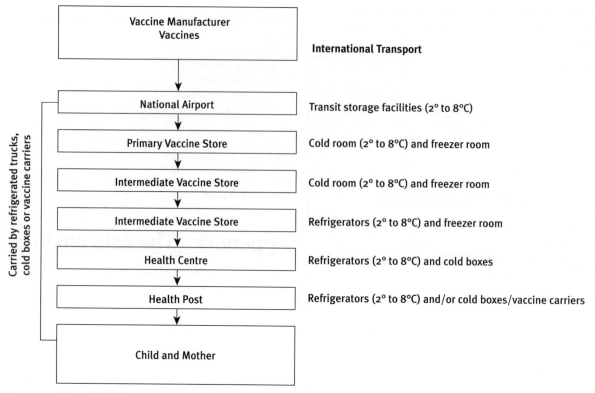

Figure 10.2 *The cold chain.*

1. *Refrigerator with freezing compartment*, or if the power or fuel supply is not always available an ice-lined refrigerator. There are special rules for using all of these refrigerators and you must read and follow these carefully (e.g. sticker on ice-lined refrigerator).

2. *Cold boxes.* A cold box is an insulated container (i.e. lets heat in or cold out very slowly), which can be lined inside with ice packs and keeps vaccines at the correct temperature for between 2 and 7 days.

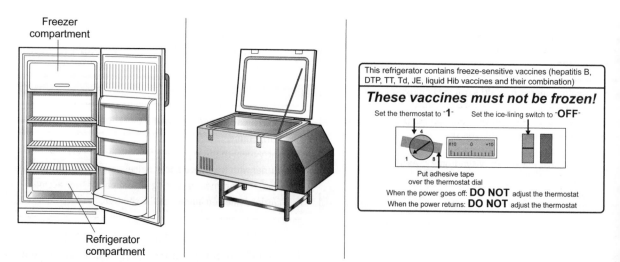

Figure 10.3 *Refrigerators.*

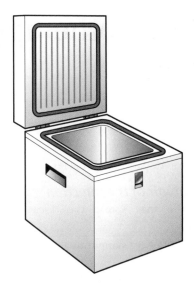

Figure 10.4 *Cold box.*

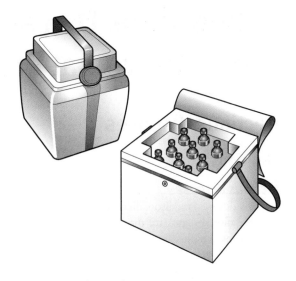

Figure 10.5 *Vaccine carrier.*

Cold boxes are used to carry larger amounts of vaccine from health centre to health centre or to store vaccine for a few days.

Boxes of the most suitable type and size should be sent to you.

3. *Vaccine carriers.* These are like cold boxes, except smaller, so that they can be carried on a bicycle or by hand when taking to actually give immunisation. They keep vaccines cold for at most 2 days, even with the lid closed all the time.

4. *Foam pad.* This is a piece of insulating foam which fits on the top of the ice packs in the vaccine carrier. Put the vaccines being used into the cuts in the foam. This keeps the vaccines being given and also the vaccines stored in the box at the correct temperature.

The vaccine carrier and foam pads allow vaccines to be taken to the place where they are to be used and the unused vaccines to be taken back to the health centre with the vaccines kept at the proper temperature all the time.

There are many important details you must know and carry out so that there is no break in the cold chain, which will mean that the vaccines will not work. See your immunisation textbooks, WHO publications and the directions which come with your equipment.

11 Infectious Diseases, Chemotherapy and Universal Precautions

Infectious diseases

Definitions

Infectious disease

Infectious diseases are also called contagious or communicable diseases, and are diseases caused by harmful organisms which can spread from one person to another.

These harmful organisms can:

1. exit from (or leave) some reservoir of infection (a person, animal or place);
2. transfer to (or spread to) susceptible persons (persons who can get the disease);
3. penetrate (or enter) susceptible persons;
4. be pathogenic (cause disease by either multiplying or making toxic products in the body).

Endemic disease

A disease is *endemic* in an area if it happens continuously (or all the time) in the area.

Sporadic disease

A disease has a *sporadic incidence* when it does not happen continuously in the area.

Epidemic

An *epidemic* of a disease is when large numbers of people are affected in a short period of time and this causes a temporary increase in the frequency of the disease.

How diseases can be caused

(see Figure 11.1)

Organisms

The specific agent or cause of a disease is a living organism which is a parasite. These include:

- prions,
- viruses,
- rickettsiae,
- bacteria,
- fungi,
- protozoa,

- worms, and
- insects.

See Chapter 10 page 40 for details of these organisms.

The reservoir of the infection

People who may spread the disease include the following:

1. people who have symptoms and signs of the disease ('cases');
2. people who are incubating the disease;
3. people who have an infection which cannot be diagnosed clinically (no symptoms and signs) (also called 'subclinical cases' or 'asymptomatic cases');
4. people who have the disease and are getting better ('convalescent carriers');
5. people who have the disease chronically (all the time) ('chronic carriers').

Animals, dirt, dust, etc. can also be reservoirs.

The exit of organisms from the reservoir

If the reservoir is a person, the organisms can go out (exit) through:

1. the respiratory tract through the mouth or nose;
2. the gastrointestinal tract in faeces or vomitus;
3. the urogenital tract by semen, vaginal or urethral discharges or in urine;
4. the skin and other mucous membranes (e.g. eyes) by discharges or bleeding.

The communicable or infectious period

This is the time during which the organism can be transferred directly or indirectly from an infected person to another person (or from an infected animal to a person).

The means of transfer of organisms

Infection (infectious organisms) can be spread by:

1. Direct contact (i.e. by touching and directly transferring the organisms).
   Some epidemiologists include as direct contact also:
   - droplets (see below),
   - some vehicles (e.g. a towel used to wipe an infected eye or nose immediately passed to another person and used to wipe the uninfected person's eye or nose),

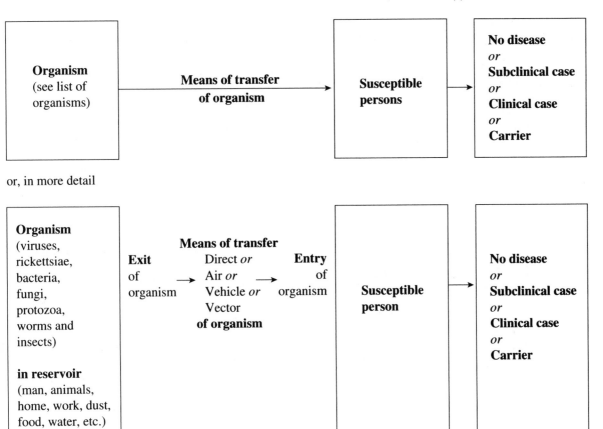

or, in more detail

Figure 11.1 *Diagrams showing how disease may be caused.*

- some vectors (e.g. an insect that stands on or feeds from a person's infected eye secretions and then soon after stands on an uninfected person's eye).
2. Airborne spread (when organisms in the air are breathed in):
   - Droplets of respiratory tract secretions containing organisms are coughed or sneezed (or talked) out into the air and inhaled; although if not inhaled, these droplets soon fall to the floor or ground.
   - Droplet nuclei containing organisms may be formed when the fluid in droplets dries before they fall, and the material left is very small and can float in the air for hours or longer and be inhaled.
   - Dust containing organisms may be formed when organisms on the floor or ground do not die but are blown into the air by sweeping or the wind, etc. with soil and other particles. This 'dust' can stay in the air for hours or longer and be inhaled before settling to the ground again.
3. Vehicles (i.e. things not infected and usually not alive but which can carry organisms):

- fingers,
- food and drink,
- water,
- instruments,
- blood-contaminated injections,
- clothing, toys, books, etc. (sometimes called 'fomites').
4. Vectors (animals which are usually infected and often are part of the life cycle of an organism and carry the organism from an infected host to a new uninfected host):
   - usually insects, e.g. mosquitoes transmitting malaria, filariasis, arboviruses, etc.

The entry of the organism (into a susceptible person)

Organisms can enter a person by:

1. inhalation (breathed into the respiratory tract),
2. ingestion (swallowed into the gastrointestinal tract),
3. inoculation (injected or passed through the mucous membranes or the skin).

The susceptible person

A person has defences against infection (see Chapter 10 page 41):

1. skin and mucous membranes covering the body surfaces,
2. the body's defence cells,
3. the body's immune systems.

If an organism enters the body, the defences usually cause an inflammatory reaction.

The time that passes after a person gets an infection and before the signs and symptoms of the disease start is known as the *incubation period*.

Means of control and prevention of infectious diseases (see Figure 11.2)

1. Kill or inactivate the organism in the original reservoir (man, animal, dust, etc.).
2. Stop the means of transfer.

   If the infection is spread by *direct contact*, then:
   * avoid exposure to carriers and persons with the disease,

* disinfect discharges,
* improve personal hygiene,
* give barrier nursing to the patient.

If the infection is spread by *droplets,* etc. in the air, then:
* cover mouth during coughing and sneezing,
* avoid overcrowded rooms and crowds,
* have good ventilation in all rooms.

If the infection is spread by *vehicles*, then:
* if instruments – improve personal hygiene, sterilisation of instruments, give barrier nursing to the patient;
* if other people (fingers) – improve personal hygiene, give barrier nursing to the patient;
* if food – supervise preparation, handling and hygiene of food;
* if water – protect and/or purify the water;
* if needles or syringes – sterilise syringes and needles properly.

If the infection is spread by *vectors* then:
* control or eradicate the insects,
* personal protection from insects (insect repellants, use of protective clothing, use of (preferably insecticide impregnated) mosquito nets at night).

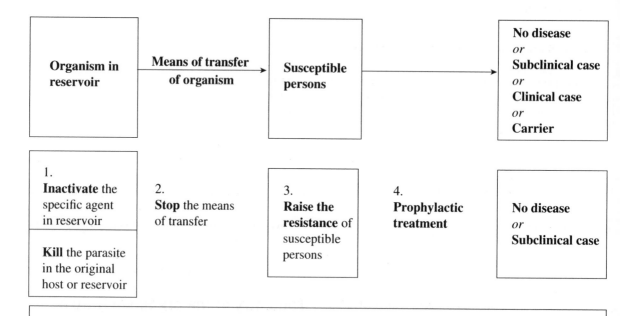

Figure 11.2 *Diagrams to show the means of spread of infectious disease (upper diagram) and the means of control and prevention of infectious disease.*

3. Raise the resistance of susceptible persons.
   • immunise these people – use active immunisation if possible, and passive if no active immunisation is available,
   • improve general health.
4. Prophylactic treatment (or 'chemoprophylaxis'). Give drugs to persons who are probably infected before the organisms cause disease. This is not often possible.
5. Use the occurrence of a case of the disease to give health education on the means of control and prevention of the disease.

Chemotherapy

Chemotherapy is giving a person a chemical that attacks the cause of the disease; in infections, it damages an organism. The chemical is absorbed into the body and kills or stops the growth and multiplication of the organisms which are infecting that person. If possible, the chemical will not harm the body of that person.

Chemotherapeutic drugs can sometimes cure an infection alone; but usually other treatment is needed too. Chemotherapeutic drugs are of three kinds:

1. natural plant products (e.g. quinine, etc.);
2. antibiotics made by bacteria or fungi to kill other bacteria or fungi (e.g. penicillin, tetracycline, chloramphenicol, etc.) (now made in the laboratory);
3. chemicals first made in the laboratory (e.g. sulfadimidine, isoniazid, dapsone, chloroquine, metronidazole, diethylcarbamazine, etc.).

A chemotherapeutic drug is usually effective against only one of the groups of pathogenic organisms as shown in Table 11.1.

A chemotherapeutic drug is also usually effective against only some of the members of that group. Table 11.2 shows some examples for antibacterial drugs.

Infecting organisms that are killed or cannot grow or multiply in the presence of a chemotherapeutic drug are 'sensitive' to that drug. Organisms that are not killed and can grow and multiply in the presence of a chemotherapeutic drug are 'resistant' to that drug.

Some organisms have always been resistant to certain drugs. Some organisms which were sensitive to

Table 11.1 Examples of different types of drug.

Antiviral drugs	Antibacterial drugs	Antifungal drugs	Antiprotozoal drugs	Antihelminthic drugs
Aciclovir	Penicillin	Griseofulvin	Quinine	Diethyl-carbamazine
Zidovudine (AZT)	Streptomycin	Nystatin	Chloroquine	Ivermectin
No antiviral drugs apart from anti-HIV drugs usually available in health centres	Doxycycline	Clotrimazole	Amodiaquine	Thiabendazole
	Chloramphenicol		Pyrimethamine	Albendazole
	Sulfadiazine		Metronidazole	Praziquantel
	Isoniazid		Mefloquine	
	Rifampicin		Artesunate	
	Dapsone		Doxycycline	

Table 11.2 Effectiveness of some antibacterial drugs.

	Penicillin	Chloramphenicol	Isoniazid	Dapsone
Pneumococcus (Pneumonia)	Effective	Effective	Not effective	Not effective
Salmonella typhi (Typhoid fever)	Not effective	Effective	Not effective	Not effective
Mycobacterium tuberculosis (Tuberculosis)	Not effective	Not effective	Very effective	Not effective
M. leprae (Leprosy)	Not effective	Not effective	Slightly effective	Effective

a chemotherapeutic drug can *develop resistance* to that drug and the drug no longer stops them growing or kills them. Development of resistance depends on the organism and the drug. Development of resistance can often be stopped by:

1. using the correct drug in the proper dose for long enough (although this no longer always applies), *and,*
2. using at least two drugs to which the organism is sensitive at the same time.

Rules for using antibacterial chemotherapeutic drugs

1. Do not give a patient with an illness or a fever for which no cause can be found antibacterial chemotherapeutic drugs, unless he becomes 'sick' (see Chapter 36 page 586).
2. Use only the 'correct' antibiotic for that illness. Others may not work or may do more harm than good. This book tells you which antibiotics to use for which illnesses.
3. Always use the proper dose of chemotherapeutic drugs – never use less.
4. Always give chemotherapeutic drugs for the full course; but for no longer. For chemotherapeutic drugs used for bacterial infections,
   (a) this is for 2 or 3 days after the patient seems cured or
   (b) – mild infections – at least 5 days;
   – severe infections – at least 7–10 days, whichever is the longer.
   – tuberculosis – at least 12–18 months unless rifampicin is used for the first 2 months, when it will be at least 9 months; unless both rifampicin and pyrizinamide are used for the first 2 months and rifampicin continued for the whole course, when it will be at least 6 months;
   – leprosy – at least 1 year for multibacillary (lepromatous) disease and at least 6 months for paucibacillary (tuberculoid) disease.
   – some infections (e.g. gonorrhoea) only one dose.
5. Do not stop antibacterial chemotherapeutic drugs in less than 48 hours because they do not seem to be effective. If the patient is getting worse *add* another drug before the 48 hours are finished. If the drug has no effect after 48 hours, then try another drug. However, if the patient gets very sick and looks as if he will die, change to chloramphenicol (see Chapter 12 page 64).

Notes on some antibacterial chemotherapeutic drugs

Sulfonamides and trimethoprim (SMX + TMP or co-trimoxazole)

Sulfonamides (e.g. sulfadiazine, sulfadimidine, sulfamethoxazole and sulfadoxine) were effective against many bacteria in all parts of the body. Now many bacteria have become resistant to them. Sulfonamides alone are not used much now for bacterial infections (except for urinary tract infection and they are still effective for trachoma) as other drugs are more effective.

The dose of sulfadiazine or sulfadimidine is 1 g four times a day and sulfamethoxazole 400–800 mg twice daily for 5–10 days.

Possible side effects include the following:

1. Formation of crystals in the urine if the patient does not drink enough when the drug is taken. Always make sure the patient drinks enough to pass a lot of urine when he takes a sulfonamide.
2. Allergic reactions, such as fever, skin rashes and jaundice, which can be serious.
3. Diarrhoea.

Sulfonamides also have an antimalarial effect. This is a weak effect, but if it is combined with another drug such as pyrimethamine or trimethoprim, the effect of both drugs together is powerful. For malaria a long acting sulfonamide, i.e. sulfadoxine is used with pyrimethamine (see Chapter 13 page 97).

Trimethoprim acts in a similar way but at a different place to sulfonamides to stop many organisms growing, but fewer organisms have become resistant to it and its side effects are fewer. It is also mildly effective against malaria. It can be used to treat respiratory infections and urinary infections. The dose is 100–200 mg twice daily or 300 mg once daily best taken with meals.

SMX/TMP or co-trimoxazole is a combination of sulfamethoxazole and trimethoprim as tablets (100 mg and 20 mg, 400 mg and 80 mg, 800 mg and 160 mg), oral suspension (200 mg and 40 mg in 5 ml) and injection (80 mg and 16 mg in 5 and 10 ml ampoules). The drug is given twice daily. It was thought that this combination was more effective than either drug alone. Its side effects are mainly due to the sulfonamide. However, the more it is used the more organisms become resistant to it. However, because it has become very cheap and because it has actions against many bacteria, it is used in some places as the first treatment for many infections including upper and lower respiratory infections, urinary tract infections, gastrointestinal tract infections, skin infections and even septicaemia. Because it has actions against many protozoa including those which cause infections in patients with HIV infection, it is used for treatment and prophylaxis of protozoal infections in HIV infected patients.

Problems with SMX/TMP or co-trimoxazole:

1. It depends on the patient understanding and remembering to continue to take it after the first dose even if he feels cured (which he is not) until the whole course in finished.
2. Side effects can occur.
3. Organisms can quickly start to get resistant to the drugs.

SMX/TMP is now given as prophylactic treatment to almost all patients with HIV infection as it stops many opportunistic infections occurring (see Chapter 19 page 239).

If it is given to many people in a community, SMX/TMP may well not be very effective for respiratory, skin and other infections in that community as many of the organisms causing these infections will have become resistant to it. If SMX/TMP is widely used in your community, discuss with your Medical Officer if you should choose alternative antibiotics for usual infections.

In pregnancy, SMX/TMP is needed for HIV infected patients and sulfadoxine with pyrimethamine is used for intermittent treatment of malaria. If other drugs were available, it would be best not to use sulfonamides, trimethoprim and pyrimethamine in the first 14 weeks of pregnancy or the last month of pregnancy. If at all possible, do not give in the last few days before delivery.

The dose of SMX/TMP for usual bacterial infections is two 400 mg/80 mg tablets or one 800 mg/160 mg tablet twice daily for 5 days (or shorter or longer depending on the condition treated), but much higher (up to 4 of the 400/80 mg tablets four times a day) for many protozoal infections.

Penicillin

Penicillin acts by stopping bacteria making cell walls, so that if they grow or multiply they break open and die.

Benzylpenicillin is effective against most organisms that cause infections in all parts of the body, except those that cause bowel or urinary tract infections. A few of the organisms that cause severe infections (including meningitis, septicaemia and pneumonia) are also resistant to penicillin. Some organisms which were sensitive have now developed resistance to penicillin.

Newer penicillins are also available which can kill most (but not all) of those organisms which are naturally resistant or have become resistant to benzylpenicillin, e.g amoxicillin, (di)cloxacillin, etc.

Benzylpenicillin is given for most infections except bowel and urinary tract infections. If the infection does not improve, SMX/TMP or doxycycline/tetracycline can be used instead. If the infection is a serious one which threatens life (e.g. meningitis, peritonitis, severe pneumonia, etc.) or an essential body part (e.g. eye, bone or joint, etc.), one of the special penicillins or chloramphenicol is used instead.

Treatment is given for 5 days for mild infections and at least 10 days for moderate or severe infections.

The main side effects are allergic reactions including skin rashes, asthma, shock and fever with arthritis. If allergy happens the patient should not be given penicillin again. You must tell him he is allergic to penicillin and that he must never have penicillin again. You must tell him to tell this to any health worker who ever treats him. You must also write it on the outside of both his outpatient and inpatient notes. Penicillin is otherwise safe during pregnancy.

Benzylpenicillin (also called crystalline penicillin), 1200 mg or 2,000,000 units IVI or IMI each 3 hours is given for infections which threaten life or an important body part; and 600 mg or 1,000,000 units each 6 hours is given for moderate infections.

Procaine benzylpenicillin, 1 g or 1,000,000 units by IMI daily is given for mild infections or severe or moderate infections which have improved after benzyl (crystalline) penicillin has been given for some days. Give procaine benzylpenicillin only by IMI, never by IVI.

Phenoxymethylpenicillin 250 mg and 500 mg tablets and usually 250 mg each 5 ml mixture is absorbed after being taken by mouth. It must be taken every 4–6 hours. It is not used much because you cannot know if the patient will remember to take it regularly. It is never used for moderate or severe infections. Normally use 250–500 mg four times daily.

Benzathine benzylpenicillin is a long acting penicillin which produces low levels of penicillin in the blood for a long time (a little up to 3–4 weeks). It is used for a 'one dose treatment' for syphilis and once each month for preventing rheumatic fever. The dose is usually 1.44 g or 2,400,000 units, usually in 5 ml by IMI.

Ampicillin and amoxicillin are newer penicillins. These are often not available as they are more expensive. They can be given by IVI, IMI or by mouth. They kill many pathogenic organisms in most parts of the body including the respiratory, urinary and gastrointestinal tracts. If they are combined with clavulanic acid, when they are sometimes called co-amoxiclav (e.g. amoxicillin 500 mg and clavulanic acid 125 mg tablet), this makes them kill even more organisms. Clavulanic acid, however, can occasionally cause liver damage and may best not be used in pregnancy (especially early pregnancy, but there is no evidence it causes problems). They can be used instead of benzylpenicillin, especially in serious infections of pneumonia, meningitis, septicaemia, etc. Most gonorrhoea organisms are now resistant. Chloramphenicol is safer in a very dangerous infection such as meningitis or septicaemia, and also for severe urinary tract and severe gastrointestinal infections (as resistance is less likely). They have the same side effects as other penicillins. In places where these drugs are scarce they are mainly used instead of tetracycline when a patient is pregnant.

The dose is 250–500 mg orally three to four times a day – larger doses are given by injection for severe infections.

Cloxacillin, flucloxacillin and *dicloxacillin*, etc. are penicillins which kill an organism called *Staphylococcus aureus* which can become resistant to other penicillins and cause serious skin and bone (osteomyelitis) infections and at times lung and other infections. These drugs are used by tablets or injection only for these infections where staphylococci are known, or are very likely, to be present, as they are not as effective as other penicillins against other organisms and are more expensive and have more side effects (including hepatitis).

Cephalosporins

Cephalosporins are a group of antibiotics, some of them being like benzylpenicillin (though one, cephalothin, being very effective against staphylococci), some of them being like amoxycillin and others, such as ceftriaxone being more like chloramphenicol. Some can be given orally but others including ceftriaxone only by IM or by IV injection. However, they are usually expensive, bacteria can become resistant and are not usually available in health centres. Ceftriaxone may be made available for serious infections, especially pneumonia and meningitis. Side effects are few but allergy can occur, especially in people allergic to penicillin. These and also other organisms in the body not causing disease and not being treated can become resistant to the cephalosporin and also other antibiotics not even being used. Then these very antibiotic resistant organisms can later cause dangerous (MRSA) skin or (VRE)

gastrointestinal and other infections. The dose for adults is 1–2 g daily by IM or IV injection in one dose daily or half the dose twice daily. It is usually continued until the infection seems cured and then for 2 more days. Ceftriaxone can be used in one dose of (125–)250 mg once only for gonorrhoea.

Chloramphenicol

Chloramphenicol comes usually as a 250 mg capsule, 150 mg/5 ml oral suspension, 1 g powder in vial for injection after mixing for IVI or IMI. (There is also an oily suspension already mixed in a 2 ml vial and containing 1 gram for IMI – do **not** give this by IVI.)

Chloramphenicol is a very powerful antibiotic effective against most (but not all) infecting bacteria in all parts of the body. Chloramphenicol enters all parts of the body.

Chloramphenicol, however, can cause death in a few patients by stopping the body making blood, and is used therefore only for serious infections. It can cause shock in newborn infants and is therefore not given to them or to women just before delivery or when breastfeeding infants. Other side effects are minor, e.g. nausea, diarrhoea, headache.

It is therefore used only for:

1. severe infection which immediately threatens life (e.g. septicaemia, meningitis, peritonitis, severe pneumonia, etc.);
2. severe infection which threatens an essential body part (e.g. eye, bone or joint, etc.);
3. infection which does not respond to other antibiotics (e.g. pneumonia, urinary tract infections, etc. which have not improved on penicillin, co-trimoxazole, tetracycline or amoxicillin);
4. infection for which no other treatment is available in the health centre (e.g. typhoid fever).

Penicillin or SMX/TMP (co-trimoxazole), or if one of these is not effective, doxycycline or tetracycline (erythromycin if pregnant), are almost always effective for the treatment of infections. However, if chloramphenicol is needed for an acute severe infection which is threatening life or a vital body part (and the risk of disease is more than the risk of the drug), then the proper large dose of chloramphenicol should be used, i.e. 100 mg/kg daily or 25 mg/kg every 6 hours. When the patient is apparently cured, the dose of chloramphenicol is reduced to half ($\frac{1}{2}$) of the above, i.e. 50 mg/kg daily or 12.5 mg/kg every 6 hours to complete the treatment course. *For adults of ordinary size 1 g (1 bottle of 1 g injection or 4 caps) every 6 hours is the usual dose.* When the patient is apparently cured (or when a patient who needs long treatment improves), the dose is reduced to 750 mg (3 caps) for large adults (> 50 kg) and 500 mg (2 caps) for small adults (< 50 kg) each 6 hours.

Chloramphenicol is well absorbed from the intestine after it is given by mouth. Chloramphenicol is therefore always given by mouth unless:

1. The patient cannot swallow it because:
   (a) he is unconscious and there is no intragastric tube;
   (b) he is unco-operative.
2. The patient cannot absorb it from the bowel, because of:
   (a) shock (little blood will be going to the bowel);
   (b) vomiting;
   (c) severe diarrhoea.
3. The patient is very sick and you cannot be sure that the drugs will be given by mouth because:
   (a) the staff are not dependable enough (staff are usually more dependable with injections than with oral drugs);
   (b) the patient is not dependable (he may refuse it or spit it out or vomit without telling the staff this);
   (c) of the other usual reasons that *very* sick patients are given injections.

Chloramphenicol acts quickly after IV injection. It acts only after some delay if given by IM injection. If it is given regularly every 6 hours this delay is not a problem after the first injection, because the effects of the previous dose will still be present. IM chloramphenicol is given if chloramphenicol by mouth is not possible (see above) and IV chloramphenicol is not needed or not possible. If IM chloramphenicol is given, it is best to give an extra injection IV with the first IM dose, if possible. If the IV injection is not possible, give the extra dose by IMI also.

See Chapter 12 page 66 for chloramphenicol resistant organisms.

Tetracycline group (normally use doxycycline)

Tetracycline, oxytetracycline, doxycycline and minocycline work by stopping organisms from using energy to make protein and they then cannot grow and reproduce. They are effective against most infecting bacteria in all parts of the body; however, some bacteria are or have become resistant to them. Therefore, they are not used for very severe infections which are threatening life or involving an essential body part. Tetracyclines are used for:

1. most infections if penicillin and/or SMX/TMP do not cure the patient or if it is best not to give (penicillin) injections or it is not possible to give penicillin or SMX/TMP (e.g. allergy);

2. gastrointestinal or urinary tract infection if other treatment (sometimes including SMX/TMP or just sulfonamides) does not cure them.

The dose of tetracycline or oxytetracycline is 20–40 mg/kg daily. For severe infections give 500 mg (2 of the 250 mg caps) four times a day and for less severe infections or after severe infections improve, give 250 mg (1 of the 250 mg cap) four times a day by mouth. Give this between meals and not with food or milk.

Doxycycline (50 or 100 mg tabs or caps) is a newer and cheaper and better form of tetracycline to use, if it is available. The dose is 2.5 mg/kg once daily, usually 200 mg for the first dose and then 100 mg daily (although 200 mg daily for severe infections). It should be taken just before a meal, as if it sticks in the oesophagus, it can cause severe ulceration and pain in the oesophagus. Patients should not lie down after taking doxycycline in case it comes back into the oesophagus.

Do not use a tetracycline and penicillin together as they do not kill organisms as well if used together.

Tetracyclines also have good activity against malaria organisms.

Tetracyclines (and erythromycin) are effective treatment for the few infections (rickettsial and some bacterial and others) which are not killed by penicillin or chloramphenicol (e.g. some 'atypical' pneumonias, Q fever, etc.).

Minocycline has activity against *M. leprae* which causes leprosy.

Side effects include vomiting and diarrhoea; discoloration of children's teeth if they are given before the teeth come through the gums, i.e. if given during pregnancy or before age of 12 years; dermatitis on skin onto which sun has shone; and doxycycline can cause oesophageal ulcers.

Do not give tetracycline to:

1. pregnant women,
2. children,
3. people with kidney (renal) failure which may be made worse.

If penicillin is not effective for these patients, you can give amoxicillin or ampicillin or erythromycin or ask a Medical Officer to supply a special drug.

Erythromycin, roxithromycin and azithromycin (macrolides)

These drugs act by stopping organisms from making protein; then they cannot grow or multiply. These effects are something between those of penicillin and tetracycline, but they have some special actions against some special bacteria that cause atypical (unusual) pneumonias. They are very safe.

Erythromycin is usually a 250 mg tablet or capsule and the dose 250–500 mg four times a day between meals. It can be used in pregnancy. Erythromycin, however, does cause nausea or diarrhoea in quite a few patients. Do not use erythromycin esteolate as it occasionally causes hepatitis.

It has to be taken 3–4 times daily and patients often forget to do this. As well as this, it is still expensive. However, erythromycin may be supplied for you to use in people who cannot be helped by SMX/TMP, who are allergic to penicillins but cannot take tetracycline as they are pregnant. It may be given together with penicillin for atypical (unusual in that it does not get better with any penicillins) pneumonia. IV erythromycin quickly blocks up veins.

Roxithromycin has similar actions but causes little nausea or vomiting and 300 mg has to be taken only once daily; however, it is still expensive.

Azithromycin stays for some days in the body and a short course is often very effective. It is very expensive. It is used for single dose treatments of some sexually transmitted diseases and trachoma.

Clindamycin

Clindamycin is somewhat similar to the above macrolides. The dose is 150(–300) mg four times daily. It is often used in pregnant patients instead of tetracycline for treatment of malaria. It also has other uses.

It can cause severe or fatal diarrhoea; however, if the patient is treated with metronidazole, the diarrhoea usually stops and the patient recovers.

Ciprofloxacin and ofloxacin (quinolones)

This group of drugs contains these and many other drugs which are very effective against a large number of bacteria and protozoa. They can usually be given by injection or orally, often once or twice daily, do not have many side effects, but as yet are very expensive. They are very unlikely to be available for some years in health centres except perhaps ciprofloxacin, which may be used for urethral discharges and ofloxacin, which is a good treatment for leprosy.

Ciprofloxacin 250, 500 or 750 mg tablets exist. The usual dose is 500 mg once only for urethral discharge or cervicitis but twice daily for other infections. Side effects occasionally occur:

- rash – in parts of the skin exposed to the sun;
- CNS – dizziness or confusion if elderly;
- damage to tendons and joints (tendons can suddenly break);

- not given to pregnant or breastfeeding women or children;
- gastrointestinal – nausea, etc.

Organisms causing STD and GI and other infections can become resistant.

Streptomycin (an aminoglycoside)

Streptomycin is effective against a number of bacteria including TB organisms. However, organisms soon develop resistance to streptomycin. Therefore, you must:

1. Use streptomycin only with other drugs. Do not use streptomycin alone. National guidelines for streptomycin use must be followed.
2. Use streptomycin only for TB in adults and children (and then only with isoniazid or another TB drug), or for neonatal infections before TB infection is possible (and then only with penicillin).

Do not use streptomycin for any other infections (unless you are told to use it for other specific infections).

See Chapter 14 page 114 for dose of streptomycin.

Gentamicin

Other aminoglycosides, e.g. gentamicin, are also very powerful antibiotics. However, all these drugs can cause deafness and kidney failure in the large doses needed to treat severe infections with ordinary bacteria and can be used safely only in a hospital where the laboratory can accurately measure the amount in the blood each 2–3 days. All need to be given by injection to get into the blood. If taken orally, they kill organisms in the bowel but are not absorbed. A once only IMI dose is safe and used for gonorrhoea.

Metronidazole

Metronidazole is a chemical which is very effective in treatment of bacteria which live in the mouth and also anywhere in the body where there is little or no oxygen, e.g. in the sinuses, bowel or abscesses not open to the air. It also kills many protozoa, e.g. amoeba in the bowel, trichomonal infection in the genital tract, etc.

It can be a tablet, suspension, suppository or IV infusion. Different strengths are available. Check the dose in mg and the strength of the preparation you are giving before actually giving it.

Side effects include a taste like metal in the mouth, nausea or even vomiting in about 20% of patients; and often severe malaise, vomiting, etc. if taken at the same time as alcohol.

The dose is usually 200–400 mg three times a day; but for some conditions just one large dose of 2000 mg.

Summary of choice of antibacterial drug

For mild or moderate infection

1. In all places except the gastrointestinal or urinary tracts use benzylpenicillin[1] (SMX/TMP[2] second choice or doxycycline[3]; see page 59).
2. In the urinary tract, except sexually transmitted urethritis, use trimethoprim or sulfamethoxazole[2] or SMX/TMP[2] (tetracycline[3] as second choice or amoxicillin if pregnant).
3. In the gastrointestinal tract – antibacterial drug usually not needed.

For severe bacterial infection which threatens life or a vital body part

In all places in adults (but not for newborn babies) use chloramphenicol in the correct *large* dose.

Remember in the newborn to use chloramphenicol in only the correct *small* dose.

Ceftriaxone is a very effective, safe, easily given IVI or IMI alternative; but is much more expensive.

If chloramphenicol is not effective, see Chapter 12 page 66 about possible resistant organisms.

For mild or moderate infections which do not respond to penicillin or SMX/TMP

In all places use doxycycline or tetracycline.[3]

If the infection is likely to come back many times and the *patient is likely to need long or repeated courses* of antibacterial drugs, it is very important to USE *doxycycline or tetracycline*; *DO NOT USE chloramphenicol* (unless the infection threatens life or a vital body part).

In some places ampicillin or amoxicillin (preferably with clavulanic acid) may be available to use at this stage. If the condition could be an atypical pneumonia or rickettsia infection, etc., erythromycin would also be needed.

In pregnant women and children use erythromycin or ampicillin or amoxicillin (preferably with clavulanic acid if not pregnant); but both erythromycin and amoxicillin may be needed.

For moderate infections which do not respond to either penicillin (or SMX/TMP) or tetracycline

First look for causes of failure to respond to treatment. There is probably a cause which needs other treatment rather than changing antibiotics.

If you can find no cause then: in all places – chloramphenicol.

> Use streptomycin in adults for only TUBERCULOSIS and ONLY TOGETHER WITH isoniazid or another anti-TB drug. Do not use streptomycin in any other way.

Continue the antibacterial drug for:

1. 2–3 days after the patient seems cured *or*;
2. mild infections   – 5 days,
   moderate infections   – 7 days,
   severe infections   – 10 days,
whichever is longer.

For special infections

None of the above is correct for these special infections:

- urethritis – see Chapter 19 page 204,
- tuberculosis – see Chapter 14 pages 112–122,
- leprosy – see Chapter 15 pages 142–145.
- atypical pneumonia – see Chapter 20 pages 289–291.
- some rickettsia and other infections.

Do not use the following antibiotics together

Some antibiotics act in the same way. Two together are no better than one dose, but would have more side effects.

Some antibiotics stop the other antibiotic working properly (e.g. patients with meningitis treated with both penicillin and tetracycline together die much more often than patients treated with penicillin alone or tetracycline alone; we would use chloramphenicol). Such combinations as penicillin and tetracycline are said to be 'antagonistic' (working to fight each other).

DO NOT USE TOGETHER:

1. Penicillin and tetracyclines (including doxycycline).
2. Tetracyclines (including doxycycline) and/or erythromycin and/or clindamycin.
3. Chloramphenicol and erythromycin.

Universal precautions

Universal precautions are ways to stop the spread of infection to yourself and other people.

---

1 Penicillin. Do not give if the patient is allergic to penicillin.
2 It may not be very effective if many people in the community are taking it for prophylaxis when HIV infected. Do not give if allergic to sulfonamides or if late pregnancy.
3 Tetracyclines. Do not give if the patient is pregnant or a child or has kidney failure.

A number of infections can be spread from patient to health worker or to other patients if these precautions are not followed. Hepatitis B and C viruses and HIV are incurable infections that are easily transmitted by reuse of contaminated sharps (needles, cutting instruments, etc.), as some people with these infections may have no symptoms at the time. It is not possible to know which patients have an infection. For this reason, universal precautions should be followed for all patients, regardless of whether they are thought to have an infection or not.

1. Use precautions with every person you see. Every time you have to cut the skin or touch body fluids, follow the advice below. This includes any time you do an operation, give an injection, stitch skin or tissue, help with childbirth or examine a vagina or rectum or even mouth.

   If you follow these rules there is no risk of spreading infection from one person to others, or of being infected yourself.

   • Do not let any body fluids such as blood, semen, vaginal secretions, discharges from sores, vomit, stool and urine touch your skin or mucous membranes. NEVER let any of them through your skin or mucous membrane.

   • Always put on a pair of clean gloves before touching any of the above. Wear gloves when collecting blood or putting in an IV needle or cannula. Label any bottle or sample of blood collected as dangerous.

   • Do not share anything that could touch blood. This includes razors, needles, any sharp instruments that cut the skin, and toothbrushes. If you must share such things, disinfect them before another person uses them.

   • Keep wounds covered with a clean bandage or cloth.

   • Do not do resuscitation using mouth to mouth unless you also use a face shield with filter.

   • Clean up spilled blood or body fluids quickly using 1% gluteraldehyde if available for blood; otherwise 1% sodium hypochlorite or phenol.

   • Wear an apron, if needed polythene tubing over arms, and goggles or other eye covering, mask, cap, as well as sterile gown and gloves when doing an operation or assisting with childbirth.

   • Put sharps (needles, etc.) into a 'sharps box'. Do not put the cap back onto a needle.

2. Wash your hands before and after examining or treating every patient. It is the most important way to kill organisms on your skin. You need to wash your hands even more thoroughly and for a longer time:

   • before and after helping someone give birth;

   • before and after touching a wound or broken skin;

   • before and after giving an injection, or cutting or piercing a body part;

   • after touching blood, urine, stool, mucous, or fluid from the vagina;

   • after changing sheets, bed clothes or patients' clothes;

   • after removing gloves.

   Use soap or other disinfectant to remove dirt and germs.

   Count slowly to 30 seconds as you scrub your hands all over with the soapy lather. Use a brush or soft stick to clean under your nails. Then rinse, using running water. Do not reuse this water.

   If handwashing is not possible, an alternative is to rub an antiseptic solution (e.g. chlorhexidine 'hand rub') all over both hands. Although this may be satisfactory between examining patients, it is not satisfactory for preparation ('scrubbing up') for any kind of surgical procedure.

3. Sterilise (or at least high level disinfection for) all equipment and instruments to be used to:

   • cut or pierce skin,

   • give an injection,

   • cut the cord during childbirth

   before use.

   Sterilisation kills all living organisms. Effective 'high level' disinfection kills all fungi, bacteria and viruses but not all spores.

   Before sterilisation or disinfection, all equipment must be properly soaked and cleaned.

   (a) *Soaking.* Soak instruments for 10 minutes. If possible, use a 0.5% solution of sodium hypochlorite or bleach (chlorine) (see below). Soaking instruments in bleach solution will help protect you from infection when cleaning them. If you do not have bleach, soak your instruments in water.

   (b) *Washing.* Wash all instruments with soapy water and a brush until each one looks very clean, and rinse them with clean water. Be careful not to cut yourself on sharp edges or points. Wear gloves when washing instruments; if possible use heavy gloves.

   (c) *Sterilisation* for things that can be heated. If possible use an autoclave. A properly used pressure cooker is, however, effective and usually available. The instruments must be kept properly packed after pressure is reached at 121°C (250°F)–131°C for the correct time, which depends on how high you are above sea level, i.e. altitude.

Altitude	Minutes
Sea level	20
1000 m	30
2000 m	35
3000 m	45
4000 m	50
5000 m	60
6000 m	70
7000 m	80

(d) *Disinfecting.*
- *Use chemicals for things which cannot be heated.* Soak in 2% gluteraldehyde for 20 minutes after cleaning (following all the safety rules when you use gluteraldehyde). Soak cups, nasogastric tubes, etc. in 0.5% sodium hypochlorite for 20 minutes.
- *Steam or boil things which can be heated* for 20 minutes.

  To steam them you need a pot with a lid. The water does not need to cover the instruments, but use enough water to keep steam coming out of the sides of the lid for the needed time. Do not overload. No instruments should be above the rim of the pot.

  To boil them, you do not need to fill the whole pot with water. But you should make sure the water covers everything in the pot for the entire time. Put a lid on the pot. Boil for the needed time.
- For both steaming and boiling, start timing after the water with the instruments in is fully boiling. Do not add anything new to the pot once you begin to count. The time needed depends on how high you are above sea level, i.e. altitude.

Boil or steam clean items as follows.

Altitude	Minutes
Sea level	10
1000 m	10
2000 m	10
3000 m	20
4000 m	20
5000 m	30
6000 m	45
7000 m	60

How to make a disinfection solution of 0.5% bleach.

If the label on your bleach says:
- 2% available chlorine – use 1 part bleach to 3 parts water;
- 5% available chlorine – use 1 part bleach to 9 parts water;
- 10% available chlorine – use 1 part bleach to 19 parts water;
- 15% available chlorine – use 1 part bleach to 29 parts water.

Mix just enough solution for one day. Do not use it again the next day. It will no longer be strong enough to kill germs.

12 Septicaemia and Other Acute Severe Bacterial Infections; and HIV Infection

Septicaemia is present when organisms get into the blood in the blood vessels and grow and multiply in the blood.

Septicaemia occurs only in special circumstances:

1. Organisms are pushed straight into the blood, e.g.:
   - injection of contaminated drugs or blood transfusion (with organisms in them);
   - an operation where a cut is made through an infected area;
   - passage of an urethral catheter, especially when there is infection in the urethra;
   - changing or leaving in too long an infected intravenous needle or cannula;
   - doing a burns dressing.
2. The body is in a state of weakened immunity or resistance, e.g.
   - HIV infection;
   - malnutrition;
   - anaemia;
   - certain chronic illnesses, e.g. diabetes mellitus or kidney (renal) failure or liver (hepatic) failure, etc.;
   - after operation or childbirth;
   - if another infection is present in the body;
   - if the patient has cancer or leukaemia, etc.;
   - if the patient is taking drugs which decrease immunity, e.g. prednisolone or anti-cancer drugs.
3. There is a particularly severe or widespread infection in the body, e.g. certain types of pneumonia.
4. The attacking organism is particularly virulent, e.g. certain types of organisms which can cause meningitis and septicaemia.

If a patient in any of these situations suddenly gets worse, always think of septicaemia.

The first group of conditions is of particular importance in the health centre. Septicaemia can follow simple procedures. A very common cause of septicaemia is putting in or taking out an urethral catheter. In all these procedures in Group 1, virulent organisms may be pushed straight into the blood where they start to grow and produce septicaemia.

If septicaemia develops, the patient may have any of the following:

1. Rigor(s) (high temperature with shivering or shaking).
2. General symptoms and signs of infection which could include:
   - severe malaise and weakness;
   - nausea, vomiting, diarrhoea;
   - being not fully conscious or being psychotic or even fitting;
   - dyspnoea (shortness of breath) and fast breathing;
   - raised temperature.
3. Fast pulse, low blood pressure, cold, cyanosed, low urine output ('cold shock').
4. Fast pulse, low blood pressure but skin warm (due to dilation of blood vessels in the skin) ('warm shock').
5. Haemorrhages into the skin, pinpoint haemorrhages (petechiae), or larger areas of bleeding (echymoses) or bruises.

Any patient who has an infection and gets worse, or any patient with weakened immunity who gets suddenly very sick or any patient who has had any type of procedure carried out on him and then gets very sick should be thought of as having septicaemia.

Management of septicaemia

If a patient has a condition which makes it likely for him or her to develop septicaemia, and he or she then develops symptoms and signs suggesting septicaemia, immediately manage as follows:

1. chloramphenicol in the correct large dose (usually 1g each 6 hours);
2. antimalarial drug as indicated, usually an artemisinin drug or quinine and a companion drug;
3. IV drip – but only if needed for shock or dehydration, etc.;
4. treatment of any heart failure;
5. treatment of any infected body part in the usual way;
6. consult a Medical Officer if necessary;
7. do not reduce the chloramphenicol dose unless the patient seems to be cured very quickly;
8. continue chloramphenicol for *at least* 10 days.

1. Chloramphenicol (25 mg/kg each 6 hours). For an adult of average weight give 2 g immediately, then 1 g every 6 hours.

   Give by IVI *if*
   • shock (essential), or
   • IV drip needed for another reason and is running.

   Give by IMI *if*
   • IV drip not needed, or
   • IV drip not possible.
   and if
   • oral drugs are not reliable enough (as very sick), or
   • oral drugs are not effective (as not able to swallow or vomiting or severe diarrhoea).

   Give orally (1 g usually 4 × 250 mg caps) *only if*
   • is not very sick; or after improves (when oral drugs are reliable enough), and
   • can swallow, and
   • has no vomiting or severe diarrhoea, and
   • is not shocked.

2. Antimalarial drug for all patients if malaria possible.

   Give by IVI if patient
   • is shocked, or
   • is unconscious, or
   • is very sick.

   Artesunate 2.4 mg/kg (or other artemisinin drug) IVI immediately and further doses, OR if not available quinine base 20 mg/kg (900 mg for a small adult or 1200 mg for a large adult) by IMI or by a SLOW (over 4 hours) IV infusion (drip).

   See Malaria Chapter 13 pages 79–87 for further treatment; or treatment if IV treatment not possible.

3. Set up an IV drip; but only if needed, i.e. if shock, severe dehydration, unconscious, very sick, not able to take oral fluids and drugs.

   Do not give more fluid than is really necessary (or this may cause cerebral oedema, convulsions and death).

   • When shock – see Chapter 27 pages 468–470.
   • When dehydration – see Chapter 23 pages 364–365.
   • When maintenance fluids only needed – give 0.18% sodium chloride in 4.3% dextrose, 1 litre each 8–12 hours.
   • When drip for IV injections only needed – give 0.18% sodium chloride in 4.3% dextrose, 1 litre each 12(–24) hours.

4. Look for heart failure. Treat if present.
   Give intranasal oxygen 2–4 litres/minute.
   Give frusemide 20–40 mg IVI or 40–80 mg orally; or if not available, any other diuretic.
   Give digoxin 0.5 mg (½ mg) or 500 µg (mcg) IVI slowly immediately or, if injection not available, 0.5 mg (½ mg) orally immediately.
   Give only maintenance fluids (see 3 above) (do not give 0.9% sodium chloride).
   Then see Heart failure (Chapter 27 pages 464–466).

5. Treat any infected part or any other complication in the usual way.

6. Consult a Medical Officer urgently about further management if you are not sure of the diagnosis or treatment or if transfer for surgery is likely.

7. Do not quickly reduce the chloramphenicol dose. *If the patient is apparently cured very quickly*, 12.5 mg/kg (12½ mg/kg) each 6 hours could be given, i.e.
   • 750 mg (3 of the 250 mg caps) each 6 hours for a large adult (> 50 kg) and
   • 500 mg (2 of the 250 mg caps) each 6 hours for a small adult (< 50 kg).
   However, *most patients* should continue 1 g (4 of the 250 mg caps) each 6 hours.

8. Continue the chloramphenicol for at least 10 days. Some infections may need longer treatment; however, use the reduced dose (see 7) *after* clinical improvement and 10 days high dose treatment.

9. Always think of HIV infection when a patient has septicaemia or any other severe bacterial infection (see below and Chapter 19).

HIV infection, septicaemia and severe infections

Septicaemia and other acute severe bacterial infections, especially pneumonia, meningitis, abscesses in soft tissues, etc., are often the first indication that a person has decreased immunity and this is usually due to HIV infection (see Chapter 19). Of course, not all patients with these illnesses have HIV infection. These illnesses, however, are many more times as common in patients with HIV infection than other people (pneumonia up to 100 times more common). If a patient gets more than one attack of these diseases it should make us even more suspicious of HIV infection.

Severe bacterial infections should make us:

1. ask the patient about possible HIV infection and do the counselling and take blood for HIV testing (see Chapter 19 pages 233–236);

2. ensure that the universal precautions to stop the spread of HIV and other illnesses are being carried out properly (see Chapter 11 pages 61–63).

If a patient with HIV infection does have septicaemia, the most common bacteria causing this are as follows.

1. *Streptococcus pneumoniae* (pneumococcus). Pneumococcal infections occur early in HIV infection, especially sinusitis, otitis media, pneumonia, and can then get into the blood and also cause septicaemia, meningitis and abscesses in soft tissue. There are often repeated and severe attacks of these after previous successful treatment. Many pneumococci are still killed by benzylpenicillin, but almost all are killed by chloramphenicol. These infections in HIV infected patients may be reduced by drug treatment of the HIV itself, pneumococcal vaccine and possibly prophylactic SMX/TMP. Always check for TB by sending three sputum samples for examination for AFB (see Chapter 14 page 108).

2. Salmonellae (although not those which cause typhoid fever), i.e. non-typhoid fever salmonellae (NTS) or other similar bacteria from the bowel. Salmonella (NTS) and other bowel bacterial infections with septicaemia usually come later in HIV infection. The only way of diagnosing them for sure is by culturing the blood, which is not possible in the health centre. We have to suspect it and treat it as such if it is likely. Only one third of the patients have gastrointestinal symptoms (e.g. diarrhoea, abdominal pain, etc.). About one third of the patients have lung symptoms and signs but these are (more often) due to pneumococcal pneumonia or TB. About one half of the patients have enlarged livers and spleens but these can also be due to malaria. This condition is more common where people also have bowel schistosomiasis.

   NTS are always resistant to benzylpenicillin and may have developed resistance to SMX/TMP, amoxicillin, tetracycline and even chloramphenicol. In some places only very expensive drugs such as third generation cephalosporins or quinolones will kill them; however, these drugs are very expensive and if used a lot the bacteria become resistant to them too. Your Health Department and Medical Officer will tell you if culture and sensitivity tests mean you should use a different antibiotic to the chloramphenicol as above. Unfortunately, these NTS infections also tend to come back often, even after treatment and also cause abscesses in soft tissues. Prophylactic antibiotics may help, but they are very expensive and lead to the NTS becoming resistant to the antibiotic and spreading to other people, causing infections we cannot treat. Drug treatment of the HIV infection itself, however, does reduce the number of times the infection comes back.

If any patient has septicaemia, pneumonia, meningitis, or acute severe bacterial infection, especially if it comes back after treatment, always think of decreased immunity due to HIV infection.

Chloramphenicol resistant organisms

All antibiotics (including chloramphenicol) have organisms which are resistant to them. Chloramphenicol is still the most effective, most available and cheapest drug for treatment of septicaemia or severe infections in a health centre.

Infections which are not killed by chloramphenicol include:

1. Some non-typhoid salmonellae (NTS) (see above).
2. Some organisms causing atypical pneumonia (see Chapter 20 pages 288–289 and Chapter 19 pages 224–225). These are usually killed by erythromycin or tetracycline as well as some newer antibiotics, but not penicillin.
3. Some organisms causing particular infections which may or may not occur in your area, e.g. leptospirosis. These are usually killed by penicillin ± erythromycin (or tetracycline) and some newer antibiotics.

Your Medical Officer will know which, if any, of the above organisms occur in your area and what you should do because of them to change the above treatment of severe infections. He (or you while waiting for advice) should consider:

1. If NTS are common, as above.
2. If atypical pneumonia is common in the area or suspected, treatment would start as usual with penicillin but erythromycin 500–1000 mg 6 hourly is added. If the pneumonia is severe when diagnosed, treatment may start with amoxicillin and clavulanic acid (co-amoxyclav) or related newer penicillin and erythromycin. The patient would then not get worse and need chloramphenicol. Of course, if pneumocystis pneumonia was suspected as the patient has, or may have, HIV infection, then a high dose of co-trimoxazole would also be given (see Chapter 19 page 224).

3. If leptospirosis or other chloramphenicol resistant infection is common in the area or suspected, then benzylpenicillin 1200 mg each 6 hours may be started with chloramphenicol from the beginning of the treatment.

4. If other infections are a problem, your Medical Officer should advise you.

5. Do not use together:
   • chloramphenicol and erythromycin.
   • erythromycin and tetracycline/doxycycline.
   • tetracycline/doxycycline and penicillin.

13 Malaria

See *Guidelines for the Treatment of Malaria* (2006 or later edition), WHO, Geneva for more detailed but still very clear, up-to-date clinical as well as treatment information about malaria.

Definition

Malaria is a disease caused by infection of the red blood cells by a protozoal organism called *Plasmodium* of which four types infect humans. Infection causes both acute and then chronic disease with fever, anaemia, enlargement of the spleen and other conditions. Infection sometimes causes very severe acute complications with disorders of the brain, kidneys, liver, blood and many other parts of the body. Malaria often causes death.

Frequency

Malaria is the most common important parasitic disease in the world. Malaria affects many of the people living between the latitudes of approximately 60°N and 40°S (see Figure 13.1). One person in five in the world is at risk. Malaria, each year, affects 300 million people and causes over 1 million deaths.

Cause

Malaria is caused by infection with one or more of four protozoal (one-celled microscopic organism) parasites (other malaria parasites affect animals):

1. *Plasmodium falciparum* is the most common in hot, wet climates.
2. *Plasmodium vivax* is the most widespread of the parasites in the world (but does not occur in West Africa) and is more common than *P. falciparum* in places which have cool or dry seasons (as well as the hot and wet seasons).
3. *Plasmodium malariae* is not common.
4. *Plasmodium ovale* is very uncommon.

Epidemiology

Man is the only host of the above malaria parasites.

Transmission of these parasites is usually from the blood of an infected person to a female *Anopheles* mosquito and then to susceptible new persons.

Occasionally, transmission is from infected blood through the placenta to a baby; by blood transfusion or use of needles, etc. contaminated with blood that has malaria parasites in it.

See Figure 13.2 for details of the life cycle of the malaria parasite.

The incubation time for the mosquito (from when it sucks up blood with malaria gametocytes in it until these develop into infective sporozoites which the mosquito injects into people when it bites) is at least 10 days. The gametocytes can develop into sporozoites only if the temperature is above 15°C (60°F) and below 34°C (93°F).

The incubation period in man (from the bite of an infected mosquito until the start of symptoms and signs of malaria) is usually about 2 weeks. However, it is often much longer (in cold climates *P. vivax* may take nearly a year). It cannot be shorter than 8 days.

Transmission of malaria can occur only if the following four conditions are present:

1. There are human gametocyte carriers present in the area.
2. *Anopheles* mosquitoes are present in the area.
3. The temperature and humidity is right for the parasite to develop in the mosquito.
4. There are susceptible human hosts (especially babies and children in endemic areas).

Partial or incomplete immunity to malaria (due to antibodies and cellular immunity and also by becoming tolerant to the parasite) can develop after 4–10 years of continuous exposure to malaria (if the person does not die from chronic malaria or one of the acute attacks of malaria during this time). This means that older children or adults, who have lived continuously for years in places where malaria is present all the time, develop partial immunity. They are often called 'semi-immune'. However, to develop and keep this semi-immunity, a person has to be repeatedly infected with malaria, and as well as being often sick is likely to die from anaemia or severe malaria in the first 4–6 years (unless treatment for acute attacks is always immediately available).

Other than these persons who have developed semi-immunity to malaria, all persons of all ages and both sexes are susceptible to malaria.

The persons most commonly affected by malaria are:

1. babies and children in areas where malaria infection is going on all the time (an area of continuous or high transmission or 'stable malaria');

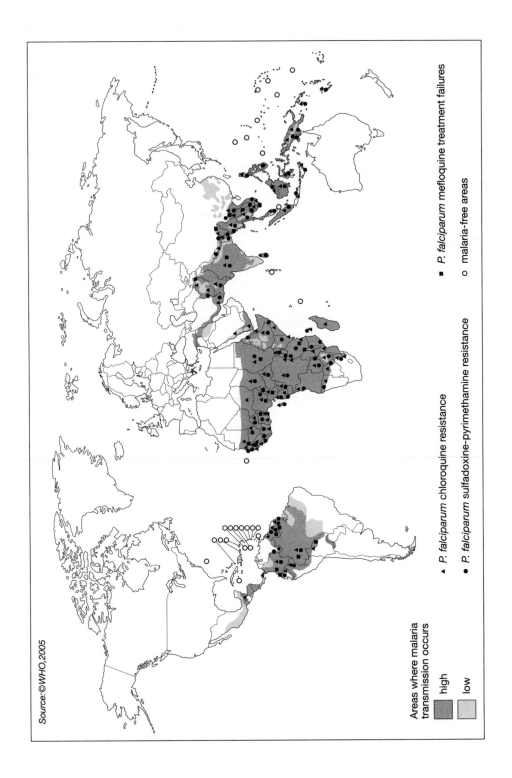

Figure 13.1 *The distribution of malaria. (Source: http://rbm.who.int/wmr2005/html/map5.htm by permission of the WHO)*

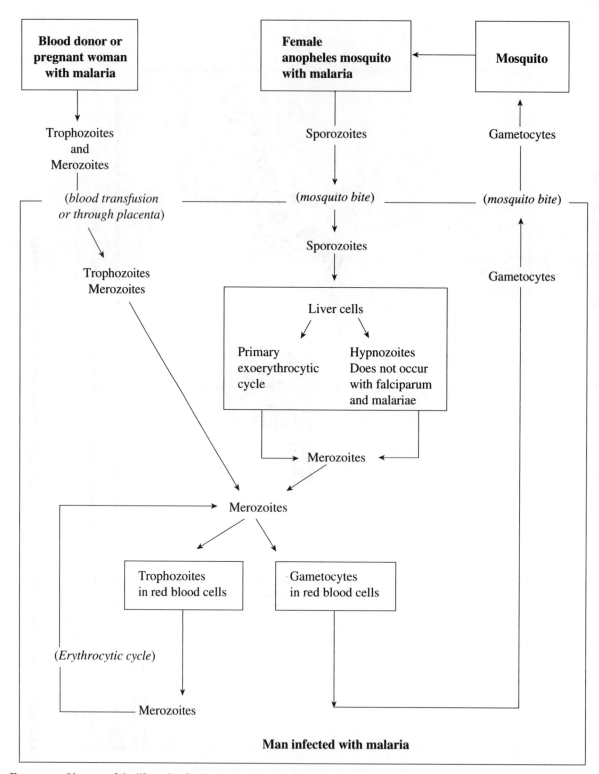

Figure 13.2 *Diagram of the life cycle of malaria parasite as it affects man.*

2. persons of all ages who come to malarial areas;
3. persons of all ages in areas where malaria can occur but where malaria is not present all the time but does occur if conditions suitable for transmission of malaria occur (e.g. temperature and rainfall change). This is an area of intermittent transmission or 'unstable malaria'.

Immunity to malaria may be overcome by the malaria parasites in the following situations:

1. during pregnancy (especially the last 3 months of pregnancy and especially in the first pregnancy);
2. during another illness;
3. if a person goes for a while with no malaria parasites present in his blood (e.g. the person has been taking antimalarials and stopped them; the person has been living in a screened house or dormitory; the person has been away from a malarial area, etc.);
4. if a person shifts to a place where there is more malaria or a different type of malaria;
5. if a person is given anti-inflammatory drugs (such as cortisone or prednisolone) or anti-cancer drugs (which stop immunity working properly);
6. if the patient has his spleen removed (which decreases immunity);
7. if the patient develops HIV infection (which decreases immunity).

Symptoms and signs, course and complications

Infection with malaria parasites can cause many different symptoms and signs and clinical states. Common clinical states include:

1. An acute attack of vivax (or malariae or ovale) malaria in a non-immune person.
2. An acute attack of falciparum malaria in a non-immune person. One or more of the common severe complications of acute malaria is likely to develop in non-immune patients with falciparum malaria.
3. Severe or complicated malaria.
4. Chronic malaria (in the years from the first infection until good semi-immunity has developed).
5. Malaria in semi-immunes.
6. Late complications of malaria.

Acute attack of vivax, malariae or ovale malaria in non-immune people

There may be a few hours to a few days of vague ill health (e.g. feeling cold, aches and pains, nausea, etc.) before any fever and severe disease. Attacks of fever then occur.

At first the patient is cold for $\frac{1}{4}$–1 hour and the temperature is not raised. The patient then starts to shiver and has a rigor and the temperature rises quickly up to about 40°C. The skin is cold and pale, the pulse fast and the BP often higher than normal. Vomiting, diarrhoea and urinary frequency are common.

Next, a hot stage comes for about an hour. The rigor stops, the patient feels hot, the skin feels hot and dry, the pulse is fast and the BP is often low. Headache, delirium, thirst and vomiting are common.

After this a sweating stage comes. The patient sweats a lot, the temperature falls, the pulse and BP become normal. After an hour or two the patient often goes to sleep. After waking the patient may feel reasonably well.

An attack may last up to 10 hours.

Attacks of fever occur irregularly but sometimes after a week or so attacks of fever may come each third (or fourth if *P. malariae*) day if the first day of the illness is counted as Day 1.

Jaundice may be seen after attacks of fever.

Anaemia, which causes pallor, gets worse after each attack of fever.

The spleen becomes enlarged.

The liver enlarges but does not become very big.

If correct treatment is given, there is a good response to treatment within a few hours. Even without treatment the attacks of fever get less frequent. However, relapses occur (when a liver hypnozoite makes merozoites) after treatment of an acute attack.

Severe and fatal complications (see page 72) do not usually occur.

Chronic malaria (see page 74) then develops.

Acute attacks of falciparum malaria in non-immune people

The incubation period is usually 2 weeks. It can be longer; but it can also be as short as 8 days.

There may be some hours to a few days of vague ill-health (e.g. feeling cold; headache, backache and pains all over; nausea, vomiting and diarrhoea).

The attack then occurs. The attack may be like other forms of malaria. However, more often the attack does not have the three definite stages.

- In an attack the patient may appear to be very sick (as in any febrile illness).
- Pains in the head, bones and muscles are severe.
- Vomiting and diarrhoea are common.

- Mental confusion and delirium are common.
- The temperature is usually raised but rigors may not occur. Sometimes the temperature is normal. Most commonly, the temperature is raised but it does not go away after an attack and may be continuous.
- Sweating is often severe.
- Pulse is usually fast.
- Blood pressure is often low.
- Breathing rate is usually fast.
- Anaemia develops quickly.
- Jaundice is sometimes present.
- The spleen is usually enlarged and tender.
- The liver is often enlarged.

If correct treatment is given there is usually a good response to it after a few hours.

If treatment is not given or if the treatment given is not correct or if the treatment is not given quickly enough, one or more of the following complications can occur and the patient is said to have 'severe' or 'complicated' malaria.

Chronic malaria (see page 74) then develops if the patient does not die from an acute attack or from a complication.

Severe/complicated malaria

One or more of the following indicates severe or complicated malaria has developed:

1. febrile fits (only in children), hyperpyrexia (complications of fever) (see right);
2. convulsions, unconsciousness, paralysis, psychotic behaviour, etc. (cerebral malaria) (see right);
3. hypoglycaemia (low sugar (glucose) in blood) (see page 73);
4. acute anaemia and hypoxaemia ('anoxia') (see page 73);
5. severe vomiting, diarrhoea and sometimes even dysentery (gastrointestinal malaria) (see page 73);
6. shock (see page 73 and Chapter 27 pages 466–470);
7. kidney failure (see page 73);
8. malarial haemoglobinuria ('blackwater fever') (see page 73);
9. respiratory symptoms and signs (pulmonary oedema) (see page 73);
10. acidosis (see page 74);
11. abnormal bleeding (see page 74);
12. complicating bacterial infection (especially pneumonia, urinary tract infection or septicaemia);
13. 5% or more of the RBCs infected with parasites (hyperparasitaemia) (see page 74).

1. Complications of fever. Febrile fit. Hyperpyrexia

Fever occurs in almost all cases of malaria.

In children, if the temperature rises very quickly from any cause, a febrile fit may occur. If the child with a febrile fit due to malaria is given an injection of an antimalarial drug and anti-convulsants and is cooled, the fitting will stop and the child will become fully conscious again. (Occasionally, another fit can occur and the child not be fully conscious for an hour or so.) This is different from cerebral malaria (see below).

> Remember that all children who fit must have a lumbar puncture in case they have meningitis (as well as a blood slide taken for malaria parasites and an injection of an effective, preferably artemisinin group, antimalarial drug).

Fever alone does not cause fitting in adults. *Adults do not have febrile fits.* All adults who fit must have a lumbar puncture in case they have meningitis (as well as a blood slide taken for malaria parasites, and an injection of preferably an artemisinin antimalarial drug).

Occasionally, in children and adults, the temperature rises above 40°C and stays there. This is called 'hyperpyrexia'. This is particularly dangerous if the patient stops sweating and the skin becomes dry. Cyanosis and mental disturbance may occur. The patient needs urgent cooling or he will become shocked and die.

Remember that sometimes the temperature taken at the surface of the body is normal in malaria and other severe infections, when in fact the patient's inside temperature is high (high enough to cause severe damage to the body, or hyperpyrexia or death). Always measure the inside body temperature with a rectal thermometer if an illness due to a high temperature is a possibility.

2. Cerebral malaria

The blood vessels going to the brain may be partly blocked or made to leak by the malaria parasites, which may also poison the brain with their toxins. All this causes an encephalitis (see Chapter 25 page 415). This condition is called cerebral malaria.

Cerebral malaria may cause all sorts of brain and mental symptoms and signs. These include those of depression of the brain functions such as severe headache, drowsiness, paralysis and unconsciousness. They also can include those of irritation of the brain functions such as restlessness, irritability, confusion, abnormal (psychotic) behaviour, arching of the back, twitching and fitting, etc. On examination, the patient is usually febrile, is not fully conscious (and this lasts for 1 hour or more), the back may be arched backwards and the neck even seem a little stiff and the mental state is usually abnormal. Any or all of the above signs may be found.

> All patients in a malarious area
> - with a severe febrile illness for which no cause can be found, or
> - who are not fully conscious, or
> - who have had a fit, or
> - with a stiff neck, or
> - with an acute psychosis when not known to be previously psychotic
>
> must have:
> 1. full doses of injected antimalarials, preferably an artemisinin drug (or quinine), and a companion drug, and
> 2. a blood smear for malaria parasites made, and
> 3. a lumbar puncture done, and
> 4. blood sugar (glucose) measurement done (see below).

The loss of consciousness from cerebral malaria may last for some days. Even after this, the patient may still make a full recovery. Some patients, however, will have permanent brain damage.

3. Hypoglycaemia
The blood sugar or glucose may become low (less than 2.2 mmol/litre or less than 40 mg/100 ml) in acute malaria. This happens especially if the malaria is severe or if the patient is pregnant or a child, or if treatment is given with quinine.

The low blood glucose can cause loss of consciousness, fitting, permanent brain damage or death. Check blood sugar with the diabetes blood glucose test equipment each 2 hours if the patient is very ill and also at any time the patient gets worse.

4. Acute anaemia and hypoxia
Acute severe anaemia with hypoxia (symptoms and signs of a low oxygen level in the brain and the rest of the body) can occur in those who have a low haemoglobin level (usually below 5 g/dl) and who then develop an acute attack of malaria. More red blood cells are destroyed and the anaemia rapidly becomes worse. Poisons from the malaria parasites stop the body cells using what little oxygen is brought by the anaemic blood ('hypoxia' – little oxygen in the tissues'). Death can occur quickly from lack of oxygen in the brain and other tissues of the body.

> Any patient in a malarious area who is very pale and develops acute malaria needs urgent, preferably artemisinin, treatment for the malaria and possibly an urgent blood transfusion.

5. Gastrointestinal malaria
The patient with malaria may develop repeated vomiting, diarrhoea with large volumes of watery stools, or even rarely dysentery. This loss of fluid may lead to dehydration and death.

> Any patient in a malarious area who develops gastroenteritis or dysentery needs a smear for malaria parasites taken, an injection of an antimalarial drug, preferably artemisinin, as well as fluids orally or IV.

6. Shock ('algid malaria')
The patient with malaria may become shocked with a fast pulse and a low blood pressure. The skin may feel cold but the body temperature, if taken with the thermometer in the rectum, is usually high. This may occur with or without vomiting and diarrhoea.

7. Kidney failure
The urine volume in 24 hours is less than 400 ml even if shock, dehydration, etc. are correctly treated (see Chapter 26 pages 439, 447, 453).

8. Malarial haemoglobinuria ('blackwater fever')
Malarial haemoglobinuria is very rare. It can occur in persons who have recently moved into the malarious area or have come back to the area, or persons who have had irregular antimalarial drugs, especially quinine. It can, however, occur in persons without any of these. Due to an abnormal immune reaction, many red blood cells are haemolysed (i.e. broken open and destroyed). Haemoglobin from inside the broken red cells is then free in the blood. This haemoglobin is also passed in the urine, which becomes red or brown or black (see Chapter 26 page 454).

The patient may become very anaemic because the red cells are destroyed. Also, haemoglobin free in the blood (and not in the red blood cells) is very poisonous to the body and especially the kidney. The patient may become shocked and develop kidney failure (when he will pass only a very little urine which is red or brown and has a lot of protein in it). Unless he is given urgent treatment, he will die of the anaemia, the shock or later the kidney failure.

9. Pulmonary oedema
The breathing rate is usually raised in malaria. In severe cases there may be some respiratory distress. As well, a cough may occur and some crackles may be heard in the chest due to fluid from inside the blood vessels

leaking through damaged blood vessels into the alveoli (pulmonary oedema). Make sure you are not giving too much IV fluid and causing heart failure (see Chapter 27 page 461) or the patient does not have pneumonia.

Never assume that lung symptoms are due to malaria alone. Always, also (1) treat them as due to bacterial infection and give antibiotic as well as antimalarial drugs and (2) check for heart failure.

---

10. Acidosis

Acidosis is when too much lactic acid collects in the body and blood. The body cells normally use oxygen and break down glucose to get energy. The glucose is first broken down to lactic acid; and then later to carbon dioxide. The malaria parasites can stop the cells getting enough oxygen to break down the lactic acid and the amount of this builds up in the body and can cause death.

Acidosis cannot be diagnosed in a health centre. It can be suspected if the patient is sick and has deep but not rapid breathing and there is no other cause. Treatment is by treating the malaria and any dehydration, shock, low blood sugar, or hypoxia (low oxygen) by giving intranasal oxygen.

11. Abnormal bleeding

Bleeding for no obvious cause from the nose, gums, IV sites, urinary tract, etc. can come if the malaria parasites make the body use up the blood clotting proteins inside the blood vessels. It is uncommon but does occur in malaria.

12. Complicating bacterial infections

Malaria makes it more likely for the patient to develop infection. Especially common are:
1. pneumonia,
2. urinary tract infections (especially if a urinary catheter has been used),
3. salmonella and other bowel organisms in the blood.

13. Hyperparasitaemia

If the percentage of red blood cells with malaria parasites is 5% or more in a person without semi-immunity, or more than 20% in any person anywhere, even if that person is not at that time sick, there are so many parasites that within hours the patient may get quickly worse and even die. Hyperparasitaemia is more dangerous if most of the parasites are not young and are *P. falciparum* (when most of the parasites may be in the deep organs and not in the peripheral blood).

Watch carefully for evidence of severe or complicated malaria in:

1. children from birth up to 6–10 years in age in areas where malaria is present all the time (area of stable malaria);
2. people of all ages in areas where malaria is not present all the time (area of unstable malaria);
3. travellers from areas of no or little malaria or residents who have been away for some years who come to a malaria area;
4. pregnant women (especially first pregnancy and the last 3 months of any pregnancy);
5. HIV infected people.

Chronic malaria

Chronic malaria occurs in persons from the time they are infected with malaria until the time they become semi-immune, i.e. until they develop enough immunity against malaria to overcome most of the malaria parasites and most of the effects of the malaria parasites, most of the time.

Development of semi-immunity may take 4–6 or even 10 years in areas where there is regular reinfection by *P. falciparum* (and other types of malaria), i.e. in areas of stable malaria. Development of semi-immunity to *P. falciparum* would not usually happen where there is not regular reinfection, i.e. in areas of unstable malaria. Semi-immunity could develop to other types of malaria in areas of unstable malaria because of regular infections from the hypnozoites in the liver, even if there is no regular infection from mosquitoes.

Semi-immunity is due to making effective antibodies against and cellular immunity against and developing 'tolerance' to (not being badly affected by) the parasite.

Some people never develop enough immunity and continue to have chronic malaria all their lives.

Symptoms and signs of chronic malaria include:

1. recurrent attacks of acute malaria,
2. anaemia,
3. enlarged spleen (often very enlarged),
4. enlarged liver,
5. poor appetite and other gastrointestinal symptoms and signs,
6. wasting of muscles (in comparison, abdomen often very enlarged due to large spleen and liver),
7. reduced resistance to other diseases, especially recurrent attacks of bacterial infections and gastroenteritis.

The above are especially severe in children and often lead to death.

If a person with no immunity to malaria but infected with malaria leaves and goes to an area where there is no malaria transmission, as long as he does not die from a complication of an attack, i.e. severe or complicated malaria (although this is likely with falciparum infections), the following happens. The patient has chronic malaria and repeated attacks, but eventually the parasite dies off and the patient is cured. This may happen (if he does not die) if infected with falciparum malaria in a year or so; if infected with only vivax or ovale malaria in 5 years or so; but if infected with malariae malaria at times not until after 30 years.

In falciparum and malariae infections, the attacks are caused by parasites in the blood and these could all be killed and the infection cured by proper treatment of the attack. In vivax and ovale infection, the attacks are caused not only by parasites in the blood but also by the hypnozoites in the liver; not only is treatment needed to kill all the parasites in the blood but also treatment is needed to kill the hypnozoites in the liver. Only then will the patient be cured.

Malaria in persons with immunity ('semi-immunes')

In areas of stable malaria these persons will be repeatedly reinfected. Because of their immunity, only the following occur:

1. Irregular short attacks of malaise, headaches, backaches, loss of appetite, fever and sweating occur.
2. Mild anaemia may be present all the time.

Malaria may, however, overcome this immunity in certain circumstances (see page 71).

If a previously semi-immune person develops a severe or complicated case of malaria, always think of the possibility that the patient has now been infected by HIV.

Late complications of malaria

After many years a few patients may develop the following:

1. hyperreactive malarious splenomegaly or tropical splenomegaly syndrome (see Chapter 21 page 319), or
2. nephrotic syndrome (see Chapter 26 page 447), or
3. Burkitt's lymphoma (see Chapter 22 page 338).

Tests

1. Make a blood smear for malaria parasites from all patients with fever or suspected malaria (see Appendix 1 page 90).

2. If the result of a blood smear cannot be available in 2 hours, if available use one of the Rapid Diagnostic Tests (RDTs; see Appendix 2 page 91).
3. Do a haemoglobin estimation on anyone who is pale (see Chapter 21 page 324).

Some further terms used about malaria

Clinical or parasitological diagnosis

A clinical diagnosis of malaria is made on history and examination.

If in an area where risk of malaria is high, there is
- fever in the last day,
- anaemia, especially if a child,
- no other cause obvious,
then malaria is likely but not certain.

If in an area where risk of malaria is low, there is
- history of possible mosquito bites in an area where malaria occurs,
- fever in the last 3 days,
- no other cause for the fever,
then malaria is likely but not certain.

A parasitological diagnosis is made from a blood smear or Rapid Diagnostic Test.

If a parasitological diagnosis is not available within 2 hours, it is not much help for patient treatment and the patient has to be treated on the clinical diagnosis only.

If in an area of stable malaria where risk of malaria is high, a parasitological diagnosis is not as important for children aged less than 5 years, as treatment for malaria is given to *all* children less than 5 with fever and no other cause likely.

A parasitological diagnosis is more important the older the patient is over 5 as, in semi-immunes, malaria is less likely to be the cause (see below), and

1. expensive malaria treatment should not be given if the patient does not have malaria;
2. if the patient does not have malaria, other causes of the illness should be looked for;
3. if the patient has HIV infection, it is even more important to look for the many other causes this patient could have for fever;
4. if the patient is pregnant it is not good to give a drug if not needed.

A parasitological diagnosis is important in an unstable malaria area where risk of malaria is low, as, if negative, other causes for fever need to be found.

In all non-immune adults who could have malaria, and in all suspected cases of severe or complicated malaria, a parasitological diagnosis is best. If, however, the result is not immediately available, start treatment for malaria immediately as patients can get worse and die in only a few hours.

Stable malaria

Stable malaria is said to exist where people are repeatedly infected with malaria by mosquitoes for at least 6 months of the year (usually more than 10 infections a year).

Such places are in Africa south of the Sahara and in many countries in the Pacific area.

The following would be expected.

1. Children after a few months in age get repeated attacks of acute malaria when the passive malaria immunity they got through their mother's placenta has gone, develop chronic malaria with anaemia, and many die of severe complicated malaria unless quick effective treatment of the attacks is given. If these children do not die, they slowly develop semi-immunity to malaria by the age of 4–6 (but sometimes up to 10) years. Before this, most of the children would have enlarged spleens ('spleen rate' 75% or more) and most of the children would have malaria parasites in their blood ('parasite rate' 90% or more). The 'mortality rate' is high.
2. Older children and adults who are semi-immune may still have malaria parasites in their blood and may still get occasional acute attacks of malaria, but these attacks are mild and are rarely complicated or severe. Attacks may be more common when infections increase, such as when the wet season starts (when many children are severely affected). Semi-immune adults would have a low 'spleen rate' and low 'parasite rate' and a low 'mortality rate', although these could increase when malaria infections increase.
3. Pregnant women, especially in the first pregnancy, and people who become infected with HIV and people whose immunity is decreased by drugs or removal of the spleen or severe illness, can all develop severe malaria, even when previously semi-immune. The pregnant woman is likely to have a miscarriage, stillbirth, premature labour, a child of low birthweight (as the placenta is affected) and the child is more likely to die than normally.
4. People who have been away from the area for years and have lost some of their immunity and who then return can get repeated acute attacks.

5. Visitors, or even whole populations in times of war or famine, etc. who come to an area of stable malaria from areas where there is no stable malaria and who are therefore not semi-immune, will get acute malaria, chronic malaria and severe complicated malaria and take 4–6 years to develop reasonable semi-immunity. Meanwhile, many will die unless effective treatment of acute attacks is given.

Unstable malaria

Unstable malaria is said to exist in areas where people are not repeatedly infected with malaria for most of the year, but only in a certain (usually wet) season when mosquito numbers greatly increase (and this can change from year to year). Such places are Asia, Latin America, etc.

Infections are not frequent enough for the population to develop significant immunity.

When mosquito numbers do increase, there is a sudden increase in malaria in people of all ages. Complicated or severe malaria and death can occur in people of all ages unless quick effective treatment is given.

In these areas the 'spleen rate' and 'parasite rate' is low in times of low transmission and high in times of high transmission. The 'mortality rate' can be high in all ages when transmission rate rises.

Malaria epidemics

A sudden large increase in malaria attacks in large numbers of the population can occur any time mosquitoes increase in areas of unstable malaria, or if people who are not semi-immune go to areas of stable malaria transmission.

Diagnostic features

1. Fever (*all* patients with fever who could have malaria must be treated with antimalarials unless there is evidence that they do not have malaria and they do have another cause for the fever).
2. Anaemia (*all* patients who could have been infected with malaria and have anaemia must be treated with antimalarials unless it can be proved that they do not have malaria).
3. Splenomegaly (in non-immunes).
4. Positive blood smear or RDT.
5. No other cause found on history and examination for illness.

Management
Management of a patient with malaria

Management may include five things:

1. Give **two** antimalarial drugs.

   If usual case where P. falciparum *possible:*
   - artemisinin drug for 3 days and long acting companion drug orally, or
   - artemisinin drug and short acting companion drug both for 7 days orally.

   If unconscious or fitting or vomiting or diarrhoea or shock, use, in order of preference:
   - IVI artemisinin drug, or
   - IV infusion quinine (double the first dose), or
   - IMI artemisinin drug (unless shock, when IV treatment essential), or
   - IMI quinine (double the first dose), or
   - rectal artemisinin drug, or
   - rectal quinine, or
   - nasogastric artemisinin drug, or
   - nasogastric quinine, **and also**
   - companion antimalarial drug (see page 80).

   If pregnant see pages 80, 81, 86.

   If HIV infection see page 86.

   If case where P. falciparum *does not occur see page 80 and page 83.*

   If treatment does not cure the patient see page 85 and page 86.
2. Treat symptoms (see page 81).
3. Treat complications (see page 81).
4. Give primaquine in special areas (if the Health Department tells you to) (see page 84).
5. Give drugs for prophylaxis only if needed (see page 88).

Resistance of malaria parasites to antimalarial drugs

It is important that we do have effective drugs which kill malaria parasites. When all the parasites are gone the patient should get better (as long as damage has not already been done from which he cannot recover). There have been many, and still are a number of drugs which do kill malaria parasites well. However, by 2006, *P. falciparum* had developed at least some resistance in some areas to all drugs which used to kill them except drugs of the artemisinin group. *Plasmodium vivax* had developed resistance to sulfadoxine and pyrimethamine in many areas and to chloroquine in Indonesia, Papua New Guinea and other islands in the Pacific and Peru. *Plasmodium malariae* may have developed resistance to chloroquine in Indonesia.

It is important we stop the resistance developing as quickly as it is now doing or we will soon have no effective drugs left to cure malaria.

It is important that when we do give drugs to treat malaria that we do kill ALL the malaria parasites in the patient's body for the following two reasons.

1. *Drugs to which the malaria parasites are only partly sensitive may help a person who is semi-immune quickly recover from an attack of malaria (as his own immunity can overcome the fewer number of malaria parasites left after the drug has killed many parasites – even though there are still some left). If such drugs, however, are given to a patient (and especially a child) who is not immune, the patient may not be able to overcome even the fewer number of malaria parasites left after the drug has killed many, and would probably remain chronically unwell or possibly die.*

2. *If a patient is given drugs which do not kill all the malaria parasites in the body, the remaining parasites which stay alive are those which probably already have some resistance to the drug. This further exposure to drug treatment will allow these partly resistant parasites to 'learn' how to resist the drug even better and become more, and possibly fully, resistant. Drug treatments which do not kill all the parasites, lead to drug resistance.*

We must have and use drugs to which the malaria parasites are not even partly resistant but are fully sensitive.

It is now thought that the way to stop the malaria parasites becoming resistant to what effective drugs we have left (especially the artemisinin group) and to any new drugs that are discovered, is to use antimalarial drugs in combinations of two (or more) together; just as more than one drug is always used for treatment of TB, HIV infection, leprosy, etc. In all populations of organisms, although almost all may be killed by a certain drug, some in that population will be resistant to that drug but will not be likely to be resistant to another drug which works in a different way. If just one drug is given, all the sensitive organisms will be killed, but the resistant ones will grow and cause another infection which cannot be treated with that first drug. This infection will then be passed to others who cannot be treated with that first drug.

If, however, two drugs which work in different ways are used together from the start, all the organisms should be killed and resistant infections will not occur. Of course, malaria parasites are able to change themselves to become resistant to a drug, but it is much harder for them to do this when two (or more) drugs are used at the same time. From now on we should ALWAYS TREAT MALARIA WITH TWO DRUGS at the same time AND THESE DRUGS MUST WORK IN DIFFERENT WAYS (it is no good giving two drugs which work in the same way). Some antimalarial treatments do contain more than one drug, but each drug damages the same process of the malaria parasite. These two drugs which work in one way are considered as only one drug treatment, e.g.

- sulfadoxine-pyrimethamine
- proquanil-dapsone
- atovaquone-proguanil.

Also, drugs such as chlorphenamine, which make some antimalarial drugs more effective, are not able to be used as a second drug.

If we always use two antimalarial drugs as above, we will continue to have drugs which will kill malaria parasites. Otherwise, we may find we cannot treat malaria.

Resistance of the malaria parasites to the drug is shown by doing blood smears from the day the patient is given the treatment at regular intervals for *at least* 28 days. Special tests may be needed after 2 weeks to tell if any parasites seen are from a new infection or from the original malaria organism treated. No parasites of the original infection treated should be seen again after they disappear from the slides after the first few days. In the past, we used to define parasites according to the different amount of resistance they had to the drug (e.g. R1, R2, R3). Now we know any resistance is dangerous. The parasite will become more resistant if treated with that drug again. We should kill all malaria parasites when we give treatment so none can survive and become resistant.

For any single drug to be suitable for use in a two-drug combination, at least 95% of the tests should show it killed all the parasites (although in some countries a 90% or even 80% cure is accepted).

If a patient has drug resistant malaria organisms:

- treatment of an acute attack may not be successful (and the patient could die);
- chronic malaria, especially anaemia, is more likely if the patient survives and the patient's malaria is not cured;
- use of one drug to which the malaria is resistant together with another drug to which the malaria is sensitive, will result in the malaria becoming resistant to the second drug. *Two effective drugs need to be given together to stop malaria becoming resistant to drugs.*

Artemisinin-based combination therapy (ACT) is now considered by the World Health Organiza-tion to be the correct treatment in all places, but especially where falciparum malaria occurs. All countries have or will soon include this in their national malaria programme. In the meantime, you will need to follow what your national malaria programme tells you to do and use the drugs that are supplied to you.

The reason an artemisinin drug is in every combination is that it is the only safe drug at present available to which there probably are (at the time of writing) no known resistant malaria parasites.

The artemisinin family at present includes:

- artemisinin itself (which is less active than the others);
- dehydroartemisinin (the active drug into which all except artemisinin are changed in the body);
- artemether (has been made into an easy-to-use IMI and into a combined tablet with lumefantrine);
- artesunate (very effective except that the injection is difficult to make up);
- artemotil (not used much);
- others, yet to be developed or proven to be safe and effective.

These drugs have been prepared in different ways, but not all drugs are available for administration in all ways. There are preparations for IVI, IMI, oral and rectal (suppository) use. See Appendix 3 pages 98–99 for details of those at present available.

You will need to get to know those your Health Department chooses for you to use (which, if used correctly, should be as good as the ones discussed below). If you do not have the drugs recommended as follows in the book, see Appendix 3 to see what alternative member of the artemisinin family you have which you could use.

See Appendix 3 pages 98–99 for details of how these drugs work and other very important things to understand about them.

A companion drug has always to be given with the artemisinin drug so that the malaria parasite is treated with at least two drugs, i.e. artemisinin-based combination therapy (ACT) so that all the malaria parasites are destroyed and resistant parasites cannot develop.

An artemisinin drug can be *given for only 3 days **only** if* a long acting companion drug is given with it, e.g.:

- lumefantrine,
- mefloquine, but possibly not suitable for children in parts of Africa,
- sulfadoxine with pyrimethamine, but only in the few areas where the malaria parasites are still sensitive,

- amodiaquine, but only in the few areas where the malaria parasites are still sensitive,
- others, see Appendix 3 page 100.

The companion drug may need to be given for 1–3 days.

An artemisinin drug will need to be *given for 7 days* **only** *if* a short acting companion drug is given with it, e.g.:
- doxycycline,
- tetracycline,
- clindamycin.

The companion drug will also need to be given for 7 days.

When tablets or capsules with both drugs in the same tablet or capsule (called co-formulations) are available, always use these combination preparations (then it is not possible for single drug and not combination drug therapy to be given). At the time of writing, the only one commonly available is artemether (20 mg) + lumefantrine (120 mg) in one tablet. However, others are being made, including artesunate + mefloquine (50 mg + 150 mg and 50 mg + 250 mg) tablets; and artesunate + amodiaquine (50 mg + 150 mg and 50 mg + 250 mg). Write which of these and their doses and any new co-formulations and their doses into the book when they become available to you.

Patients who have acute malaria, especially children and non-immune adults, can become very quickly worse and develop severe or complicated malaria within a few hours. These patients need immediate treatment. This means they need treatment in the village or near where they live. Some government Health Departments have set up treatment centres where oral drugs or, if the patient is vomiting, IM injections or suppositories, can be given by a specially trained person who lives in that place (who need not be a health worker). This saves many lives and prevents much sickness. It is absolutely essential that these patients get the whole 3 or 7 day course of treatment even if they get better very quickly and long before the treatment ends. It is essential that they get a two-drug treatment. Otherwise, not only may the malaria return, the malaria parasites may become resistant to the drugs. This is of particular importance if one of the artemisinin group of drugs is used.

Drugs which may be supplied for this pre-referral treatment of severe malaria include:
- artesunate or artemether for IMI;
- quinine for IMI;
- artesunate or artemisinin suppositories for rectal treatment;
- quinine for rectal retention enema,

but a companion drug is also needed.

Note on management of malaria

All patients with a fever who are in or who are from areas where malaria occurs are assumed to have malaria unless it can be proved otherwise. *But always look for other causes,* especially severe infections. Always do a full history and examination and test the urine.

Even if there appears to be another cause of fever, *treat all such patients with a fever with a full treatment course of antimalarials unless it can be proved that they do not have malaria.* Treat any other cause as well.

Admit if a severe attack or a complication.

Treat as outpatient if a mild attack.

However, if the patient is in the group likely to get a complication, admit if possible for at least the first day of treatment.

Give antimalarial drugs
Usual attack if P. falciparum *possible, but:*
No vomiting. No diarrhoea.
Not in the first 14 weeks of pregnancy

Best treatment is:
artemisinin drug orally for 3 days AND ALSO
long acting companion drug orally (usually for 3 days).
Use both drugs in one co-formulated tablet or capsule
or blister pack if available.

Give artemether 20 mg + lumefantine 120 mg tablets:
　4 tablets if weight > 34 kg each dose
　3 tablets if weight < 34 kg each dose
　first dose immediately
　one dose twice daily for 3 days but the second dose on Day 1 after 8 (not 12) hours if possible.

OR

Give artesunate 4 mg/kg each dose:
　first dose immediately, then
　one dose daily on Days 2 and 3
AND ALSO
mefloquine; but only if recommended in your area:
　none immediately
　first dose 15 mg/kg on Day 2
　second dose 10 mg/kg on Day 3
　if not in co-formulation tablet or blister pack with artesunate
　or
　8 mg/kg each dose
　first dose immediately, then
　one dose daily on Day or Days 2 and 3
　this is the dose in some blister packs and co-formulation tablets with artesunate (in which 8 mg of mefloquine to each 4 mg of artesunate).

OR

Give any artemisinin drug in its dose for 3 days
and also

any long acting companion drug but only if it is also
effective,

e.g. lumefantrine

e.g. mefloquine (only if recommended in your area)

e.g. amodiaquine; but only if cure rate for amodiaquine alone is greater than (80–)90% (see page
79)

e.g. sulfadoxine/pyrimethamine; but only if cure
rate for sulfadoxine/pyrimethamine alone is
greater than (80–)90% (see page 78).

Other very effective treatment is:
artemisinin drug orally for 7 days AND ALSO
short acting companion drug orally for 7 days.
Use both drugs in one co-formulated tablet or capsule
or blister pack if available.

Give artesunate 4 mg/kg orally immediately, then
(2–)4 mg orally daily for 6 more days
OR
Any other artemisinin drug in its proper dose immediately and for 6 more days
AND ALSO
doxycycline 3.5 mg/kg daily;
usually 100–200 mg
daily for 7 days

} but not if pregnant or a child

or
tetracycline 4 mg/kg; usually
250 mg/qid for 7 days
OR
clindamycin 40 mg/kg/day; usually 150 mg qid or
300 mg bd for 7 days (e.g. if pregnant)
OR
other effective drug.

After any artemisinin drugs are given, as long as no vomiting
occurs, give milk or fatty food to increase the absorption of
the drug.

Treatment which is not recommended unless the malaria
parasites are (80–)90% sensitive to both amodiaquine
and to sulfadoxine-pyrimethamine would be:
amodiaquine for 3 days (see page 85) and also
sulfadoxine-pyrimethamine one dose (see page 97).

Usual attack as above, but: In first 14 weeks of pregnancy

Use alternative drug to artemisinin if available; but if
not available use artemisinin drug.

Use alternative long acting companion drug to
lumefantrine if available, e.g. amodiaquine or sul-

fadoxine + pyrimethamine but only if (80–)90% of
malaria parasites sensitive to any of these.

Use alternative short acting companion drug to
doxycycline or tetracycline, e.g. clindamycin 150 mg
qid for 7 days.

After 14 weeks of pregnancy, use usual drugs except
not doxycycline or tetracycline.

Usual attack in area where P. falciparum malaria does not occur (i.e. only P. vivax, malariae or ovale area)

Give artemisinin drug for 3 days (as above),
BUT ALSO
If (80–)90% of malaria parasites are sensitive:
Give amodiaquine 10 mg/kg base each dose
small adult 450 mg
large adult 600 mg
immediately and for 2 more days
OR
Give chloroquine in the same dose.

See page 84 about primaquine.

Severe or complicated malaria

Immediate treatment is needed. Give whatever you can
give the most quickly.
Give immediately artemisinin drug by IVI or IMI;
or if not available:
Give quinine by IV infusion or IMI
AND ALSO
Give, as soon as improves, a companion drug.

Give artesunate 2.4 mg/kg by IVI immediately; but if
unable to do so, give by IMI, then
1.2 mg/kg by IVI or IMI after 12 hours then
(1.2–)2.4 mg/kg daily to complete 7 days of treatment or until can take oral artemisinin drug.
OR
Give artemether by IMI (not IVI) 3.2 mg/kg immediately, then 1.6 mg/kg daily for 7 days or until can
take oral artemisinin drug.
OR
Give other artemisinin drug by IVI or IMI.
OR
If artemisinin drug not available:
Give quinine *not by* IVI but by
• controlled rate IV infusion in 5% dextrose at
5 mg/kg/hour (see Appendix 3 page 94), or by
• IMI.
First dose only:
• 20 mg base/kg (i.e. double dose).

- If unable to weigh patient:
  small adult – 800 mg
  large adult – 1200 mg.

All doses after first dose:

- 10 mg base/kg each 8 hours until the patient can take oral quinine to complete 7 days.
- If unable to weigh patient:
  small adult – 400 mg
  large adult – 600 mg.

If injection not possible, use rectal treatment.

Give artesunate 10 mg/kg/dose or artemisinin 40 mg/ kg/dose immediately rectally by suppository, then

Give artesunate 10 mg/kg/day or artemisinin 20 mg/ kg/day once each day until can take orally.

OR

Give other artemisinin rectally administered drug.

OR

Give quinine (but only if artemisinin drug not available), preferably quinine gluconate:

20 mg/kg first dose, then

10 mg/kg each 8 hours until can take oral quinine.

If rectal drug is expelled within 15–30 minutes, repeat the same dose of the drug and strap the buttocks together.

If injections and rectal treatment not available or possible, give oral drugs (see page 79) crushed and through nasogastric tube; but only if IVI or IMI or rectal drug treatment not possible.

Give first IMI or through the nasogastric tube
metoclopramide 10 mg
or if not available and not shocked chlorpromazine 0.25 mg/kg (maximum 12.5 mg).

After the drugs are given, and after ensuring no vomiting likely, give milk or fatty food through the tube to increase absorption of artemisinin drugs.

If liver disease or kidney failure is present (especially if urine volume less than 400 ml in 24 hours if well hydrated) or if patient does not improve after 1–2 days (as the liver and kidneys would then not be working properly), reduce the dose of quinine to two-thirds or 66% of its usual dose, but do not reduce the dose of the artemisinin drug.

Once the patient has improved and can swallow and does not have vomiting or diarrhoea, do the following.

1. Change IV or IM or rectal drugs to oral drugs and finish 7 days of treatment. Remember to

give artemisinin drugs with milk or some fatty food.

2. Start doxycycline 100 mg daily which needs to be continued for 7 days (i.e. it will finish after the artemisinin drug or quinine) unless the patient is pregnant, or a child, when give clindamycin 125 mg qid for 7 days;
   or if neither of these are possible:
   Give the full oral course for 3 days of artemether and lumefantine or other oral combination used for acute malaria, except avoid mefloquine if possible if the patient had cerebral malaria or fitting. (see Appendix 3 page 95).

3. Also, if it is the policy to do so, start primaquine.

Treat the symptoms

New research suggests blood platelets may help kill malaria parasites. It may be best not to give acetyl-salicyclic acid to malaria patients as this drug stops platelets working properly.

- Rest
- Pain – paracetamol 500–1000 mg 4 hour orally or rectally by suppository if vomiting; no more than 4 g in any 24 hours.
- Fever – paracetamol as above. Sponge or wrap in wet sheet and fan.
- Vomiting many times – metoclopramide 10 mg IVI or IMI 4 hourly. If no metoclopramide, chlorpromazine 0.25 mg/kg IMI once maximum 12.5 mg, but do not give if systolic blood pressure < 80.

Treat any complications

1. Very high fever

Give *immediately* artemisinin drug or quinine (by IVI or IMI if temperature above 40°C).

Up to 40°C:

- Paracetamol 500–1000 mg as above.
- Sponge or wrap in wet sheet and fan.

Above 40°C:

- Emergency treatment needed.
- Paracetamol as above.
- Wrap in a wet sheet; repeatedly wet the sheet and fan vigorously.
- IMI chlorpromazine 0.25 mg/kg (maximum 12.5 mg).
- Watch carefully for shock and treat if it occurs (see Chapter 27 pages 468–469).
- When improved, temperature falls and treatment stopped, still watch carefully for rise in temperature again which needs the same treatment again.

- Give IVI or IMI, not oral, artemisinin (or quinine) antimalarial drug (see page 80 and see page 81).

2. Cerebral malaria (see also Chapter 25 page 413)

Give immediately by IVI or IMI artemisinin drug (or quinine) and see page 80.

Also *immediately* do blood glucose test. If glucose less than 2.2 mmol/litre or 40 mg/dl or if test not available, give 1 ml/kg of 50% dextrose or glucose by IVI. Repeat blood glucose test each hour.

Also *immediately,* if temperature above 39°C, give paracetamol suppository 500–1000 mg and see page 81.

Also *immediately,* if available, give oxygen 2 litres/minute by nasal prongs.

Also *immediately,* if convulsions,
give diazepam IVI 5–10 mg slowly over 5–10 minutes or 0.5 mg/kg rectally (maximum 20 mg), or
give paraldehyde 5–10 ml by deep IMI, but must use only glass syringe.
(Then see Chapter 25 pages 424–426.)

Do lumbar puncture *always.*

Treat for meningitis also if CSF is not clear or is bloody or rapid diagnostic tests are suggestive of meningitis or is not obtained (failed LP) (see Chapter 25 pages 409–413).

Care of unconscious patient (see Chapter 25 pages 422–424).

If not improved in 24 hours do a repeat lumbar puncture. If CSF still clear, continue treatment. If CSF not clear, or rapid diagnostic tests suggest meningitis, or is bloody or is not obtained (failed LP) treat for meningitis also.

When unconsciousness lasts more than 24 hours and the patient is not improving, transfer to Medical Officer care.

3. Hypoglycaemia (low blood glucose)

Emergency treatment is needed.

Treat if present or suspected. Give oral sugar or jam or honey 20 g (20 ml or 1 tablespoonful), etc. if able to swallow; or IVI 50 ml of 50% dextrose or glucose if unable to swallow.

Recheck the blood glucose each hour and give glucose if needed until the blood glucose and the patient improves. (Very important if the patient is pregnant or being treated with quinine.)

4. Acute severe anaemia

Give immediately injection of artemisinin (or quinine) antimalarial drug (see page 80).

Also immediately, if available, give oxygen 2 litres/minute by nasal prongs.

Transfer urgently (emergency) for blood transfusion if Hb less than 5 g/dl and malaria (fever).

Give IV or IM antimalarials first if vomiting of oral antimalarial drugs may occur during transfer.

5. Gastroenteritis or dysentery

Give oral or IV fluids for dehydration (see Chapter 23 pages 364, 366).

Give IV or IM artemisinin group antimalarial drug (see page 80).

6. Shock

Give IV artemisinin antimalarial drug (see page 80).

Give IV fluids for shock (see Chapter 27 page 468).

Start IV antibiotics for septicaemia if suspect infection (see Chapter 12 page 65).

7. Acute kidney failure

Give IVI or IMI artemisinin group antimalarial drug rather than quinine (see page 80).

Look carefully for dehydration or shock. If present, treat with IV fluids (see Chapter 27 page 468).

If still no increase in urine output and especially if signs of heart failure develop:
1. reduce total of all IV fluids to 500 ml of 5% dextrose in 24 hours,
2. try a dose of diuretic, e.g. frusemide 80 mg preferably IVI.

If still no increase in urine output see Chapter 26 pages 447 and 453 and transfer urgently (emergency) to Medical Officer care.

8. Haemoglobinuria (blackwater fever)

Do *not* give quinine. Give instead IV or IM or rectal artemisinin antimalarial drug (see page 80).

Start immediately treatment for shock or acute kidney failure if present (see Chapter 27 page 468 and see 7 above).

Transfer urgently (emergency) to Medical Officer care.

9. Pulmonary oedema

Give IVI or IMI artemisinin group antimalarial drug rather than quinine (see page 80).

Prop up (e.g. on pillows) at 45 degrees (45°) from the waist up.

Give oxygen if available at 2 litres/minute by nasal prongs.

Stop IV fluids except essential drugs in no more than 500 ml 5% dextrose in 24 hours.

Give a diuretic, e.g. frusemide 40–80 mg preferably IVI.

Treat as for heart failure (see Chapter 27 pages 464–466).

If suspect infection, start treatment for septicaemia (see Chapter 12 page 64).

Transfer urgently to Medical Officer if does not improve.

10. Acidosis

Give IV or IM artemisinin group antimalarials rather than quinine (see page 80).

Give oxygen at least 2 litres/minute by nasal prongs.

Give IV glucose if blood glucose low or cannot measure blood glucose (see page 82).

Treat dehydration or shock if present (see Chapter 27 page 468).

Transfer for blood transfusion if very anaemic and Hb less than 5 g/dl.

11. Abnormal bleeding

Treat with IV artemisinin antimalarial drug rather than quinine (see page 80).

Give vitamin K 2.5–25 mg if available.

Transfer urgently (emergency) to Medical Officer for transfusion with fresh whole blood or other blood product.

12. Complicating bacterial infection

Look carefully for and treat if present;

• pneumonia,
• meningitis,
• septicaemia.

Bacterial infection is even more likely if the patient also has HIV infection.

If the patient on correct malaria treatment is getting worse for no other reason, start treatment with antibiotics as in Chapter 12 page 65.

13. Hyperparasitaemia

Treat urgently with an IV (or IM) artemisinin drug (or quinine) and companion drug and observe the patient for 48 hours for other complications needing treatment. Especially, if the parasite rate is 20% or higher, do not just give oral drugs and allow the patient to go home.

If a patient on correct treatment for severe or complicated malaria gets worse always check for and treat:

1. low blood sugar;
2. infection/septicaemia;
3. fitting which has not been noticed and needs very careful examination to be seen;
4. too little IV fluid and dehydration;
5. too much IV fluid and pulmonary oedema;
6. hyperpyrexia (measure rectal temperature).

Treatment of malaria where *P. falciparum* is not present (i.e. caused only by *P. vivax*, *P. ovale* or *P. malariae*)

In some areas, transmission rates are low, there is unstable malaria, and the malaria there is caused by one of the above, especially *P. vivax*. If you are in one of these areas, you will have been told this by your Health Department.

In these areas of unstable malaria, although transmission of infection from mosquitoes can occur for only part of the year, attacks can occur at other times of the year. These attacks are due to previous infections which were not treated until all the parasites were gone, or drugs were not given to kill the hypnozoites of *P. vivax* and *P. ovale* (which from time to time release merozoites from the liver into the blood to start a new infection in the red blood cells).

Attacks from these parasites (i.e. other than *P. falciparum*) do not often cause severe or complicated malaria (although they occasionally can); but they do cause acute attacks, anaemia, low birthweight babies and general poor health in children and adults.

People living in areas of unstable malaria do not develop semi-immunity to malaria as people in areas of stable malaria do; and people of all ages are at risk.

Resistance of *P. vivax* and *P. malariae* parasites to antimalarials occurs, but is much less a problem than with *P. falciparum*.

*Sulfadoxine with pyrimethamine, however, is **not** effective in many areas.*

Chloroquine is effective in many but not all areas – especially not in Oceania, Indonesia and Peru. If the malaria is sensitive to it, chloroquine is the drug of first choice.

Amodiaquine is effective in most areas and is the drug of second choice.

Artemisinin drugs, mefloquine and quinine are all effective.

A second or companion drug is, however, needed to go with chloroquine, amodiaquine, artemisinin or any other drug to stop resistance developing.

A drug is also needed to be given with the treatment to kill the hypnozoites in the liver to stop relapses (or the malaria coming back again) even if all the merozoites in the blood have been killed.

Primaquine

Primaquine is a drug which can be a companion drug AND is a drug to stop relapses as it kills:

1. merozoites of *P. vivax* but not *P. falciparum* (although not as effectively as the artemisinin drugs);
2. hypnozoites of *P. vivax* and *P. ovale* (*P. falciparum* and *P. malariae* do not have hypnozoites).

For details of primaquine see below and Appendix 3 page 96.

Alternative companion drugs which help stop development of resistance (but which do not stop relapses as they do not kill hypnozoites) (if primaquine is not used) include artemisinin drugs and doxycycline/tetracycline and clindamycin; however, not usually sulfadoxine + pyrimethamine (as resistance already exists or is likely).

Primaquine is not normally given if reinfection is very common, as in stable malaria areas; semi-immunity normally develops.

Primaquine, however, in low transmission areas of unstable malaria, may allow people to be well for long periods without recurrent attacks when transmission of malaria is not occurring. This would be of particular benefit to patients such as children under 5, pregnant women, HIV infected persons, etc.

Primaquine can cause haemolysis (breaking down of the red cells in the blood), mainly in people with a condition called glucose 6 phosphate dehydrogenase deficiency (usually called G6PD). In areas where G6PD is common, primaquine causes less trouble if given in half the usual dose but for twice the usual length of time (the total dose of primaquine is not reduced). If severe G6PD is present in a patient or is common in a population, then primaquine cannot be used.

Primaquine can cause abdominal discomfort. Give it with food to try to stop this.

Primaquine kills merozoites of *P. vivax* (but not *P. falciparum*) and by giving it with the usual full dose of treatment for *P. vivax*, two drugs are being used; this helps to prevent resistance to the drugs developing.

Primaquine is used together with a full treatment course of drugs for 'radical cure', i.e. getting rid of all of the malaria parasites from the body if the patient has left the area where malaria occurs.

The dose of primaquine is as follows.

1. Usual cases: 0.25 mg base/kg/day (usually 15 mg daily for adults)
   for 14 days (shorter courses are not effective).
2. In SE Asia, Indonesia and Oceania (where the Chesson strain of *P. vivax* is more resistant):
   0.5 mg base/kg/day (usually 30 mg daily for adults) for 14 days.
3. In areas where G6PD deficiency is common:
   0.75 mg base/kg on one day each week (usually 45 mg for adults weekly) (**not each day**) for 8 weeks.
4. If G6PD deficiency is common and severe in a population, primaquine cannot be used.

Choice of drug treatment for *P. vivax*, *P. ovale* or *P. malariae*

1. In an area of chloroquine sensitive malaria see below.
2. In an area of chloroquine resistant but amodiaquine sensitive malaria see page 85.
3. In an area of chloroquine and amodiaquine resistance see pages 85 and 79.
4. If severe complicated attack see page 85 and page 80.
5. If the patient is not cured by the above or is very sick see pages 85 and 80.

1. Chloroquine for usual attack in chloroquine sensitive area

No vomiting. No diarrhoea:
Give oral chloroquine

- Give 10 mg/kg of the base immediately;
      if cannot weigh patient
      small adult (< 50 kg) – 400 mg
      large adult (> 50 kg) – 600 mg.
- Give 5 mg/kg of the base 6 hours later;
      if cannot weigh patient
      small adult (< 50 kg) – 200 mg
      large adult (> 50 kg) – 300 mg.
- Give 5 mg/kg the following day – see above.
- Give 5 mg/kg the following day – see above.
- Give therefore 25 mg/kg over 3 days.

If the patient immediately vomits the tablets, give the same dose again; but do not repeat the dose if the patient vomits more than $\frac{1}{4}$ of an hour later; but if nausea still present when the next dose is due, start with the first dose of IM chloroquine.

In some health centre areas the dose of chloroquine as above may be too complicated for your staff and your patients to remember. A very simple dose (Table 13.1) was used for many years in Papua New Guinea and has been effective and safe and easy for staff and patients (although the dose is 30 mg/kg over 3 days).

Table 13.1 Simplified chloroquine dosage.

Using 150 mg base/tablet

Size of adult	Dose on Day 1	Dose on Day 2	Dose on Day 3
Small (less than 50 kg)	3 tablets	3 tablets	3 tablets
Large (more than 50 kg)	4 tablets	4 tablets	4 tablets

You, however, will have to follow the rules laid down by the Health Department where you work. Start also oral primaquine.

Vomiting or diarrhoea:
Give IM chloroquine.

> When possible use oral instead of IM chloroquine.
> Do not give both oral and IM chloroquine at the same time to a patient.
> If the patient is very ill it is safer to give an IV or IM artemisinin drug.

Give 3.5 mg chloroquine base/kg patient's body weight (maximum dose 200 mg) each dose.

The dose, if you cannot weigh the patient, is:
• small adult (< 50 kg) – 150 mg
• large adult (> 50 kg) – 200 mg.

After 6 hours if the patient cannot take oral chloroquine, repeat the *same* dose of IM chloroquine. However, if the patient can take oral drugs, give the first dose of the three daily doses of chloroquine tablets instead (see above).

If the patient still cannot take oral chloroquine, then, instead of the once daily dose of tablets, give IM chloroquine each 6 hours. Use the *same* IM dose (see above). As soon as possible change to oral chloroquine.

Stop chloroquine after a total of 25 mg/kg of treatment, i.e. after 7th dose or after 36 hours.

If the chloroquine has to be given by injection, it would be better to give an artemisinin drug or quinine instead to most patients who are this sick.

As soon as the patient can swallow and has no diarrhoea or vomiting and is not shocked, change to oral chloroquine. Oral chloroquine is just as effective and is safer and easier than injection.

Give also primaquine or alternative companion drug see page 84 and page 80.

Amodiaquine treatment in a chloroquine resistant but amodiaquine sensitive area

Give amodiaquine 10 mg base/kg daily for 3 days.

If using the 153 mg base tablets the dose will be the same as for chloroquine 150 mg base tablets (Table 13.1); but if using the 200 mg base tablets the number of tablets is different – 3 (instead of 4) and 2 (instead of 3). See also Appendix 3 page 93.

No injectable amodiaquine is available.

If vomiting means oral amodiaquine cannot be used, then use an IM or IV artemisinin drug.

Give also primaquine or alternative companion drug see page 84 and page 80.

Drugs if chloroquine and amodiaquine resistance

Treat as for *P. falciparum* (see page 79) unless other drugs have been supplied to you.

Drug treatment if patient is not cured by this course or is very sick

Treat as for severe complicated malaria due to *P. falciparum* (see page 80).

Give also primaquine (if it is Health Department policy).

If antimalaria treatment does not cure patient or there is deterioration within a month

Causes include the following.

1. The diagnosis was wrong – malaria was not the cause of the patient's illness (even if malaria parasites were in his blood). Look for all other possible causes.
2. The dose of the antimalaria drugs was incorrect. Check the dose.
3. The patient did not take the full 3 or 7 day treatment. Find out if possible from others (as well as the patient) what the patient took.
4. The patient did not absorb the drugs as he had vomiting or diarrhoea or did not take artemisinin drugs with milk or fatty food. Find out about this.
5. The drugs given were poorly made or stored and therefore not effective. They may even have been counterfeit or 'fake' drugs. Check this and discuss the matter with your Medical Officer.
6. The malaria parasite is resistant to the drugs given.
7. The patient has a new malarial infection (he could get sick from a new infection after only 2 weeks).

Unless you find a cause for the patient's illness, transfer the patient to the Medical Officer for help.

If transfer is not possible and the patient is not very sick:

1. Give the full treatment again, watching to make sure the patient swallows every dose of every drug.
2. Do thick and thin blood smears before starting treatment and each 2(–3) days for 28 days, saving them to be sent for examination in the laboratory and the results to come back to you.
3. If the patient remains well and no parasites are seen in blood smears after the first and second lot of blood slides, the patient is cured and no further action is needed.
4. If the patient is not well or the blood slides are positive after the first or second lot of tests, it is essential to send the patient and the results to the Medical Officer, as the patient seems to have drug resistant malaria.
5. If there is a delay in sending the patient to the Medical Officer, use an effective and different treatment while waiting, i.e. artemisinin and doxycycline or clindamycin; or quinine and doxycycline or clindamycin.

Treatment of pregnant women

A woman when pregnant is more likely to develop malaria even if semi-immune; and if she has an attack it is more likely to become complicated.

In areas of stable malaria, even if the woman does not develop acute malaria, the baby is likely to have a low birthweight and be more likely to die.

Attacks should be treated with a full course of effective drug treatment.

Safe drugs include:

• sulfadoxine with pyrimethamine, but this may not be effective;
• chloroquine, but this may not be effective;
• proguanil, but this may not be effective unless given with another drug;
• quinine, but best not used after 14 weeks, as can cause low blood glucose;
• artemisinin, but this is not certain before 14 weeks; however, if given accidentally (e.g. the patient did not know she was pregnant) there is no reason as yet to think it will cause problems;
• clindamycin.

Unsafe drugs include:

• tetracycline,
• doxycycline,
• primaquine.

It is not yet known whether other drugs not included here are safe or not.

In the first 14 weeks of pregnancy, an acute attack could be treated with:

quinine OR if not available an artemisinin group drug } for 7 days

AND

sulfadoxine + pyrimethamine } if there is not more than 10–20% resistance to it; but not in the last week before delivery

OR
clindamycin
OR
mefloquine if there is no other effective drug available.

Low blood sugar is a dangerous complication of malaria and also of quinine treatment in a pregnant woman. Check the blood sugar every 2–4 hours when severely ill and immediately at any time if the patient gets worse. Give IVI glucose (e.g. 50 ml of 50% dextrose) if needed.

During breastfeeding all drugs are safe except dapsone, tetracycline and probably doxycycline.

Treatment of patients with HIV infection

These patients are more likely to get malaria and also get serious or complicated malaria. Pregnant women are very likely to have problems (see left).

Give the usual drug treatment.

Do not, however, use sulfadoxine + pyrimethamine if the patient is already taking sulfamethoxazole + trimethoprim (SMX + TMP) as these drugs have similar actions and the sulfadoxine with pyrimethamine almost certainly will not be effective.

Treatment of hyperreactive malarious splenomegaly or tropical splenomegaly syndrome

See Chapter 21 pages 319–321.

> *If* any patient being treated for malaria is very ill or shocked and has some history or some signs that suggest he may have an acute severe bacterial infection, *then* treat for septicaemia also (see Chapter 12).

Transfer to Medical Officer care

This is required *if* severe or complicated malaria occurs *and if* it is not possible to treat the complications properly in the health centre, e.g.

1. cerebral malaria with unconsciousness which has lasted more than 1 day and is not improving on treatment;
2. acute anaemia (Hb less than 5 g/dl and fever);
3. shock which cannot be corrected;
4. blackwater fever;
5. acute kidney failure;
6. pulmonary oedema which does not improve;
7. abnormal bleeding which continues after malaria treatment.

Transfer also if

1. drug treatment is not effective;
2. hyperreactive malarious splenomegaly and pregnancy or haemolysis, etc.

Prevention and control

Eradication is not possible in most areas.

The best methods of control for your area will have been worked out by your Health Department. You need to follow their policy. The following will have been considered.

Kill all parasites in the bodies of all the original hosts

Give antimalarial drugs to kill all trophozoites and all hypnozoites, and if possible all gametocytes. These drugs would have to be given to the whole population until all the mosquitoes carrying malaria have died. This has been found to be not possible in almost all areas.

However, the new treatment regimens do reduce the reservoir. Artemisinin-based combination therapy (ACT) given for the proper length of time will get rid of all of the merozoites from the body of the treated person. Also, the artemisinin drug will kill *P. falciparum* gametocytes so that the patient will not infect the mosquito. In areas where *P. vivax* and others are the main problem, a proper treatment course will kill all the trophozoites and by adding primaquine will cure the patient by stopping relapses from hypnozoites (and also kill the gametocytes of any *P. falciparum* also present). In some situations these treatments will help in malaria control. More importantly, however, these treatments will help prevent drug resistant malaria from developing.

Stop transmission

A previous eradication programme was carried out based on the idea that if all anopheles mosquitoes which had bitten people (and who could therefore develop and pass on malaria) were killed, then malaria could no longer spread. All indoor surfaces of all dwellings were sprayed regularly with DDT or another residual (long-lasting) insecticide (poison for insects). Anopheles mosquitoes bite at night when most people are indoors or near a house. After feeding, the mosquito likes to rest on a wall, which should have been covered with insecticide. Before there was time for the malaria to have developed in the mosquito, the insecticide should have killed the mosquito. The aim of spraying was to kill all anopheles mosquitoes that had bitten human beings in their houses (the aim of spraying was not to kill all mosquitoes).

Unfortunately, for many reasons, this method alone failed in most areas. Together with use of insecticide-treated nets (ITNs) and other means, however, this method is now being used again.

Bites from anopheles mosquitoes, which usually bite at night, can be greatly reduced by the following:

1. Cover the body with clothing, e.g. long-sleeved shirts and long trousers to be put on as daylight goes. Most bites are usually near the floor; so covering the legs is most important.
2. Use insect repellents (e.g. DEET or permethrin) on uncovered areas, e.g. face and hands.
3. Use the insect screens on windows and doors to keep mosquitoes out. Otherwise, treat curtains over them with permethrin to kill mosquitoes which come in, or at least make them less likely to bite (see Appendix 4 page 100). DDT treatment of the house also does this.
4. Use insecticides in the house or at least burn 'mosquito coils'. Do not spray DDT into the air.
5. Use insecticide-treated nets to cover people at night when sleeping. Good nets would stop people being bitten by mosquitoes, but mosquitoes do get under them. If nets are treated with permethrin or deltamethrin, mosquitoes which do get under the net but touch the insecticide will be less likely to bite and many will die. These have been shown to be very effective in reducing malaria. Long lasting insecticidal nets (LLIN) are made with insecticide in the material and this lasts for 5 years, even when the net is washed up to 20 times. The net can be either coloured or white. At present, there are only three which WHO has approved. Factory treated nets other than these may not be reliable. WHO may approve others later. Ordinary nets can be treated at home with insecticides (see Appendix 4 page 100). White nets hold the insecticide much

better than coloured nets. However, home treated nets need retreating with more insecticide after three washes and if possible every 3 months or at least once a year. Use of these nets is so effective that this is one of the three essential things to do in trying to reduce the morbidity and mortality of pregnant women and their newborn children in places with malaria. ITNs also reduce other diseases carried by insects, e.g. leishmaniasis, viral encephalitis, lymphatic filariasis and Chagas' disease. They also reduce head lice and bed bugs.

6. Put beds as high as possible above the floor, as in many areas mosquitoes bite more in low areas near the floor than in higher areas.

In some areas, methods may be able to be used to decrease the number of mosquitoes, e.g. drain breeding sites, introduce fish which eat mosquito larvae, put things on the surface of the water to kill larvae, etc.

In areas of high transmission and stable malaria, measures other than preventing mosquito bites are unlikely to help a lot. Also, unless completely successful, all they may do is change a stable area into an unstable area and semi-immune people would lose their immunity and be liable to get attacks of severe malaria. In areas of unstable malaria, however, it may be possible to use these methods, including stopping mosquitoes breeding at the time of rain, etc. together with the new treatment regimens for patients, to greatly reduce malaria. If this is possible, your Health Department will ask for your help in giving the correct drug treatment.

Raise the resistance of susceptible persons

This is not yet possible, but immunisation with a malaria vaccine is the main hope for control of this disease for the future. At present a number of vaccines are under trial. Results so far suggest one of these may be successful.

Prophylactic treatment

Regular prophylactic antimalarial drugs will stop the development of malaria parasites in the blood (trophozoites). They will therefore prevent clinical malaria. But they will also prevent the development of semi-immunity to malaria. And after a variable period of time (often about a year) they will cause the loss of any existing semi-immunity to malaria.

Regular prophylactic antimalarial drugs are therefore given only to certain groups of people.

1. People who
   • have no immunity to malaria, *and*
   • have come to a malarious area, *and* who
   • do not need to develop semi-immunity to malaria (e.g. they will not live in the malarious area for the rest of their lives or for many years), *or*
   • do not wish to suffer the ill-health needed to develop semi-immunity to malaria, i.e. chronic malaria with repeated acute attacks of malaria for 4–10 years (see pages 74–75); although the danger and severity of this ill-health can be greatly reduced by quick correct treatment of any acute attack which occurs.

   This group will include:
   (a) adults from areas where malaria does not occur,
   (b) adults from areas where the same kind of malaria is not present all the time,
   (c) children under 6 years; but only in *some* countries (after the age of 6 the children can clearly complain of the symptoms of malaria and be given quick drug treatment of the acute attack and are then allowed to develop chronic malaria and semi-immunity).

   These people are usually travellers or expatriates who will not permanently reside in the area. Doxycycline, mefloquine, atovaquone and proguanil ('Malarone') are often used, but really only a combination of drugs (to stop resistance developing) such as atovaquone and proguanil should be used but is expensive.

2. People who do have some immunity to malaria but this immunity is reduced for a while due to another condition.

   This group will include:
   (a) women when they are pregnant (pregnant woman are the largest group of semi-immune adults who could be helped by intermittent prophylactic treatment (IPT), which will greatly reduce disease and death in these women and their children). (See pages 86, 89.)
   (b) people sick from another illness, e.g. pneumonia (stop antimalarials as soon as the pneumonia is cured) or anaemia (stop antimalarials as soon as haemoglobin is 10 g/dl).

3. People who cannot develop or who have permanently lost normal immunity to malaria. This group will include:
   (a) patients with HIV infection;
   (b) patients who are taking prednisolone or anti-cancer drugs;
   (c) patients with hyperreactive malarious splenomegaly or tropical splenomegaly syndrome;

(d) possibly people who have had their spleens removed.

Chloroquine was used for this, but resistance has made it of no help in most places where there is *P. falciparum*. Sulfadoxine with pyrimethamine was then used, but again development of resistance has made this also of little help in many places, not only where there is *P. falciparum* but also *P. vivax*. It should now not be used for prophylaxis except in pregnant women until a better drug combination is found for them too. Your Health Department will tell you the best combination of drugs to use in your area for preventative treatment.

For most people who live all their lives in areas where malaria is endemic and stable because of high transmission, they are best to develop semi-immunity by not taking prophylaxis all the time. Any acute attack of malaria should be treated fully and immediately before it becomes severe or complicated. By doing this, they can slowly build up their immunity and not risk dying from an acute attack in the meantime. If people live far from health care, they will need to have a nearby supply of drugs and someone who is taught when and how to give them. These drugs will need to be a combination treatment of more than one drug and it is essential the patient takes the whole course and does not stop as soon as he feels well. The drugs may include artemisinin suppositories for treatment of those too sick to swallow. Your Health Department will give you instructions about this.

Special note about pregnant women

Pregnancy decreases what immunity a patient has to malaria. During pregnancy malaria parasites (especially *P. falciparum*) infect the placenta and stop some of the nutrition, oxygen, etc. getting to the baby and they may release toxins which are carried to the baby.

In areas of high malaria transmission, i.e. stable malaria, most adult women have enough immunity that they do not often get attacks of acute malaria. They do, however, get more anaemia, which makes it more likely for them to die at delivery if they have a haemorrhage. The placental infection causes more miscarriages and stillbirths, more premature births, more low birthweight babies and more deaths of the children soon after birth.

In areas of epidemic or unstable malaria, most adult women do not have significant immunity and have a two or three times greater risk than non-pregnant women of getting severe or complicated malaria and dying from this or anaemia. The baby is also affected as above.

In Africa alone, where there are 30,000,000 pregnancies in malarious areas each year, 10,000 of these women and 200,000 of their children die because of malaria.

If the following three things are done for pregnant women, this will greatly decrease disease and death.

1. Pregnant women, and also their newborn children, should sleep under insecticide treated nets (ITNs).
2. Treatment of any attack of acute malaria, should be early and effective (certainly before 24 hours). If a treatment centre is not nearby, the pregnant woman should be supplied with the correct treatment drugs for her area to take home and taught when and how to take them and to finish the whole course (see also pages 86 and 80).
3. Give intermittent preventative treatment during pregnancy (IPTP) (a special type of prophylactic treatment).

It has been shown that if every pregnant woman is given two full curative treatment courses in the second and third trimester of pregnancy (usually starting after the woman feels the baby's movements), then anaemia, attacks of malaria, abortions or still births, low birthweight children and deaths of newborn children are greatly reduced.

The drug used in these trials has been the combination of sulfadoxine with pyrimethamine. Unfortunately, both *P. falciparum* and *P. vivax* have been rapidly becoming resistant to this drug combination as in many places it is being used alone (without a companion drug to stop resistance developing). Fortunately, despite this resistance, it does still seem to be helpful, probably because many patients do have some immunity. Trials of other drugs are being done and the results should shortly tell us if the present sulfadoxine with pyrimethamine should continue or if we should use one of the ACTs or another combination. Meanwhile, if sulfadoxine and pyrimethamine are no longer used as a single drug treatment, this drug may continue to be an effective treatment for pregnant women. (Of course, theoretically, it should not be used alone in pregnant women; but the tests which showed it worked were done before this was known.)

Two courses of sulfadoxine with pyrimethamine should be given to all pregnant women. This should be part of normal antenatal care; but if the patient does not get antenatal care, give these drugs when she is seen for any other reason.

Appendix 1 Malaria blood smear

You really should take a blood smear for examination for malaria parasites ('MPs') from all patients who have a fever. Even though you usually cannot examine the slide in the health centre you should still take one. At the end of the month you should send all the slides to the Malaria Control Office. This will help them tell how much malaria and what kind of malaria is occurring in the area. However, your Health Department will tell you if you should do this or not.

Blood smears are also used to help diagnose and treat individual patients.

Method of making malaria blood films

Both thick and thin blood films are used to detect and identify malaria parasites. These are usually made on the same frosted ended slide. See Chapter 6 page 27 for details.

1. For best results make a spreader. Break off the corners of a glass slide making sure that the edge of the slide is smooth. It must not be chipped or rough because this will spoil the thin blood film.

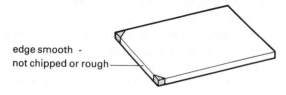

edge smooth -
not chipped or rough

2. Imagine that the non-frosted area of a standard clean slide is composed of three equal parts.

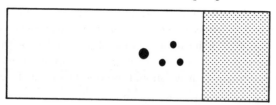

3a. Put one large or preferably three small drops of blood in the middle of the part nearest the frosted end.
3b. Put one small drop of blood at the beginning of the next part.

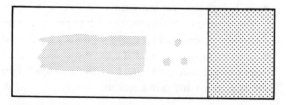

4. Bring the edge of a second slide to contact the surface of the blood slide just in front of the one drop of blood – push this spreader slide backwards until it just touches the drop of blood, which will then spread along its edge.

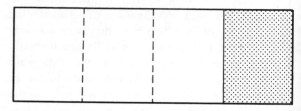

5. Hold at an angle of 45° and spread the drop of blood by pushing the spreader forward. (See Chapter 6 page 28 for details.)

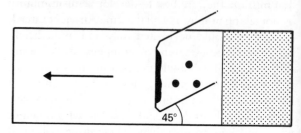

45°

6. With the corner of the spreader slide, spread the 3 drops to form a circular thick film about 1 cm in diameter. Spread the blood evenly. If you can just see the print of a newspaper through it, the smear is the right thickness.

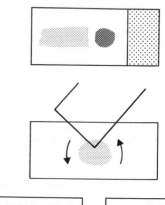

IF YOU CAN READ THE TYPE. THEN THE BLOOD FILM IS TOO THIN

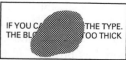

IF YOU CA... THE TYPE. THE BL... TOO THICK

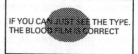

IF YOU CAN JUST SEE THE TYPE. THE BLOOD FILM IS CORRECT

7. Leave the slide flat so that the thick film will dry evenly. Use a pencil to write the slide number on the frosted end of the slide.

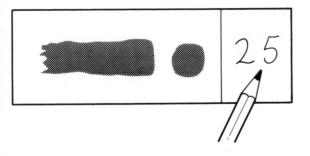

Interpretation of reports of malaria smears

A report of 'negative' means that after the examination of 100 high power fields under the microscope, no malaria parasites were seen. Therefore, it is very unlikely that the patient's illness is caused by malaria.

If malaria parasites are found, the number of parasites per field is counted and recorded in the following way.

1. If the number of parasites in an average field is higher than 20 (e.g. 43) only one field is counted and the total number of parasites reported (e.g. 43/1).
2. If the number of parasites present in an average field is between 3 and 19 (e.g. 14), then ten fields are counted, and the total number of parasites reported (e.g. 140/10).
3. If the number of parasites present in an average field is less than 3 (e.g. 1 or 2) in most fields, then 100 fields are counted and the total number reported (e.g. 120/100).

If mixed infections are found, then each species is reported separately.

Trophozoites and *P. falciparum* gametocytes are reported separately.

Another method of recording parasite density is as follows.
- Fewer than 10 parasites in 100 fields.   +
- More than 10 parasites but fewer than   + + 100 parasites in 100 fields.
- More than 100 parasites in 100 fields   + + + but fewer than 10 parasites in 1 field.
- More than 10 parasites in one field.   + + + +

Again, mixed infections are reported separately and trophozoites and *P. falciparum* gametocytes are reported separately.

A more accurate method of estimating parasite density is to estimate the number of parasites present in 1 cubic mm of blood (1 microlitre of blood). When examining the film, the laboratory worker counts 200 white cells and all the parasites present in the fields which contained the 200 white cells. He then multiplies the number of parasites by 40 (as there are about 8000 white cells per cubic mm) to give the number of parasites per cubic mm. Again mixed infections are reported separately, and trophozoites and *P. falciparum* gametocytes are reported separately.

A quick and easier but less accurate way is using the thick film and reporting the number of red blood cells seen which have parasites in them as a percentage. At a thin part of the film where the RBCs are in a single layer and just touching each other, using a ×100 objective lens 2000 RBCs are counted. The number of these with parasites inside is also counted. The percentage parasites = number of infected red blood cells × 100/2000. Gametocytes are counted separately.

The presence of trophozoites or gametocytes shows infection with malaria parasites. But only trophozoites harm humans. Trophozoites indicate the patient's illness *may be* caused by malaria. Gametocytes do not harm humans. The presence of gametocytes in the blood does *not* suggest that the patient's illness may be caused by malaria. Some drug treatment may cure a patient of falciparum malaria and trophozoites will disappear from his blood within 1 week. However, if these drugs do not kill *P. falciparum* gametocytes, the smear may show gametocytes for another 3–4 months, although the patient is cured. The gametocytes are, however, infectious for mosquitoes.

Trophozoites ('Troph' or 'T') present in a slide mean the patient **may be sick with malaria.**

Gametocytes ('G') **do not mean the patient may be sick with malaria** (but the patient can pass on the disease to mosquitoes).

Appendix 2 Malaria Rapid Diagnostic Tests (RDTs)

These tests may be available if microscopic tests are not available.

RDTs take these forms – a dip stick or a strip which is put on to a plastic cassette or a card.

RDTs show only the presence of proteins which are only in or only made by malaria parasites. These proteins will be in the blood of only people who are or who have recently been infected with malaria parasites. If the proteins are in the blood tested, the stick or strip shows a particular colour change. Some RDTs show only *P. falciparum* parasite proteins; but others may show this and one or more or all of the three other malaria parasites. A good RDT can show as few as 100 parasites/microlitre – about the same as the microscope. The RDT may not be this accurate, depending on the number and types of parasites present, how well the manufacturer made the test, how well the test has been looked after before the test was done (see below) and the training and skill of the person who does the test.

As the RDTs are expensive, one should be used only where the result will mean something and change the management/treatment of the patient.

You need training to use the RDT correctly. Do not allow the blood to get on you. Follow the instructions exactly (as different RDTs have different directions). The RDT must never be allowed to get too hot (>30°C) or have the packet it is in punctured or broken. The unopened packet should get to room temperature before it is opened. The RDT must be used immediately it is opened and it must be read at the correct time.

Remember that a negative test does not mean the patient could not have malaria, e.g.:

- there may be too few parasites in the peripheral (surface) blood collected to show a positive result (but there may be many in the blood vessels of the internal organs and brain);
- the RDT may have been damaged or not used properly;
- the patient's illness may be due to a malaria parasite the RDT does not test for.

Remember also that a positive test does not always mean the patient's illness is due to malaria, e.g.:

- the protein from the parasite may still be in the blood after all the trophozoites have died (or gametocytes are present which do not cause human illness);
- other chemicals or substances in the blood may have caused a 'false positive' test;
- malaria parasites in the blood (especially if the patient is semi-immune) do not mean the patient's illness is necessarily due to malaria.

Appendix 3   Drugs used for treatment of malaria

Quinolone related drugs

Chloroquine

Chloroquine is a 4 amino quinolone.

It is quickly absorbed from the gastrointestinal tract and after IMI.

It is excreted very slowly (over months) by the kidneys.

An overdose is dangerous as it stops the heart and there is no antidote.

Side effects in proper doses include itchiness, which can be severe in dark-skinned people and not helped by antihistamines, and other skin reactions and hair loss; nausea or vomiting or diarrhoea; headache and other CNS effects.

Chloroquine previously very effectively stopped malaria merozoites growing; but unfortunately most *P. falciparum* and some *P. vivax* organisms have become resistant to it.

It is still used in areas where *P. falciparum* does not occur and the other malaria organisms are still sensitive to it.

In places of unstable malaria, mainly *P. vivax* malaria, it should be combined with primaquine to give a two-drug treatment of the merozoites; the primaquine will stop relapses of *P. ovale* and *P. vivax* by killing hypnozoites. If primaquine is not given, then an artemisinin or other companion drug should be given with the chloroquine to try to stop resistance developing.

Chloroquine is available as tablets, syrup and injection.

The dose is ordered in mg of chloroquine base (not in mg of sulfate or phosphate salt).

- Tablet – usually 100 mg and 150 mg base, but others too of chloroquine base as phosphate or sulfate
- Syrup – usually 10 mg base/ml as phosphate or sulfate
- Injection – usually 40 mg base/ml as sulfate, phosphate or dihydrochloride.

Many different strengths and sizes of tablets or injections are available.

Chloroquine dose for usual attack. No vomiting. No diarrhoea

Give oral chloroquine.

- Give 10 mg/kg of the base immediately;
      if cannot weigh patient
      small adult (< 50 kg) – 400 mg
      large adult (> 50 kg) – 600 mg.

- Give 5 mg/kg of the base 6 hours later;
  if cannot weigh patient
  small adult (< 50 kg) – 200 mg
  large adult (> 50 kg) – 300 mg.
- Give 5 mg/kg the following day – see above.
- Give 5 mg/kg the following day – see above.
- Give therefore 25 mg/kg over 3 days.

If the patient immediately vomits the tablets, give the same dose again; but do not repeat the dose if the patient vomits more than $\frac{1}{4}$ of an hour later; but if nausea still present when the next dose is due, start with the first dose of chloroquine by IMI.

In some health centre areas the dose of chloroquine as above may be too complicated for your staff and your patients to remember. A very simple dose, as in Table 13.1, has been effective and safe and easy for staff and patients, although the overall dose was 30 and not 25 mg/kg.

Table 13.1 Simplified chloroquine dosage.

Using 150 mg base/tablet

Size of adult	Dose on Day 1	Dose on Day 2	Dose on Day 3
Small (less than 50 kg)	3 tablets	3 tablets	3 tablets
Large (more than 50 kg)	4 tablets	4 tablets	4 tablets

You, however, will have to follow the rules laid down by the Health Department where you work.

Usual attack but vomiting or diarrhoea

Give IM chloroquine. (If any possibility *P. falciparum* could be present also, treat for *P. falciparum* malaria with injection of artemisinin drug or quinine.)

Give 3.5 mg chloroquine base/kg patient's body weight (maximum dose 200 mg) each dose.

The dose if you cannot weigh the patient is:
- small adult (< 50 kg) – 150 mg
- large adult (> 50 kg) – 200 mg.

After 6 hours if the patient cannot take oral chloroquine, repeat the *same* dose of IM chloroquine. However, if the patient can take oral drugs, give the first dose of the three daily doses of chloroquine tablets instead (see above).

If the patient still cannot take oral chloroquine, then, instead of the once daily dose of tablets, give IM chloroquine every 6 hours. Use the *same* IM dose (see above). As soon as possible, change to oral chloroquine.

Stop chloroquine after a total of 25 mg/kg of treatment, i.e. after 7th dose or after 36 hours.

> Never give chloroquine by IVI (as this is likely to cause death).
> If antimalarial drug needs to be given intravenously (e.g. shock), then patients who are this sick should not be given chloroquine but should be given an artemisinin drug or quinine instead.

As soon as the patient can swallow and has no diarrhoea or vomiting and is not shocked, change to oral chloroquine. Oral chloroquine is just as effective and is safer and easier than injection.

Give also primaquine with the chloroquine (or an alternative companion drug)

See pages 84 and 80.

The dose of chloroquine for prevention of malaria

Chloroquine is usually not effective as many malaria parasites are resistant. If the malaria parasites are sensitive to chloroquine, give a large adult 600 mg base each week and a small adult 450 mg base each week. If given regularly for more than 5 years, some people can develop problems with their eyes and sight. It should be given with a companion drug.

Amodiaquine

Amodiaquine is similar in action and dose to chloroquine (see pages 82–83). It is more effective than chloroquine against some resistant organisms.

- Tablets contain either 153 mg of base as chlorohydrate or 200 mg base as hydrochloride. No injection is available.
- The dose is 10 mg base/kg/day. As long as the 153 mg base tablets are used, this is 3 tablets for a small adult (under 50 kg) and 4 tablets for a large adult (over 50 kg) each day for 3 days. If the 200 mg base tablets are used, the dose is 2 for a small adult and 3 for a large adult.
- If vomiting means oral amodiaquine cannot be used, IV or IM artemisinin drug or IV infusion of or IM quinine would be used.
- Give primaquine also in areas of unstable malaria; or another companion drug in all malaria areas.

If used for a long time, it can occasionally cause fatal blood disorders. It is therefore not used now for prophylaxis.

Quinine tablets and injection

Quinine used for malaria acts on the fully grown trophozoites in the RBCs but does not stop the young ones growing and does not stop the RBCs with parasites in them getting 'sequestrated' (stuck) in the blood vessels of the brain and other internal organs. It is, however, a very effective drug for severe or resistant malaria.

Quinine kills the gametocytes of *P. vivax, P. malariae* and *P. ovale,* but not all the fully grown gametocytes of *P. falciparum*; but it does help in the control of malaria.

Quinine is well absorbed from the gastrointestinal tract and after IMI. It can be given IV only by infusion (see below) and only slowly or it will cause death. It must not be given by IVI. It can also be given as a retention enema if no other way of giving it exists, but this is less likely to be absorbed reliably.

It is broken down by the liver but also excreted by the kidney. It lasts in the body for only many hours to a day or so, but it lasts longer if the patient has severe malaria or kidney failure.

Quinine dose is sometimes ordered in mg of base and sometimes as mg of salt. It is best to order mg of base.

Table 13.2 Quinine: salt–base equivalents.

	Salt (mg)	Base (mg)
Quinine sulfate	363	300
Quinine bisulfate	508	300
Quinine hydrochloride	405	300
Quinine dihydrochloride	366	300
Quinine hydrobromide	408	300
Quinine ethylcarbonate	366	300

Quinine tablets and injections can come in different strengths, although the WHO recommendations are for only tablets of 300 mg base (as phosphate or sulfate) and only 300 mg base per ml (as dihydrochloride) for injection in a 2 ml vial (which would hold 600 mg base in the 2 ml vial).

As an overdose is likely to cause death or an underdose allow malaria to cause death, make sure you write or read carefully what dose of salt or base is ordered and what strengths of tablets and injections are available to be given.

Dose for quinine is 10 mg base/kg patient's body weight, each dose every 8 hours (i.e. three times a day) for 7 days:

- small adult (< 50 kg) – 450 mg base ($1\frac{1}{2}$ of 300 mg base tabs or 1.5 ml of 300 mg/ml base injection).
- large adult (> 50 kg) – 600 mg base (2 of 300 mg base tabs or 2 ml of 300 mg/ml base injection).

If quinine is being given for treatment of severe or complicated malaria by IV infusion or by IM, the first dose (not later doses) is doubled to 20 mg/kg.

If severe or complicated malaria and artemisinin drug is not available and if quinine cannot be given by IV infusion or IMI, quinine can be given in the usual dose rectally as a retention enema in the same dose as orally or by injection, strapping the buttocks together after giving it. The gluconate salt of quinine is the best to use for this if available.

The dose of quinine should be reduced to 66% or two-thirds of the above doses if the patient is very sick or jaundiced, or has kidney failure or develops side effects of quinine. 'Cinchonism', however, with ringing in the ears, nausea, headache, dry eyes, changed sight, is a side effect, but is not dangerous and is not a reason for stopping full treatment. If vomiting, abdominal pain, diarrhoea and severe dry eyes occur, reduce the dose. Allergic type reactions can occur, including fever, asthma, bleeding due to platelet damage and haemolysis (breakdown of the RBCs in the blood vessels) and haemoglobinuria (blackwater fever).

A very important side effect is hypoglycaemia or low blood glucose. This is very common in pregnant women and in severe malaria. Do blood glucose tests every 2–4 hours and at any other time immediately if the patient gets worse for no apparent reason. If the blood glucose is low (2.2 mmol/litre or less than 40 mg/100 ml), or a blood test for glucose cannot be done, give IV glucose, e.g. 50 ml of 50% glucose, or if the patient can still swallow, give oral sugar or jam or honey 20 g (20 ml or 1 tablespoonful), as this condition is very dangerous. Check blood sugars each hour after this and give more glucose if needed.

Even if the patient is semi-immune, 3 days of treatment with quinine is not enough to cure and stop resistance developing and 7 days treatment must be given.

A companion drug must also always be given to stop quinine resistance occurring.

If the patient is not immune or is pregnant and is unable to take any other drugs, give quinine for 10, or better, 14 days.

Method of giving quinine by slow IV drip

Give quinine by a slow IV drip *only if*:

1. It has been possible to get a drip running immediately (before 15 minutes have passed). (An immediate IMI is better than a late IV drip.)
2. The staff are able to keep the drip running.
3. The staff will not let the drip run in quickly. (A rapid IVI of quinine will cause sudden death.)

If not, it is better to give the quinine by IMI.
Give quinine by IMI *when*:

1. IV drip was not started immediately (before 15 minutes have passed).
2. The staff are not capable of keeping the drip running.
3. You are not certain that the staff will not let the drip run quickly.

IM quinine is not as effective as IV quinine, especially if the patient is shocked. Also, it may cause an injection abscess.

For IV infusion use 10 ml/kg patient's body weight of 5% dextrose or 4.3% dextrose in 0.18% sodium chloride solution to dilute the quinine. Glucose is needed as both quinine and malaria can cause hypoglycaemia (low blood glucose). Let the fluid run out of a flask of dextrose saline until the required amount is left (e.g. 500 ml for an adult).

Work out the dose of quinine by the patient's weight (8–10 mg base/kg every 8 hours, but the first dose should be double this, i.e. 20 mg/kg).

Add the dose of quinine to the solution by injecting the quinine into the flask.

Mix well.

The rate of the quinine should be no more than 5 mg base/kg body weight each hour. A way of doing this, if no syringe driver is available, is to run the drip *slowly over four (4) hours.*

- Order the number of drops per minute.
- Mark on the IV flask the level for each hour.
- Then, every hour check that the fluid has fallen to the level of this mark, but *no more.* If it has gone below the level, stop the quinine and work out what time it should have been when the quinine was down to this level. Until then, give only 5% dextrose. Then start the quinine infusion again when the time you worked out before is reached.

> IMI is usually the easiest method for giving quinine in a health centre. IV infusion is, however, needed for giving quinine if the patient is shocked.

Mefloquine tablets

Tablets are either 250 mg base or 227 mg base.

Mefloquine has been used for treatment and prevention of malaria, although some *P falciparum* are now resistant to mefloquine, especially in SE Asia.

Mefloquine is reasonably well absorbed from the gastrointestinal tract but can cause nausea, vomiting, abdominal pain, loss of appetite and diarrhoea. If the treatment dose can be broken up into $\frac{1}{2}$ or $\frac{1}{3}$ of it given over 2 or 3 days there is less nausea, etc. and better absorption. It stays in the body for many weeks. It is absorbed less and stays in the body a shorter time if the patient has acute severe malaria. It is excreted by the liver and gastrointestinal tract.

Side effects other than gastrointestinal include headache, dizziness, loss of balance, sleepiness or not being able to sleep and bad dreams. At times, encephalitis (see Chapter 25 page 415) or a psychosis (see Chapter 35 pages 570, 572) can develop. Do not give mefloquine to patients who have had encephalitis or fitting or psychotic problems.

Skin rashes, blood pressure changes, heart beating fast or irregularly, etc. occasionally occur.

Mefloquine should not be given if halofantrine has been given in the previous 4 weeks as this can cause death.

Mefloquine may be unsuitable for use in some areas of Africa for children.

The treatment dose is from 15 mg base/kg in areas of low resistance to 25 mg base/kg in areas of higher resistance to mefloquine; but 25 mg/kg is probably the best to use everywhere. It is not necessary to give on the first day of treatment of an acute attack if an artemisinin drug is also being given (as artemisinin drugs are very effective in the first few days and it is best not to risk causing gastrointestinal side effects). Also, the mefloquine will last longer in the body if swallowed when the malaria is less severe. Divide the dose into $\frac{1}{2}$ or $\frac{1}{3}$. Give $\frac{1}{2}$ of the dose on Days 2 and 3, or $\frac{1}{3}$ of the dose on Days 2, 3 and 4. The total dose will vary from 2 to 6 tablets, but normally do not give all in 1 day and do not give more than 4 tablets on any 1 day.

If used in a fixed dose or co-formulation tablet or in blister pack with artesunate 4 mg/kg daily for 3 days, then the dose of mefloquine would be 8 mg/kg/day for 3 days (i.e. 24 mg/kg).

The preventive dose is 5 mg/kg each week – usually one tablet each week.

Mefloquine should always be given together with another drug (usually an artemisinin drug for acute severe complicated attack (but not until after 12 hours after the last dose of quinine)) to lead to cure and stop resistant malaria developing.

It is expensive.

Halofantrine

- Tablet 250 mg
- Syrup 100 mg/5 ml

Halofantrine can be used for treatment of malaria, although some malaria organisms are now becoming resistant to halofantrine.

It is expensive.

It can have serious side effects.

It would not normally be given in a health centre.

The dose is 8 mg/kg usually 2 tablets of 250 mg every 6 hours on an empty stomach for 3 doses. Repeat these 3 doses after 1 week.

Do not give within a month of mefloquine or death from heart problems may occur.

Atovaquone

Atovaquone is not well absorbed from the gastro-intestinal tract but is better absorbed if taken with fatty food. It lasts in the body for about 7 days. It is excreted unchanged in the faeces.

Atovaquone stops the malaria parasite using energy to grow and multiply.

Atovaquone is effective against all *Plasmodium* species. It also stops liver cycle development and oocyst development in the mosquito.

Atovaquone is not used alone, as parasites can quickly develop resistance to it. If used with proguanil hydrochlorate it is very effective in prevention of malaria and in treatment. However, in treatment it is best used with also an artemisinin drug.

Tablets contain:
- atovaquone 250 mg and proguanil 100 mg for adults
- atovaquone 62.5 mg and proguanil 25 mg for children.

The treatment dose is 15–20 mg/kg/day for atovaquone and 3.5–8 mg/kg/day for proguanil, i.e. 4 tablets daily for adults over 40 kg for 3 days with an artemisinin drug.

The dose for adults for prophylaxis is one 250 mg atovaquone/100 mg proguanil daily with food.

Proguanil

Proguanil and chlorproguanil are similar. Both are easily absorbed from the gastrointestinal tract and changed to an active drug in the liver; but some people are not good at making this change (especially Asians and those from the Pacific Islands). It lasts in the body some days and about half is excreted in the urine and the rest in the faeces.

Proguanil stops the malaria parasite making protein properly and
- may stop liver stages developing;
- slowly stops trophozoites growing;
- makes gametocytes non-infective;
- kills sporozoites.

Proguanil is best used with other drugs:
- Proguanil 100 mg with atovaquone 250 mg for treatment of malaria. Use with artemisinin drug.
- Proguanil 25 mg with atovaquone 62.5 mg for treatment of malaria in children. Use with an artemisinin drug.
- (Chlor)proguanil with dapsone and artesunate is used for treatment of drug resistant malaria.
  For doses see atovaquone (left).
  Side effects of proguanil are few.

Primaquine

Primaquine is an 8 amino quinolone.

Primaquine is quickly absorbed from the gastro-intestinal tract and stays in the body for a number of hours. It is destroyed by the liver.

Primaquine:
- kills trophozoites (especially important are those of *P. vivax*) but not as effectively as the artemisinin drugs;
- kills all malaria parasites in the liver and therefore the hypnozoites of *P. vivax* and *P. ovale*;
- kills the gametocytes of *P. falciparum*.

Side effects include the following.
1. Abdominal pain, nausea and vomiting, which usually do not occur if it is taken with food.
2. Cyanosis or blue colouring of the blood (best seen in the mucosa of the tongue) which is not serious.
3. Haemolysis (red blood cells broken open inside blood vessels) and the haemoglobin is released into the blood and passed in the urine (which becomes dark or brown or black) and the patient becomes anaemic (pale). This is not serious if there is only a little; but serious if there is a lot of haemolysis. Haemolysis occurs mainly if patients do not have much of a special enzyme or chemical called glucose 6 phosphate dehydrogenase (shortened to G6PD) in their body and this is mostly determined by race and family inheritance. In some areas of the world it is of little importance and in other areas of such great importance that this drug cannot be used. Your Health Department will tell you what the situation is where you work.

Primaquine is used as follows.
1. As a companion drug to kill merozoites for the treatment of acute malaria to stop resistant organisms developing. It is used mainly to treat *P. vivax* together with chloroquine or amodiaquine.
2. As a drug to kill hypnozoites of *P. vivax* and *P. ovale* in the liver and therefore together with a drug which kills all the merozoites to 'cure' a patient

with *P. vivax* or *P. ovale* malaria (often called a 'radical cure'). This is not needed for *P. falciparum* or *P. malariae,* which do not have hypnozoites.

If reinfection is very common, as in stable malaria areas, semi-immunity would develop. There is no point in giving primaquine.

In low transmission areas of unstable malaria, its use may allow people to be well for long periods without recurrent attacks when transmission of malaria is not occurring. This would be of particular benefit to such patients as children under 5, pregnant women, HIV infected persons, etc.

The dose is 0.25 mg base/kg daily, usually 15 mg base for 14 days for adults.

Lower total dose courses are not effective, but the same total dose can be given over a longer period.

In some areas, especially SE Asia, Indonesia and Oceania, the Chesson strain of *P. vivax* is more resistant and the dose is 0.5 mg base/kg/daily usually 30 mg base for 14 days.

In areas where G6PD is common, primaquine causes less trouble if given in a dose of 0.75 mg/kg base once each week, usually 45 mg daily for adults for 8 weeks. (The total dose of primaquine is not reduced.) If severe G6PD is present in a patient or common in a population, then primaquine cannot be used.

Antifolate drugs

These include:

- sulfonamides or sulfones, usually sulfadoxine tablets or injection, but also sulfamethoxazole and dapsone,
- pyrimethamine tablets,
- pyrimethamine 25 mg with sulfadoxine 500 mg tablets and injection,
- pyrimethamine 12.5 mg with dapsone 100 mg (Maloprim) was used for prophylaxis against malaria but now not used because of side effects,
- proguanil tablets,
- proguanil with atovaquone tablets,
- chlorproguanil tablets,
- trimethoprim (TMP) tablets,
- trimethoprim with sulfamethoxazole tablets and injection (TMP/SMX) (co-trimoxazole).

See Chapter 11 pages 56–57.

Sulfadoxine and pyrimethamine

Sulfadoxine is a sulfonamide which is excreted only slowly over many days by the kidneys. It is well absorbed from the gastrointestinal tract or after IMI.

Pyrimethamine is well absorbed from the gastrointestinal tract or after IMI. It is broken down in the liver but excreted from the body by the kidneys over many days.

Sulfadoxine stops malaria parasites (and many bacteria) from making the proteins needed for their growth and reproduction; and the organisms cannot reproduce and later die. Malaria organisms can very quickly become resistant to sulfadoxine. It is therefore combined with another drug pyrimethamine (for malaria), which acts in a different place but still prevents the making of proteins, although the malaria organisms can also soon become resistant to the pyrimethamine. If both drugs are given together, resistance takes a lot longer to develop. Unfortunately, many *P. falciparum* and *P. vivax* organisms have learned or are learning how to develop this resistance. If the malaria organisms are not resistant to this combination in some places it can still be used; but it should now always be used together with another drug, which acts in a different way to these two drugs on the malaria organism, to stop resistance developing.

Side effects of sulfadoxine include nausea, vomiting, diarrhoea, etc. and allergic type reactions, the most worrying being 'Stevens Johnson Syndrome' where the skin blisters and peels off and the patient often dies.

If a patient who has taken sulfonamides gets a rash, the sulfonamide should be stopped immediately; if the rash is serious it should never be given to the patient again. Do not give sulfonamides if the patient has severe liver or kidney disease.

Do not give sulfadoxine with pyrimethamine to a patient who is already taking trimethoprim with sulfamethoxazole (TMP/SMX), e.g for HIV infection prophylaxis (as these drug combinations have similar effects).

Side effects of pyrimethamine are rare but it can cause blood, skin, gastrointestinal and nervous system (headaches and dizziness) symptoms, etc.

Tablets contain 500 mg sulfadoxine and 25 mg pyrimethamine; ampoules of 2.5 ml for IMI containing 500 mg sulfadoxine and 25 mg pyrimethamine are available.

The dose for treatment of malaria is:
- small adult < 50 kg 2 tablets once or 5 ml (2 ampoules) once
- large adult > 50 kg 3 tablets once or 7.5 ml (3 ampoules) once.

Sulfadoxine and pyrimethamine should always be given together with another antimalarial drug which acts in a different way (although it is still used as a single drug for intermittent preventative treatment during pregnancy (IPTP)) (see page 89).

Artemisinin/Qinghaosu group

Artemisinin is one of a family of related drugs all with the same actions against malaria and all with no significant side effects except for a very occasional person who has an allergic reaction to them.

The artemisinin group of drugs:

1. Act by killing the parasite by destroying the protein of the organism.
2. Act quickly – about 10–100 times more quickly than other drugs in reducing parasite numbers.
3. If given for only 3 days the malaria parasites are killed in just two of their reproductive cycles (of 2–3 days) and there are remaining parasites which need to be killed by another companion drug which has to be long lasting.
4. If given for 7 days, most, but not all, of the malaria parasites would be killed and any not killed could develop resistance. These organisms need to be killed by the companion drug in this time. If a short acting companion drug is added, less than 7 days would not be enough for either drug. Both drugs have to be given for 7 days.
5. Kill *P. falciparum* as well as *vivax, ovale* and *malariae* trophozoites (i.e. all human malaria parasites).
6. Kill also many *P. falciparum* gametocytes and therefore make the person less infectious to mosquitoes and therefore to other people and helps malaria control.
7. Have few side effects:
   • urticaria or hives or a type 1 allergy reaction occur in 1 in every 30,000 people given the drug;
   • gastrointestinal upsets occur but are not serious.
8. Companion drugs *always* have to be given with the artemisinin group of drugs.
9. If an artemisinin drug is given for only 3 days one of the following long acting companion drugs must also be given.
   • *Lumefantrine* 120 mg in the combined tablet with artemether 20 mg 3 tablets if weight 25–34 kg and 4 tablets if weight > 34 kg immediately and then again in 8 hours and then bd for 2 more days.
   • *Mefloquine* either in a separate tablet or in a fixed dose co-formulation tablet or in a blister pack (see pages 95, 79–80).
   • *Sulfadoxine* 500 mg with pyrimethamine 25 mg in 1 tablet, 2 tablets if small adult or 3 tablets if

large adult only once on Day 1 or Day 2 (but see below).
   • *Amodiaquine* 153 mg base in a separate tablet 3 tablets if weight under 50 kg or 4 if above 50 kg daily for 3 days (but see below).
   • *Atovaquone and proguanil* (at present too expensive).
   • *Piperaquine* (but at present not available).
   However, use any companion drug only if 80% or preferably 90% of the malaria parasites are sensitive to it.
10. Artemisinin drugs will need to be given for 7 days if the following short acting companion drugs are given and these also need to be given for 7 days:
    • doxycycline 100–200 mg daily
    • tetracycline 250 mg qid
    • clindamycin 150 mg qid or 300 mg bd.

Unfortunately, as yet, many of the drug combinations are not available as one tablet and this makes it:
• harder for health workers to work out the dose;
• harder for patients to take when there is more than one lot of tablets per dose;
• easier for health workers to give and patients to take just one of the two needed drugs and this can lead to ineffective treatment and drug resistant malaria.

If combination tablets such as the one tablet containing artemether (20 mg) + lumefantrine (120 mg) (already widely available) are available to you, always use these combination tablets. Combination tablets of artesunate + mefloquine (50 mg + 250 mg or 200 mg + 250 mg) and tablets of artesunate + amodiaquine (50 mg + 150 mg or 50 mg + 250 mg) are available in some areas; but tablets with other dose ratios may become available.

The World Health Organization at present makes the following recommendations, but these will change as conditions change and the drugs available change. You must follow your government Health Department recommendations.

In areas of multidrug resistance (SE Asia but also other areas), although this would be preferable in all areas use:
• artemether and lumefantrine, *or*
• artemether and mefloquine.

In Africa, use:
• artemether and lumefantrine,
• artesunate and ★amodiaquine,
• artesunate and ★sulfadoxine with pyrimethamine
(★only if more than 80% or preferably 90% of the parasites in that area are sensitive to the companion drug).

Remember, in no part of the world give any single anti-malarial drug (or combinations of drugs which act in the same way). Always give **two** antimalarial drugs which act in different ways in the correct doses.

Remember, every patient (even if appears cured in a short time) must take the whole 3 or 7 day course of the treatment. Use the drug combinations recommended by your Health Department.

Artemisinin (250 mg tablets or capsules)

10 mg/kg bd on Day 1, then

10 mg/kg daily on Days 2 and 3 + long acting companion drug,

or

10 mg /kg daily on Days 2–6 + short acting companion drug also given for 7 days.

Artemisinin suppositories (100, 200, 300, 400 and 500 mg)

Dose not yet certain, but at present use:

40 mg/kg bd on Day 1, then

20–40 mg/kg daily, but as soon as possible change to oral or IM or IVI treatment.

Dihydroartemisinin (20, 60 and 80 mg tablets)

2 mg/kg bd on Day 1, then

2 mg/kg daily on Days 2 and 3 + long acting companion drug,

or

2 mg/kg daily on Days 2–6

not recommended alone but with short acting companion drug for 7 days.

Dihydroartemisinin (80 mg suppositories)

Dose as for oral administration.

Dihydroartemisinin + piperaquine tablets

May be very effective, but are not generally available.

Artemether (40 mg capsules and 50 mg tablets)

2 mg/kg on Day 1, then

2 mg/kg on Days 2 and 3 + long acting companion drug

or

2 mg/kg on Days 2–6 with short acting companion drug for 7 days.

Artemether (40 mg/ml and 80 mg/ml injection) for IMI only (NOT for IVI)

3.2 mg/kg Day 1, then

2 mg/kg on Days 2 and 3 or change to oral drug and long acting companion drug,

or

1.6 mg/kg on Days 2–6 or change to oral drug with a short acting companion drug also for 7 days.

Artemether + lumefantrine (a long acting companion drug) (20 mg + 120 mg in same tablet)

4 tablets if weight > 34 kg immediately, then

4 tablets after 8 hours, then

4 tablets for Days 2 and 3, i.e. 6 doses in all.

But for multidrug resistant malaria 4 tablets bd on Days 2 and 3, i.e. 8 doses in all.

Artesunate (50 mg and 200 mg tablets)

200 mg (4 mg/kg) Day 1, then

100–200 mg (2–4 mg/kg) on Days 2 and 3 with long acting companion drug,

or

100–200 mg (2–4 mg/kg) on Days 2–6 with short acting companion drug for 7 days.

Artesunate (50, 100 and 400 mg suppositories)

10 mg/kg/day PR, repeated if expelled in less than $\frac{1}{2}$ an hour and strap buttocks together.

As soon as possible change to oral or IM or IV treatment.

Artesunate (60 mg powder for IV or IM injection; 5% sodium bicarbonate solution for mixing)

2.4 mg/kg IVI or IMI; 1.2 mg/kg 12 hours later

1.2–2.4 mg/kg IVI or IMI on Days 2 and 3 with long acting companion drug, or

(1.2)–2.4 mg/kg IVI or IMI on Days 2–6 but as soon as possible change to oral drug + short acting companion drug for 7 days.

Artemotil or artemether (150 mg in 2 ml vials for IMI)

Dose as for artemether.

Lumefantrine

Lumefantrine is absorbed from the gastrointestinal tract well if taken with fatty food. It remains in the blood for some days. It works in a similar way to quinine.

It is used as a long acting companion drug to artemether.

Tablets contain 20 mg artemether and 120 mg lumefantrine in the same tablet.

The usual dose is 1.5 mg/kg artemether together with 9 mg/kg lumefantrine each dose.

Adults less than 34 kg usually take 3 tablets and above 34 kg 4 tablets each dose.

Doses are taken immediately and then 8 hours later, then daily for Days 2 and 3 for routine cases, but twice daily for Days 2 and 3 if multidrug resistant malaria.

Take the drugs with fatty food or milk.

Side effects of lumefantrine have so far not been significant.

Other drugs likely to be used

Piperaquine

Like lumefantrine, piperaquine was developed in China.

It is active against multidrug resistant *P. falciparum*.

The mode of action is not yet clear.

It has so far no recorded significant side effects.

It has been used as a companion drug to dihydroartemisinin (and also trimethoprim and primaquine).

The dose is one 80 mg tablet or capsule immediately, then 8 hours later and once daily on Days 2 and 3 together with dihydroartemisinin in the usual doses.

More information is needed before its place in treatment is known.

Pyronaridine

Pyronaridine has been developed in China.

It is related to amodiaquine but kills multidrug resistant *P. falciparum*.

It has been used in a dose of 1200–1800 mg daily for an adult for 3 days, but there have been problems with its absorption.

It is a drug, however, that is being tested for use with artesunate and if these trials are successful may be used.

Antibiotic drugs with antimalarial activity

- Sulfonamides (e.g. sulfadoxine and sulfamethoxazole).
- Sulfones (e.g. dapsone).
- Tetracyclines (e.g. tetracycline, doxycycline).
- Macrolides (e.g. erythromycin, roxithromycin).
- Clindamycin.
- Quinolones.

See Chapter 11 pages 56–60.

Appendix 4 Method of making insecticide-treated bed nets (ITNs)

Permethrin can be purchased as a 5% emulsifiable concentrate or a wettable powder.

Each square metre of net (m^2) will need 0.5 g of permethrin. A 6 m^2 net will therefore need 3 g permethrin or 6 ml of 50% emulsifiable concentrate or 12 g of wettable powder. Mix this with 150 ml of water.

Place the net in a large plastic bag.

Pour the diluted insecticide on top of the net in the bag, making sure none spills.

Screw up the top of the plastic bag in your hand so that no liquid can come out of the bag.

Squash the net and the fluid in the bag until all the fluid is absorbed into all parts of the net.

Then take the net out and hang it up to dry.

Store the dry net in a plastic bag when it is not being used so that the insecticide stays in it.

A net treated like this will give a lot of protection for 3 months (but only until washed for the third time) from mosquitoes which bite at night.

See also pages 87–88.

If curtains over windows and doorways are also treated like the nets, these will give more protection to those in the house.

14 Tuberculosis

For further information about tuberculosis see:
- *Tuberculosis Care with TB-HIV Co-management* (IMAI), 2007, WHO.
- *TB/HIV. A Clinical Manual*, 2nd edn, 2004, WHO.
- *Treatment of Tuberculosis. Guidelines for National Programs*, 3rd edn, 2003, WHO.
- *Tuberculosis Infection Control in the Era of Expanding HIV Care and Treatment*, 2006, CDC (US), USAID, US PEPFAR, The Union and WHO (addendum to *WHO Guidelines for the Prevention of Tuberculosis in Health Care Facilities in Resource Limited Settings*, 1999, WHO).
- *Guidelines for the Programmatic Management of Drug Resistant Tuberculosis*, 2006, WHO.

Definition, cause, pathology and epidemiology

Tuberculosis (shortened to TB) is a disease which most commonly affects the lungs, but can affect other parts of the body. Man, and sometimes other animals, are affected. It is usually a chronic disease but can be acute.

TB is caused by an infection by a bacterial bacillus called *Mycobacterium tuberculosis,* or occasionally by *M. africanum* or *M. bovis* or other Mycobacteria. When the *M. tuberculosis* bacillus is stained in the laboratory and then covered with acid, it keeps the colour of the stain. Most other organisms lose their colour. *M. tuberculosis* is therefore called an 'acid-fast bacillus', shortened to AFB. (*M. leprae* is also an AFB. See Chapter 15 page 127.)

Infection by *M. tuberculosis* is controlled by the body's immune system and other defences in 90–95% of infected people and the infected person does not develop TB disease. Infection by *M. tuberculosis* is not controlled by the body's immune system, etc. in 5–10% of infected people; the *M. tuberculosis* grows and spreads and damages the body and causes TB disease. If the body's immune system is damaged (e.g. by HIV infection), then 30–50% of these people infected by *M. tuberculosis* develop TB disease before they die.

TB is very common in developing and tropical countries. It is especially common in urban areas and especially where there is poor general health, malnutrition and overcrowding in housing. It is more common if there are not enough public health services to quickly diagnose and treat infectious cases of TB. TB has recently become very common in places where HIV infection is common.

There are about 9 million new infections with *M. tuberculosis* each year (about one each second), about 90% of these being in the developing world. About 30% of the world's population has been infected with *M. tuberculosis*. About 5–10% of healthy people infected with *M. tuberculosis* organisms will develop TB disease from the *M. tuberculosis* organisms during *their whole lifetime*, most (but not all) in the first few years after infection. However, in people who have HIV infection as well as the *M. tuberculosis* infection, about 5–10% will develop TB disease from the *M. tuberculosis* organisms *each year they live*, most (but not all) in the last few years of life with the HIV infection when immunity is greatly decreased; and 50% develop TB disease before they die. In some areas of the developing world, up to half of all new cases of TB are found to have HIV infection also. TB now causes almost 2 million deaths each year.

M. tuberculosis is nearly always spread by persons with TB of the lungs who are not being treated. On average, a person with infective TB infects 10–15 other people each year. Untreated TB patients cough out *M. tuberculosis* organisms in droplets into the air (up to 3000 can be made by one cough), although talking and spitting, etc. can also spread them. When some of the liquid dries off these droplets, they become very small 'droplet nuclei' which can float in the air for hours. The organisms would be killed by sunlight in 5 minutes, but they live for a long time in the dark. These droplets or droplet nuclei can then be inhaled into the respiratory tract of another person. The *M. tuberculosis* organisms then start to grow if the person does not have some immunity to the organism. The greater the number of droplet nuclei in the air and the longer the person breathes the air in which they are present, especially out of sunlight, the greater the number of *M. tuberculosis* organisms that get to the lungs. Sleeping in a closed room at night with a coughing TB patient is therefore very dangerous.

Some immunity against infection with *M. tuberculosis* organisms can be given by previous infection with *M. tuberculosis* from which the person has recovered; or by deliberate immunisation using weak mycobacterial organisms that are able to cause only a skin sore for a couple of weeks but no more disease that this (e.g. BCG).

If *M. tuberculosis* organisms grow in the lungs, they cause a small area of bronchopneumonia. The organisms then spread to the lymph nodes in the chest. They are then carried by the lymph into the blood. Then the blood spreads the organisms to the whole body. In the 1–2 months while this is happening, the body is slowly developing cellular immunity to the organisms (see Chapter 10 page 41). If this immunity develops properly, the body usually then kills the *M. tuberculosis* organisms and the infection heals. This is called '*primary tuberculosis*'. A few organisms may remain alive (in the lungs or any other part of the body to which they spread) for many years or the rest of the person's life and are said to be 'dormant' or are called 'persistors'. But these organisms are usually surrounded by scar tissue and are not able to cause disease. The person has *infection* with tuberculosis but does not have *disease* from tuberculosis (the disease is called TB). His tuberculin test (page 109) would be positive.

'*Post-primary TB*' happens if the organisms start to grow again and escape from their surrounding scar tissue. This can happen at any of the places they spread to in primary tuberculosis. It happens most commonly in the lungs; but it can also happen in lymph glands, meninges, bones and joints, kidneys, etc. This patient then has TB *disease* as well as tuberculosis *infection*.

Post-primary TB becomes less likely as the years after infection go by. It usually occurs in the first 5 years, especially in children. It occurs in 5–10% of infected people.

In post-primary TB, as the patient usually has some immunity to the organisms, the disease is often kept in one organ, but in the fight between the organism and the body's immune system, that organ is often severely damaged, and parts or all of it can be destroyed, forming thick pus (called 'caseation') and leaving holes (called 'cavities') in the organ, especially the lung.

Post-primary TB could also happen if the patient was infected again by an infective TB patient.

Sometimes in primary or post-primary TB, when the organisms get into the blood and spread to many or all organs of the body, they continue to grow and multiply in all these places and cause '*miliary tuberculosis*'.

During primary or post-primary TB, the *M. tuberculosis* organisms can grow without being stopped by the body's defences if the cellular immunity is decreased by malnutrition, another disease such as measles, certain drugs, especially adrenocorticosteroids (e.g. cortisone or prednisolone), and anti-cancer drugs, but most especially if cellular immunity is damaged by HIV infection. The *M. tuberculosis* infection could be just in one organ or miliary TB could occur. These things can happen at any time of a person's life if immunity is decreased.

Figure 14.1 shows the stages of infection with organisms.

Symptoms and signs

Symptoms and signs of TB are caused by:

1. disease of the organ infected by the *M. tuberculosis* organisms – destruction of the organ and the formation of pus in it; and
2. toxins made by the *M. tuberculosis* organisms – causing general symptoms and signs of infection.

The symptoms and signs of primary TB, post-primary TB and miliary TB are outlined in this section.

As explained (see page 101), TB occurs much more commonly in patients with HIV infection. If a patient has symptoms and signs which could be due to TB, look for symptoms and signs which could be due to HIV infection and if possible do counselling and an HIV test. HIV infection can change the symptoms and signs usually caused by TB, as explained in this chapter and Chapter 19.

Primary tuberculosis

The body's defence system usually wins the fight against *M. tuberculosis* before any organ is badly damaged. Usually, there is only a mild febrile illness, the cause of which is not found out by the health worker.

Post-primary tuberculosis

Pulmonary tuberculosis

Symptoms include the following:

1. Chronic cough, almost always. The cough stays and does not go away even after treatment with antibiotics. *Anyone who has a cough for more than 3 weeks and any possibly HIV infected patient who has a cough for more than 2 weeks must have sputum examined for AFB.* Often a cough is the only symptom or sign of TB.
2. Sputum, usually – usually made of pus.
3. Haemoptysis (coughing up blood), sometimes – it can be a large or small amount.
4. Pain in the chest, usually of pleuritic type; but this is not common.
5. Shortness of breath, sometimes. This comes early in the disease if the disease is severe (e.g. miliary

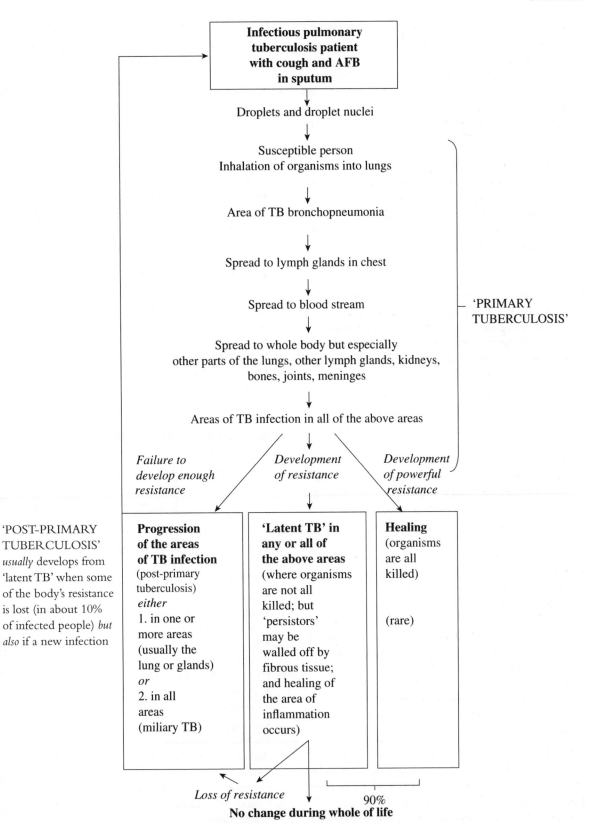

Figure 14.1 *Diagram showing the stages of infection with tuberculosis organisms.*

TB or there is a large pleural effusion); otherwise it comes only after years when most of the lungs are destroyed.

6. Fever, sweating, etc. especially at night. (i.e. general symptoms of infection) – not very common until later in the disease (unless HIV infection).

7. Loss of weight – only if acute severe disease or late disease (unless HIV infection also).

Signs include the following:

1. Sometimes fever; usually only in severe or late disease (more common if HIV infection also).

2. Sometimes wasting and weight loss; usually only in acute severe or late disease (more common if HIV infection).

3. Sometimes anaemia; usually only in acute severe or late disease.

4. Sometimes abnormalities on chest examination; but often not. If abnormalities in the lung are present, they are most likely to be those of upper lobe disease or of pleural effusion. However, patients who also have HIV infection may have pneumonia from TB in the lower lobes of the lung.

Patients with TB can also get ordinary pneumonia or acute bronchitis. When you ask how long patients have had a cough, they often say for only as long as their acute chest infection. They think the previous chronic cough (for more than 2–3 weeks) was normal. Therefore, always ask all patients with acute chest infections if they also had a chronic cough before the start of this present infection. Send sputum from all patients with a chronic cough for AFB tests.

Pneumonia or other chest infection which is unusual or not 'typical' in any way, may be caused by *M. tuberculosis*. Suspect pneumonia of being caused by TB if *any* of the following are true:

1. it is in an upper lobe of the lung, but if the patient has HIV infection the lower lobes may be affected;

2. the signs in the chest are much worse than you expect (possibly because of pleural effusion) because the patient does not seem very 'sick';

3. the pneumonia does not get better as quickly as it should with proper treatment; or

4. the patient had a chronic cough before the start of the pneumonia.

Send three sputum samples or slides from such patients for AFB tests. If the patient is still not cured after 2 weeks of proper treatment, send three more sputum slides for AFB tests (see page 108).

If the patient has these repeated sputum tests negative for AFB and is not cured by proper treatment, then see Chapter 19 pages 225–226 and Chapter 20 pages 290–291 and discuss the case with the Medical Officer. Non-urgent transfer for chest X-ray and other tests may be needed for diagnosis and special treatment may be needed. These conditions include the following:

1. Pneumonia:
   • not properly treated;
   • with complication – pleural fluid, empyema, lung abscess.

2. Unusual lung infection:
   • legionella or mycoplasma or chlamydia or Q fever causing 'atypical pneumonia' needing tetracycline or erythromycin;
   • *Staphylococcus aureus,* especially after influenza needing (di-)cloxacillin;
   • nocardia needing SMX/TMP;
   • aspergillus needing intraconazole;
   • histoplasmosis needing special antifungal treatment.

3. Unusual lung infection present only in certain areas:
   • melioidosis needing special antibiotics;
   • lung fluke needing praziquantel;
   • fungal infections in North America needing special antifungal treatment;
   • brucellosis needing special antibiotics.

4. Opportunistic infections in patients with decreased immunity, especially HIV infection:
   • pneumocystis needing high dose sulfamethoxazole and trimethoprim;
   • cryptococcus
   • penicilliosis
   • candida
   • histoplasmosis } needing special antifungal drugs.

5. Other non-infectious lung diseases:
   • asthma;
   • COPD or chronic bronchitis and emphysema;
   • bronchiectasis;
   • inhaled foreign body;
   • cancer of lung;
   • Kaposi's sarcoma;
   • industrial lung disease.

6. Irritation from worms traveling through lungs:
   • hookworm;
   • roundworms;
   • strongyloides;
   • schistosomiasis, etc.

7. Aspiration (inhaling, breathing in saliva, drink or food):
   • nervous system disease, e.g. stroke with some paralysis of swallowing muscles or not being fully conscious;
   • alcoholism or drug overdose;

- oesophageal disease, e.g. gastro-oesophageal reflux or block from cancer or nerve or muscle disorder.
8. Chronic sinusitis: post-nasal drip.

> Everyone who has had a cough for more than 3 weeks (2 weeks if has HIV infection) *must* have samples of sputum sent for AFB (TB) tests even if the person has no other symptoms or signs (see exception later).

Lymph node (gland) tuberculosis

(see also Chapter 22 pages 334, 340)
Usually children or young adults are affected, but anyone of any age, especially if HIV infected.

Usually neck nodes are affected; but nodes in other areas can be affected (see Figure 14.2).

Usually the only symptom is a lump which does not go away, but gets bigger.

Usually the only sign is enlarged firm lymph nodes which are matted (or joined) together and which are not tender or red or hot. Sometimes there may be a sinus (hole) discharging pus over the nodes.

> Any chronic enlargement of cervical lymph nodes with no obvious cause (e.g. infection in the ENT or face or scalp) which does not improve after antibiotics for 3 weeks, must be aspirated (or biopsied) to look for TB (especially if the tuberculin test is positive).

In HIV infected patients, lymph gland TB may be acute and may look like acute infective lymphangitis.

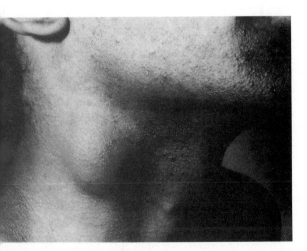

Figure 14.2 *Tuberculous cervical lymphadenitis. An aspiration or biopsy must be done.*

Kidney or urinary tract tuberculosis

(see also Chapter 26 pages 451, 454)
Symptoms are those of an urinary tract infection (pain when, or frequency of passing urine; or kidney pain; or blood in the urine).

Signs are often not present; but there may be kidney tenderness or epididymitis (inflammation of the tubules at the back of the testis).

Tests in the health centre usually show pus or blood or protein in the urine. (Urine collected first thing in the morning on 3 days and sent to the hospital laboratory for examination for AFB and culture for *M. tuberculosis* may show the organism.)

Treatment with trimethoprim and then tetracycline or chloramphenicol does not cure the patient. Refer or non-urgently transfer such patients to a Medical Officer for definite diagnosis and treatment.

> Any patient with a urinary tract infection, which is not cured by proper treatment, must be transferred to a Medical Officer for diagnosis and treatment.

Vertebral tuberculosis

(see also Chapter 29 pages 490–491)
Symptoms and signs include the following.

The patient has back pain and stiffness which lasts for months, which never improves but instead becomes steadily worse.

When you examine the back it is stiff (i.e. it will not bend normally). When you feel (or gently hit with the side of your hand) all along the spine, you will find a tender part.

If no treatment is given the infected bones of the spine collapse and a lump or deformity occurs in the line of the spinal bones (see Figure 14.3).

If treatment is not quickly given, weakness or paralysis or loss of sensation in the legs may occur and the patient may not be able to pass urine (because of pressure on the spinal cord).

Suspect vertebral TB if there is chronic increasing backache with tenderness and stiffness.

Transfer such patients for X-ray and definite diagnosis. If transfer is not possible, start and complete treatment for TB.

> Any patient who has chronic backache which is becoming worse and who has a stiff spine with a tender part, must be transferred for examination for spinal tuberculosis.

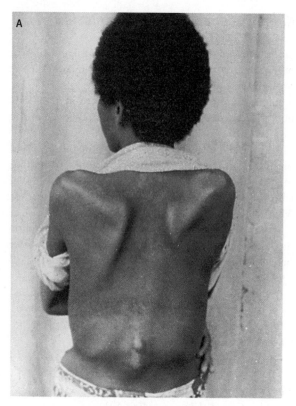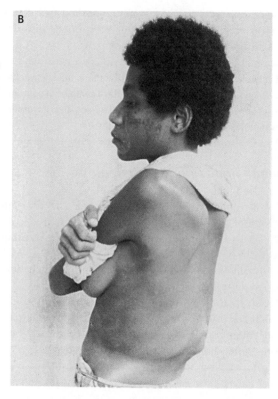

Figure 14.3A and B *Tuberculosis of the spine. Note the deformity of the spine (often called a 'gibbus'). Tuberculosis of the spine is often called 'Pott's disease'. This patient needs urgent transfer for treatment before she becomes paraplegic.*

Tuberculous arthritis (see also Chapter 29 page 489)

The hip or knee joints are most often affected, but any joint can be affected.

Children or young adults are most often affected, but anyone can be affected.

Symptoms are usually chronic continuous pain and stiffness of the joint or a limp which slowly becomes worse.

Signs include:

1. *chronic arthritis which slowly becomes worse* (swelling, tenderness, warmth, pain on moving joint, limited movement of joint, not able to use joint properly, etc.);
2. *wasting of muscles* which move the joint is typical and is *usually* severe (wasting is a very important sign suggesting TB);
3. nearby lymph nodes are usually enlarged;
4. a sinus discharging pus may be present over the joint late in the disease.

Any chronic arthritis which becomes progressively worse over months should be suspected of being tuberculous arthritis.

Transfer all such patients for definite diagnosis.

> Any chronic arthritis (i.e. with inflammation of the joint), which becomes progressively worse over months, should be suspected of being tuberculous arthritis. TB is even more likely if only one joint is involved, nearby muscles are wasted and especially if the tuberculin test is positive. Such cases should be referred or transferred for tests.

Meningeal tuberculosis (see also Chapter 25 page 414 for more details)

Most often the patient is a child, but the patient can be any age.

Symptoms and signs are somewhat like acute bacterial meningitis (see Chapter 25 page 409), but the disease develops much more slowly and is much less severe at first. The history is usually much longer (i.e. days or weeks or months, not a few hours or a day or so). A headache which slowly gets worse (over days or weeks) is usual. A contact may have TB or a chronic cough not yet diagnosed as TB – check the family. The condition is much more common in patients with HIV infection – check for HIV.

At first the patient is not as sick and febrile as you would expect for bacterial meningitis. Symptoms and signs are often even less if the patient has HIV infection also (as body defence and inflammation is less). The patient may have symptoms and signs (including wasting) of TB or HIV elsewhere in his body. Other symptoms and signs of brain damage slowly develop. Alertness decreases, irritability or depression or psychosis may develop, paralysis of eyes, mouth or face muscles can occur, vomiting may develop, walking may become difficult and even paralysis develop and eventually coma leading to death.

The patient, meanwhile, would not have improved, even if proper treatment for bacterial meningitis had been given.

The CSF is sometimes yellow or forms a web after standing; but it can seem normal to naked eye examination. The protein, however, is high and the blood sugar low (see Chapter 25 page 436).

A contact may have TB or a chronic cough not yet diagnosed as TB – check the family. The condition is much more common in patients with HIV infection – check for HIV.

Transfer urgently:

1. all cases with the above history, examination and tests;
2. all cases diagnosed as meningitis or encephalitis or cerebral malaria which do not improve after 2 days of proper treatment; as these patients need definite diagnosis and special drug treatment as TB or cryptococcus or nocardia or toxoplasma or other chronic meningeal infection is likely.

Abdominal (peritoneal, intestinal or lymph node) tuberculosis

Symptoms include: swelling of the abdomen, usually; bowel colic, sometimes; general symptoms of infection, e.g. weight loss, fever, malaise, often.

Signs include: abdominal ascites, usually; masses or tenderness, sometimes; general signs of infection, e.g. fever, weight loss, anaemia, often.

Suspect abdominal tuberculosis in a patient with ascites if:

- no oedema of the back or legs, or
- no response to treatment with diuretics, or
- abdominal masses or tenderness are also present, or
- general signs of infection are present.

Transfer all suspected cases for diagnosis and treatment.

Miliary tuberculosis

This occurs when *M. tuberculosis* organisms spread in the blood throughout the body and then grow in these many places in the body.

The patient may have a family or contact history of TB, suggesting a recent primary infection or he may have a past history of a chronic cough or another condition which suggests post-primary TB. Be very suspicious of this condition if the patient has HIV infection.

Symptoms are usually not specific but are severe – malaise, fever, sweating, weakness, nausea, vomiting, diarrhoea, cough, shortness of breath, headache, etc.

Signs are usually not specific but are severe – not fully conscious, fever, fast pulse, dyspnoea, weight loss, anaemia, large liver or spleen, etc.

Antibiotics and antimalarials do not help the patient who quickly becomes worse.

Transfer such cases urgently if they do not improve with proper treatment for septicaemia (see Chapter 12) and malaria (see Chapter 13 pages 79–86) within 48 hours, as chest X-ray or other tests may be diagnostic and treatment may cure.

Prognosis of untreated tuberculosis

If patients with pulmonary tuberculosis are not treated, within 5 years 50% will be dead, 25% will be alive and well, having overcome the disease themselves by their cellular immunity, and 25% will be alive but sick from the disease and be spreading tuberculosis.

HIV infection and tuberculosis

TB may occur at any stage of an HIV infection (see pages 101–102 and Chapter 19 page 225).

Many people have been infected with *M tuberculosis* but their cellular immunity has stopped the *M. tuberculosis* growing and causing disease, though there are still 'persistors' in the body. If a person like this then gets an HIV infection, once the HIV infection destroys enough of the body's cellular immunity, the 'persistors' can start to grow again and cause TB disease. At other times, a patient may have HIV infection and have poor cellular immunity when infected for the first time with *M. tuberculosis* organisms. This sort of person would not be able to stop these organisms growing and they would quickly cause TB disease. Whereas only 5–10% of people infected with *M. tuberculosis* go on to develop TB disease in their lifetime, if a person has HIV infection, 5–10% of people infected with *M. tuberculosis* develop TB disease each year and 50% in their lifetime.

If the HIV infected person still has some cellular immunity, the TB infection may be just like TB infection in non-HIV patients and is most often in the upper part of the lungs or as described above.

If the HIV infected patient has very poor cellular immunity, then the TB infection may spread quickly into many parts of the body and be different in the following ways:

1. Lung disease may be unusual. It may be more in the lower rather than the upper lung. Sputum for AFB may be negative; but sputum culture may still grow *M. tuberculosis*.
2. Lung disease may be little or none and most of the TB infection may be in other parts of the body. Sputum for AFB may be negative.
3. Lymph node, bowel, meningeal and miliary TB are likely.
4. Meningeal TB may have fewer signs and even fewer CSF changes than expected that suggest meningitis especially early in the condition.
5. The tuberculin test (Mantoux) is often negative.
6. Unusual mycobacterial organisms, which usually do not cause infection and could be resistant to the usual anti-TB drugs can infect these patients.
7. Reactions to anti-TB drugs, especially thioacetazone, are much more common and severe.

If a patient with HIV infection develops a new cough and sputum, which becomes chronic, and it is not due to pneumonia or empyema, these symptoms are often due to TB. If these symptoms do not respond to treatment for pneumonia (see Chapter 20 pages 289–291) and the sputum examination is negative for AFB, then see Chapter 19 pages 224–226 and Chapter 20 pages 290–291 for other possible diagnoses. Also find out from your Medical Officer if you should send these patients to the hospital for a chest X-ray and further investigation, or whether you should start them on anti-TB treatment. If anti-TB drugs are started, unless another diagnosis for the cough and sputum is proven, the whole treatment for TB *must* be given until it is all finished.

Always suspect HIV infection and do counselling and blood tests in:

1. all new patients with TB;
2. all patients with TB when it is not pulmonary or is unusual for TB in any way;
3. any patient with symptoms or signs or conditions suspicious for HIV infection (see pages 107–108).

Tests

Sputum tests for AFB

This is how to do the sputum test for AFB:

1. *Saliva* from the mouth is of *no use* for this test. *Sputum* coughed up *from inside the chest* and spat out is essential.
2. Give the patient a container (such as a bottle or plastic bag), or if one of these is not available, something such as a banana leaf. Get the patient to stand either outside in the open air or alone in a room facing an open window (and never in a closed room, e.g. a toilet). Ask the patient to breathe deeply three times, then to cover his mouth and then to cough deeply when he feels ready to cough. When he coughs deeply to produce sputum, tell him to spit the sputum into the container, holding it close to his mouth.
3. Now look to see if the specimen is suitable for examination. A proper specimen is thick with solid pieces of pus or yellowish material and at least 2–5 ml in volume.
4. If the sputum is not suitable, ask the patient to repeat the process until a good specimen is obtained. At times, it is necessary to give physiotherapy (hit the patient on the back when he coughs or make him bend or lie down with the head lower than the chest and hit his back while he coughs) to get a proper specimen. In the hospital the patient may be given hypertonic (strong) 3% saline (salt) solution nebulised to breathe in to help him cough up the sputum.
5. This first specimen, which you collect when you first see the patient at the health centre, can be called specimen or sample 1 or 'A'.
6. Tell the patient to collect another specimen or sample of sputum in the same way at home immediately when he wakes the next morning and then return with it. This can be called specimen or sample 2 or 'B'.
7. When the patient comes back the next day with the specimen or sample 2 or 'B', collect the third specimen or sample at the health centre. This can be called specimen or sample 3 or 'C'.
8. To make a smear from the sputum specimen, take a clean slide and mark it on the rough end with the patient's name, address, etc. With an applicator stick (or any kind of stick), lift out one or two thick yellow solid pieces of sputum. Then spread this sputum around the other two-thirds of the slide thickly and evenly.

Allow the slide to dry in the air (for about 15 minutes). Make sure it is protected from flies and insects. After it is dry, 'fix' it by passing it three times through the flame of a spirit lamp (or over any non-smoky flame, e.g. over a hurricane lamp if a spirit lamp is not available), until it is just hot enough to be uncomfortable if held on the back of the other hand. Make sure the patient's sputum and name are facing upwards. Place the slide into a slide box, or protect it with another slide tied to it but separated from it by broken applicator or match-sticks. It must be kept away from cockroaches or other insects. Burn the specimen containers and applicator sticks.

Stain the slide for acid-fast bacilli (AFB) by the Ziehl–Neelsen method or other method as taught. Examine under the microscope with oil immersion lens for AFB. Otherwise, send the fixed slide to the laboratory for staining and examination.

The sputum smear will show AFB in almost all cases on at least two of the three slides if the patient has pulmonary TB causing symptoms.

There have to be at least 10,000 AFBs/ml of sputum for any AFBs to be seen on the slides and the report would then be reported as just 'scanty'. The slide is reported as + or ++ or +++ as more and more AFBs are seen and the patient is more and more infectious.

In some early cases, before a bronchus is broken open by the disease, the sputum will be negative. Patients with HIV infection as well as *M. tuberculosis* infection also can have negative sputum tests for AFB (see Chapter 19 pages 224–226). The most common other causes of slides being negative, when, in fact the patient does have pulmonary TB, are:

1. saliva but not sputum was put on the slide,
2. errors were made in the laboratory.

In places where TB is common any patient who has a cough which has lasted for more than 3 weeks (2 weeks in places where HIV infection also common), or who has any other symptoms or signs suggesting pulmonary TB, should have his sputum tested for AFB three times (see above).

If a patient has negative slides for AFB and you still strongly suspect pulmonary TB, do the sputum tests for AFB again. If sputum culture for *M. tuberculosis* is available, send a sputum sample in a bottle for culture. Always remember to counsel and test for HIV infection. Treat with antibiotics for a possible chest infection.

If the patient has these repeated tests negative for AFB, discuss the case with the Medical Officer as non-urgent transfer for chest X-ray and other tests may be needed.

Other causes for chronic cough may need diagnosis and treatment (see Chapter 20 pages 303–304).

If a patient has had a cough for more than 2–3 weeks think of:

1. TB,
2. TB and HIV infection, and
3. HIV infection with unusual organisms causing pneumonia (see Chapter 19 pages 224–226).

Gastric aspirate examination for AFB

This is done for children and adults who are not able to produce sputum. Collect the contents of the stomach aspirated (sucked out) through a nasogastric tube.

Collect three (3) fasting morning specimens.

This test is not as accurate as sputum (false negative and false positive results can occur) and the test is not often used.

Tuberculin test (also called 'Mantoux' test)

Part of dead *M. tuberculosis* organisms called tuberculin or purified protein derivative ('PPD') can be injected intradermally (into the skin). If the body's defence cells have learned to fight mycobacterial organisms, there will be an acute inflammatory reaction in the skin at the site of the injection within a couple of days.

Give PPD 5 units or 0.5 ml by *intradermal* injection only into the front (palm of hand side) of the forearm, where the upper third and middle third would meet. This should raise a small lump in (not under) the skin which should have gone away by 2 hours.

At 48–72 hours, measure and write down on the patient's chart the diameter in mm of the swelling (not the redness).

- 0–9 mm negative except as follows;
- 5–10 mm negative except in patient infected by HIV when probably positive;
- 10+ mm positive (especially if patient has not had BCG).

If the reaction is negative, there is no immune reaction to *M. tuberculosis* organisms; and, as long as the PPD was active and the test was done properly, infection with *M. tuberculosis* is unlikely (but still possible).

A positive reaction means that the body has tried to develop some cellular 'immunity' against mycobacterial organisms: organisms have been in the body in the past or are there at present.

But, remember that:

1. The tuberculin test may be negative when the patient does have active TB disease. Times when this occurs include:
   (a) when the TB infection is very severe, e.g. miliary TB or tuberculous meningitis;
   (b) when another illness is present (especially viral infections such as measles or chickenpox, but also other severe infections);
   (c) when the patient has malnutrition;
   (d) when the patient has HIV infection;
   (e) when the patient is taking certain drugs (especially prednisolone or cortisone-like drugs);
   (f) when the patient has some cancers;
   (g) when the PPD was not reliable, or the test was not done properly.

2. The positive tuberculin test does *not* mean that the patient is sick with TB disease. It means only that *M. tuberculosis* or other very similar mycobacterial organisms are or were alive in his body (i.e. the body has had an infection). Do *not* diagnose TB disease just because the tuberculin test is positive.

3. The positive tuberculin test does not mean the patient is immune to *M. tuberculosis*. It means only that the body has tried to develop some immunity to the mycobacterial infection.

BCG immunisation, which causes an ulcer in a few days (instead of the usual few weeks), has the same meaning as a positive tuberculin test and is called an accelerated BCG reaction.

Lymph node aspiration

This is nearly as accurate (70%) as a biopsy (80%) in diagnosing TB in a lymph node.

Inject local anaesthetic, e.g. 1% lignocaine (lidocaine) into the skin over the node and on top of the node.

Put a large, e.g. 18(–21) gauge needle onto a 5–10 ml syringe. Hold the node between the finger and thumb, or, better still, get an assistant to hold it. Make sure if the needle goes too far, it cannot go into any important structure such as an artery, trachea or especially lung. Push the needle through the skin until it is in the middle of the node held between the finger and thumb. Suck out any material possible into the syringe. If needed, squeeze the node and move the needle in and out of the centre of the node. After taking the needle out of the skin, take it off the syringe, draw 2–3 ml of air into the syringe, put the needle back on the syringe and use the air to push the aspirated fluid out of the needle on to a glass slide. If it is not possible to suck out

any material, put 2–3 ml of sterile 0.9% saline into the syringe, inject the saline into the node and then suck this back. Use this with any other material in the needle or syringe to make a slide. Make the smear on the slide just as you would for sputum for examination for AFB and send this to the laboratory. If pus is aspirated, make a slide for Gram stain. If culture is available, send the aspirate in a closed bottle for culture.

Lymph node biopsy

Lymph nodes near the body surface, i.e. just under the skin and which can be easily held between the finger and thumb – the biopsy can be done at the health centre. However, do not try to do this unless you have been taught to do it and have done it previously under supervision (it is harder to do than it looks).

Deep lymph nodes – refer or transfer to a Medical Officer, for biopsy.

Chest X-ray

A chest X-ray is not possible at most health centres and is usually not necessary for diagnosis.

A normal chest X-ray makes pulmonary TB unlikely.

An abnormal chest X-ray means further tests (mainly sputum for AFB) are needed to see if the abnormality on the X-ray is caused by TB or another disease.

Ask your Medical Officer about a chest X-ray for the following patients.

1. TB suspected in a patient without HIV infection as cough for more than 3 weeks but sputum for AFB × 3 negative on two (or more) occasions;
2. TB suspected in a patient with HIV infection as cough for more than 2 weeks but sputum × 2–3 for AFB negative on one (or more) occasion;
3. TB suspected in a patient without HIV infection but only one sputum smear positive for AFB (and not the required two (or more) smears positive for definite diagnosis) (although only one needed if HIV infection);
4. TB present and a complication develops which you are not able to properly manage in the health centre, e.g. pneumothorax or pleural fluid or heart failure or coughing up of a lot of blood, etc.;
5. TB possible but sputum for AFB x 3 negative on two more occasions, but also other conditions needing diagnosis and treatment likely (see page 104).

HIV counselling and testing

It is best that these be done whenever the diagnosis of TB is considered or made.

These must be done in all patients with TB if the following apply.

1. History and examination makes it possible the patient may have HIV infection (see below);
2. The patient comes from an area where HIV infection is common (HIV prevalence 5% or more, or HIV prevalence in pregnant women 1% or more);
3. The patient has any illness that could be TB which is altered in the way HIV can alter TB (as described in this chapter and Chapter 19).

Diagnostic features

1. A cough that has lasted for more than 2–3 weeks.
2. A chronic cough is especially suspicious when there is also sputum, or haemoptysis, or chest pain, or night sweats or fever or weight loss.
3. Swollen lymph glands in the neck with no obvious cause (especially no ENT or scalp infection) which do not go away after treatment with antibiotics.
4. Tuberculin test usually (but not always) positive. The positive tuberculin test diagnoses only infection (past or present), not disease.

Possibility that patient with tuberculosis also has HIV infection

Whenever a patient has TB diagnosed, always ask yourself if the patient could also have HIV infection.

HIV infection is likely especially if he has a history of, or present evidence of, any of the following:

1. a sexually transmitted disease of any (other) type and/or unsafe sexual practices (see Chapter 19 pages 193–196);
2. previous blood transfusion;
3. non-sterile skin piercing (tattooing, etc.);
4. intravenous drug abuse;
5. persistent generalised lymphadenopathy;
6. itchy macular skin rash of unusual type;
7. minor injuries in the skin causing large infections;
8. herpes zoster, especially if it is in a young person or if it is affecting more than one nerve or if it comes back again soon after it goes;
9. pneumonia, meningitis, septicaemia or other severe bacterial infection, especially if it comes back again after treatment;
10. high fever for which no obvious cause can be found;
11. chronic diarrhoea which does not respond to the usual treatment; and/or

12. progressive weight loss of more than 10 kg or 20% of original weight;
13. candida infection in the mouth or unexplained pain on swallowing which suggests candida of the oesophagus in anyone; and severe and recurrent candida of the vagina in a woman who is not a diabetic;
14. oral hairy leukoplakia;
15. herpes simplex which spreads further than usual, lasts longer than usual or comes back again after it settles;
16. kala azar in someone not expected to get it;
17. Kaposi's sarcoma;
18. burning sensation in the feet from peripheral neuropathy for no obvious cause;
19. unexplained change in behaviour or organic psychosis or unexplained nervous system changes especially without a stiff neck.
20. chronic meningitis or symptoms like a cerebral tumour.

If any history or symptoms or signs suggest that the patient has HIV infection, see Chapter 19 page 236 about counselling and page 233 about doing a blood test for HIV antibodies.

If a patient who has TB also has HIV infection, his TB treatment is not changed and is exactly as if he did not have the HIV infection apart from three things.

1. An HIV positive patient is not given thioacetazone as this drug often causes severe skin rashes in patients who have HIV infection.
2. If trials now being done show that longer treatment (e.g. 8 rather than 6 months for DOTS) is better, then increase the length of the anti-TB treatment (follow your national guidelines).
3. If the HIV infected patient is given anti-retroviral drug treatment, rifampicin can cause significant reactions with some of these drugs and immune reconstitution inflammatory syndrome (IRIS) can occur (see Chapter 19 page 248). If at all possible, anti-retroviral therapy should not be started until after the first 8 weeks of intensive rifampicin containing anti-TB treatment has finished. If this delay is not possible, try to delay at least until after the first 2 weeks of the anti-TB therapy. As well, special anti-HIV drugs may be chosen. (See Chapter 19 page 244.)

If the patient is still alive after the first 2 months of DOTS treatment, it would be expected that his chance of cure of the TB by continuing DOTS treatment would be as good as non-HIV infected patients, although his weight gain will be less. He is, of course, more likely to die than other TB patients. In fact, about 20–30% will die before the TB is cured, but many of these deaths are from other complications of the HIV infection and not due to the TB or its treatment.

If a patient with HIV infection is cured of his TB by DOTS treatment, he is still more likely to get a relapse of the TB (the infection coming back) or a new infection of TB from an infectious TB patient than other TB patients without HIV who are treated. Tests are being done to see if a longer DOTS treatment or isoniazid prophylaxis treatment or other things can help this or not.

Treatment

Special anti-TB drug treatment but only:
• in the correct combination of drugs; and
• in the correct dose; and
• for the correct length of time; and
• as long as all doses are swallowed,

is able to
• cure the patient of TB; and
• stop further damage to the organs of the body; and
• stop the disease coming back; and
• stop the infection spreading to other people; and
• stop the development of drug resistant *M. tuberculosis* organisms.

Unfortunately if the drugs are not given or taken as above:
• the patient is not cured; and
• severe organ damage or death can occur while on treatment; and
• the disease can come back again after apparent cure; and
• others continue to be infected as the *M. tuberculosis* organisms are not all killed; and
• *M. tuberculosis* organisms develop resistance to the drugs and these very dangerous organisms can then spread to others.

The main reason that anti-TB drugs will not work unless given correctly is that in all populations of *M. tuberculosis* organisms, there are occasional organisms which will be resistant to one drug but not to other drugs. If only one drug is used, all the sensitive ones will be killed, but later the resistant one will grow and cause the disease. If two drugs are given, it is unlikely, but possible, there will be some organisms which are resistant to both drugs, and when all other organisms are killed these organisms may grow and

cause disease. If three, and if particularly four drugs are given, this is very unlikely to happen.

If, however, not every single dose of the drugs is taken, organisms which are sick but not killed by the drugs may recover and then be resistant to those drugs from then on; and after all the other organisms are killed, these resistant organisms can grow to cause the disease again. This patient's disease and anyone else who is infected by him, will then not be helped by the drugs to which the *M tuberculosis* organism has become resistant.

To stop the above problems occurring, treatment must be with more than one drug (it is best to give four at the beginning of treatment); and treatment must never be stopped and started and stopped and started, etc. As well as this, various combinations of drugs have been tried out and found to work. Only these combinations should be used. It is not possible to make up a treatment of your own, as there may be a reason you do not know about why your treatment will not work.

The most important things in the treatment of the patient therefore are:

1. Give only the recommended drugs in the recommended combinations. Three or four drugs will be given at the beginning of treatment. Never fewer than two drugs are used even for the continuation of treatment.
   • Never give only one anti-TB drug by itself for treatment of TB disease – at least two are always given together.
   • Never add only one new drug if the patient is not being cured by his drugs. (Two or more new drugs are needed.)
   • Never change the drug combinations or any drug yourself except as specified in your National Anti-tuberculosis Programme.
2. Give only the correct doses which will depend on the patient's size (weight) and other factors.
3. Give these drugs *regularly* for *at least* the shortest amount of time that is needed for them to cure the disease. If rifampicin is not used, this means at least 12 months. If rifampicin is used, this means 9 months. If rifampicin and pyrazinamide are both used, this means 6 months. If HIV infection is also present, tests may later show that these may need to be longer (and never less than 8 months).
4. Make sure that every dose of every drug is taken – you or someone else reliable must watch the patient swallow every dose of every drug for the whole course (i.e. Directly Observed Treatment or 'DOT').

Treatment is divided into two parts:

1. Initial short-term intensive chemotheraphy to try to kill most of the *M. tuberculosis* organisms during this time. Give daily for 8 weeks or, if any drug resistance possible, 12 weeks. Give four (or at least three) drugs; or if any drug resistance possible, five drugs.

2. Continuation or maintenance treatment for 4 or 6 or 10 or more months (depending on what drugs are available for initial short-term intensive chemotherapy and for maintenance therapy) to kill the rest of the organisms, especially the 'persistors'.

This treatment should be:

1. fully supervised treatment every day *or*, in some cases in maintenance treatment, three times weekly: where a health worker watches the patient swallow each drug (i.e. DOT);

2. only very occasionally, and only for some very special reason and only in the maintenance phase, unsupervised home treatment daily where the patient gives the drugs to himself.

WHO and other trials have shown that if a health worker watches to make sure that all patients swallow all doses of the drugs for the whole length of the treatment (directly observed treatment or 'DOT'), then almost every patient is cured by the recommended drugs. These trials have also shown that if a health worker does not watch that all doses of all drugs are swallowed by all patients for the whole course, then many patients are not cured. Some patients who do not have DOT do forget to take some doses or some drugs or stop the drugs before all the course is taken, and are not cured.

The combination of drugs now recommended by WHO is called short-course treatment ('S') because although the length of treatment is still 6(–12) months, this is much shorter than the old 'standard' treatments which were 12–18 or more months. Modern treatment is therefore called 'Directly Observed Treatment Short Course' or 'DOTS'.

Treatment aims to:

1. Cure the patient.
   DOTS does this more quickly.

2. Kill the *M. tuberculosis* organisms as soon as possible before they do further damage to the body.
   DOTS does this more quickly.

3. Kill the *M. tuberculosis* organisms as quickly as possible so that there is less chance of them spreading to other people.
   DOTS does this more quickly.

4. Prevent *M. tuberculosis* organisms becoming resistant to the drugs used.
   DOTS treatment does this best.

Only certain antibiotics kill *M. tuberculosis*.

See Table 14.1 for those antibiotics which are most commonly used.

There is a 'Standard Code' for TB treatment regimens.

The abbreviation for each drug is used (see Table 14.1 page 114).

The initial intensive phase usually 2(–3) months is separated by a '/' from the follow-up continuation phase, usually 4–6 months.

The number before each phase is the length of that phase in months.

The number after each drug abbreviation is the number of times each week the dose of that drug is given. In most cases there is no number, and this means the drug is given every day. If the number is 3, this means the drug is given three times a week (usually Monday, Wednesday and Friday).

Examples;

2SHRZ/6HR

The initial phase is before the '/'.

The initial intensive phase is for 2 months as there is a '2' before the drugs.

The drugs used are streptomycin (S), isoniazid (H), rifampicin (R) and pyrazinamide (Z).

The drugs are given daily as there is no number after each drug.

The continuation phase is for 6 months as there is a '6' before the drugs.

The drugs used are isoniazid (H) and rifampicin (R).

The drugs are given daily as there is no number after each drug.

2SHRZ/4H3R3

The initial phase is as above.

The continuation phase is different.

The continuation phase is for 4 months as the number '4' is before the drugs H and R.

The continuation phase is with isoniazid (H) and rifampicin (R).

The isoniazid is given three times a week as there is a '3' after the H (H3) and the rifampicin is given three times a week as there is a '3' after the R (R3).

Fixed dose combinations (FDC) are when there is more than one drug in each tablet or capsule. In the Standard Code, these drugs are put between brackets, e.g. (HR) – a FDC of isoniazid and rifampicin. Use FDC whenever possible.

FDC makes it easier for the health worker to work out doses.

FDC makes it easier for the patient to take as there are fewer tablets or capsules.

FDC makes it impossible to take just one of the important drugs above (especially rifampicin) (taking just one drug or not taking drugs in the proper combination leads to the *M. tuberculosis* organisms being resistant to that drug).

FDC is most important if direct observation of the patient swallowing the drugs is not completely reliable.

All countries have a National Tuberculosis Programme (NTP) and usually an NTP Manual (book) or policy papers.

In these will be details of:

1. Which patients are to have anti-TB drug treatment;
2. How Directly Observed Treatment is to be carried out;
3. What drugs and doses are to be used in the initial intensive phase;
4. What drugs and doses are to be used in the follow-up phase;
5. What Fixed Dose Combinations (FDC) are to be used;
6. What administrative action is to be taken about registering patients and recording their clinical progress, sputum tests, how well they are taking their drugs, what is being done if patients do not take the drugs, etc.

> YOU MUST FOLLOW YOUR OWN NATIONAL TUBERCULOSIS PROGRAMME.

The following is a management plan for patients with TB. However, if your NTP is different, you must follow your NTP

1. Find out the part or parts of the body infected by TB and if *M. tuberculosis* bacteria were seen (smear for AFB positive) or *M. tuberculosis* grown (culture positive):
   • Pulmonary (lungs). Bacteriologically positive or negative.
   • Extrapulmonary (organs other than the lungs). Bacteriologically positive or negative.
2. Find out if the patient has ever had TB treatment (for a month or more):
   • No previous treatment.
   • Previous treatment; but
   treatment default – patient has missed 2 or more months of treatment in a row,

treatment failure – sputum is still positive after 5 months of treatment,
relapsed – treatment completed and patient 'cured'; but again bacteriologically positive,
other – all other bacteriologically positive cases who have had more than 1 month of TB treatment.

3. Find out:
   • HIV status (if the patient has HIV infection or not);
   • ART (anti-retroviral therapy with drugs for HIV) being taken or not.
4. Choose:
   • Depending on the above.
   • Treatment at the health centre or referral or transfer to Medical Officer for treatment.
   • Which anti-TB drugs to give and for how long they should be given.
5. Remember, with all anti-TB drug regimens:
   • Always give pyridoxine 10 mg daily to all patients to prevent peripheral neuritis and encephalitis from isoniazid.
   • If rifampicin given, oral contraceptives may not be effective and condoms should be used.
   • If pregnant, do not give streptomycin as this may cause deafness in the baby – use ethambutol instead.
   • In all cases, but especially if pregnant, offer HIV testing after counselling as proper management of any HIV infection present will improve the prognosis.
   • If breastfeeding, continue the anti-TB treatment; but give the baby isoniazid for 6 months and when isoniazid ceased, then BCG.
   • Do not start treatment in the health centre, if already taking ART.
   • If any new symptoms, always ask yourself if these could be due to side effects of the anti-TB drugs.

Table 14.1 Drugs used for the treatment of TB.

Anti-TB drug (abbreviation)	Recommended dose in mg/kg (maximum adult daily dose)	
	Daily	Intermittent 3x/week
Isoniazid (H)	5 (300 mg)	10 (600 mg)
Rifampicin (R)	10 (600 mg)	10 (600 mg)
Pyrazinamide (Z)	25 (2 g)	35 (3 g)
Streptomycin (S)	15 (1 g)	15 (1 g)
Ethambutol (E)	15 (1.2 g)	30 (2 g)
Thioacetazone (T)	2.5 (100–150 mg)	not given

Note: abbreviations for 'Standard Code' in brackets; doses, maximum dose in brackets.
See also Table 14.3 page 116 for further details; also Table 14.7 for sizes of tablets used and when not to give these drugs and side effects.

Table 14.2 The usual combination of drugs used in DOTS treatment for tuberculosis.

2 months initial intensive chemotherapy	4–6 months continuation chemotherapy
Isoniazid (H) daily *and* Rifampicin (R) daily *and* Pyrazinamide (Z) daily *and* Ethambutol (E) (or streptomycin (S)) daily	Isoniazid (H) and ethambutol (E) daily for 6 months *or* Isoniazid (H) and rifampicin (R) daily 3 times a week for 4 months *or* Isoniazid (H) and rifampicin (R) daily for 4 months *or* Isoniazid (H) and thioacetazone (T) daily for 6 months (now rarely used)

Note:

1. Only if both rifampicin and pyrazinamide (as well as isoniazid) are used for the first 2 months can the whole course be short (6–8 months).
2. Only if rifampicin (as well as isoniazid) is used for continuation therapy (and only after the above drugs are all used for the first 2 months intensive chemotherapy) can the continuation course be as short as 4 months (and the whole course be as short as 6 months).
3. If the patient has also HIV infection, you may later be told to make these courses longer (and at least 8 months), but this will depend on the results of trials at present being done.
4. Patients with less severe cases of extrapulmonary TB, e.g. lymph node, joint (but not spine), pleural effusion (but only one side and sputum negative) may have only three drugs in the initial 2 months, i.e. HRZ (called WHO category III regime).

IF

1. pulmonary TB
   i.e. pulmonary AFB positive or
       pulmonary AFB negative but
           likely to die before transfer possible AND
2. new patient (i.e. no previous TB drugs) AND
3. HIV negative or positive but not on ART,

THEN

1. treat in the health centre
2. treat with
   2 (HRZE)/4(HR)3, i.e.
   WHO category I regime (Table 14.4)
       and Table 14.3 for doses of drugs
       according to weight.

IF

1. pulmonary AFB positive TB, BUT
   previous treatment and { default, or
   failure, or
   relapse, or
   other previous
   treatment, OR

2. pulmonary AFB negative TB AND
3. HIV negative; or positive not on or on ART,

THEN

1. send sputum for culture and sensitivity for *M. tuberculosis,*
2. transfer or refer the patient to the Medical Officer for treatment
   (except relapses; or AFB positive lymph gland TB but no other TB; and not on ART – these may be started on treatment at the health centre – relapses, category II regime; lymph nodes, category I regime),
3. the usual drug regime is;
   2(HRZE)S/1(HRZE)/(5HR)3E3 or 5(HR)E, i.e. WHO category II regime (Table 14.4 (see page 117) and Table 14.3 page 116 for doses of drugs according to weight).

IF the patient is already on ART for HIV infection,
THEN

1. do not start TB drugs in the health centre;
2. transfer to Medical Officer.
   (See page 121 for reasons why this is so important.)

IF the patient has possible multidrug resistant TB (MDR-TB) or extensively drug resistant TB (EDR-TB),
THEN

1. isolate the patient (see pages 124 and 35),
2. send sputum for *M. tuberculosis* culture and sensitivity test,
3. urgently transfer the patient to Medical Officer care.

IF the patient has TB and also HIV infection,
THEN

1. the patient may or may not need drug treatment for the HIV infection (ART) (see chapter 19 page 244),
2. do **not** start HIV treatment in the health centre – transfer to Medical Officer care,
3. but do start TB treatment as above urgently.

Table 14.3 Recommended treatment regimens for each diagnostic category. (World Health Organization. *Treatment of Tuberculosis. Guidelines for National Programmes,* 3rd edition, Geneva, 2003. See Table 14.4 for patient category.)

Category I regimen

Regimen:	Initial phase (2 months)	Continuation phase (4 or 6 months)	
	2(HRZE)	4(HR)$_3$	6(HE)**
	Daily 56 total doses	3 times per week 48 total doses	Daily 168 total doses
	(Isoniazid 75 mg + rifampicin 150 mg + pyrazinamide 400 mg + ethambutol 275 mg)	(Isoniazid 150 mg + rifampicin 150 mg) for 4 months	(Isoniazid 150 mg + ethambutol 400 mg) for 6 months

Patient's weight:			
30–39 kg	2	2	1.5
40–54 kg	3	3	2
55–70 kg	4	4	3
Over 70 kg	5	5	3

Category II regimen

Regimen:	Initial phase (3 months)		Continuation phase (5 months)	
	2(HRZE)S/1(HRZE)		5(HR)$_3$E$_3$	5(HR)E
	Daily 84 total doses of HRZE plus 56 doses of S		3 times per week 60 total doses	Daily 140 total doses
	(Isoniazid 75 mg + rifampicin 150 mg + pyrazinamide 400 mg + ethambutol 275 mg)	Streptomycin (vials, IM) 2 months	(Isoniazid 150 mg + rifampicin 150 mg) + ethambutol 400 mg	(Isoniazid 150 mg + ethambutol 400 mg) + ethambutol 400 mg

Patient's weight:				
30–39 kg	2	0.500	2 + 2	2 + 1.5
40–54 kg	3	0.750	3 + 4	3 + 2
55–70 kg	4	1 g*	4 + 6	4 + 3
Over 70 kg	5	1 g*	5 + 6	5 + 3

*750 mg for patients aged over 60 years

Category III regimen

Regimen:	Initial phase (2 months)	Continuation phase (4 or 6 months)	
	2(HRZ)	4(HR)$_3$	6(HE)**
	Daily 56 total doses	3 times per week 48 total doses	Daily 168 total doses
	(Isoniazid 75 mg + rifampicin 150 mg + pyrazinamide 400 mg)	(Isoniazid 150 mg + rifampicin 150 mg) for 4 months	(Isoniazid 150 mg + ethambutol 400 mg) for 6 months

Patient's weight:			
30–39 kg	2	2	1.5
40–54 kg	3	3	2
55–70 kg	4	4	3
Over 70 kg	5	5	3

**Regimens in grey with 6 HE daily in the continuation phase may be associated with a higher rate of treatment failure and relapse compared with the 6-month regimen with rifampicin in the continuation phase.

Table 14.4 WHO recommendations for selecting patient TB category. (World Health Organization. *Tuberculosis Care with TB-HIV Co-management* (IMAI), 2007, page 26.)

Disease site	Laboratory results	Type of patient		Recommended treatment category
Pulmonary	Sputum smear-positive[a]	New		CAT I
		Previously treated	Relapse	CAT II
			Treatment after failure	CAT II
			Treatment after default	Usually CAT II
			Chronic or MDR-TB	CAT IV
	Sputum smear-negative[b]			CAT I or III[c]
Extrapulmonary[b]				CAT I or III[c]

A doctor/Medical Officer diagnoses and prescribes treatment for cases in the shaded boxes. Either a health worker or a doctor/Medical Officer can select the treatment category for the other cases (unshaded). This is based on the disease classification (site), laboratory results, type of patient, HIV status and recommendations in National Guidelines.

a If only one sputum sample is positive, the HIV positive patient is considered to be smear-positive. The HIV negative patient should be referred to a clinician for diagnosis.

b Pulmonary sputum smear-negative cases and extrapulmonary cases may rarely be previously treated (treatment after failure, relapse, treatment after default, chronic). Diagnosis should be based on bacteriological and pathological evidence.

c As recommended by WHO, category III treatment may be the same regimen as for category I. Each country will decide whether category I and III are different drug regimens or not. If they are different, the selection of a regimen for a particular patient will depend on the severity of the disease.

Drugs given to kill *Mycobacterium tuberculosis* are powerful drugs, which sometimes have side effects.

Some side effects are mild and will be ignored by the patient if they are explained to him. Other side effects are serious and can be fatal (Figure 14.4). If serious side effects occur, you must talk to your Medical Officer about changing the treatment (see Tables 14.5 and 14.6).

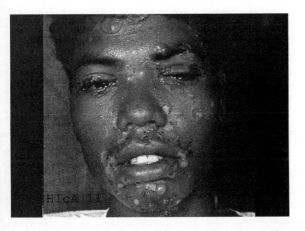

Figure 14.4 *A typical case of the severe, life-threatening skin rash (Stevens–Johnson Syndrome) that can be caused by thioacetazone. It seems to be more common in some populations than others. It is much more common if the patient also has HIV infection. Do not give thioacetazone to patients who may have HIV infection. (Source: TALC)*

Table 14.5 Symptoms which may be side effects of anti-TB drugs and what to do about them. (Adapted from A.D. Harries and D. Maher (1996) *TB/HIV: A Clinical Manual.* Geneva, WHO)

Side effects	Drug(s) probably responsible	Management
Minor		**Continue anti-TB drugs**
Loss of appetite, nausea, abdominal pain	Rifampicin	Give tablets last thing at night but still without food
Joint pains	Pyrazinamide	Acetylsalicylic acid or non-steroidal anti-inflammatory drug
Burning sensation in feet	Isoniazid	Pyridoxine 50 mg daily
Orange/red urine	Rifampicin	Reassurance
Itch but no rash	Thioacetazone, streptomycin, or others	Stop thioacetazone and streptomycin
Major		**Stop drugs responsible**
Skin rash	Thioacetazone, streptomycin, all others if not these	Stop all anti-TB drugs and transfer to MO urgently
Deafness (no wax blocking canal)	Streptomycin	Stop streptomycin, use ethambutol instead
Dizziness/vertigo/nystagmus	Streptomycin	Stop streptomycin, use ethambutol instead
Jaundice (other causes excluded)	Most anti-TB drugs	Stop all anti-TB drugs and transfer to MO urgently
Vomiting and confusion (possible drug-induced early severe hepatitis, before jaundice)	Most anti-TB drugs	Stop all anti-TB drugs, transfer to MO urgently, if no other cause found able to be treated (e.g. malaria, meningitis, etc.)
Difficulty seeing or loss of colour vision	Ethambutol	Stop ethambutol and transfer to MO
Generalised, including shock and bleeding	Rifampicin	Stop rifampicin and transfer very urgently to MO

Table 14.6 Anti-TB drugs and common side effects to watch for and what action to take. (Tables from *Guidelines to Rational Drug Use* by Fr von Massow & R. Korte © 1997, reprinted by permission of Macmillan Education)

Drug/Tablet size	Do not give if	Side effects	Notes
Isoniazid 50 mg alone tablet 100 mg alone tablet 300 mg alone tablet	• Allergy to it • Hepatitis	• Encephalitis/fits • Peripheral neuritis (loss of feeling or movement in legs and arms) • Jaundice/hepatitis	• Pyridoxine prevents (stops) nervous system side effects • Stop if hepatitis and transfer to MO
Rifampicin 150 mg alone 300 mg alone (can be tablet or capsule)	• Allergy to it • Hepatitis	• Jaundice/hepatitis • Fever/flu like symptoms • Bleeding due to platelet damage (rare) • Shock (rare) • Red urine and tears always • Stops oral contraceptives working • GI symptoms	• Stop if jaundice or hepatitis or bleeding or shock and transfer to MO • Advice about contraceptives • Give dose at night if nausea, abdominal pain, etc.

Table 14.6 *(continued)*

Drug/Tablet size	Do not give if	Side effects	Notes
Pyrazinamide 400 mg tablet 150 mg dispersable tablet 150 mg tablet	• Allergy to it • Hepatitis	• Nausea/vomiting • Joint pain/gout • Hepatitis	• Anti-nauseants p.r.n. and/or give at night • Give aspirin for mild arthritis • Stop if severe gout and transfer to MO • Stop if hepatitis and transfer to MO
Streptomycin powder to be dissolved for IMI injection 1 g vial	• Allergy to it • Already deaf • Pregnancy • Not able to ensure needles and syringes sterilised properly • Kidney damage/renal failure	• Dizziness and 'pins and needles' at time of injection not important • Dizziness all the time especially if eyes closed or in dark, important • Deafness • Kidney damage	• Stop if getting dizzy or unsteady on feet (e.g. heel toe walking in a straight line) or any loss of hearing and change to ethambutol • Check with MO about reduced dose if any kidney disease
Ethambutol 100 mg tablet 400 mg tablet	• Allergy to it • Poor vision even if wears spectacles • Kidney damage/renal failure • Young children who are not able to tell you if sight affected	• Rashes • Nausea/vomiting • Loss of vision	• Stop if sight getting worse – check vision with chart before starting treatment and each review • Check with MO about reduced dose if kidney disease
Thioacetazone 50 mg 150 mg 150 mg with 300 mg isoniazid	• Allergy to it • It has been proven to have a lot of side effects in your population • Patient has also HIV infection	• Nausea/vomiting • Rashes which can be severe and damage all skin and mucous membranes of mouth, etc.	• Stop if itch or rash and transfer to MO if rash gets worse • Use ethambutol instead if patient has HIV infection
Rifampicin + isoniazid tablets 60 mg + 30 mg 150 mg + 75 mg 300 mg + 150 mg 60 mg + 60 mg 150 mg + 150 mg	• See both rifampicin and isoniazid	• As for both rifampicin and isoniazid	• For daily treatment • For three times a week treatment
Isoniazid + ethambutol tablets 150 mg + 400 mg	• See both isoniazid and ethambutol	• As for both isoniazid and ethambutol	
Rifampicin + isoniazid + ethambutol tablet 150 mg + 75 mg + 275 mg	• See rifampicin and isoniazid and ethambutol	• As for rifampicin and isoniazid and ethambutol	

Table 14.6 *(continued)*

Drug/Tablet size	Do not give if	Side effects	Notes

Rifampicin + isoniazid + pyrazinamide tablet
  60 mg + 30 mg + 150 mg
  150 mg + 75 mg + 400 mg
 	
  150 mg + 150 mg
  + 500 mg
	• See rifampicin and isoniazid and pyrazinamide	• As for rifampicin and isoniazid and pyrazinamide	
			
			• For daily treatment
			
			• For three times a week treatment

Rifampicin + isoniazid + pyrazinamide + ethambutol tablet
  150 mg + 75 mg +
  400 mg + 275 mg
	• See rifampicin and isoniazid and pyrazinamide and ethambutol	• As for rifampicin and isoniazid and pyrazinamide and ethambutol	

Remember the following important points about treatment of all tuberculosis patients

1. Do not start drug treatment unless:
   • sputum is positive for AFB; *or*
   • lymph gland (or other) aspirate or biopsy is positive for TB; *or*
   • patient has suspected severe TB and would die before test results could be obtained or transfer was possible (diagnosis *must* later be confirmed in these cases or the full length of treatment completed); *or*
   • TB has been diagnosed by a Medical Officer in another way.
2. Always do a full medical history and physical examination and test the urine first.
   Diagnose and treat any other conditions present, especially anaemia, other bacterial chest infections, malnutrition, etc. but especially HIV infection.
3. Choose drug treatment only according to your National Tuberculosis Programme.
   Make sure you arrange the patient's DOTS
   • at a place which is close to his home (or work) and easy and quick for him to get to;
   • with a health worker or other person who is acceptable to the patient;
   • in a way which does not keep him from working a long time (although he may be admitted first for the initial short-term intensive treatment).
4. Register the patient and do all the administrative duties required by your NTP.
5. If the patient is a woman in the child bearing years, tell her that rifampicin is likely to stop oral hormonal contraceptives from working and that she should use other means of contraception (usually condoms) until the treatment of TB is finished.
6. Start patient and family education about TB. See page 122.
7. Arrange for contact education, examination, tests and treatment. See page 122.
8. Check the patient's attendances for DOTS treatment each month.
   If he is not having DOTS, when he comes back for a new supply of drugs, remember to check the number of pills left over. This will tell you whether he has taken all the doses. If he has not, ask him in a sympathetic way, why. This will help you to give him the right advice about taking his full treatment. However, it would be best to have him changed to DOTS.
9. Arrange for a home visit if the patient does not attend for every treatment or does not return for review. This must be done in a sympathetic and friendly way to persuade the patient to take his treatment or come back for review. This can be done by a specially trained non-health worker as well as a health worker. It is important to know the patient's correct address. An illiterate patient may need the postman to write it down. It is best to also know the name and address of a relative who lives nearby or a shop which the patient uses regularly.
10. Make sure you never stop any or all of a patient's anti-TB treatment and do nothing more about it. The patient must have other drugs put in the place of any drugs stopped and you should always talk to your Medical Officer about this. If all anti-TB drugs have to be stopped, urgently transfer the patient to the Medical Officer for further care, unless the patient is about to die and shortly does die.

11. Make sure each month, by reviewing your records, that none of your patients stop their treatment and do *nothing more about it*.

    If not sure, arrange for a visit to solve any problem that is stopping regular treatment.

12. Make sure that you do or send progress sputum tests from those patients who had a positive sputum at the beginning of the treatment:
    - at 2 months (at the end of the intensive phase of treatment),
    - at 3 months if the test at 2 months was not negative,
    - at 5 months,
    - at the end of treatment.

    If the sputum is still positive at the end of the initial intensive phase, many programmes recommend continuing the intensive phase for 4 more weeks and then repeat the sputum tests; they then go to the continuation phase no matter what the sputum results.

    If the sputum is not negative at the end of 5 months the treatment has failed. The most common cause is that the patient is not taking the treatment correctly. The most serious cause is that the tuberculosis organisms are resistant to the drugs. It is essential that you immediately report such cases to your Medical Officer, who must organise sputum culture and drug sensitivity tests and organise for the patient to be treated as a category II or IV patient. See also page 123 about multidrug resistant TB (MDR-TB) and extensively drug resistant TB (EDR-TB).

    If the sputum smears are negative at the end of treatment and on one other previous occasion, the patient is said to be 'cured'. All other patients should be discussed with your Medical Officer.

13. Make sure that you do all the recording and reporting needed by your Health Department.

    They can then see how your patients are doing and give you help if needed. It also shows how the tuberculosis control programme in the country is going and what changes may need to be made.

Note the following special things about tuberculosis and HIV infection

If the patient with TB also has HIV infection the following things must be done.

1. Watch for reactions to anti-TB drugs as these are more common; but most occur in the first 2 months.

2. Do not use thioacetazone as HIV positive patients have more skin reactions to it.

3. Consider the following patients for anti-HIV treatment (anti-retroviral therapy or ART).

    If no CD4 count possible:
    - Stage 4
    - Stage 3
    - Stage 2 and total lymphocyte count less than 1200/mm^3.

    If CD4 count available:
    - Stage 4; any count
    - Stage 3; if count <350 mm^3
    - Stage 2; if count <200 mm^3
    - Stage 1; if count <200 mm^3,

    unless the patient also has some kidney or liver disease or other incurable disease, but see also 5 below.

4. There are problems using ART and anti-TB drugs together.
    - Rifampicin and NNRTIs especially NVP together can cause liver and skin side effects.
    - Immune reconstitution syndrome (IRIS) can occur (see Chapter 19 pages 244 and 248).
    - Isoniazid and d4T can both cause peripheral neuropathy and are best not used together.

5. If it is not essential to treat the HIV infection immediately, if the patient is unlikely to die during the 6–8 months of anti-TB treatment with disseminated TB or stage 4 or 3 HIV infection, it is usually best to treat the TB infection first and treat the HIV infection later.

    If at all possible, try to at least get the initial 2 months intensive anti-TB chemotherapy given when rifampicin is used, before starting anti-HIV treatment; and if this is not possible, at least the first 2 weeks. This delay will decrease the chance and severity of the drug interactions and IRIS (see Chapter 19 page 248).

6. If ART and anti-TB treatment are both immediately needed by the patient, consider drug combinations such as EFV rather than NVP with two NNRTIs or 3 NRTIs together with his anti-TB treatment.

7. If the patient is already on ART when a sputum smear for AFB is positive or when a smear-negative TB is suspected, transfer the patient to Medical Officer at the hospital for the treatment plan. This is because there are many possibilities and potential problems, e.g. ART treatment failure; TB reinfection or reactivation; active TB causing symptoms and signs as the result of immune reconstitution inflammatory syndrome

(IRIS); drug interactions; and ART may need to be switched.

8. The patient with HIV is also likely to get other infections, especially pneumococcal respiratory (and other) infections and non-typhoid salmonella gastrointestinal and blood infections (see Chapter 19). If a patient with HIV on treatment for TB becomes worse, always look for other infections and treat them with penicillin and, if needed, chloramphenicol.

9. The patient with HIV infection would need chemoprophylaxis with co-trimoxazole, i.e. trimethoprim 160 mg and sulfamethoxazole 800 mg daily if:
   • no CD4 count available but clinical stage 4 or 3 or 2;
   • CD4 count available and <350 mm³ and stage 1 or 2; but any count if clinical stage 3 or 4.

10. *If a patient has HIV infection but does not have TB, he is very likely to develop TB if infected with M. tuberculosis.* Try to prevent this happening.
    • Diagnose and treat patients with infectious TB (sputum positive) as quickly as possible. This is the best way of stopping TB spreading;
    • Health workers with HIV infection should not work in TB or medical wards where there may be infectious TB patients;
    • Patients with HIV infection should never be admitted to a TB ward unless they have been diagnosed as suffering from TB and are immediately started on anti-TB treatment;
    • Good ventilation and a lot of sunlight will reduce infection;
    • If patients with infectious TB wear face masks until they have become non-infectious (2 weeks after starting anti-TB therapy) when near HIV patients, this will decrease infections (the wearing of face masks by health workers and HIV patients does not give much protection against TB);
    • Patients with TB should cover their mouths when coughing, not spit on the ground or floor, and they should use tissues or sputum containers with lids which are later buried or burned.

Note on health education and contact tracing

The patient

Always be kind, friendly and patient.

Teach the patient about the disease and also the need for regular treatment until it is all finished. Show the patient the kind of pills he will take and how to take them. Get the patient to remember the month and the year he should finish treatment (if all goes well). Use the local calendar if this is understood better. You may need to explain about local beliefs about TB and its treatment.

Tell him if he does not take treatment the disease will destroy his lungs and infect others. Tell him if he takes regular treatment he will be cured and he will not infect others.

Tell him to come to the treatment centre immediately if he gets itch, rash, blisters, nausea, fever, jaundice, etc. Explain why he must not just stop the drugs. Explain how you can help.

If possible, give him a leaflet or book explaining all the above for him to take home to read.

Tell him to tell the treatment centre if he intends to move to another place or go on holiday.

Ask if he has any worries or questions, and answer them.

Family, other contacts and community education

Contact follow-up is done once the health system is able to give early diagnosis and proper treatment to most infectious TB patients.

All contacts (family, those who live in the same house, friends, workmates, schoolmates, etc.) should be seen.

Educate them about the symptoms of the disease and tell them that drugs cure it and tell them to come back if symptoms develop.

Question and examine them for cough, enlarged lymph glands and wasting, etc. Any who have chronic cough or other symptoms or signs should have sputum tested for AFB, and aspirate (or biopsy) of any enlarged lymph nodes.

If tuberculin testing is available, do this in children aged 5 years or less. If X-rays are available, do these in children who cannot produce sputum; or adults with a cough who do not produce sputum or have sputum for AFB × 3 negative; or other things suggestive of TB.

Give any child under 5 years who has a positive tuberculin test but is otherwise well, prophylactic isoniazid for 6 months. Give newborn (and probably all young children), who are close household contacts of infectious sputum-positive pulmonary TB patients, prophylactic isoniazid 5 mg/kg even if the tuberculin test is negative (especially if the patient is the mother). *(Make sure that the child does not have TB disease, as then the child needs not just one anti-TB drug but needs proper 3 drug treatment for TB disease.)*

Give BCG to other well children who have a negative tuberculin test.

Educate everyone to come to the health centre if symptoms develop.

Explain to all the family and contacts how TB can be treated and how they can help the patient and make sure he or she gets regular treatment.

Transfer

Transfer to Medical Officer care any of the following:

1. patients who are strongly suspected of having TB, but you cannot prove the diagnosis at the health centre;
2. patients who develop serious drug reactions (urgent);
3. patients with complications, especially significant haemoptysis (urgent);
4. patients with suspected drug resistant infection, i.e. patients who continue to have positive sputum for AFB after 5 months supervised regular treatment which you know has been given and taken (non-urgent);
5. Patients with HIV infection and also TB if ART is likely to help (see page 121). You should not start ART at the health centre. Meanwhile, immediately start anti-TB treatment.

Control and prevention
Get rid of the reservoir of infection

Persons with infectious pulmonary TB who are not on drug treatment spread the disease by coughing. Each such patient infects about 10–15 other persons each year.

Almost as soon as a patient starts on effective anti-TB drugs (certainly by 2 weeks), he becomes non-infectious.

If all pulmonary cases of TB could be found and kept on treatment, the disease could no longer spread.

The WHO aim or target adopted by many countries is:

1. to detect (or find and diagnose) at least 70% of those people with TB disease and sputum smear positive for AFB.
2. to cure 85% of the sputum positive cases found – the most important aim. If this is done (even though not perfectly), there will be:
   • rapid decrease of TB prevalence (total number of infected people) and mortality (number of people dying) and transmission (spread of the infection);

• gradual (or slow) decrease in TB incidence (number of new cases);
• less drug resistance.

Make certain, therefore, that you always do the following:

1. Every time you see any patient for any reason, ask if he has a cough. If it has been present for more than 3 weeks (2 weeks if the patient has, or is likely to have, HIV infection), send sputum for AFB;
2. Make sure every patient you know about with TB is put on effective anti-TB treatment.
3. Make sure that anyone in your care who is started on anti-TB treatment takes every dose until the sputum becomes negative and the course is finished and the patient is cured.
4. Once a case is found, as long as you are going to make certain this person takes all his treatment until he is cured, examine all the patient's contacts to find who gave him the disease and to whom he has given the disease, before they spread it further (see above).

The most dangerous *M. tuberculosis* organisms are those which have become resistant to one or more of the anti-TB drugs, **i.e. multidrug resistant TB organisms (MDR-TB)**. At present, in most places there are still other drugs which can kill these MDR-TB organisms; but these drugs are expensive and have many side effects and may need long (18–24 months or more) treatment and the patients need Medical Officer care and possibly hospital care, i.e. DOTS Plus Strategy.

If all of these things are not done, the MDR-TB may become resistant to all our anti-TB drugs, **i.e. become extensively drug resistant TB (EDR-TB)**. This has happened in some places such as eastern Europe and probably many developing countries. Such EDR-TB organisms are likely to kill most patients they infect and also kill many of the family and friends and health workers to whom they spread the EDR-TB. It is possible these could spread all over the world and cause a pandemic. We must therefore find patients with the MDR-TB and cure them while the MDR-TB organisms are still sensitive to the drugs we have.

Besides making sure you do all of the above four things to stop the spread of MDR-TB, make sure that if a patient still has sputum positive for AFB after 5 months of DOTS (or other treatment):

1. never let him continue to do as he is doing (taking treatment regularly or irregularly or not at all);
2. always find out if he is taking his treatment regu-

larly and in the correct dose; and if he is not, take action to get him to do so;

3. always arrange for sputum to be collected and sent to the laboratory for *M. tuberculosis* culture and sensitivity tests and if possible blood for an HIV test;

4. always get the Medical Officer to see the patient (transfer the patient if needed) to give whatever drugs are needed to kill these possibly dangerous organisms and to decide whether other treatment such as surgery (to cut out the part of the lung containing the MDR-TB) is needed.

Stop the means of spread of the organisms

Help educate the public about ways to stop droplet and airborne spread in the community.

1. Educate everyone to cover their mouth (and nose) when coughing (or sneezing), with a tissue or handkerchief or at least the inside of their arm (not their hands). Educate everyone not to spit onto the ground but into a tissue or handkerchief or container with a lid. Tissues and containers should later be burned and handkerchiefs boiled or disinfected.

2. Encourage people to make houses with good ventilation (airflow through the house) to carry droplets and droplet nuclei out of the house, i.e. with a lot of windows which are left open. Encourage people to have as few persons as possible sleep in any one room.

Make sure droplet and airborne spread is as little as possible in your health centre.

1. If possible get all patients to wait under cover but not inside a room, i.e. wait on a verandah or in a building with a roof but no walls.

2. Get a health worker to ask all patients as they arrive if they have had a cough for more than 2–3 weeks. If so, get these patients to sit in another well-ventilated area away from other patients and see them as soon as possible.

3. Tell patients with a cough to cover their mouths when coughing and not to spit. Supply the patients with tissues or give them a surgical mask to wear to make the patients less infectious. (If staff or other patients wear a mask, this mask is not very effective in stopping the staff or patients getting infected.)

4. Immediately do sputum tests for AFB or other tests needed for the coughing patients. Give counselling about HIV infection and recommend, and if possible immediately do, HIV testing. Diagnose and treat also any other condition the patient has. As soon as possible send the patient home with an appointment for follow-up for the AFB and HIV test results.

5. In the health centre wards, keep possible TB patients and known TB patients who have not had 2 weeks of treatment and become non-infectious away from other patients in a well-ventilated area. Most importantly, do not put these patients together in the same room or ward with patients who do, or may have, decreased immunity from HIV infection.

6. Start TB treatment immediately the diagnosis of TB is made.

7. Make sure that the place where health workers see patients is well ventilated. Airflow should be from behind the health worker toward the patient and then to the outside of the building where no other people will be. Use the usual wind or airflow. If needed, put a fan in a window behind the patient, to make the air flow in the best direction. See Figure 14.5.

Make sure that special groups of people do not spread *M. tuberculosis* in your health centre. Health workers:

1. Teach all workers that if they get a cough which lasts for more than 2–3 weeks, they must send sputum tests for AFB (regular chest X-rays, etc. are not as helpful).

2. Encourage all workers to get an HIV test. If the test is positive, give them work where they are less likely to be infected by *M. tuberculosis* and get them seen by the Medical Officer about HIV drug treatment and prophylactic isoniazid treatment.

Patients who have or may have multidrug resistant TB (see page 121):

1. Keep these patients apart from all other patients in a well ventilated area and stop other people sleeping in the same room.

2. Send these patients urgently to the Medical Officer for assessment and special drug treatment.

Raise the resistance of susceptible persons

The resistance of the general population can be raised by general public health measures (malaria control, prevention of malnutrition, treatment of anaemia, prevention of measles and whooping cough by vaccination, and especially prevention of HIV infection). Do all you can to stop HIV infection spreading in your community. HIV infection is the main reason TB is becoming more and more common today. See page 101.

The resistance of some individual persons may be

O = patient
X = health worker

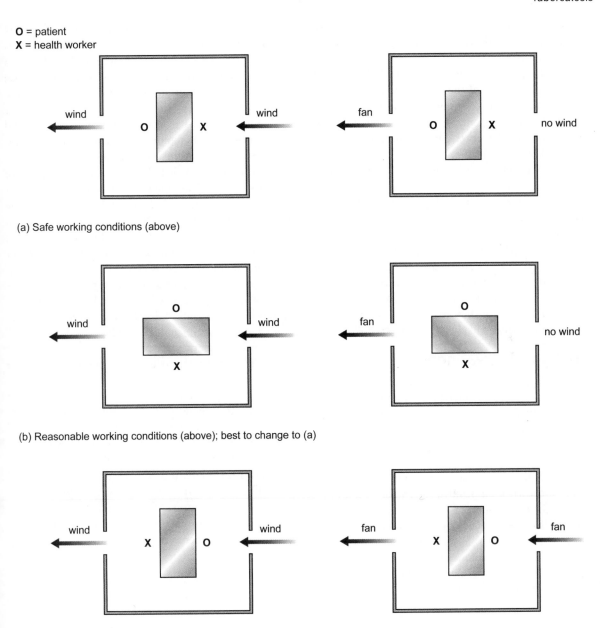

(a) Safe working conditions (above)

(b) Reasonable working conditions (above); best to change to (a)

(c) Unsafe working conditions (above); must change (preferably to (a))

Figure 14.5 *How to arrange rooms to see patients safely (see (a) above). Do not allow rooms to be arranged unsafely (as in (c)). (Reproduced from Tuberculosis Infection Control in the Era of Expanding HIV Care and Treatment, Appendix B Information on ventilation and fans 2006, by permission of WHO.)*

greatly increased by BCG immunisation given before TB infection usually happens.

BCG (bacillus Calmette-Guérin) is the name given to a type of *Mycobacterium bovis* organism. When these are injected into the skin they usually cause only a skin sore which is overcome by the normal body's cellular immunity and heals in some weeks. The body's cel-lular immunity system may partly learn how to fight *Mycobacterium tuberculosis* when it is learning to fight the BCG mycobacteria and the person is then less likely to get TB *disease* after tuberculosis *infection*.

Surveys have suggested it has little effect in adults. They also suggest that it may not reduce the number of infections in children but does stop the organisms spreading as early in the body and there are fewer cases of miliary and meningeal TB in children who have had BCG.

Complications are very rare. They include it spreading onto other parts of the skin if the child has dermatitis or eczema (do not give to children with more than mild eczema). It only very occasionally spreads to the lymph nodes or other parts of the body (but can be treated by anti-TB drugs).

Give BCG 0.05 ml intradermally to all newborns and those under 3 months of age and 0.1 ml intradermally to other children. The risk of complications is less than the risk of TB in countries where TB is common even in children with HIV, unless the HIV is stage 3 or 4 when BCG is not given.

Make sure all children have all their expanded programme of immunisation vaccines. Preventing measles and whooping cough will stop the reduction in cellular immunity these diseases cause (when the child would be more likely to get TB disease).

Prophylactic treatment

Give prophylactic treatment to particular people who have been contacts of infectious patients, and therefore may have been infected. This treatment is to kill the few organisms in any infected contact before the organisms multiply and produce clinical *disease*.

In most places prophylactic treatment is given only to children under 5–7 years of age with *M. tuberculosis* infection shown by a positive tuberculin test and no evidence of TB disease.

It is also given to newborn children (and probably best given also to all children under the age of 3) who are household contacts of sputum-positive TB patients (especially if this person is the mother) even if the tuberculin test is negative.

These children are given isoniazid 5 mg/kg daily for 6 months. Do not give isoniazid alone if there is any evidence of TB disease (as well as *M. tuberculosis* infection); give instead full treatment for TB. If the child was tuberculin negative, give BCG after the course of isoniazid is finished.

Do not treat with isoniazid adults who are well and have a positive tuberculin test (as this would mean in some places most of the population would need treatment, although only 5–10% of patients with a positive Mantoux from *M. tuberculosis* infection would ever get TB disease during their lifetime and most of these would have got it in the first 5 years after infection – not in adult life). A more worthwhile use of the effort and money would be to find infectious patients and treat them all with DOTS.

There are reasons for and against giving prophylactic isoniazid to patients with HIV who have been infected or may be infected with *M. tuberculosis* (but do not have TB disease) and those who have been 'cured' after anti-TB therapy. At present, the reason for not giving it in many countries is that the patient has not had X-rays and other tests to make sure he does not have TB infection and need full treatment and not just isoniazid. Also, many patients may not continue the drug. Both of these things could lead to *M. tuberculosis* becoming resistant to isoniazid. Special groups (e.g. health workers with HIV infection who may be exposed to TB patients and who are assessed by a Medical Officer) possibly should be offered prophylactic isoniazid. More groups of patients will possibly later be given this treatment. (See the recommendations in your National Tuberculosis Programme.)

15 Leprosy

Definition

Leprosy is a chronic bacterial infection of man. It is common only in parts of the world where infectious patients are not diagnosed and treated quickly (and continue to spread the organisms), and where there is poverty, overcrowding (with more contact with infectious patients) and poor general health (with less resistance by the immune system once infection has occurred). The infection causes chronic inflammation and destruction of the skin and the peripheral nerves. Sometimes it can also cause inflammation and destruction of the eyes, the mucous membrane of the upper respiratory tract, the muscles, the bones, the testes and other organs. Multidrug therapy is able to cure the infection in 6–12 months. Patients also need to be taught how to care for parts of their body already damaged or made anaesthetic (before cure of the infection) to prevent deformities and ulcers. Cure of infectious cases by drugs stops leprosy spreading.

Cause, pathology

Leprosy is caused by an infection with *Mycobacterium leprae*, a bacterial bacillus. If you stain the *M. leprae* bacillus in the laboratory and then cover it with acid, it keeps the colour of the stain. (Most other organisms lose their colour.) *M. leprae* is therefore called an acid-fast bacillus. This is shortened to AFB. (*M. tuberculosis* is also an AFB, see Chapter 14 page 101.)

M. leprae grows very slowly inside body cells. It likes to grow in skin and in nerve cells more than in other cells. It also likes to grow in cool areas of the body more than in warm areas of the body. It therefore grows best in the skin and in nerves which are cool near the surface of the body. It also grows well in the cool nasal mucosa and testes. However, if there is not much body defence against the organism, *M. leprae* can grow in all organs of the body.

The body defends itself against *M. leprae* by its immune cells (see Chapter 10 page 41). The body also makes antibodies against *M. leprae*; but these do not kill the organism or stop it growing.

In most people, the body has very powerful cellular immunity. This destroys all the *M. leprae* organisms before any damage is done to the body. The infected person does not get the disease. Probably 95–99% of infected people 'cure' themselves.

If the body has bad cellular immunity (or none), the *M. leprae* organisms grow and multiply and spread through all parts of the body and cause disease. This is called 'multibacillary leprosy' ('multi' means 'many'; and 'bacilli' refers to *M. leprae* bacilli) or 'lepromatous leprosy'.

If the body has good cellular immunity but not enough to kill all the M. leprae organisms, the body fights the organisms and keeps them in 1–5 places in the skin and/or in probably just one of the nerves. But the skin and nerves can be severely damaged in the fight. This is called 'paucibacillary leprosy' ('pauci' means 'few') or 'tuberculoid leprosy'.

There are also people with intermediate cellular immunity, which is neither good nor bad. They can get disease and features of both lepromatous and tuberculoid leprosy. The organisms grow and multiply, but the intermediate strength cellular immunity stops them spreading to all of the body. Disease occurs in many parts of the skin and many nerves. This is still 'multibacillary leprosy' and is also called 'borderline leprosy'.

Table 15.1(a) and (b) show the relationship between cellular immunity and the outcome of *M. leprae* infection.

Epidemiology

Organisms can spread only from patients with multibacillary lepromatous and borderline leprosy. The organisms spread mainly from their upper respiratory tract secretions; and only possibly from lepromatous ulcers and ulcerated erythema nodosum leprosum (ENL) lesions.

Spread is mainly by droplets from the respiratory tract. *M. leprae* organisms can stay alive outside the body for days, weeks and possibly up to 5 months.

Organisms enter another person through the respiratory mucous membrane when breathed in and only possibly through the skin.

The incubation period is usually 2–5 years, but it can be shorter or longer than 20 years.

All persons are susceptible, but children and males more commonly get the disease. However, most people (95–99%) infected with *M. leprae* organisms overcome the organisms by powerful cellular immunity and get no leprosy disease.

Those people who do not overcome the infection probably have a special abnormality of just one part of

Table 15.1(a) This table shows how the body's resistance (cellular immunity) to *M. leprae* organisms determines what happens after the body is infected with *M. leprae*.

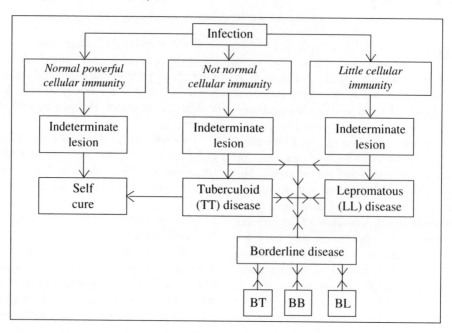

Table 15.1(b) and in more detail

Body resistance to organism	Little	Between little and good	Good but not quite normal	Normal powerful
Number of M. leprae which grow in skin	Many	Many; but not as many as lepromatous, but more than tuberculoid	Some but not many	None
Where M. leprae grow	Everywhere in all organs	In skin – in many areas In nerves – in many	In skin – in 1–5 areas In nerves – in usually only 1	Nowhere

Clinical classification	Multibacillary	Multibacillary	Paucibacillary	No leprosy
Medical classification	Lepromatous (L)	Borderline (B)	Tuberculoid (T)	No leprosy
Specialist classification	(LL)　　　　　(BL)	(BB)	(BT)　　　　　(TT)	No leprosy
Number of people in the population	Very few	A few	A few	Most
	Of the few people infected with *M. leprae* who develop leprosy disease (about 1%), only 10–20% of these few (1%) develop this lepromatous type of leprosy	Of the few people infected with *M. leprae* who develop leprosy disease (about 1%), most of these few (1%) develop these kinds of tuberculoid or borderline leprosy		Most of the people infected with *M. leprae* (95–99%) do not develop leprosy disease

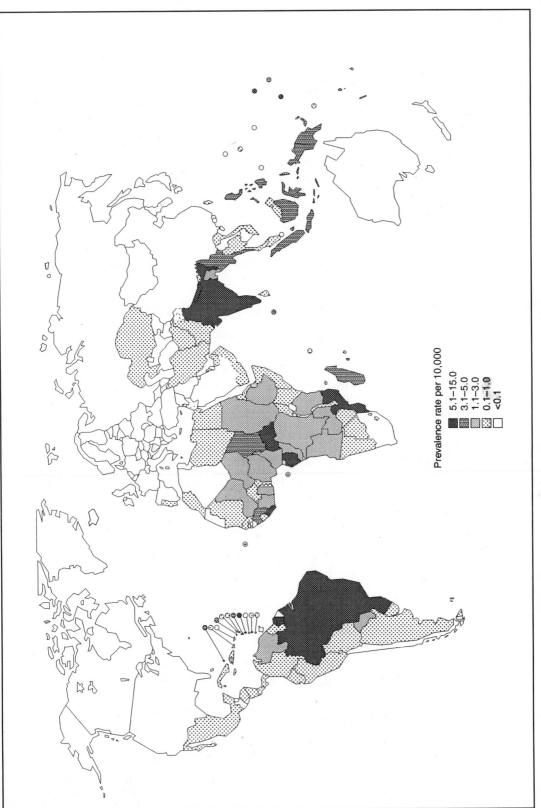

Prevalence rate per 10,000

5.1–15.0
3.1–5.0
1.1–3.0
0.1–1.0
<0.1

Figure 15.1 *The distribution of leprosy. (Source: WHO Technical Report Series No. 874, 1998). See, however, page 130.*

their cellular immune system which does not kill the leprosy organisms. Other parts of their cellular immunity may be normal. This may explain why, so far, it has not been shown that people with HIV infection develop leprosy more often than non-HIV infected people.

Leprosy occurs in communities where people hide their illness and do not come for diagnosis and treatment (because of fear of the illness), or where the health service does not quickly diagnose and treat cases. More and more *M. leprae* grow in these persons, who therefore become more and more infectious. It also occurs in areas where there is poverty, especially where a lot of people live crowded together with bad ventilation in houses and in poor general health. It is then easy for *M. leprae* to spread from an infected to an uninfected person and then grow in them.

The places in the world which have in recent decades been affected by leprosy are shown in **Figure 15.1 on page 129 and recent changes are discussed below.**

Remember, however, that although the registered cases of leprosy have been falling and are now only a quarter of a million, some leprosy experts disagree with this and estimate between 2 and 2.5 million people have leprosy which was not diagnosed, registered and treated between 2000 and 2005. They think there may be now 1 million people needing diagnosis and treatment. This would explain the 500,000–800,000 new cases each year estimated by some to occur.

Leprosy is considered a public health problem at rates of 1 or more per 10,000 population.

The prevalence rates of 21 cases per 10,000 population in the 1980s dropped to the above rate in the 1990s and to less than 1 by the year 2000.

The number of cases in the world dropped from 5,000,000 to now only $\frac{1}{4}$ of a million.

This dramatic improvement was due to:

1. diagnosis of people with the disease, and
2. effective treatment of patients with multidrug therapy so that they were cured (and in 3 days after starting treatment were no longer infectious).

However, India, Brazil, Madagascar, Nepal, Mozambique and Tanzania and other countries still have a significant number of cases.

New cases are still occurring, including in children in many of the areas shown on the map. This means that there must therefore still be undiagnosed untreated infectious patients in these communities.

There are still over 2,000,000 people living with severe disabilities caused by leprosy before it was cured. We need to stop more of these from happening.

It is important that:

1. we need to keep looking for people with
   - skin patches or dermatitis, or
   - nerve pain or swelling, or
   - typical changes of paralysed muscles due to nearby nerve damage, or
   - ulcers on the hands or feet which are not painful;
2. if examination shows these people have leprosy, we should cure them of the infection and stop them infecting others by giving multidrug therapy;
3. we provide proper education and care of cured leprosy patients who can still have problems, especially due to nerve damage;
4. we continue health education about the symptoms and signs of leprosy, encouraging people to come for examination and cure if they have leprosy before any permanent damage is done.

Symptoms and signs

Leprosy causes:

1. Skin patches or infiltration (see below).
2. Nerve enlargement and/or tenderness and/or loss of function (motor and/or sensory) (see page 133).
3. Anaesthesia (loss of sensation) of areas supplied by affected nerves. Injuries, burns, ulcers and destruction occur in anaesthetic areas.
   The parts affected are especially the hands and feet and eyes (see page 135).
4. Weakness, wasting, paralysis of muscles supplied by affected nerves. Deformities of affected areas can then occur.
   The parts affected are especially the hands and feet and eyes (see page 135).
5. Changes in other organs (only in multibacillary lepromatous leprosy) – the eyes, upper respiratory tract, bones, muscles, joints, testes, etc. (see page 138).
6. 'Reactions' (see page 138).

Look for skin patches or infiltration

Look at all the skin of the body. Remove as many clothes as possible. Ask the patient to stand in good even natural light or sloping sunlight.

Look very carefully at the face. Examine especially the ears, eyebrows, forehead, cheeks and nose for infiltration and nodules.

Firstly, look for all lesions present. Find out their type (see page 131), number, size, if they are all the same, and if they are symmetrical (same number on both sides) or not symmetrical.

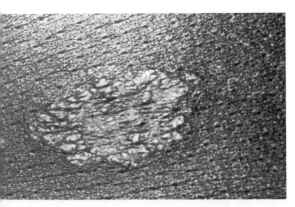

Figure 15.2 *Close up view of an early paucibacillary tuberculoid type skin lesion.*

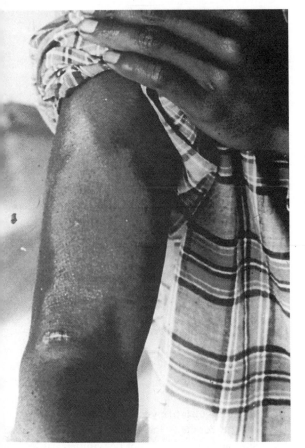

Figure 15.3 *A typical large paucibacillary tuberculoid type skin lesion of the arm.*

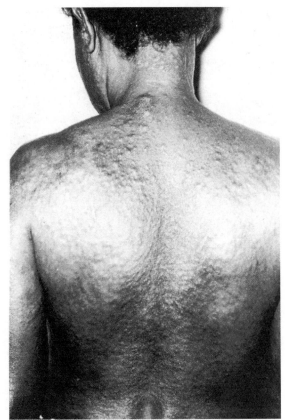

Figure 15.4 *Well advanced multibacillary lepromatous leprosy.*

Next, look at the individual lesions and find out what type they are. Find out if they are flat or raised, if the edges are definite or not definite, the appearance of the centre, the appearance of the surface, the colour, and if the lesion is anaesthetic.

If: the lesions are 1–5 patches of any size, are not all the same and are not symmetrical, *and*

if: the individual lesions are raised with a distinct edge, healing in the centre, dry, pale, without hair, and anaesthetic,

then: the patient has *paucibacillary* or *tuberculoid type skin lesions* (see Figures 15.2 and 15.3).

If: the skin lesions are very many (too many to count), small, all the same and symmetrical, *and*

if: the individual lesions are flat, without a clear edge, the same all over, shiny (red, not pale) and not anaesthetic,

then: the patient has *multibacillary or lepromatous type skin lesions* (see Figure 15.4).

If: there are no individual lesions and all the skin is affected, so that the skin of the whole body is thick with deep lines, folds and nodules, which are shiny and perhaps anaesthetic at the ends of the limbs,

then: the patient has *late multibacillary or late lepromatous type skin changes* (see Figures 15.5, 15.6 and 15.7).

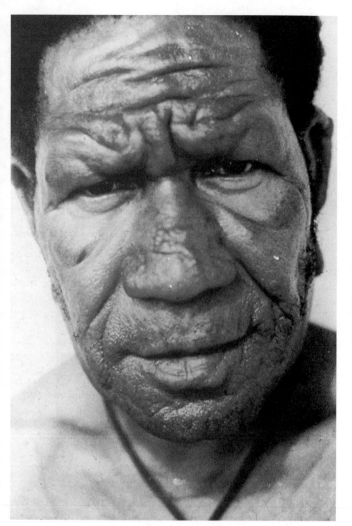

Figure 15.5 *Late multibacillary or lepromatous leprosy.*

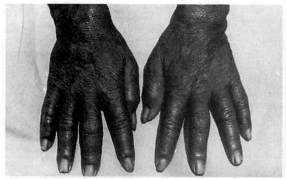

Figure 15.7 *Late multibacillary or lepromatous leprosy. Swelling of all the skin of the body is often more easily seen in the swelling of the fingers and hands, as in this patient.*

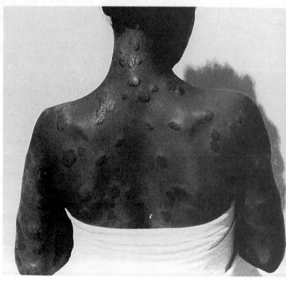

Figure 15.8 *Multibacillary borderline leprosy.*

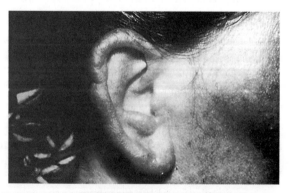

Figure 15.6 *Late multibacillary or lepromatous leprosy with nodules on the ear. Nodules are more easily seen on the ear than other places. You can see nodules on the ear even more easily if you examine the patient from behind.*

If: the patient has many patches (but the number can still be counted) and the patches are of various sizes and may or may not be symmetrical, *and*

if: the individual patches are different (some looking like tuberculoid patches and some looking like large lepromatous patches),

then: the patient has multibacillary *borderline type skin changes* (see Figures 15.8 and 15.9).

Sometimes in borderline type skin changes the patches merge into normal skin and this normal skin merges into other patches. It is then difficult to see which is normal and which is abnormal skin, and the skin looks like a relief map in an atlas. These changes are characteristic of borderline leprosy.

Test any skin patches for loss of sensation (anaesthesia) with cotton wool or a pin (see Figure 15.10). First touch some normal skin with a piece of cotton wool when the patient has his eyes open. Ask the patient to put a finger on the same place as you touched. Then ask the patient to close his eyes. Touch normal skin again. Ask the patient to put a finger on the place you touched. Do this several times on normal skin with the patient's eyes closed until you are sure that he understands what to do. Then touch the skin in places where there may be loss of sensation as well as places where there is normal skin. If the patient does not put his finger on places you touch, then he feels nothing in these areas. He has anaesthesia in these areas. Repeat this several times on places which appear to be anaesthetic. Check the opposite side of his body in the same places.

Make sure the patient has leprosy and does not have dermal leishmaniasis (see Chapter 18 page 178) or a fungus infection of the skin (see Chapter 32 page 527) or other skin conditions mentioned in Chapter 32.

Skin patches from leprosy have *not* been there since birth, do *not* itch, are *not* white, black or dark red, do *not* peel and do *not* come and go quickly.

Skin patches with loss of sensation, no sweating and no hair, especially if there are also enlarged nerves in the body, *are likely* to be due to leprosy.

Examine for nerve damage – enlargement and/or tenderness and/or loss of function

The important nerves most commonly affected by leprosy which can be palpated (felt) are the ulnar, median and radial in the arms, lateral popliteal and posterior tibial in the legs and the great auricular nerves in the neck (see Figure 15.11).

Feel for enlargement or tenderness of the:
- ulnar nerves at inside of elbows (Figure 15.12),
- posterior tibial nerves behind the inside of the ankle joints (Figure 15.13),

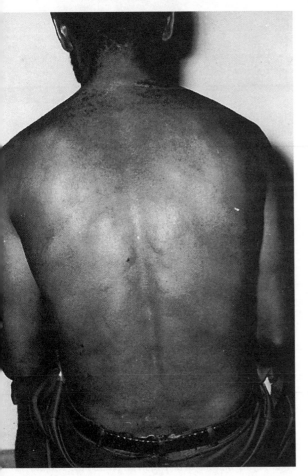

Figure 15.9 *Multibacillary borderline leprosy.*

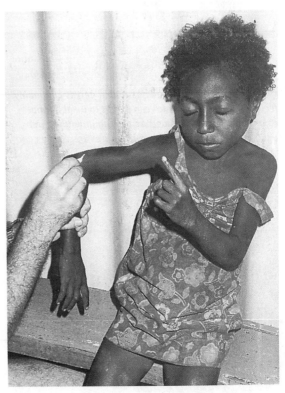

Figure 15.10 *Testing for anaesthesia of a patch in the skin. (See text for description.) Compare with testing for anaesthesia in hands and feet. (See Figure 15.15.)*

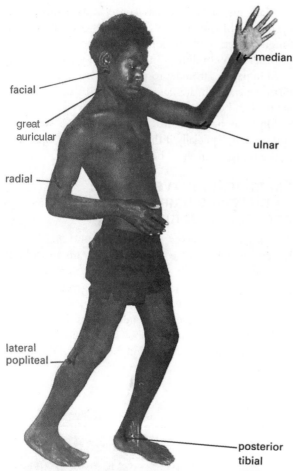

facial

great
auricular

radial

lateral
popliteal

median

ulnar

posterior
tibial

Figures 15.11a and b *show the position of nerves commonly affected in leprosy and which can be felt to be abnormal – enlarged or tender. The method of examining the three most important areas are shown in Figures 15.12, 15.13 and 15.14.*

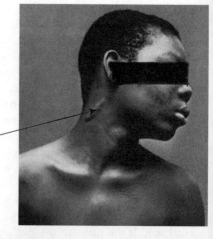

enlarged great
auricular nerve

Figure 15.11b

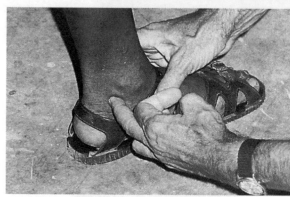

Figure 15.13 *Method of palpating for tenderness and/or enlargement of the posterior tibial nerve.*

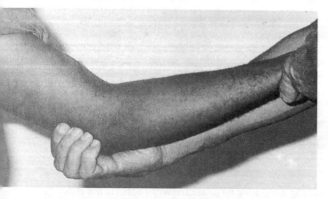

Figure 15.12 *Method of palpating for enlargement and/or tenderness of the ulnar nerve.*

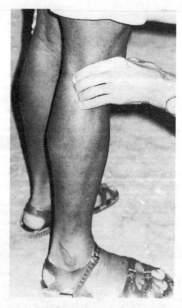

Figure 15.14 *Method of palpation for tenderness and/or enlargement of the lateral popliteal nerves.*

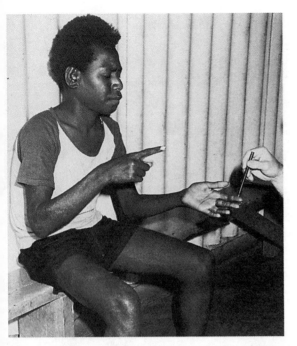

Figure 15.15 *Testing for anaesthesia in the hands and feet. Note the difference from testing for anaesthesia in a skin patch (see Figure 15.10). Gently but firmly touch the palms of the hands and soles of the feet with the tip of a pencil or a piece of wire. With his eyes closed, the patient must put a finger close to the place you have touched. If he puts his finger more than 2 cm away from the place you touched, he has lost enough sensation for him to severely damage this part of his body without knowing it.*

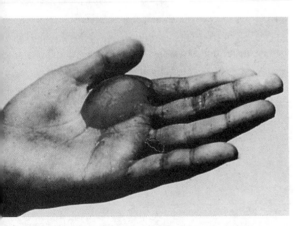

Figure 15.16 *Blister from burn due to loss of sensation.*

- lateral popliteal nerves at the outside of the knees (Figure 15.14).

Nerves in the skin near a patch may be enlarged.

Nerves going to the face and the eye may be affected; but these cannot be felt easily.

Test for anaesthesia of areas supplied by affected nerves (hands, feet and eyes)

Ulnar nerve damage causes anaesthesia in the little finger and half of the next finger.

Median nerve damage causes anaesthesia in the rest of the hand.

Lateral popliteal nerve damage causes anaesthesia in the outside part of the leg.

Posterior tibial nerve damage causes anaesthesia underneath the foot.

Damage to the nerve going to the eye causes anaesthesia of the cornea of the eye.

1. Test the hands, feet and eyes for anaesthesia (see Figure 15.15 and below).
2. Look and feel for burns, blisters, cuts, ulcers, swellings, hot areas, etc. on the hands and feet. These can be present in anaesthetic areas without the patient noticing them (see Figure 15.16).
3. Look for severe destruction of the hands or feet which can be caused by the anaesthesia and injuries which the patient does not notice because there is no pain (see Figures 15.17 and 15.18).
4. Test for anaesthesia in the eye by getting the patient to look upwards and towards his nose and then touch the cornea with a small piece of cotton wool from the side of his face. If the patient still has sensation, the eye will blink.

Test for weakness, wasting or paralysis of muscles supplied by affected nerves (hands, feet and eyes)

Ulnar damage causes a claw hand, affecting mostly the little finger and the finger next to it. The patient cannot straighten or bend these fingers properly (see Figure 15.19).

Median damage causes claw hand of the other fingers which the patient cannot bend or straighten properly, and paralysis of thumb so that the patient cannot pinch or lift it away from the palm of the hand (see Figure 15.20).

Radial damage causes wrist drop or the wrist cannot bend backwards (see Figure 15.21).

Lateral popliteal damage causes foot drop or the foot cannot bend up at the ankle (see Figure 15.22).

Posterior tibial damage causes paralysis of small muscles of the foot, and claw toes.

Facial damage causes paralysis of eyelid – the patient cannot close his eye properly (lagophthalmos) (see Figure 15.23).

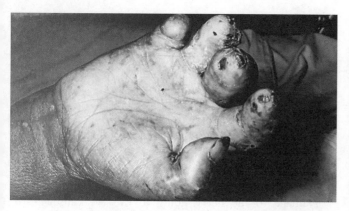

Figure 15.17 *Hand destroyed because of loss of sensation and lack of special care of the anaesthetic hand. The patient has trauma including burns, cuts, blisters, etc., as the patient has in Figure 15.16, but they did not hurt and as he did not know how to look after his hand, this is what happened.*

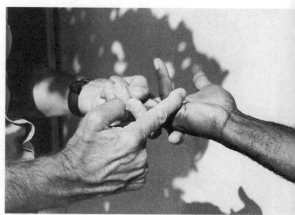

Figure 15.19 *Testing for weakness of one of the muscles supplied by the ulnar nerve.*

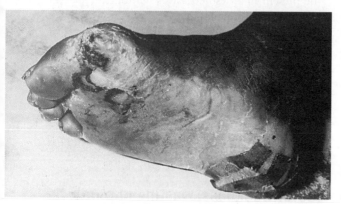

Figure 15.18 *Photograph of plantar ulcers (i.e. ulcers on the sole of the foot). These ulcers were caused by injuries (such as cuts and bruises) which the patient did not worry about or care for because there was no pain. If the patient had cared for his feet properly (see page 146), he need not have got these ulcers. If the ulcers had been treated properly they would have healed. The dressings used by the health worker for this patient were useless. For proper treatment of plantar ulcers see page 147. Note that these ulcers are NOT caused by the leprosy organisms in the ulcer. These ulcers are caused by nerve damage with loss of sensation under the foot.*

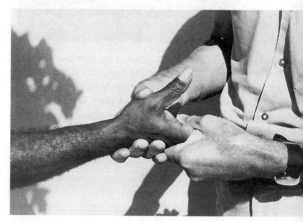

Figure 15.20 *Testing for weakness of one of the muscles supplied by the median nerve.*

A quick test for paralysis of hand muscles is as follows (see also Figure 15.24):

1. Ask the patient to hold his hand like the hand on the left of Figure 15.24 (wrist up, fingers straight but bent to 90° where they join the palm, and thumb across the palm).
2. Look for clawing of little and next finger (both of patient's hands) from ulnar weakness.

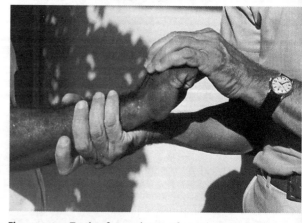

Figure 15.21 *Testing for weakness of muscles supplied by radial nerve.*

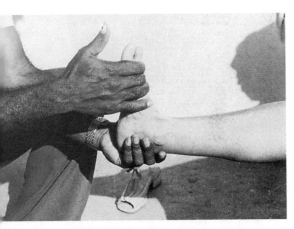

Figure 15.22 *Testing for weakness of muscles supplied by the lateral popliteal nerve.*

3. Look for clawing of other fingers (patient's left hand) for median weakness.
4. Look for wrist drop (not present) from radial weakness.
5. Check if the thumb cannot go across the palm (not present) from median weakness.

Later effects

Fixed deformities occur later in the disease if treatment is not successful. The joints become stiff in the position in which they are paralysed and cannot be straightened even with another hand helping.

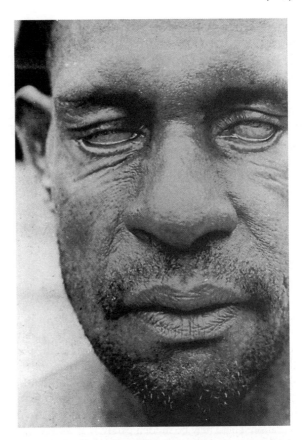

Figure 15.23 *Bilateral lagophthalmos. The patient is trying to close both eyes. The eyes turn upwards, but the eyelids will not close.*

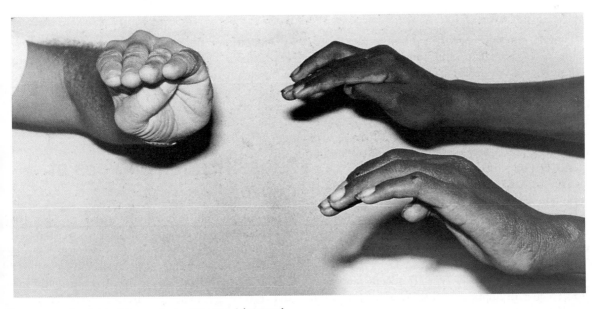

Figure 15.24 *A quick test for paralysis of the hand (see text).*

Look for damage of other organs – occurs only in multibacillary lepromatous leprosy

Nose – swollen mucous membrane causes blocked up nose which can bleed. Later, the bone collapses and the nose becomes flat.

Bones of hands and feet – these become weak and easily crushed, and the fingers and toes, etc. become shorter.

Testes – these become smaller, and sterility and gynaecomastia (swollen breasts) develop.

Eyes – iritis with loss of vision can occur (see Chapter 31 page 515).

Look for 'reactions'

There are two types of reaction and 'neuritis'. It is more important to recognise that a reaction is occurring and treat it than to remember which type it is.

Type I reaction occurs in multibacillary borderline leprosy and affects the nerves and the parts of the skin that are already affected by leprosy. The edges of the skin patches may become swollen, painful and tender. More seriously, the affected nerves may become swollen, painful and tender. There may be a sudden loss of sensation. There may be sudden paralysis. It is caused by 'delayed hypersensitivity' cellular immune reaction to the *M. leprae* proteins. (The tuberculin reaction is also a delayed hypersensitivity reaction but to *M. tuberculosis* antigens.) It occurs most often in the first 2 months after treatment starts (probably as there is a lot of protein left from *M. leprae* organisms dying) and can occur in women after childbirth.

Type II reactions occur in multibacillary lepromatous leprosy. Small, painful lumps called erythema nodosum leprosum (ENL) may develop in the skin, so this reaction is often called an ENL reaction (Figure 15.25). There may be also acute inflammation of any of the organs involved in lepromatous leprosy. Especially important are acute iritis (painful red eye with some loss of sight), acute orchitis (painful swelling of a testis or both testes) or painful swelling of nerves with sudden loss of sensation or paralysis. The joints or hands and feet may become very swollen. This reaction is due to 'immune complexes' or collections of parts of *M. leprae* and antibodies causing 'allergic' type reactions wherever the blood carries and then releases them.

If a reaction (especially Type II) occurs, there may also be general symptoms and signs of inflammation – fever, fast pulse, etc.

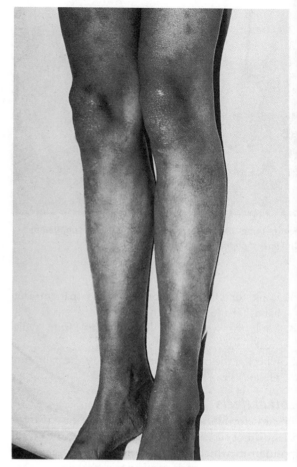

Figure 15.25 *Leprosy reaction with ENL. ENL are inflamed tender nodules, most common on the front of the legs and the backs of the arms and on the face.*

Neuritis or nerve damage is probably due to a reaction but without the other signs of reaction. It can occur at any time before or when on treatment. Look for new paralysis or loss of sensation in all patients when seen. Treat for a reaction if any new paralysis or loss of sensation has occurred.

Classification of types of leprosy

The simple clinical classification of just two types of leprosy (multibacillary or paucibacillary) is the one you are most likely to use. (See after next two paragraphs for more details.)

But **leprosy also can be divided clinically into five types** (see Table 15.1 page 128 and Table 15.2 page 139):

1. indeterminate,
2. tuberculoid,
3. borderline,
4. lepromatous, and
5. neural.

Leprosy can also be divided into two types by the results of skin smears for bacillary index (BI) or results of biopsy.

1. *Multibacillary.* These patients have many AFB in skin smears. (For leprosy experts they will usually be LL, BL, BB or at times BT cases.) They are called 'multibacillary' as 'multi' means 'many' and 'bacilli' refers to AFB.
2. *Paucibacillary.* These patients have so few AFB in skin smears or biopsy that they are not seen. (For leprosy experts they are, clinically, usually TT and indeterminate cases, although some may be BT.) They are called 'paucibacillary' as 'pauci' means 'few'.

Clinical multi- or paucibacillary leprosy

Leprosy can be divided into the number of bacilli *likely* to be there just by clinical examination of the skin (and nerve) lesions. This is particularly useful where there are no laboratories to do examinations for AFB. This classification is good enough to indicate what type of treatment to give (see page 142).

1. Paucibacillary (PB) leprosy of two types:
   PB as only one single skin lesion;
   PB as only two to five (2–5) skin lesions.
   No more than one nerve would be affected.

2. Multibacillary (MB) leprosy:
   MB as more than five skin lesions.
   More than one nerve could be affected.

Indeterminate leprosy

Indeterminate leprosy may occur soon after the leprosy organisms have entered the body and started to grow, but before it can be told if the body's defences or the organisms will win the fight.

One (or a few) flat (or slightly raised), indistinct, slightly pale, sometimes slightly anaesthetic patch in the skin may be found. Skin smears (see page 141) may show a few AFB, but may be negative.

Unless the smear is positive for AFB, do not diagnose indeterminate leprosy. Either biopsy the lesion (see page 141) (*but* do *not* biopsy a lesion on the face), or see the patient each 6–12 weeks until either the lesion goes away, or the lesion is obviously leprosy, or the lesion is examined by a Medical Officer. Many people with a clinical diagnosis of 'indeterminate leprosy' do not have leprosy at all.

Tuberculoid, borderline and lepromatous leprosy

See Table 15.2.

Neural leprosy

Some cases only involve nerves and have no skin lesions.

Some cases may have had skin lesions which healed, and only nerve changes remain.

These are both called 'neural' leprosy, or, if many nerves are involved, 'polyneuritic' leprosy.

Table 15.2 Main features of the main types of leprosy.

	Type of leprosy			
	Tuberculoid TT Type Paucibacillary	Borderline BB Type Multibacillary	Lepromatous – early LL Type Multibacillary	Lepromatous – late LL Type Multibacillary
1. Skin				
(a) Lesions				
• type	Patches	Patches	Patches	The patches join; all the skin is affected
• number	1–5	Many – but can be counted	Many – cannot be counted	
• size	Small or large	Vary	Small	
• all the same	No	No	Yes	
• symmetrical (i.e. same both sides	No	Sometimes	Yes	

Table 15.2   *(continued)*

	Type of leprosy			
	Tuberculoid *TT Type* *Paucibacillary*	*Borderline* *BB Type* *Multibacillary*	*Lepromatous – early* *LL Type* *Multibacillary*	*Lepromatous – late* *LL Type* *Multibacillary*
(b) Individual lesions				
• flat or raised	Raised at edge	Some flat; some raised	Flat	⎤
• edge distinct or indistinct	Distinct	Some distinct; some indistinct	Indistinct	⎥ The skin is all
• appearance of centre	Healing and scarring	Some healing; some not	All the same	⎬ thickened with folds and nodules
• appearance of surface	No sweating; no hair	Some normal; some not sweating; no hair	Sweating; hair	⎥
• colour	Pale at edge	Some pale; some shiny	Shiny (red) not pale	⎦ Shiny (red) not pale
• anaesthesia	Anaesthetic	Some anaesthetic but not complete	No anaesthesia	Anaesthesia
2. Nerves				
Cutaneous (skin) (sensory)	Only nerves going to a patch	Nerves going to patches	Hands and feet both sides	Much of arms and le[g] both sides
Peripheral and cranial number	1(–3)	Many	None to all	All
Symmetrical (i.e. same both sides)	No	Sometimes	Yes	Yes
• swollen	Yes (very)	Yes	Only a little	Yes
• tender	No	No; yes if in reaction	No; yes if in reaction	No; yes if in reactio[n]
3. Anaesthesia				
of area supplied by affected nerves	Yes (usually)	Yes	No	Yes
4. Paralysis				
and wasting of muscles supplied by affected nerves	Yes (usually)	Yes	No	Yes
5. Other organs affected				
(a) mucous membranes of URT	No	Not marked	Yes	Yes
(b) bones	No	Not marked	Yes	Yes
(c) muscles	No	Not marked	Yes	Yes
(d) testes	No	Not marked	Yes	Yes
(e) general symptoms and signs	No	Not marked	Yes, especially if reaction	Yes, especially if reaction
6. Reactions	No	Yes (Type 1) and neuritis	Yes (Type 2) and neuritis	Yes (Type 2) and neuritis

URT, upper respiratory tract

Tests

Skin smear for BI and MI

Do a skin smear if:

1. a case of suspected lepromatous or borderline leprosy but you are not sure of the diagnosis;
2. leprosy seems to have come back again in a patient who was previously treated for leprosy;
3. at the end of 12 months of multidrug therapy (earlier in some cases) the leprosy does not appear to be cured.

How to make a skin smear

Take smears from the ear lobes, the eyebrows and any suspicious skin lesions. Pinch the skin firmly between your thumb and forefinger so that it cannot bleed. With a sharp scalpel, make a slit in the skin 2–3 mm deep and 5 mm long. Then scrape the tissues from the bottom of the wound with the point of the scalpel blade. Use the material on the scalpel blade to make the slide. Warm the slide over a flame until it is just too hot to hold on the back of the hand ('to fix it').

Pack the slide where no insects can reach it, and send it to the laboratory with a request form asking for examination for AFB, including both BI and MI (see Figure 15.26).

Bacillary index (BI) tells how many *M. leprae* organisms there are in the slide. The bacillary index is high (e.g. BI 6 +) in lepromatous cases. Some bacilli may be seen in borderline cases (e.g. BI 1–4 +). No bacilli are seen in tuberculoid cases (BI negative or 0). If originally high, the BI takes years to become negative, even after successful treatment.

Morphological index (MI) tells the percentage of the *M. leprae* organisms that are seen which are morphologically normal (or solid staining or in one piece). The morphological index therefore shows what percentage of organisms are alive. Before treatment MI may be up to 60%. (It is never much more than 60% and never 100%.) MI should fall to 0% after 6 months of successful treatment. The MI should stay at 0% if treatment is effective.

Skin biopsy

Do a skin biopsy if the diagnosis of tuberculoid or borderline leprosy is not certain.

Take a skin biopsy from the edge of the patch. The bigger the biopsy the better the report can be; but an oval piece of skin about 1 cm in length is enough.

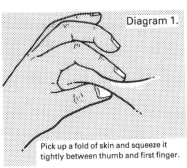

Diagram 1.
Pick up a fold of skin and squeeze it tightly between thumb and first finger.

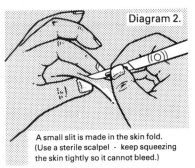

Diagram 2.
A small slit is made in the skin fold. (Use a sterile scalpel - keep squeezing the skin tightly so it cannot bleed.)

Diagram 3.
The base of the skin slit is scraped with the tip of the scalpel. (Keep squeezing the skin fold to prevent bleeding.)

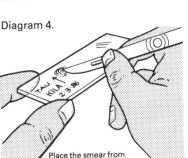

Diagram 4.
Place the smear from the patient onto a properly labelled glass slide.

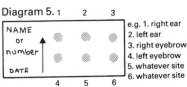

Diagram 5.
1   2   3

NAME or number

DATE

4   5   6

e.g. 1. right ear
2. left ear
3. right eyebrow
4. left eyebrow
5. whatever site
6. whatever site

This is how to label and place the patient's smears on the slide. Use a diamond pencil or sticking plaster to label. Do NOT use pencils or paper labels which can rub off. The arrow is to show where you start numbering the smears. Place the smears ON THE SAME SIDE of the glass as the LABELLING. On the requisition slip - use the same numbering as shown in the diagram. Give the actual site from which each smear came.

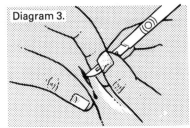

Diagram 6.
match sticks

rubber band

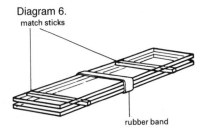

Slides can be packed in pairs like this. The smears must face inwards.

Figure 15.26 *Diagrams 1–6 show how to make skin smears for AFB (see text). Wear gloves to do this test.*

Infiltrate the area with local anaesthetic. Mark a narrow oval of skin 1 cm in length to be cut out. With a sharp scalpel cut along the mark you have made, down to the *fat* under the skin. Lift the biopsy up by the fat underneath the skin *very carefully* (with the smallest forceps you have), and cut through the fat to remove the skin biopsy. Do not squeeze the skin with the forceps because this will make it difficult to examine under the microscope. Drop the biopsy into 20–30 ml fixative solution or formal-saline. Stitch up the skin. For best results, ask your laboratory to send you Ridley's FMA for fixative solution. Leave the biopsy in this solution for 2 hours; then rinse it with water and put it in 70% alcohol. If you do not have this special fixative, use formalin and leave the specimen in the formalin.

Course and complications

Paucibacillary indeterminate leprosy cures itself without treatment in three out of four cases. Treatment will cure the other types.

Paucibacillary tuberculoid leprosy will often cure itself without treatment. But before this happens, severe nerve damage can occur. Treatment will kill the infection and soon stop more nerve damage occurring.

Multibacillary lepromatous leprosy never cures itself but becomes worse. Reactions are common. Many organs are damaged. Treatment can cure the infection. After some time of regular correct treatment, reactions become less common and then stop.

Multibacillary borderline leprosy without treatment will later become like either tuberculoid or lepromatous leprosy. Meanwhile, severe nerve damage occurs. Treatment can cure the infection and after some time the reactions will stop.

When multidrug therapy has killed all *M. leprae* organisms and when no further reactions occur, no further damage can be done by the leprosy (the patient is no longer a 'case' of leprosy). If, however, permanent damage has been done to the nerves or eyes, etc., this cannot get better. The patient can then get further damage to hands, feet, eyes, etc. if they do not feel injuries happening, and the injuries therefore become severe; or, if muscle paralysis stops them moving muscles and joints, and muscles and tendons become scarred and shortened and joint deformities occur. There are ways the patient can prevent this further damage being done. Early effective multidrug therapy, however, before any permanent damage to nerves or eyes, etc. is done, is much better.

Treatment of *M. leprae* infection

The most important thing in the management of the patient is treatment of the infection.

1. Give anti-leprosy multidrug therapy (MDT) according to the type of leprosy the patient has and using the drugs recommended by your Health Department for as long as they say to give them. It is also essential to do the following.
2. Give the patient education about:
   (a) the need for regular treatment for 6 or 12 months,
   (b) the care for hands/feet/eyes if these are anaesthetic or weak or paralysed, and
   (c) the need to come for quick and proper treatment of reactions and neuritis if these occur later.
3. Start treatment for any complication the patient already has (especially hands, feet and eyes).
4. Look for any other condition the patient has, especially TB or HIV infection. Send sputum for AFB × 3 if the patient has a chronic cough. However, if the patient has multibacillary leprosy the sputum may be positive for AFB because *M. leprae* and not *M. tuberculosis* are in the sputum. Some patients will therefore need a chest X-ray and check by the Medical Officer. It is most important to diagnose TB, as leprosy treatment contains rifampicin, which is used also for TB treatment. This rifampicin dose for leprosy is not enough to cure TB and the *M. tuberculosis* would soon develop resistance to rifampicin, which is a terrible problem (see Chapter 14 page 123). Also, if the patient has HIV infection and is on anti-retroviral therapy, some of these drugs can interact with rifampicin and the patient needs review by the HIV staff.

Until the early 1980s treatment was by giving dapsone alone for 5 years for tuberculoid disease and for life for lepromatous disease. Patients often did not take the drug, so they were not cured. Dapsone resistant organisms started to occur.

In 1982, WHO recommended multidrug therapy.

The reasons for this are similar to the reasons multidrug therapy is also given for infections with TB, malaria, HIV organisms and others. (See Chapter 14 page 112 and Chapter 13 pages 77–79.)

Multidrug therapy has reduced the number of registered cases of leprosy from over 5 million in 1985 to now only a $\frac{1}{4}$ of a million.

Multidrug therapy (MDT) for leprosy is as follows.

Multibacillary (MB) leprosy:
  Rifampicin 600 mg once monthly
  Clofazimine 300 mg once monthly **and** 50 mg daily
  Dapsone 100 mg daily
  Duration of treatment 1 year.

Paucibacillary (PB) leprosy:
  Rifampicin 600 mg monthly
  Dapsone 100 mg daily
  Duration of treatment 6 months.

Paucibacillary (PB) leprosy with definitely only one skin lesion (indeterminate leprosy):
  Rifampicin 600 mg
  Ofloxacin 400 mg
  Minocycline 100 mg
  Duration of treatment is only one dose once.

Multidrug therapy is supplied free of charge for all leprosy patients in the world by the WHO.

The drugs come in a 'blister pack' with 4 weeks' or 1 month's supply in it. The dose of drugs for the day is to be pushed out of one of the blisters, then swallowed (see Figure 15.27).

The first dose each month is the most important dose as it contains the only dose of rifampicin 600 mg given in each month for all patients and the only large dose of clofazimine 300 mg given each month for multibacillary patients as well as dapsone. Always get the patient to take the first dose when you give him the blister pack and watch that he swallows it. It is best if you can get the patient to come back each month so that:

1. you can directly observe the patient swallow the most important first dose of the month each month when you give him the next blister pack;
2. you can check by looking at the blister pack if he has taken all other doses;
3. you can check for Type I and Type II and neuritis reactions and for side effects of drugs, and how well he is caring for his hands, feet and eyes and check for any other health problem he has.

The other drugs in the blister pack will be:

dapsone 100 mg dose daily for both paucibacillary and multibacillary leprosy
clofazimine 50 mg daily for only multibacillary leprosy.

If the patient is unable to come back each month, you can supply the number of blister packs needed

MDT Regimens   Each blister pack contains treatment for 4 weeks.

PB adult treatment:

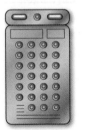

Once a month: Day 1
  – 2 capsules of rifampicin (300 mg × 2)
  – 1 tablet of dapsone (100 mg)
Once a day: Days 2–28
  – 1 tablet of dapsone (100 mg)
Full course: 6 blister packs

PB adult blister pack

PB child treatment (10–14 years):

Once a month: Day 1
  – 2 capsules of rifampicin (300 mg + 150 mg)
  – 1 tablet of dapsone (50 mg)
Once a day: Days 2–28
  – 1 tablet of dapsone (50 mg)
Full course: 6 blister packs

For children younger than 10, the dose must be adjusted according to body weight.

PB child blister pack

MB adult treatment:

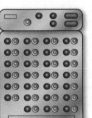

Once a month: Day 1
  – 2 capsules of rifampicin (300 mg × 2)
  – 3 capsules of clofazimine (100 mg × 3)
  – 1 tablet of dapsone (100 mg)
Once a day: Days 2–28
  – 1 capsule of clofazimine (50 mg)
  – 1 tablet of dapsone (100 mg)
Full course: 12 blister packs

MtB adult blister pack

MB child treatment (10–14 years):

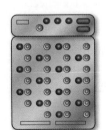

Once a month: Day 1
  – 2 capsules of rifampicin (300 mg + 150 mg)
  – 3 capsules of clofazimine (50 mg × 3)
  – 1 tablet of dapsone (50 mg)
Once a day: Days 2–28
  – 1 capsule of clofazimine every other day (50 mg)
  – 1 tablet of dapsone (50 mg)
Full course: 12 blister packs

MB child blister pack For children younger than 10, the dose must be adjusted according to body weight.

Figure 15.27 *MDT regimens. Patients must understand which drugs they have to take once a month and which every day.*

until he can return (even up to the full treatment); but it would be best to see him regularly. If the patient cannot return monthly, it is better to supply further blister packs to a relative or friend who will carry them to the patient for him to take until the patient can return (even up to the full treatment); but it would be better to see him regularly.

When you give the patient blister packs of drugs, make sure he knows the following.

1. About leprosy:
   - The patient will be cured of leprosy if he takes all of the drugs in all the blister packs as advised, preferably an hour or so before any food.
   - He must complete a full course of treatment: 6 blisters for PB patients and 12 blisters for MB patients.
   - The drugs stop the disease from spreading 3 days after the first dose as long as the patient continues the treatment.
   - Patients can lead normal lives. They can live at home, go to school, work, play, get married, have sex, have children, participate in social events, etc.

2. About their treatment:
   - The MDT blister packs are free of charge.
   - The blister packs should be kept in a dry, safe and shady place and out of the reach of children.
   - If the drugs are spoiled (changed colour, broken), the health worker will replace them.

3. About possible problems:
   - The medicines will turn urine red and skin darker. Patients should not worry: both will return to normal once the treatment is completed.
   - Oral contraceptives may not work.
   - Other drug side effects are as below.
   - The patient must go immediately to a health centre if he has any problems or other illness (drug side effects, reactions, pain, fever, malaise, new lesions, muscle weakness, etc.).
   - He should return either each month to get a new blister pack, take the first dose and for a check up; or if this is not possible, at the latest after he completes the treatment.
   - If he already has disabilities, tell and show him how to protect himself from injuries and supply what treatment and apparatus is needed.

Important facts about MDT

1. MDT is very safe and effective in curing leprosy.
2. MDT is safe during pregnancy.
3. MDT is safe for patients being treated for TB as well as those who are HIV positive.

4. Rifampicin is in both the treatment of leprosy and TB. The dose in MDT for leprosy is not enough to treat TB. Give the full dose of rifampicin in the TB treatment. Otherwise, just give both treatments at the same time.
5. Rifampicin may have interactions with drugs used for HIV infection, i.e. anti-retroviral therapy (ART). Do not start MDT leprosy treatment until the patient is reviewed by the HIV staff if the patient is on ART.
6. If the patient cannot take dapsone because of severe side effects, refer the patient to the Medical Officer. It may be omitted in MB disease and clofazimine put in its place in PB disease.
7. If the patient cannot take rifampicin because of side effects or drug interactions, refer the patient to the Medical Officer. Special regimens including ofloxacin, clarithromycin or minocycline and longer courses of the treatment will need to be organised.
8. If clofazimine will not be taken by patients because it makes their skin too red, refer the patient to your Medical Officer regarding the use of another drug. These drugs cause other side effects. Try to convince the patient that clofazimine is the better drug for him to use, and that the side effects will all go away after the drug is ceased.
9. If the morphological index (MI) is not zero at the end of 6 months, it is most likely that the patient has not been taking the drugs regularly. It is possible, although very unlikely, that the patient's organisms are resistant to the drugs. All such cases must be seen as soon as possible by the supervising Medical Officer. (The BI may take years to become zero.)

Side effects of anti-leprosy drugs

Rifampicin

1. Red brown urine, tears and sputum colour. If this does not occur, the patient is not taking his rifampicin. Warn the patient about the colour of his urine and explain that it is a good sign.
2. Gastrointestinal upsets. Even if these occur, rifampicin must be taken on an empty stomach, and no food must be eaten for half an hour after the rifampicin. At home, if first thing in the morning causes too many side effects, try last thing at night. In supervised treatment, tell the patient not to eat for 2 hours before he is seen, when he will be given the drug.
3. Influenza-like reaction after the dose.
4. Hepatitis is the most serious side effect. The rifampicin, but also other anti-leprosy drugs, should

be stopped and the patient immediately sent to the Medical Officer's care. Do not just stop the rifampicin.

5. Oral contraceptives may not work. Tell the patient to use other forms of contraception while taking rifampicin, i.e. usually use condoms.

Clofazimine

1. The skin becomes red and later darker but always fades when the clofazimine is ceased.
2. The skin on the forearms and shins may become dry, shiny and scaly.
3. Gastrointestinal symptoms, mainly abdominal pain – this usually occurs only if the dose is larger than 100 mg.

Minocycline

1. Gastrointestinal problems.
2. Central nervous system upsets including dizziness.
3. Discoloration of the teeth in children (not therefore given to pregnant women or children).

Fluoquinolones, e.g. ofloxacin

1. Gastrointestinal upsets.
2. Central nervous system upsets including dizziness.

Dapsone

1. Gastrointestinal upsets.
2. Blood abnormalities including anaemia.
3. Skin rashes.
4. Psychiatric conditions.

Before treatment

Do not start treatment unless:

1. the diagnosis is certain because of typical symptoms and signs, or
2. the diagnosis was not certain but is now confirmed by a test (skin smear or biopsy).

If the diagnosis is not certain:

1. do a skin smear for AFB if you suspect lepromatous or borderline leprosy;
2. do a skin biopsy if you suspect tuberculoid or borderline leprosy (but do not biopsy face);
3. if a biopsy is not possible, then review the patient each 6–12 weeks instead;
4. wait for the results before starting treatment.

Always do a full medical history and physical examination and test the urine. Diagnose and treat any other conditions you find, especially anaemia or TB.

Diagnosis and drug treatment of leprosy

Multibacillary (MB) leprosy
Diagnose as:
- more than 5 skin patches;
- more than one nerve may be affected;
- if done, skin smear shows AFB organisms.

Treat with 3 drugs in the adult multibacillary blister pack for 12 months.

Paucibacillary (PB) leprosy
Diagnose as:
- no more than 5 skin patches;
- no more than one nerve affected;
- if done, skin smear shows no organisms or biopsy shows changes of tuberculoid leprosy.

Treat with 2 drugs in the adult paucibacillary blister pack for 6 months.

Paucibacillary (PB) leprosy with just one skin patch only
If in doubt treat as above for PB for 6 months.
If no doubt treat with one dose only of rifampicin and ofloxacin and minocycline.

Treatment of the infection only is not the proper management of a case of leprosy. Remember the other things needed in the management of the patient. (See box below.)

Management of a patient with leprosy

Management includes not only MDT but in all ten things:

1. Register the patient. Fill in any books, cards, treatment cards, etc. needed. Arrange for a treatment centre and for follow-up of the patient.
2. Start multidrug therapy; supervised, if possible, each month.
3. Educate patient and carers about drugs and reactions and the care of any anaesthetic or paralysed hands, feet or eyes and the use of footwear.
4. Arrange contact tracing.
5. Treat any reactions quickly and effectively.
6. Arrange physiotherapy for weak, paralysed or deformed feet, hands, eyes.
7. Plaster of Paris casts, footwear, etc. for plantar ulcers.
8. Arrange surgery if needed.
9. Visit the patient if he is not taking the treatment.
10. Transfer to Medical Officer care if needed.

Do all necessary administrative procedures

1. Confirm the diagnosis (if the diagnosis was made by another health worker).
2. Fill in details of the patient in the register book or card and any report you have to send to the Health Department.
3. Fill in details of the treatment plan on any treatment card needed for the patient to carry if he is to get treatment at another centre.
4. Check attendances and if the patient has taken all the drugs from the previous blister back, preferably each month but otherwise when you see him again.
5. Notify the Health Department regularly as you have been told to do.

Start anti-leprosy multidrug therapy (preferably supervised)

See page 143.

Educate the patient and carers

See page 144 about drugs, pages 138 and this page about reactions and pages 146–148 about care of hands, feet and eyes.

Arrange contact tracing

See page 149.

Treat any reaction quickly and effectively

Give health education to the patient about the symptoms and signs of reactions. Tell him that he should immediately come to the health worker if he gets any of these symptoms or signs – lumps in the skin; swelling of skin patches; nerve pain; sudden paralysis; sudden loss of sensation; painful eyes; any loss of sight; painful and swollen testis.

Treat reactions as follows:

1. Treat anything which may have caused the reaction (e.g. illness, accident, anxiety, etc.).
2. Make the patient rest in bed if possible. Support any affected part in a sling or a well padded splint.
3. Continue the full dose of all anti-leprosy drugs.
4. Give effective anti-inflammatory drugs.
   If the reaction is severe (e.g. new loss of sensation, new paralysis, eye affected, etc.) prednisolone is needed urgently. Transfer the patient to the Medical Officer urgently unless you have been taught how

to use prednisolone. It can have severe side effects. It can allow other infections to develop and the patient usually needs to have prophylactic isoniazid 5 mg/kg/day (max. 300 mg) daily with pyridoxine 10 mg/day to stop TB reactivating. Prophylactic antimalarials may be needed. The dose of prednisolone is large 1 mg/kg/day (max. 50 mg/day) until the condition settles and then reduced by 5 mg each week so that the prednisolone course lasts for about 12 weeks.

5. While waiting for transfer or if the reaction is mild (see above), give the mild anti-inflammatory drugs available in the health centre:
   - Acetylsalicylic acid 900–1200 mg four times a day regularly or if this is not effective, then instead ibuprofen 1200–1600 mg daily in 3–4 doses a day regularly with food.
   - Chloroquine 300 mg base (2 tablets of 150 mg base) daily. Stop if not helping in 1–2 weeks and stop even if helping in 3 weeks. Give only if Type II (ENL) reaction (not Type I reaction),
   - Clofazimine 100 mg three times a day with food, but reduce to 100 mg twice daily after 1 month and 100 mg daily after 2 months and 100 mg three times a week after 3 months and then stop after this month.

   Do not, however, try to treat a severe reaction or a reaction which does not quickly settle with these drugs. The patient needs prednisolone and further assessment regarding other possible treatment and must be transferred.

6. Transfer any cases as recommended above and on page 149 as they may need not only prednisolone but also tests for other possible diagnoses and (if not a woman of child-bearing age) thalidomide or even surgery for decompression of inflamed nerves.

If the patient has anaesthetic hands or feet or eyes, give education about their care and supply protective footwear

Give a copy of a suitable booklet in the patient's own language for him to read.

Special care for anaesthetic hands usually includes:

1. Soak in room temperature water every day. Rub off any thick lumps of skin (calluses) with a flat stone or 'nylon pot scourer or scraper' (usually green or blue) but do not rub right through the skin. Then apply any oil to keep the water in the skin (not vegetable oil as cockroaches will come to eat it).

2. Precautions to stop burns.

3. Precautions to stop injuries.

4. Every night and morning look at both sides of the hands for burns or injuries, and feel for hot areas.

5. Wash, dress and splint any burn or injury.

6. Get medical treatment if the burn or injury does not improve quickly (dressings, splint, antibiotics, etc.).

Special care for anaesthetic feet includes:

1. Soak in water, remove calluses and oil every day (as above).

2. Always wear footwear to stop injuries or burns to the outside of the foot.

3. No running, jumping, long steps, long walks, etc. to try to prevent injuries to the inside of the foot.

4. Every night and morning: look for lumps, wounds or ulcers; feel for hot areas; feel for deep tenderness.

5. Wash and dress any injury and do not walk on the foot until it is better (i.e. go to bed or use a crutch or stick).

6. Ask for medical treatment if the injury does not improve quickly (usually a plaster of Paris (POP) cast is necessary).

Special care for anaesthetic eyes includes:

1. Look at the eye every night and morning.

2. If the eye becomes red, ask for medical help, i.e. to remove any foreign body (not felt by the patient), to treat any infection and to treat any reaction (iritis especially) if necessary.

If the patient has weakness or paralysis or deformity of hands, feet or eyes:

1. Transfer the patient for special drugs, special plasters and special exercises if any of these are recent; as if occurred in the last 6 months, they were probably caused by a reaction.

2. Transfer for treatment with special plasters and special drugs if any foot drop which has started in the last 6 months; as probably caused by a reaction.

3. Ask the patient to do the special exercises (start physiotherapy) in all other cases.

Treat any plantar ulcer with a plaster of Paris (POP) cast and footwear:

> Plantar ulcers are not caused by leprosy organisms in the ulcerated areas. These ulcers do not happen without a definite cause. These ulcers are always caused by an injury to or pressure on part of the foot.

Because of anaesthesia, the patient does not feel the cause of the injury. He therefore does nothing about the cause. The injury becomes worse and worse. Even when he does know of the injury he continues to walk on the foot. This makes the damage worse and stops healing. (A person with normal sensation would have too much pain to walk.)

Abnormal positions of parts of the foot due to muscle weakness or deformity cause a lot of pressure on some areas of the foot. This can damage the skin and other tissues in this area, and ulcers then form.

Secondary bacterial infection usually occurs and makes the ulcer worse.

Note that the ulcer is *not caused* by leprosy organisms or bacterial infection but *is caused* by anaesthesia and injury.

It is important that you tell the patient how to prevent ulcers. Treatment for ulcers includes the following:

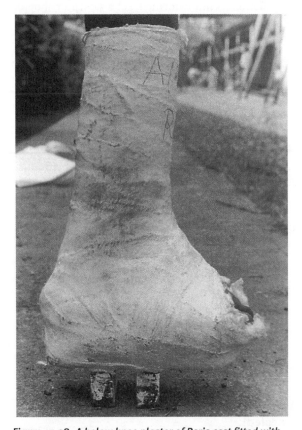

Figure 15.28 *A below knee plaster of Paris cast fitted with a 'home made' walking rocker made out of scrap wood and an old car tyre. The whole job was done by an orderly, and although it was not perfect, the ulcer was completely healed in 6 weeks.*

If there is secondary bacterial infection

(i.e. if the foot is hot, red, swollen, etc. or pus is discharged from the ulcer):

1. Rest the foot:
   - Rest in bed with the foot end of the bed raised, i.e. foot higher than the rest of the body.
   - Use crutches to walk (to toilet, etc.).
   - The foot must *not* be put on the ground.
   This is the most important part of the treatment.
2. Antibiotics – give penicillin at first; give tetracycline if penicillin is not effective.
3. Do dressings with Eusol (see Chapter 32 page 524).
4. Cut away any thick dead skin. Do not cut any living tissue (which will bleed).
   Do not cut out bone from inside the ulcer. Remove *loose* pieces of bone or any foreign body with forceps.

Prepare suitable footwear (before POP applied):

1. If the foot is not deformed, get a sandal or shoe of the patient's size. Get a soft rubber insole and stick it inside the sandal or shoe.
2. If the patient's foot is deformed, take a POP cast of the foot. Send the cast to the leprosy shoe workshop. They will make a suitable shoe with an insole shaped to fit the patient's foot and send it back to you.

When infection is controlled:

1. Apply a below knee POP cast (see Figure 15.28).
2. When the cast is dry apply a wooden rocker or walking iron to the POP (see Figure 15.29).
3. The patient can then walk on the POP.
4. The patient may be kept in the health centre or discharged and checked every week, to make sure the POP is not damaged.
5. Remove the POP (and apply a new one) if there is pain under the POP or any other suspicion of pressure.
6. After 6 weeks remove the POP cast. In most cases the ulcer will be healed. If it is not healed remove any dead hard skin, treat any infection, and then re-apply a POP cast.

After removing the POP cast (when the ulcer is healed):

1. Immediately tell the patient to put his new shoes on.
2. The patient must *always* wear these shoes. He must never walk anywhere without these shoes.

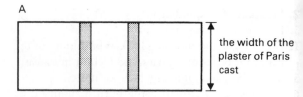

Figure 15.29 *Diagram of a simple rocker: (A) from underneath; (B) from the side. The main part or platform is made from 3- or 5-ply or a piece of wood such as the top of a packing case. The rockers are made of two pieces of wood nailed across the whole width of the platform. Underneath these, rubber cut from an old car tyre is nailed on. Apply the below knee POP one day and do not let the patient walk on it. The next day make the bottom of the cast flat with POP and then plaster the rocker on with a POP bandage. Do not allow the patient to walk on it until the next day.*

3. Allow the patient to walk only a little the first day and then a little more every day. After 3–6 weeks he can walk normal distances.
4. Get new shoes for the patient before the old ones wear out. Do not allow anyone to repair the shoes with nails or wire. These could damage the patient's foot.

Arrange surgery if needed

If physiotherapy is not successful, surgery may help. Cases which surgery may help include patients with:

1. completely wasted hand muscles and deformed hands;
2. foot drop for more than 6 months;
3. lagophthalmos for more than 6 months.

Surgery may be available for people with:

1. collapsed noses;
2. total loss of outside edge of eyebrows;
3. very enlarged breasts in men.
   Discuss these cases with your Medical Officer.

Visit the patient if needed

Visit all the patients who do not come for treatment and try to get them to take treatment regularly.

Notify the OIC of the Leprosy Control Unit if the patient does not have his treatment for 3 months.

See Chapter 14 pages 120–122 for advice on how to organise successful treatment and follow-up of patients – what applies to TB, applies to leprosy also.

Transfer to Medical Officer

Transfer the following cases:

1. All *new* cases who before treatment is started, have:
   (a) a reaction, and/or
   (b) tender nerves.
2. All cases with a *reaction* which
   (a) involves vital body parts (especially the nerves or eyes), or
   (b) is severe, or
   (c) does not stop quickly with treatment available in the health centre.

   These include patients who have:
   • tender nerves,
   • acute paralysis or loss of sensation (and foot drop starting within last 6 months),
   • acute orchitis (painful, swollen testis),
   • iritis (eye red or painful, or sight becoming worse),
   • severe general signs and symptoms,
   • mild reaction which does not stop after 3 weeks of treatment, or
   • reaction which returns after reaction treatment has stopped.
3. All patients who have drug reactions, especially hepatitis, which stops them taking their drugs; or patients who will not take a particular drug, e.g. clofazimine (do not just stop treatment and do nothing else).
4. Patients who have problems with treatment of another illness too, e.g. TB or HIV infection.
5. Patients who are already taking or need anti-retroviral therapy.

Refer to visiting Medical Officer

Any case with complications especially paralysis or deformity, for advice and assessment for possible surgery.

Control and prevention

Kill the organism in the body of the original host or reservoir

Discover and treat all the infectious, i.e. multibacillary (lepromatous and borderline) cases. When they start multidrug therapy, leprosy patients become non-infectious within probably 3 days, and as long as the patient continues the treatment cannot spread the disease.

Early diagnosis of all possible infectious cases and immediate treatment with effective drugs (MDT) so that they are no longer infective is the best way of controlling leprosy.

How to find cases of leprosy

1. Contact education and examination.
   You should see all contacts (family, those who live in the same house, friends, workmates, schoolmates, etc.) and educate them about the symptoms of leprosy and tell them it can be cured. You should then examine and test them all. You should tell them to come to the health centre if symptoms develop later.
2. You should educate and examine special groups during other health examinations – especially school children.
3. You should educate the general public.
4. You should arrange surveys in areas of known or suspected high prevalence of leprosy. (Whole population surveys are not usually as useful as using your available resources for (1) and (2).)

Follow-up of treated patients

Follow-up is not needed as a routine. If they actually took their MDT regularly for the correct time, relapse is very uncommon. It is better to teach the patients the signs of leprosy and tell them to come back for examination and tests at any time they have symptoms or signs which could be due to leprosy coming back.

Stop the means of spread of the organism

Education of all people of how to reduce droplet spread of organisms will help (see Chapter 14 page 124).

Improvement in housing (especially so that a lot of people do not live and especially sleep close together in a few rooms) will decrease transmission.

Isolation of cases is not possible and should not be tried. Isolation stops patients coming for diagnosis and treatment and they then spread the disease to many people.

Multidrug treatment of infectious patients makes them not infectious after 3 days, as long as they continue their treatment and is far more effective than isolation.

Raise the resistance of susceptible persons

1. The resistance to leprosy of the general population is raised by better housing, stopping of overcrowd-

ing, better nutrition, the prevention and treatment of other diseases and general public health methods.

2. The resistance of individual persons in some groups of people in some countries is raised by childhood BCG immunisation (see Chapter 14 pages 124–126). This resistance has then been raised even more by further BCG vaccination after childhood and in some areas up to 80% protection is gained (although this may be mainly against only tuberculoid type leprosy). In some areas it is no more than 20%. BCG may well have helped reduce leprosy in the past but now that MDT is so effective, mass vaccination with BCG just to stop leprosy would not be done.

3. Specific immunisation against leprosy is not available at present.

Prophylactic treatment

This is not given routinely or even usually. In some countries, certain people such as infants or even all household members who are contacts of an infectious patient may be given a combination of rifampicin and ofloxacin and minocycline. Follow your national health plan.

16 Some Common Infectious Diseases

This chapter covers some acute specific infectious diseases that cause fever and occur everywhere.

Measles (morbilli)

Measles virus infection causes inflammation of the skin and all mucous membranes (outside and inside the whole body). It is common, infects most children but can infect non–immune adults. It is endemic, but small epidemics occur.

Spread is from the respiratory tract of an infectious patient by direct contract or by droplets.

The incubation period is of medium length (1–2 weeks). Patients are infective from 4 days before the rash to 4 days after the rash starts.

1. At first the symptoms and signs of a fever and then a quite severe viral-type upper respiratory tract infection (URTI) and conjunctivitis develop. These last for about a week.
2. During this time Koplik spots appear in the mouth. They are like white grains of salt on the red mucous membrane, usually on the inner side of the cheek. If you see Koplik spots, the disease is not a usual URTI, but measles.
3. After about 4 days, the typical measles rash comes (see Figure 16.1). There are many slightly red and raised patches of various sizes on the skin. These start on the face and shoulders and then spread to the rest of the body. The other symptoms improve as the rash appears.
4. Severe inflammation can cause viral pneumonia, gastroenteritis, bleeding into the skin and blindness.
5. Secondary bacterial infection of the respiratory tract often occurs, especially otitis media and pneumonia. This usually happens when the rash is improving.

Treatment of measles itself is symptomatic only – rest, paracetamol, and (if in a malarious area) antimalarials. As yet no available antiviral drug helps.

Treat secondary bacterial complications with antibiotics.

Give vitamin A to protect the eyes (100,000–200,000 units) and repeat the next day if a child; or adult with malnutrition.

If otitis media occurs see Chapter 20 page 280.

If pneumonia occurs see Chapter 20 page 287.

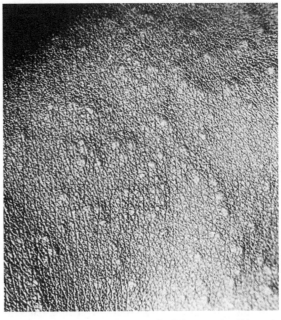

Figure 16.1 *A close-up photograph of the measles skin rash. The rash is often very hard to see on a dark skin.*

If gastroenteritis occurs see Chapter 23 page 360.

If oral thrush (candida or monilia infection) see Chapter 19 pages 226–227 for drugs to use.

> If the patient is a child, see a textbook on children's diseases.

Immunise all children at the age of 9 months and certainly before the age of 1 year with an injection of live measles virus vaccine. Give a later further dose in case the original vaccination was not effective.

Immunise any family and contacts of the patient who have not been immunised.

As a large dose of the virus causes a more severe disease than a small dose, tell non-immune people to keep away from infectious measles patients.

German measles (rubella)

Rubella is not a commonly diagnosed disease. It usually affects children and young adults.

It is endemic but small epidemics occur. The cause is the rubella virus.

Spread is by direct contact or by droplets from the respiratory tract during the infection of children and of adults, or by any discharge from an infant with congenital infection for about 1 year.

The incubation period is of medium length (2–3 weeks).

The patient is infectious from 1 week before the rash appears until 4–7 days after it appears.

The symptoms and signs are usually mild – mild fever, etc. then a rash like mild measles, enlarged lymph nodes behind the neck and in adults often arthritis of fingers, wrist and knee.

Treatment is symptomatic only.

The disease is important only because pregnant women infected in the first 4 months of pregnancy may have babies with deafness, cataracts and other severe problems.

> Patients with rubella should not be allowed to come into any type of direct or indirect contact with non-immunised pregnant women. Infectious patients include normal child or adult patients and babies born with the disease.

Young girls should be immunised if they have not had the disease before the age when they may become pregnant. One live virus vaccine contains measles and mumps as well as rubella vaccine and may be best given at the age of 9 months. It can also be given either before puberty or immediately after delivery.

Chickenpox

Chickenpox is a common infectious disease. The cause is one of the herpes group of viruses – the chickenpox or varicella–zoster virus. It usually affects children, but can also affect adults.

It is endemic, but small epidemics occur. Spread is by direct contact and by droplets from the respiratory tract of infectious patients (but not from the crusts of the sores). The incubation period is of medium length (2–3 weeks). The patient is infectious from the day before the rash appears until 1 week after it appears.

The disease causes:

1. Mild general symptoms and signs of infection (fever, malaise, etc.).
2. A typical rash (see Figure 16.2):
   • macules, papules, vesicles, pustules and crusts (see Figure 32.2),
   • mostly on the trunk and face,
   • with new lesions appearing from time to time (so that at any one time in any one place there are lesions at different stages).
3. The mucosa (conjunctiva, respiratory tract, etc.) can be affected.

In adults a severe chickenpox virus pneumonia or encephalitis sometimes occurs.

Treatment is symptomatic only, with paracetamol and calamine lotion and (if in a malarious area)

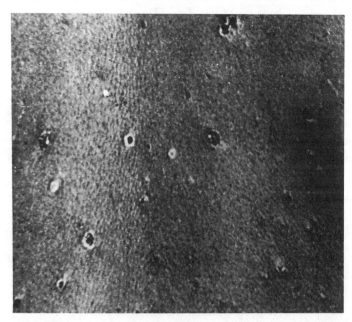
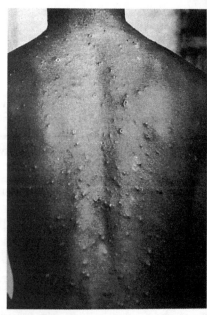

Figure 16.2 *Photographs of a patient affected by chickenpox at about the end of the first week. Note that the lesions are at different stages.*

antimalarials. Antiviral drugs are not available. If the skin lesions become infected by bacteria, give antibiotics by injection or by mouth and skin preparations (see Chapter 32 page 532).

If pneumonia occurs see Chapter 20 page 287.

> If the patient is a child, see a textbook on children's diseases.

Shingles (or herpes zoster)

Reactivation of the chickenpox (or herpes varicella zoster) virus in someone who has had chickenpox before, and some of the viruses have stayed alive in the nerve cells for up to many years, causes this condition. This can happen for no apparent reason, but it can be because the person's immunity has decreased, e.g. old age, cancer and especially HIV infection.

A rash like the chickenpox rash appears (see Figure 16.2 and Figure 16.4) *but*

- it is in the area of skin supplied by only one nerve (see Figure 16.3),
- it is usually on only one side of the body,
- it stops exactly at the midline of the body,
- it usually appears on the trunk or the face,
- there is severe pain in the affected area often before the rash appears, as well as during the rash, and sometimes for months or years after the rash goes.

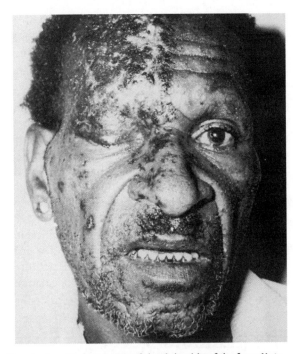

Figure 16.4 *Herpes zoster of the right side of the face. Note that the lesions stop exactly at the midline. Note that the eye is affected and the patient therefore needs urgent treatment and transfer to Medical Officer care. Note that the patient is elderly (probably got HIV infection too).*

Management is as for chickenpox. Powerful drugs, including codeine or even morphine may be needed to control pain at first, and amitriptyline 10–25 mg nocte may help. If the eye is affected put tetracycline or chloramphenicol ointment into the eye every 3 hours, keep the eye covered and transfer the patient urgently to Medical Officer care. Aciclovir 800 mg 4–hourly five times a day, but *only* if given *before* 3 days have *gone* since the rash started *may* reduce pain; but this is usually too expensive to be available.

If the patient is young (less than 50 years old) or if the infection involves more than one nerve at one time or if the infection comes back again after going, always think of an underlying HIV infection allowing the herpes zoster virus to grow and give counselling and do HIV serology. (See Chapter 19 page 231.)

Other viral diseases with skin rash

The diseases described so far have:

1. fever and other generalised symptoms and signs of infection,

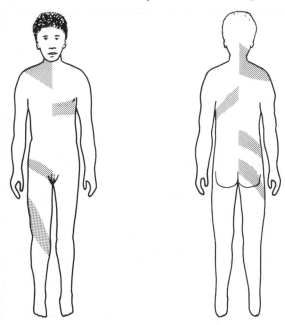

Figure 16.3 *Diagram to show some of the possible distributions of the herpes zoster rash.*

2. skin rash – which is typical of the disease, and
3. mucosa often affected (including respiratory and gastrointestinal tracts),
4. other complications.

There are many other viral diseases which are similar, except that the rash is not typical of only one disease. These viral infections cannot therefore be identified by most health workers, but this does not matter.

If the patient is not very 'sick', treat only the patient's symptoms and (if in a malarious area) give antimalarials. (See Chapter 13 page 81 and see Fever Chapter 36 page 585.)

If the patient is very 'sick' treat him for septicaemia (see Chapter 12) and malaria (see Chapter 13). If he does not improve, transfer him to Medical Officer care. If complications such as encephalitis occur, transfer the patient to Medical Officer care.

The glandular fever syndrome

Epstein–Barr virus (EBV) infection, cytomegalovirus (CMV) infection and toxoplasma infection are all very like each other in a number of ways.

1. Most infections, especially in early childhood, cause few symptoms.
2. All can cause 'glandular fever' (like EBV) (see below) as people become older.
3. After infection the organisms stay in the body for life; but with normal immunity rarely cause disease.
4. If CMV or toxoplasma infection occurs during pregnancy, this can cause severe abnormalities of the unborn child.
5. If immunity is decreased (especially if HIV infection) the infection can start to develop again and cause disease.

Epstein–Barr virus (EBV) infection

This virus infects the B lymphocytes (which make antibodies) and other organs of the body. Almost everyone is eventually infected and the virus stays in the lymphocytes for life; but normal immunity stops them producing disease. The infection usually occurs from infected material spread by close oral contact (e.g. kissing), although possibly at times through blood transfer or sexual intercourse. In developing countries, most infections occur in infancy and cause little or no clinical illness. As health standards improve, infections occur later in life in adolescence and often cause the illness called 'infectious mononucleosis' or 'glandular fever'.

Infectious mononucleosis causes fever, sore throat, neck swelling, pains in various parts of the body and malaise. On examination the tonsils are enlarged and often coated with a white material (which can look like bacterial tonsillitis), lymph nodes are enlarged especially in the neck, the spleen is usually slightly enlarged and there is often a maculopapular rash. The patient usually recovers without treatment in 6–8 weeks. Ampicillin or amoxicillin, if given, often cause a severe rash. Other complications include viral hepatitis, viral meningitis or encephalitis and blood disorders.

Diagnostic blood tests (atypical mononuclear cells in the blood smear and a positive infectious mononucleosis test) can be done in a laboratory.

EBV infection is of importance because of the following. The EBV is associated with the development of Burkitt's lymphoma, anaplastic nasopharyngeal carcinoma (malignant tumour of the back of the nose) and some lymphomas. Infectious mononucleosis has the same symptoms and signs as the 'seroconversion' reaction of HIV infection (though infectious mononucleosis is not related to HIV infection). EBV infection in HIV infected patients commonly causes oral hairy leukoplakia and lymphomas once they develop immunosuppression.

No treatment except of symptoms helps; but do not give amoxicillin or ampicillin, which may make a severe rash occur. As yet no antiviral drugs help. (See Chapter 36 page 585 about fever.) Vaccines are being tested to see if they can prevent the infection.

Cytomegalovirus (CMV) infection

This is similar to EBV except:

1. Hepatitis is more prominent.
2. The infectious mononucleosis blood test is negative.
3. If the infection occurs during pregnancy there is a significant risk of nervous system abnormalities in the baby.
4. In HIV patients CMV can start to grow again. It can cause inflammation of the whole of the gastrointestinal tract, difficulty swallowing and weight

loss. It can cause inflammation of the nervous system with encephalitis and inflammatory masses in the brain (see Chapter 25 page 415). CMV is one of the likely causes of CNS disease in patients with HIV infection.

5. In other immunosuppressed people it can cause inflammation of the lungs with pneumonia.

Toxoplasma infection

This is similar to EBV except:

1. The organism is a protozoan parasite of the small intestine of cats. Infectious cysts in cat faeces spread to other animals including man and form cysts in tissues including muscles and brain. If these cysts are eaten in undercooked meat, these also will cause infection in man.
2. Swelling of the neck lymph nodes is usually the most obvious sign of the disease.
3. The infectious mononucleosis test is negative.
4. If the infection occurs during pregnancy there is a significant risk of damage in the baby, especially the eyes and brain.
5. Treatment is not very effective for an initial infection.
6. In HIV infected patients, toxoplasma can start to grow again and cause inflammation of the brain with symptoms of encephalitis or like a brain tumour. This will often greatly improve if treated with pyrimethamine and a sulfonamide (see Chapter 19 page 229). Inflammation of the lung and pneumonia may also occur.

Mumps

Mumps is a common disease which usually affects children. It is not very infectious, so not all children get it. Many adults are therefore not immune to mumps and so it can also affect adults. The cause is the mumps virus.

Spread is from an infected patient from the respiratory tract and mouth by direct contact and by droplets. The incubation period is of medium length (2–3 weeks). The patient is infectious from a week before the salivary gland swelling appears until all the swelling goes. One attack gives immunity against mumps for life.

The disease causes the following:

1. mild general symptoms and signs of infection,
2. painful, tender swelling of one parotid gland, which lasts for about a week (see Figures 16.5 and 16.6),
3. often painful, tender swelling of the other parotid gland as the first one improves.

Complications include:

1. acute orchitis (painful tender swelling of one or both of the testes) – common in adults;
2. acute pancreatitis with upper abdominal pain and vomiting;
3. viral meningitis and/or encephalitis (see Chapter 25 page 415).

Make sure the patient does not have acute bacterial parotitis. This is an acute severe inflammation of the parotid gland with severe pain, severe tenderness and a lot of swelling as well as fever. It usually occurs in someone who is already sick and not drinking much and not keeping his mouth clean. Acute bacterial parotitis needs urgent treatment with antibiotics.

If the patient has only usual mumps, treat the patient's symptoms with paracetamol or acetylsalicylic acid and (if in a malarious area) antimalarials.

If severe orchitis occurs, transfer the patient for Medical Officer care urgently. If the patient has torsion (see Chapter 19 page 197) he needs urgent surgery, or if mumps orchitis needs prednisolone, or if a bacterial infection needs antibiotics.

Encourage boys to get mumps before puberty as orchitis is then less likely. Mumps complications may not be common enough to spend money on the live mumps vaccine for developing countries; but if measles mumps rubella (MMR) vaccine is available and given at 9 months of age or before puberty, mumps will be prevented.

Whooping cough (pertussis)

Whooping cough, an infection caused by the bacterium, *Bordetella pertussis*, is uncommon in adults. A 'whoop' is not usual in adults who have whooping cough.

But whooping cough may be the cause of some attacks of respiratory illness with severe chronic cough which last for many weeks and have little sputum and any sputum negative for AFB (see Chapter 14 pages 108–109). A blood test would be positive if a laboratory was available. Treatment with inhaled asthma drugs (see Chapter 23 page 294) and with codeine 30–60 mg each 4 hours at times when the cough is worst (often in the night) may help the cough.

> If the patient is a child, see a textbook on children's diseases.

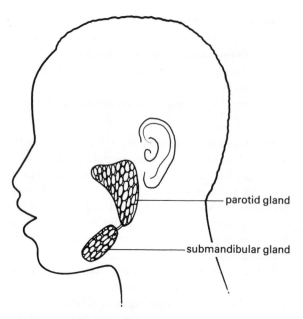

Figure 16.5 *Diagram to show the anatomical position of the parotid and submandibular salivary glands.*

parotid gland

submandibular gland

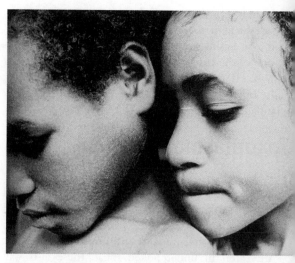

Figure 16.6 *Mumps. The child on the left has parotitis with swelling in front of and below his left ear – in the position of the parotid gland (see Figure 16.5).*

Q fever

Q fever ('Q' originally meant 'query' or 'unknown') is an infection which occurs almost all over the world caused by a very unusual bacterium which lives inside body cells (called *Coxiella burnetti*). This organism can infect most animals including domesticated animals, and can cause them to have an abortion, and lives mostly in the birth canal (including the placenta) and mammary glands. Secretions at birth or from milk get into the air, or if they get onto the ground, they survive and later get into the air in dust, and are inhaled by people who live with animals or who work with animals including those who slaughter animals (kill for meat).

After an incubation period of 3 to 30 days, the person may develop:

1. a mild non-specific influenza-like illness;
2. atypical pneumonia;
3. hepatitis;
4. encephalitis;
5. miscarriage;
   or later on
6. heart (valve) disease;
7. malaise (chronic fatigue).

Diagnosis is not possible in a health centre as it is by blood (serology) test.

Treatment is with doxycycline (100 mg bd for 2 weeks) or tetracycline; if pregnant (for the whole of the pregnancy) co-trimoxazole or erythromycin; or if chronic infection, two antibiotics for up to 2 years.

Q fever is an example of many febrile infectious diseases.

1. It is more common in some than other places. We need to find out and remember what are the common diseases in our area; and then think of these diseases when we see sick people.
2. Even though the diagnosis cannot be proven in a health centre, if thought about, the disease can often be recognised (or at least strongly suspected) by its clinical features.
3. If we recognise the disease, we are much more likely to give effective treatment. (For Q fever, penicillin (used for many mild and moderate infections) does not help; and chloramphenicol (used for many severe infections) will not help. Tetracyclines, however, which are cheap and usually available, do help; and in fact cure.)

Leptospirosis

Leptospirosis is a bacterial (*Leptospira*) infection of many animals including rats, cattle and dogs. The organisms are passed in the urine from infected animals often into water. *Leptospira* get into humans from this water, or from animal urine through close contact with animals. The *Leptospira* get through breaks in the skin but also through normal mucous membranes. Workers who have to go into water and people who handle animals are most infected. The *Leptospira* attack all organs but especially the liver, kidneys, meninges and the inside lining of blood vessels. The organ damage often gets worse when the body has made some antibodies and these damage the *Leptospira* and this causes inflammation in the infected organs.

Infection after 1–4 weeks may cause:

1. No recognised illness often.
2. A mild non-specific influenza-like illness with fever (which can last a long time).
3. A moderate to severe illness with:
   - fever; which can be high;
   - conjunctival inflammation;
   - nausea and vomiting and constipation; which can be followed by abdominal pain, liver enlargement, jaundice and significant hepatitis;
   - muscle aching; which can become severe;
   - headache; and later signs of meningitis but the CSF has findings more like a viral than bacterial meningitis;
   - bleeding with small petechial (pinpoint) haemorrhages in the conjunctiva; which can be followed by bleeding into the skin and all other organs;
   - sore chest; and later cough, chest pain, haemoptysis and shortness of breath with cyanosis;
   - iritis.
4. A severe illness. This may continue to develop from the above; or may, after a few days of apparent improvement after the above, suddenly develop again when inflammation is caused by the body making antibodies which damage the bacteria and causes inflammation in the affected organs:
   - severe hepatitis;
   - kidney failure;
   - bleeding into any part of the body;
   - heart failure;
   - shock;
   - severe pneumonia;
   - death in up to 15% of such cases.

The differential diagnoses of this severe form of the disease include most of the serious acute infec-tions in Chapter 17; but these illnesses (unlike leptospirosis) occur in only some parts of the world. See Table 17.1 page 170.

Diagnosis cannot be proven in the health centre as it needs organisms to be seen in the blood early in the disease or in the urine later, but is usually by blood (serology) tests.

Treatment is as follows.

1. Benzylpenicillin 1.2 million units 6 hourly, or doxycycline 100 mg bd (or tetracycline).
   The patient may get worse due to an inflammatory reaction when the organisms start to die 6–8 hours after treatment starts.
   Note that chloramphenicol is not effective.
   If this disease needing penicillin and other possible diseases needing chloramphenicol are suspected, give BOTH penicillin and chloramphenicol.
   Do not, however, give both penicillin and tetracycline.
2. Antimalarial drugs (see Chapter 13 page 80).
3. Treatment of any condition or bleeding caused by the infection.
4. Transfer to Medical Officer if severe disease as complications (e.g. kidney failure) may need special treatment.

Leptospirosis, like Q fever (page 156), is another example of many febrile infectious diseases.

1. It is more common in some than other places. We need to find out and remember what are the common diseases in our area; and then think of these diseases when we see sick people.
2. Even though the diagnosis cannot be proven in a health centre, if thought about, the disease can often be recognised (or at least strongly suspected) by its clinical features.
3. If we recognise the disease, we are more likely to give effective treatment. (For leptospirosis, if it is not thought about and is seen when obviously a severe infection, only chloramphenicol may be given, which would not help. If thought about, penicillin and chloramphenicol would be given, and cure of the infection expected.)

17 Some Serious Acute Infectious Diseases with Limited Distribution

This chapter is about some acute specific diseases which cause fever but which occur only in certain parts of the world:

1. Bacterial infections
   - Relapsing fever
   - Melioidosis
   - Bartonellosis
   - Plague.
2. Rickettsial infections
   - Typhus fevers.
3. Virus infections
   - Arbovirus infections in general
   - Dengue fever
   - Yellow fever
   - Haemorrhagic fever due to arbovirus infections
   - Japanese encephalitis
   - Haemorrhagic fever due to other viral infections.

Find out which of these diseases occur in your area. If any of these diseases do not occur in your area, do not learn about those diseases.

See Chapter 36, page 585 for diagnosis and management of a patient who has a fever and you are not sure of the cause of the fever.

Relapsing fever

Relapsing fever (relapse means to come back again after it seemed to have gone) is an acute bacterial infection which causes repeated attacks of acute severe fever and damage to the blood, blood vessels, liver, spleen, eyes, nervous system, lungs and heart for 2–9 days which appears to get better and then comes back again in 2–5 days.

There are two types of relapsing fever. One type is caused by a bacterium which normally lives in small animals and is spread by ticks. This is called endemic tick-borne relapsing fever (Figure 17.1). The other type is due to a bacterium which normally lives in man and is spread by lice. This is called epidemic louse-borne relapsing fever (Figure 17.2). The two diseases are clinically similar but the epidemic louse-borne type is the more severe.

Endemic tick-borne relapsing fever

There are many areas where this disease occurs (Figure 17.1). Find out if it occurs in your area.

The bacteria (*Borrelia*) which cause endemic relapsing fever normally live in small animals (such as rats and bats). Ticks bite these animals to suck their blood, and bacteria are carried from an infected animal to another animal by the ticks. These ticks like to live in the cracks of walls and floors of houses. During the night these ticks come out and bite animals and people to suck their blood. The ticks can pass on the bacteria to any person they bite. The infected tick also passes on the bacteria to its offspring through its eggs. An infected woman can pass on the disease to her child through her placenta. Figure 17.3 shows the means of spread.

The symptoms and signs of the infection include:

1. A high fever with chills, headache and confusion, body pains; often nausea and vomiting; often liver and spleen enlargement and, in severe cases jaundice. After 4–5 days the temperature goes down and the patient stays well for 4–5 days or longer.
2. Then a relapse occurs with the same signs though usually they are less severe.
3. This cycle of a fever for 4–5 days and then being reasonably well for 4–5 days may happen up to 10 times.

Complications occur. These include:

1. meningitis with CSF that is clear to naked eye examination (see Chapter 25 page 408);
2. encephalitis (with unconsciousness or fitting) (see Chapter 25 page 415);
3. iritis (see Chapter 31 page 515) and loss of sight.

Apart from loss of sight, relapsing fever can look exactly like malaria, including having similar complications as severe malaria; it is not possible to tell if the patient's condition is caused by malaria unless his blood slide is examined.

Like malaria, people who do not die from the relapsing fever, should become immune to it. The people most affected by relapsing fever are therefore (1) newcomers to the area, (2) infants and children, (3) pregnant women.

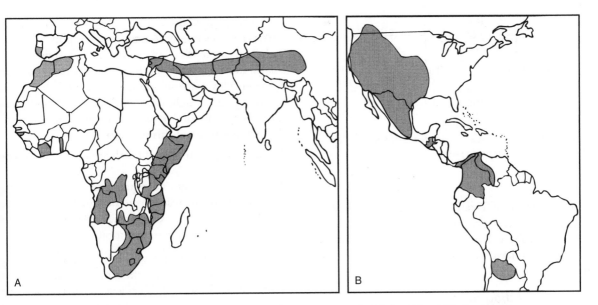

Figure 17.1 *Geographical distribution of tick-borne (endemic) relapsing fever in (A) the Old and (B) New World.*

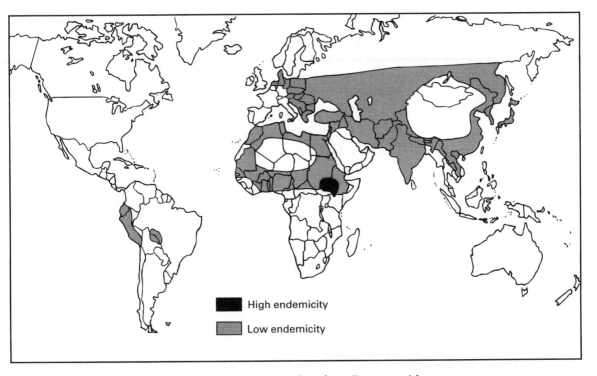

Figure 17.2 *Geographical distribution of louse-borne relapsing fever* (Borrelia recurrentis).

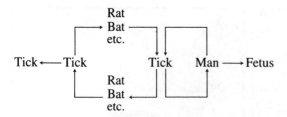

Figure 17.3 *Diagram showing the means of spread of endemic tick-borne relapsing fever.*

If women are infected during pregnancy they usually have a miscarriage, stillbirth or premature labour; but, if the baby is born alive, it can be born infected and will soon have the symptoms and signs of relapsing fever.

Differential diagnosis

This includes malaria and all the causes of fever (see Chapter 13 and Chapter 36 page 585).

If the patient is in or from an area where malaria occurs it is not possible to tell without tests if his fever is caused by relapsing fever or malaria. Always take a blood slide (see Figure 17.4). If possible have the slide examined immediately. If the bacteria (*Borrelia* or *Spirochaetes*) are seen and no malaria parasites are seen the patient has relapsing fever. If malaria parasites (plasmodia) are seen but no bacteria are seen the patient probably has malaria. If it is not possible to have the slide examined immediately you must treat the patient for both conditions.

If the patient has jaundice see Chapter 24 page 401.

Treatment

Penicillin, tetracycline and chloramphenicol all kill the bacteria of relapsing fever. However, some of the bacteria are becoming resistant to penicillin.

When antibiotics kill many bacteria quickly, the toxins from the dead bacteria often cause a severe reaction. This reaction can include a high fever, fast breathing and cough, fast pulse and low blood pressure, encephalitis, shock or heart failure and death. Do three things to avoid this reaction.

1. Keep the patient in bed for the first 2 days of treatment.
2. Make sure drugs and equipment needed for the treatment of any reaction are near to the patient (see Chapter 10 page 44, Chapter 12 and Chapter 37).
3. Give only a small dose of antibiotic at first.

Start treatment with procaine benzylpenicillin 200 mg or 200,000 units IMI. Give the same dose for the next 4 days; or on the second day change to oral tetracycline 250 mg (1 cap) four times a day for a week or doxycycline 100 mg daily. However, do not give tetracycline or doxycycline to pregnant women or to children.

Always treat with antimalarials too (see Chapter 13 page 80) unless you are certain (from history of no possible exposure and good blood slide results) that the patient does not have malaria.

Control and prevention

The only effective way is to stop the spread of the organism by getting rid of the ticks.

1. Treat the home with gamma BHC regularly. This is expensive.
2. Make better houses with no cracks in the walls, floors, ceilings in which the ticks can live.
3. Personal protection with repellents, use of insecticide-treated bed nets (see Chapter 13 page 100), and always sleep above the floor level, etc.

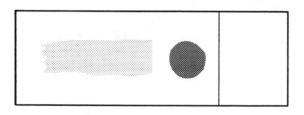

A

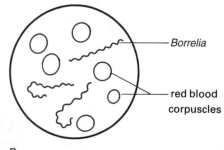

B

Figure 17.4 *Always take a thick and thin blood slide (A) from every patient with any illness and in an area where malaria and relapsing fever occur. Ask for examinations for both malaria and relapsing fever parasites. The appearance of relapsing fever parasites* (Borrelia) *under the microscope is shown in B. They are seen between the red cells; malaria parasites are seen in the red cells.*

Epidemic louse-borne relapsing fever

See page 158, Relapsing fever, first.

Cause, epidemiology, symptoms and signs

The type of bacterium (*Borrelia*) which causes epidemic louse-borne relapsing fever is a parasite of men and lice only. The lice do not pass on the disease to their offspring (see Figure 17.5). This disease starts when an infected person or an infected louse brings the disease to a group of people who are infested with lice. People have lice because they do not wash themselves or their clothes properly. Epidemic louse-borne relapsing fever is normally less common than the endemic type; but large epidemics can occur especially in times of famine or war, in refugee camps, etc.

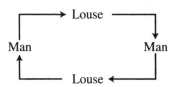

Figure 17.5 *Diagram showing the means of spread of epidemic louse-borne relapsing fever.*

The *symptoms and signs* are similar to the symptoms and signs of the endemic type (see page 158) though there are some differences:

1. The attacks are often more severe with fever and bleeding nose at first, hepatitis with jaundice, enlarged spleen, bleeding, meningitis and encephalitis, and then shock or heart failure as the attack ends.
2. The attacks last longer (up to 10 days) and there may be less time between attacks; but there are usually fewer (3 or less) attacks.
3. Half the people affected may die if they are not treated.

Treatment is the same as for the endemic type (see page 160).

Control and prevention

1. All cases must be treated to reduce the reservoir; but there will still be infected lice.
2. The main means of control is therefore to stop the means of spread. All lice both on patients and other people and in clothing and bedclothes should be killed. People should try to not get lice from other people. See page 165 for details of how to do this. As soon as possible, regular washing of their bodies and clothes should start.

3. Immunisation is not possible.
4. Prophylactic antibiotic treatment is not needed if effective precautions about lice are taken.

Melioidosis

Melioidosis is an acute or chronic infection caused by a bacterial organism (*Burkholderia pseudomallei*). This organism usually lives in soil, ponds, rice paddies, etc. in Southeast Asia but also other tropical countries and is more common in the rainy season. It gets into people by being breathed in or through cuts, etc. on the skin. It does not spread person to person.

Many infections cause no symptoms or signs. If breathed in there may, however, be acute bronchitis, pneumonia or lung abscess. At other times, a chronic infection in the lung develops with symptoms and signs like tuberculosis (but of course sputum is negative for AFB). If the organism gets in through the skin, skin infections with pus formation and lymphangitis or lymphadenitis may occur. Chronic discharging abscesses may follow. The infection can get into the blood at any time after infection through the lungs or skin and cause septicaemia and usually death follows quickly. Any part of the body may be affected with acute or chronic infection but the lungs, skin, liver and parotid glands are those parts most often affected.

People with decreased immunity from, e.g. chronic renal failure, diabetes mellitus, chronic liver disease, alcoholism, old age and possibly HIV infection are more likely than others to develop the disease and more likely to get septicaemia (see Chapter 19 page 224).

Diagnosis is difficult and is made by seeing the organism under the microscope or by special serological blood tests.

Treatment is difficult as special antibiotics such as ceftazidime as well as co-trimoxazole or amoxicillin and clavulanic acid are needed sometimes for many weeks to many months – as well as surgery to drain any collections of pus.

In the health centre the condition may be suspected if a pneumonia does not respond to correct treatment or the patient seems to have TB but the sputum is negative for AFB or a liver or parotid abscess occurs; but all such cases would be transferred urgently to the hospital for Medical Officer care.

Bartonellosis

Bartonellosis is a bacterial infection (with *Bartonella*) of the red blood cells and the cells which line the inside of blood vessels and the lymphatic system. Probably the reservoir is only man. The vector which carries the bacterium is a sandfly. It occurs only in parts of Central and South America.

The acute stage is caused by the bacteria breaking many red blood cells open (haemolysis). The symptoms and signs are: high fever, pains all over the body, vomiting and diarrhoea, enlargement of liver and spleen, anaemia and often unconsciousness and death.

If the patient does not die, he then improves for a month or so. Then many small red lumps full of blood come up on the skin (and also the lining of the respiratory, gastrointestinal and genital tracts). These are most commonly seen on the head and toward the ends of the arms and legs. These lumps go away after 2–3 months.

Treatment is by antibiotics. Chloramphenicol is best especially as secondary infections, which may be sensitive to only chloramphenicol, also occur. Usually, other treatment and often blood transfusion are needed. A severely affected patient usually needs transfer for Medical Officer care after chloramphenicol and treatment of the patient's other conditions are started. (See Chapter 12 pages 64–67.)

People who live in the area where bartonellosis occurs, and do not die from the infection, become immune. It is mostly newcomers to the area and children who are severely affected.

Prevention is by spraying sandfly breeding areas with insecticide and the use of repellents and protective clothing, insecticide-treated bed nets, etc. as well as treatment of patients. Do not transfuse any blood from people in the area unless the test for infection is negative.

Plague

Plague is an acute infection with bacteria (*Yersinia pestis*) which causes:

1. inflammation of lymph nodes,
2. septicaemia, and
3. pneumonia.

Plague occurs in parts of North and South America, Africa and Asia (see Figure 17.6).

In most of these places plague is endemic and is a disease passed from one bush animal to another, often rats, by infected fleas. The infected bush animals often do not die.

If infected fleas from bush animals infect village or town rats, these newly infected rats often die and the fleas then look for a new host and may find man. Man can also be infected when hunting among infected bush animals.

After a bite from an infected flea the person develops bubonic plague – fever, severe sickness and swelling of the lymph nodes (called a bubo) near the flea bite. He then develops septicaemia. He may also develop pneumonia and cough up many of the plague bacteria. These plague bacteria can be breathed in by other people and these people then develop a severe plague pneumonia and usually die quickly. One patient with pneumonic plague can cause an epidemic. An epidemic can also be caused by infected fleas passing from one person to another.

The clinical features are therefore as follows.

Bubonic plague

Usually fever with rigors and severe generalised symptoms and signs of infection occur.

Swelling of the lymph nodes near the flea bite, called a bubo, also occurs. The bubo may become very tender. The swelling is often the size of a chicken's egg. If the patient lives, after a week or so the bubo bursts through the skin and pus comes out.

Usually the patient gets worse with severe toxaemia, bleeding into many parts of the body, septicaemia, sometimes pneumonia and death in 1–2 weeks.

Septicaemic plague

The patient becomes so ill so quickly with the septicaemia that he dies in coma and shock within 3–5 days, before the bubo can become very big.

Pneumonic plague

This may appear in a patient who has bubonic plague or in a person who has inhaled plague bacteria coughed out by a patient.

The onset is acute with fever, rigors and marked toxaemia. There is severe shortness of breath and a cough. At first the sputum is watery but it soon becomes bloodstained. Often the clinical signs in the chest are not marked.

The patient dies in 1–2 days.

Minor plague

An occasional patient (usually during an epidemic) who has bubonic plague is not very sick and the bubo bursts and discharges pus. The patient can walk around; but his pus may infect others.

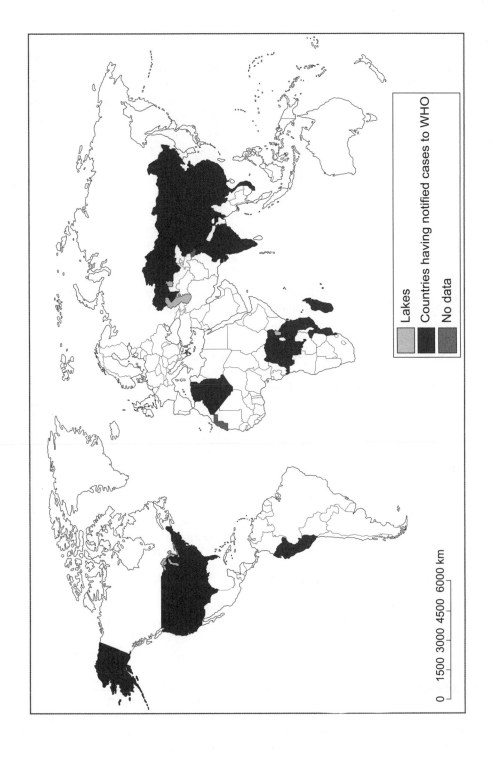

Figure 17.6 *Countries having notified human cases of plague to WHO, 2002–2005. (Source: reproduced from http://www.who.int/csr/resources/publications/WHO_HSE_EPR_2008_3w.pdf)*

Diagnosis of plague can be confirmed by the examination of:

1. fluid aspirated from a bubo,
2. 10 ml of venous blood, and
3. sputum.

Take these samples to send to the laboratory and immediately start treatment. Do not wait for any results if you strongly suspect plague.

Treatment can be with chloramphenicol, tetracycline or streptomycin. As streptomycin should not be used in a health centre except for tuberculosis and as the patient is usually very sick, treat with chloramphenicol as in Chapter 12. It is most important to give immediate treatment to try to save the patient's life and also to try to stop spread of the disease.

Control methods should start immediately, as soon as the disease is suspected.

1. Take the necessary tests from the patient.
2. Start the patient on treatment.
3. Isolate the patient (reverse barrier nursing) until 48 hours of treatment has been given and the patient is improving. Disinfect discharges of body fluids.
4. Start all contacts including yourself on prophylactic treatment (usually tetracycline 500 mg (2 caps) four times a day for a week, but sulfamethoxazole/ trimethoprim (co-trimoxazole) also effective).
5. Very urgently notify the Health or Medical Officer who will immediately confirm the diagnosis and take over control procedures.
6. Kill all fleas on the patient and his clothes and bedclothes and goods. Treat all the patient's contacts and their clothes, etc. similarly. Treat staff who care for the patients similarly. Use permethrin 1% as for lice (see page 165). Treat the whole health centre with insecticide (e.g. permethrin) to kill fleas.
7. Apply insecticides to places where rats run.
8. Kill rats and treat them with insecticides.

If you do these things you may save many lives.

Plague is an 'Event of Public Health Concern' and the Government will notify its occurrence to the World Health Organization and neighbouring countries.

Typhus fever

Typhus fevers occur only in special areas or in special conditions. Only one type is likely to occur in your area, although the epidemic type can occur anywhere if the conditions are right (see page 165). Find out if typhus occurs in your area; and if so, what type.

The typhus fevers are acute infectious diseases caused by rickettsiae (see Chapter 10 page 40). These organisms are carried to people by infected insects. These rickettsiae cause inflammation of the inside of blood vessels going to all parts of the body. The damage to blood vessels and toxins produced by the organisms cause the symptoms and signs of typhus.

The onset is usually sudden with fever and a rigor; the fever usually lasts for about 2 weeks.

Pains and weakness in the muscles are marked.

Headache is severe. Mental disturbance and deafness can occur. In severe cases encephalitis and unconsciousness follow.

The face is usually flushed and the conjunctivae are red.

A rash comes by about the fifth day but may be hard to see if the skin is black. At first the rash is like measles and is of pink macules which go pale when pressed. However, unlike measles, it starts near the axillae and spreads mainly to the trunk. Later on, it does not go away when it is pressed, as bleeding has occurred into that part of the skin.

In the second week, especially in older people, the condition may get worse and often leads to death.

• The spleen becomes enlarged.
• The pulse becomes faster and the blood pressure lower.
• The encephalitis gets worse.
• Blood vessels can be blocked and cause death of parts of the skin or the fingers or the toes, etc.
• Bleeding can occur.
• Kidney failure can occur.
• Heart failure or shock can occur.

After the second week, those who have not died usually improve slowly.

Treatment is usually very effective – as long as it is given soon enough.

1. Give tetracycline or chloramphenicol. Tetracycline is used if the diagnosis is certain. Chloramphenicol is used if the other differential diagnoses of relapsing fever, typhoid, meningococcal meningitis, etc. are not excluded.
   • Give the antibiotic as soon as possible before the serious effects of the disease occur, which the antibiotic cannot cure.
   • Give a large dose for the first dose, i.e. tetracycline 1 g, doxycycline 200 mg or chloramphenicol 2 g.
   • After the first dose give the normal dose for any severe infection, i.e. tetracycline 500 mg each 6 hours, doxycycline 100 mg bd or 200 mg daily or chloramphenicol 1 g each 6 hours.

2. Take a blood smear and start treatment for malaria. (See Chapter 13 page 80).
3. Give good nursing care and the usual treatment of any of the complications which have already occurred.

Control and prevention depend on the type of typhus that is present (see below). There are four main groups or types of typhus.

Epidemic louse-borne typhus

Epidemic typhus is carried from person to person by the human body louse (see Figure 17.7). This disease occurs in places where a lot of people are crowded together and people do not wash themselves and their clothes properly. Suspect epidemic typhus if an illness that could be typhus occurs in a group of people, e.g. famine or war refugees in a camp.

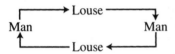

Figure 17.7 *Diagram showing the spread of epidemic louse-borne typhus.*

Control of the disease will include treatment of the patients to reduce the reservoir of infection. However, infected lice still remain. Control of epidemic louse-borne typhus is therefore best done by killing all lice on patients and on all other people, as well as on their clothing and bedclothes. This is done with a suitable in-secticide, at present 1% permethrin or malathion, and it is also helped by better personal washing and hygiene.

1. Wash the patient. Put clean clothes on the patient. Then treat the patient, the clothes and the bed-clothes with insecticide (1% permethrin or malathion powder).
2. Sterilise the patient's clothes by heat. If a steriliser is not available use a hot iron. If ironing is not pos-sible treat the clothes with insecticide powder as above and leave them for 2 weeks before they are worn again.
3. Treat the whole population with insecticide. Special blowers are available which can blow about 60 g of insecticide powder into a person's clothes without their undressing. This should be repeated 1 week later.
4. Regular washing of their bodies and their clothes should start as soon as possible.
5. Get staff to apply insecticide powder to their own clothes and, if possible, have protective clothing which is tight-fitting at neck, arms, legs, etc.

A typhus vaccine exists to raise the resistance of people to the disease. However, the vaccine is usually not available where epidemic typhus occurs.

Prophylactic treatment of close contacts and staff with doxycycline 200 mg daily is needed only before the control measures listed above are in place.

Endemic flea-borne (murine) typhus

Endemic flea-borne typhus is carried to people from fleas which have fed on infected rats (see Figure 17.8).

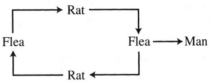

Figure 17.8 *Diagram to show the spread of endemic flea-borne murine typhus.*

Endemic flea-borne typhus is a much milder disease than epidemic louse-borne typhus and death rarely occurs. It is usually a short-lived 'fever of unknown cause'. Treatment is as described above.

Control is by control of rats (by warfarin, ratproof-ing food and burying or burning rubbish, etc.) and fleas (by insecticides). Insecticides are often put where rats are known to run. Protective clothing and insec-ticides should be used by garbage workers and staff caring for patients.

Sporadic tick-borne typhus

Tick-borne typhus is normally a disease of small animals and ticks. Occasionally an infected tick may bite a person. Infected ticks may be brought into a house by dogs which do not themselves suffer from the disease (see Figure 17.9).

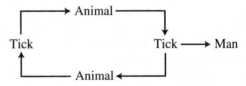

Figure 17.9 *Diagram to show the spread of sporadic tick-borne typhus.*

The disease is usually mild. However, at the place where the tick bit the person, a black ulcer (called an eschar) usually appears and the nearby lymph nodes are usually enlarged.

However, in North America a severe form of typhus called 'Rocky Mountain Spotted Fever' is car-ried by ticks.

Treatment is as described for typhus (see page 164).

Control and prevention is the avoidance of bites from ticks. Treat ticks on dogs. Do not allow dogs to sleep on beds. Wear suitable clothing and insect repellant if going to area where there are ticks. Look for and remove any ticks after possible exposure.

Sporadic mite-borne scrub typhus

Mite-borne scrub typhus is normally a disease of small animals and mites in jungle areas of Asia and the Pacific, especially where jungles have been cleared and scrub or bush is regrowing. People are affected if they are bitten by infected mites (see Figure 17.10).

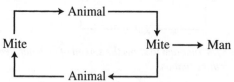

Figure 17.10 *Diagram to show the spread of mite-borne scrub typhus.*

The disease can be quite severe and cause death. Also a black ulcer (eschar) can form where the mite bit. Nearby lymph nodes become enlarged. Numerous eschars can be present and many lymph nodes enlarged if many infected mites bit the person.

Prevention is by keeping away from areas known to have infected mites or by people wearing protective clothing and repellents if they have to go to that area.

If an area where people must live becomes affected, the bush has to be cleared, small animals killed and the area treated with insecticide or burned.

Arbovirus infections

Arboviruses usually live in animals (not man, except dengue) and are carried (or borne) from one animal to another by insects (mosquitoes, sandflies, ticks). (Insects are also called arthropods and 'arbovirus' is short for '*a*rthropod-*bo*rne *virus*'.)

Man is affected by these viruses when an insect carries the virus to him instead of the normal host, although occasionally the virus can be spread another way.

Arboviruses are often localised to one area. They depend on an animal host, which may be localised to one area, and an insect vector, a particular species of which is needed for spread, possibly being localised to one area.

Most of the infections are mild and some possibly occur during infancy when the infant has partial protection from his mother's antibodies. Many local people are immune therefore to the viruses in their own area.

Human epidemics can occur:

1. at the edge of an area of endemic infection;
2. if there is a change in land use which changes the number of animal hosts or vectors (e.g. new irrigation areas allowing more mosquitoes to breed);
3. if there is a change in the human population with non-immune immigrants shifting to the area.

Symptoms and signs can include:

1. spread of the virus from the site of the bite throughout the body, with growth of the virus causing fever for some days;
2. often then an improvement for a day or more;
3. if the virus grows and damages further parts of the body, the following can occur:
   • fever again,
   • skin rash,
   • gastrointestinal symptoms with diarrhoea or vomiting,
   • hepatitis,
   • kidney damage,
   • arthritis,
   • meningitis/encephalitis,
   • immune system damage with blood platelets, blood vessel wall lining, etc. being damaged and allowing serum or even blood to leak out of the vessels and produce low blood volume, bleeding and shock ('haemorrhagic fever').

These symptoms and signs can look very like severe falciparum malaria or septicaemia as well as a number of other infections.

There are very many arboviruses and very many different languages and therefore very many names given to the diseases that they may cause. On most occasions they will not be able to be diagnosed at the health centre and would need special serology blood tests (or even viral cultures) done in a laboratory to be able to diagnose them. This, however, does not matter as most will get better. Tests will be needed only if severe cases occur or if an epidemic occurs.

Special infections are:

• *Dengue fever* – the most common and quickly spreading.
• *Yellow fever* – one of the severe types affecting liver and kidneys.
• *Haemorrhagic fever* – the possible result of either of the above but possible with any arbovirus infection, some other viral infections but also at times almost any type of infection.
• *Japanese encephalitis* – one of the severe arbovirus infections affecting the brain.

Dengue fever

Dengue occurs in most parts of the world. Four types of dengue virus can cause this disease. Dengue viruses are spread by mosquitoes (*Aedes aegypti*). Man is the only host in urban areas, although monkeys can be affected in rural areas. Dengue usually occurs in small epidemics.

Infection with one of the dengue viruses can cause:

1. no symptoms,
2. viral type fever only,
3. typical dengue fever as below,
4. haemorrhagic fever as follows.

Typical dengue fever begins with fever and headache. After this there is often mild upper respiratory tract and conjunctival inflammation, worsening of the headache, severe pain on moving the eyes, severe backache and severe joint pains. The patient may not be able to eat or sleep and may be weak and depressed. Later abdominal pain may occur.

On examination there is fever, the pulse is not fast, conjunctival inflammation, tender eyes, various rashes on the skin (at times like measles though more often red in colour and starting on the trunk and spreading to the arms and face), small vesicles (blisters) on the palate and enlarged non-tender lymph glands.

In some cases after 2–3 days, the patient improves for 1–2 days but the disease returns again and lasts for about 7–10 days in all. Often at the stage of fall of fever, small spots of bleeding (petechiae) are seen in the skin, especially on the lower legs and arms.

In some epidemics in some countries, especially in children, bleeding and shock can occur at this stage. Dengue, therefore, is one of the viral causes of 'haemorrhagic fever' (see next heading and page 170).

There is no improvement in the patient when antimalarials or antibiotics are given.

The patient may feel unwell for months.

Unless a blood slide can be examined for malaria and is negative, all cases of dengue in malarial areas must be treated with antimalarials (see Chapter 13 page 79) as well as rest and other symptomatic treatment. However, do not give aspirin which could make any bleeding worse. Use paracetamol instead. If the patient is very ill, treat for septicaemia (see Chapter 12 page 64). If bleeding or shock occurs, treat as in Chapter 27 page 466.

The means of control and prevention is to kill mosquitoes and stop mosquitoes breeding by having no still uncovered water near houses.

Vaccines to protect against all the four strains of dengue virus are being trialled.

Dengue haemorrhagic fever

This complication of infection with a dengue virus is common in all areas except Africa. It is more common in children under 16 years. It is thought to happen during a second infection with a different dengue virus. The antibodies from the first infection do not control the second infection, but in fact help to cause even more damage than ordinary dengue infection to the blood vessels (making them leak plasma and even blood) and damage to the blood clotting systems (allowing bleeding to occur).

The first 2–7 days of the illness are like (and are) ordinary dengue fever with high fever, etc. *(First point in diagnosis – fever for 2–7 days.)*

After this, there are small bleeding spots in the skin (petechiae), but these are often in the skin over all parts of the body. Bleeding from the nose, gums or gastrointestinal tract, and rarely urinary tract, can occur. If a blood pressure cuff is used on the arm after this, a number of new petechiae may be seen – especially if the cuff is left up between systolic and diastolic pressure for 5 minutes and 20 or more are seen in any 2.5 × 2.5 cm square area on the forearm. *(Second point in diagnosis – bleeding.)*

The liver can be felt enlarged and tender but soft. *(Third point in diagnosis – tender liver.)*

Soon after, the temperature drops; the patient develops cool skin; becomes restless and over the next few hours develops definite shock with fast pulse, low blood pressure, poor peripheral circulation, low urine output, decrease in level of consciousness, etc. and often is dead within 24 hours unless treated correctly. *(Fourth point in diagnosis – shock.)*

If blood tests are available, these would show a low platelet count and a high haemoglobin and haematocrit due to more plasma than red blood cells leaking from the damaged vessels. *(Fifth point in diagnosis – typical blood tests.)* Blood tests such as these and a (MAC) ELISA test to quickly diagnose the dengue virus infection are not usually available.

Treatment includes the following:

1. Give symptomatic treatment; but no aspirin which may cause more bleeding.
2. Give oral rehydration fluid if at any stage of a dengue-like illness the patient is not eating or drinking, so that they will always have adequate hydration and can withstand plasma leak better.
3. Watch carefully at the time of the temperature drop (3–7 days) for cool skin, restlessness, abdominal pain,

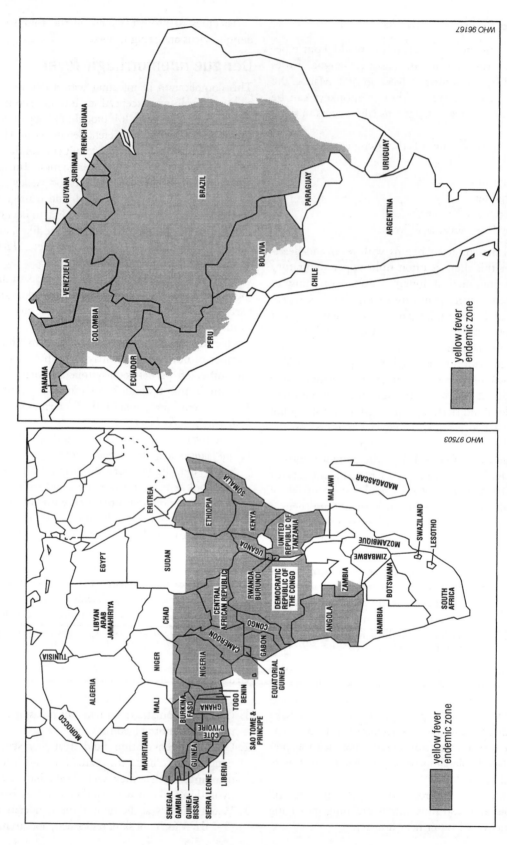

Figure 17.11 The distribution of yellow fever. (Reproduced from www.who.int/csr/disease/yellowfev/impact1/en by permission of the WHO)

low urine output and any bleeding into the skin or elsewhere which would mean development of leak of plasma from the vessels and shock developing. Immediately start intravenous rehydration to replace the fluid inside the vessels (see Chapter 23 page 368). Treatment is usually needed for no more than 48 hours.

4. Make sure not too much intravenous fluid is given, as this could cause heart failure. Once the pulse rate, blood pressure, urine output and skin circulation are normal, reduce the IV fluids to just maintenance fluid. If the jugular venous pressure becomes raised, stop the intravenous fluid until it becomes normal.

If cases occur, always urgently notify your Medical Officer, as treatment of an epidemic of patients and control of the mosquitoes causing the epidemic, may need special organisation.

Prevention will be possible only when a vaccine which produces immunity to all the four strains of dengue virus is available.

Yellow fever

Yellow fever occurs only in western and central Africa and the north part of South America. It may spread to other tropical areas (see Figure 17.11).

Yellow fever is an acute viral infection which can cause:

1. fever,
2. liver damage with jaundice (hepatitis),
3. kidney damage with protein in the urine and sometimes kidney failure, and
4. bleeding into all parts of the body.

The yellow fever virus is usually passed between monkeys and mosquitoes. A person can be infected if he is bitten by an infected mosquito in the jungle (jungle yellow fever). If an infected monkey, mosquito or person comes to a town, the disease can then be passed between people and mosquitoes in the town (urban yellow fever) (see Figure 17.12).

People who live in an area where yellow fever is common and do not die from an attack usually become immune or suffer only mild attacks. Severe attacks occur especially when people from other areas go to an infected area or the disease spreads to a new area.

A typical severe attack is as follows:

1. At first there are severe general symptoms and signs of a viral type infection, similar to dengue fever – fever; pains in the head, eyes, back and joints; red watery eyes; nausea, vomiting, etc. The pulse is usually slow, not fast.
2. After a few days the temperature falls and the patient may improve.
3. After some hours or a day or so, however, the patient may get much worse. He or she develops a high fever (although the pulse is still slow), jaundice and a tender liver and bile in the urine (hepatitis – see Chapter 24 page 393), a lot of protein in urine and also bleeding into the skin and from the nose, mouth, lungs, intestine, etc.
4. Death occurs from liver failure (page 393) or kidney failure (page 453) or bleeding (page 469). If these can be successfully treated and the patient lives for about 12 days, the patient usually recovers.

Yellow fever is therefore one viral cause of 'haemorrhagic fever'.

The differential diagnosis includes malaria, septicaemia, relapsing fever, leptospirosis and viral hepatitis. If laboratory tests are available these would help (see Table 17.1 page 170).

For management, see page 171. Notify any case as an 'Event of Public Health Concern'.

Prevention is by immunisation with living 17D strain of yellow fever virus which does not cause disease but gives immunity for 10 years.

Japanese encephalitis

Japanese encephalitis, which occurs in Asia and in the Pacific Islands as far south as Northern Australia, is one of the arboviruses which causes the most severe type of encephalitis.

Most infections, however, produce no symptoms; or a fever; or an influenza-like illness or gastroenteritis with abdominal pain; then complete recovery and immunity to reinfection. In a few, however, the virus reaches the brain and causes the neck to be arched backwards, loss of full consciousness (the patient may be sleepy, drowsy, unconscious, etc.), signs of irritation of the brain (the patient may be restless, irritable,

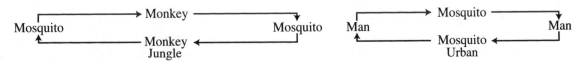

Figure 17.12 *Diagram to show how yellow fever virus spreads.*

Table 17.1 Table to show the differential diagnosis of some causes of a fever with jaundice if you have laboratory tests to help. Remember that pneumonia is also a very common cause of fever and jaundice; but there are also signs in the chest.

Causes of jaundice and fever	Proteinuria	White blood cell total	Blood slide
Yellow fever	A lot	Low	Negative
Malaria	Little or none	Low or normal	Plasmodia
Relapsing fever	Some	High	Borrelia
Septicaemia	Little or none	Variable – often high	Negative
Leptospirosis	A lot	High	Negative but see page 157
Viral hepatitis	Little or none	Low or normal	Negative

confused, delirious, psychotic, twitching, fitting, etc.) and then, within a few days the patient may become unconscious and paralysed. Many die, although some slowly recover with mental abnormality, paralysis, etc. The lumbar puncture shows clear cerebrospinal fluid (CSF). (See Chapter 25 page 415.)

Many of the other arboviruses produce much less severe encephalitis from which there may be much better or even complete recovery.

For management, see Chapter 25 page 415.

Immunisation is possible against this particular arbovirus. Your country may have chosen one of the newer safer live inactivated virus vaccines. The inactivated mouse brain-derived vaccine is given in 3 doses, the second 1 week after the first and the third 3 weeks after the second and boosters after 1 year and then 3 yearly. It is not given before the age of 9 months. As well as mild reactions, about 1 in every 1000 to 10,000 has a severe allergic reaction minutes to 9 days later. Patients should therefore stay near a health centre for 10 days after the vaccination.

'Haemorrhagic fevers' (including dengue, yellow and other viral fevers)

There are a *large number of arboviruses*, as already mentioned (page 166), which can cause symptoms and signs similar to **dengue** or **yellow fever**.

These diseases can cause fever, often with a slow pulse (which should make you suspect a viral disease or typhoid or some unusual infection), generalised aching and pains all over the body, rash, liver damage (hepatitis), kidney damage (proteinuria or kidney failure), bleeding, shock and other conditions.

There are *other groups of virus infections*, which are not arboviruses, but which can cause a similar clinical disease. The infections can also be complicated by shock from blood vessels leaking fluid or blood; or

bleeding through many blood vessels (haemorrhagic fever) with shock.

Lassa fever in West Africa and **Junin** virus in Argentina and **Mochipo** virus in Bolivia are one group of these other viruses. They are spread from man to man by body fluids or body secretions including urine, during close personal contact. They may also be spread to man from rats living in a person's house.

Hanta virus infection in Asia and Europe and America is spread from rats and can cause pulmonary oedema as well as haemorrhagic fever with kidney failure.

Marburg disease and **Ebola** fever in sub-Saharan Africa are from another group of these other viruses. The carriers of the original infection are probably fruit bats (which are not damaged by the organism), which infect gorillas and other monkeys, antelopes and other animals (even porcupines), who die. The infection is spread to humans who handle the sick or dead animals; and then to other people who contact the body secretions of sick or dead infected people.

Crimean Congo Haemorrhagic Fever and **Rift Valley Fever** may be spread by arthropods – ticks in Africa, Asia and Europe for the first group and mosquitoes in Africa for Rift Valley.

Diagnosis of any of these viral diseases is not possible (unless a known epidemic of one of them is occurring) without special laboratory tests (e.g. PCR) not available at a health centre and often not in a country. The Medical Officer must be notified so that he can make arrangements for these tests to be done. Unless a definite diagnosis is made, the best treatment, control and prevention measures cannot be carried out.

Antiviral drugs, usually ribavirin, help most (except dengue, yellow fever, Ebola and Marburg) infections, but are expensive and may not be available in the country. However, if the patient can be kept alive until his body can make enough antibodies to kill the virus, he will probably recover. In a severe case Medical Officer care in a hospital will be needed to do this.

However, there are also a **number of diseases, other than these viral diseases**, which also can cause similar symptoms and signs but are easily curable. Make sure the patient does not have one of these and die from it. Treat for all of these diseases that are treatable if they cannot be ruled out. These diseases include the following:

1. malaria,
2. septicaemia (especially meningococcal and plague),
3. relapsing fever,
4. leptospirosis,
5. typhus,
6. typhoid,
7. viral or other causes of acute hepatitis,
8. drug side effects.

Management

Management in a health centre of an unusual severe acute disease of unknown cause, which causes fever, abnormalities of many body systems, but especially haemorrhage in many places of the body, and shock, therefore includes the following. When a final diagnosis is made, those measures below that are not needed can be stopped.

1. Immediately notify the Medical Officer and the Health Officer and ask for advice and help.
2. Do *not* transfer the patient unless the Health Officer or Medical Officer tells you to do so, as epidemics can be caused by transfer. In an epidemic a special medical team should be sent to set up a proper isolation and treatment unit where the disease is occurring.
3. Isolate and barrier nurse the patient with extreme care.
   - Staff must take care not to get even the smallest amount of blood, urine, stool, saliva, or ANY body fluid onto themselves as the infection may get through normal skin.
   - Staff should wear plastic aprons and if possible tubular plastic over the arms, these things being under a gown, two pairs of gloves, waterproof mask and goggles, cap and overshoes.
   - Only if staff can be certain that no blood or secretions can possibly get on them, should IV treatment or blood (or other) tests be taken. If this is not certain (and it is probably best to wait for the Medical Officer to check this) give enough oral rehydration fluid and oral drug therapy for the conditions below.

4. The patient's clothes and bedclothes (sheets, etc.) are infected and must not be handled until sterilised or be burned or buried.
5. Staff should put insecticide (e.g. 1% permethrin powder) on their clothes if the case is possibly epidemic typhus. Treat the patient and his clothes and his bedclothes with 1% permethrin powder.
6. Treat for septicaemia (see Chapter 12 pages 64–67). (If IV treatment is not possible give oral chloramphenicol.)
7. Treat for falciparum malaria (see Chapter 13 page 80). (If IV treatment is not possible give oral artemisinin drug and companion drug.)
8. Treat shock if it occurs. (See Chapter 27 page 466.) Start IV fluids immediately. (If IV treatment is not possible give oral hydration fluids as for dehydration.)
9. Do not give acetylsalicylic acid which may make bleeding worse. Instead give paracetamol.
10. Treat bleeding if it occurs (see Chapter 27 page 469 and give vitamin K 2.5–25 mg).
11. Treat for hepatitis if it occurs (see Chapter 24 pages 393–395).
12. Treat for kidney failure if it occurs (see Chapter 26 page 453). However, until you are certain kidney failure has occurred, make sure you give the patient enough fluid (at least 2 litres a day) so that the patient has enough fluid in his body to make a normal amount of urine.
13. Nurse the patient under an insecticide-treated mosquito net (and, if possible, in a room which has insect screens on the door and windows). Treat the net and screens with insecticide (permethrin) (see Chapter 13 pages 87 and 100).
14. Have the patient's room and the whole health centre sprayed with a residual insecticide.
15. Destroy or treat any breeding places for mosquitoes around the health centre.
16. Treat the patient's room with gamma BHC if ticks occur in the area.
17. Kill any rats by warfarin or other rat poison or any other means. Also put insecticide along known rat runs and on any dead rats.
18. Take 20 ml of blood and keep it in the refrigerator at 4°C for special laboratory tests. Take and keep blood and urine for the usual laboratory tests (see Chapter 6 pages 26–29). If the patient dies, get permission to take at least a piece of liver for examination (a piece aspirated (sucked back into a syringe) through a very thick needle put into the liver through the skin is better than none).

Do these only if you can be absolutely certain no blood or fluids could get on you.

19. If a diagnosis of the cause of an epidemic is made and ribavirin is effective and is provided, it should be given as soon as possible to suspected cases.

20. Try to make sure infected dead people are buried 2 m under the ground or completely cremated (burnt) without anyone except those with full protective clothing, gloves, etc. touching the body.

21. No one should handle dead gorillas, other monkeys, antelopes or other animals who have died from an acute severe illness (as above), especially if a number of animals have died (i.e. epidemic amongst the animals).

22. All contacts of the patient should be kept separate from the rest of the community for as long as the incubation period of the illness is found to be. All should be seen twice daily. If any develop a temperature or other symptoms of the disease at any time, this person should immediately be admitted and isolated and treated as a case.

Make sure no blood or ANY tissue fluid or body secretion gets on your staff members or you. Use plastic aprons and tubular plastic over arms under gown, two pairs of gloves, waterproof mask, goggles, cap and overshoes.

18 Some Serious Subacute and Chronic Infectious Diseases with Limited Distribution

This chapter is about the following diseases:

1. Bacterial infections
   - Typhoid fever
   - Brucellosis
2. Protozoal infections
   - Leishmaniasis
   - Trypanosomiasis
3. Worm infections
   - Schistosomiasis

Typhoid fever (enteric fever)

Typhoid fever is an acute or subacute disease caused by the typhoid bacteria. At first it causes malaise, fever, abdominal pain and constipation. Later, it causes diarrhoea, rash, enlargement of the spleen and very severe toxaemia. This stage may be complicated by intestinal haemorrhage or perforation. Sometimes, mild cases may cause only a non-specific illness and fever.

Cause, epidemiology, pathology

Typhoid fever is caused by infection with typhoid bacteria *(Salmonella typhi)*. The reservoir is persons infected by the typhoid bacteria.

The typhoid bacteria in the faeces or urine of infected people may contaminate food or the water supply. This may occur if infected people handle food, or if they do not use a toilet. It may also occur if the water supply is not safe from contamination by urine and faeces or is not treated. Sometimes flies carry the bacteria from faeces to food.

The bacteria, when swallowed, multiply in the bowel and then spread through the whole body. They grow best in the lymph glands, spleen, gall bladder and parts of the wall of the intestines.

The faeces of the patient are often infectious for weeks or months; and the patient may become a carrier for life.

The incubation period is about 2 (1–3) weeks.

An attack of the infection usually produces considerable immunity.

A similar but less severe disease caused by *Salmonella paratyphi* types A, B or C is called 'paratyphoid fever'. This is occasionally also carried by domestic animals.

Symptoms and signs, course and complications

For the first week the patient has the general symptoms and signs of infection with some special features. He has malaise, headache, pains all over and fever. He may have a cough and nose-bleeds. He usually has mild abdominal pain and constipation. On examination, the patient has fever but the pulse may be slower than expected. Nothing else special is found.

During the second week the patient becomes worse. General symptoms and signs may be severe. Abdominal pain becomes more severe and diarrhoea occurs. On examination the patient may not be fully conscious. The fever and slow pulse are still present. There may be signs of bronchitis in the chest. The abdomen is usually distended and may be tender especially in the right iliac fossa. The spleen is enlarged. A rash made up of red spots, each of which lasts for a day or so, may be seen, especially on the abdomen.

During the third week, the general and abdominal symptoms and signs become worse. The patient may become unconscious and die.

During this third week two special complications may also occur.

1. The bowel may perforate (get a hole in it through to the peritoneal cavity). The pulse gets faster, the temperature falls, the abdominal pain and tenderness get worse and signs of generalised peritonitis may develop (see Chapter 23 pages 349–350).
2. Haemorrhage may occur from the intestinal wall into the intestine. The patient may pass blood from the rectum; or simply become pale and shocked (and later pass blood).

If the patient does not die he or she usually starts to recover quickly after the fourth week. However, in some cases, after about 2 more weeks, there is a return of the symptoms and signs, though usually not as severe as before.

A much milder disease often occurs. Sometimes it may be only a fever with perhaps a mild gastrointestinal upset, or some of the other symptoms or signs of the more severe disease.

Tests

None are available at the health centre.

The white cell count is usually not raised unless a complication has developed when it may be high.

Blood and faeces cultures may grow the typhoid organism.

Diagnostic features

- Generalised symptoms and signs of infection (often pyrexia of unknown origin ('PUO'), 'sick', and no response to antimalarials, see Chapter 36 page 585).
- Slow pulse despite fever.
- Constipation at first, then diarrhoea.
- Abdominal distension and tenderness.
- Spleen enlarged.
- Rash on abdomen.
- Persistence of temperature and severe toxaemia, after treatment with antimalarials, without any focal signs.
- Intestinal bleeding or perforation after 3 weeks.

Differential diagnosis

- Other causes of fever (see Chapter 36 page 585).
- Other causes of gastroenteritis have to be differentiated from typhoid (Chapter 23 page 360).
- Other causes of septicaemia (Chapter 12 page 64).

Treatment

Transfer the patient to Medical Officer care, if this is possible.

Dispose of faeces and urine carefully. Disinfect bedpan and other articles used by the patient, and carefully wash your hands after caring for the patient.

Give chloramphenicol 1 g orally (or by injection) each 6 hours. When the fever stops reduce the dose to 500 mg orally four times a day. However, continue the chloramphenicol for 2 weeks. In some areas sulfamethoxazole/trimethoprim (co-trimoxazole) or even amoxicillin/ampicillin may be more effective. (See Chapter 11 pages 56–57.) You need to find out from your Medical Officer what antibiotic and what dose to give for your area.

Treat also as for other cases of gastroenteritis. (See Chapter 23 pages 363–367.)

Treat any complication in the usual way.

Treat later with praziquantel if schistosomiasis is possible so that the worm does not become a carrier. (See Chapter 18 page 190.)

Transfer

Transfer these cases:

1. All diagnosed cases (especially if laboratory tests have shown many *S. typhi* organisms in your area to be resistant to drugs available to you in the health centre and the patient therefore needs a quinolone or third generation cephalosporin or azithromycin, etc.; or in case injected high-dose dexamethasone or a blood transfusion or an operation is needed). (Start antibiotics before transfer.)
2. The diagnosis is suspected but cannot be made and the patient is very 'sick'.
3. A complication occurs, especially intestinal perforation or haemorrhage.

Control and prevention

1. Kill the organism in the body of the host (reservoir) (patients and carriers).
   If typhoid fever is uncommon in the area, investigation is needed to find out where the infection came from. A carrier is usually responsible. A Medical Officer may be able to treat such a carrier with drugs or sometimes an operation. However, *if typhoid is common in an area,* a search would not be made for the source of infection.
2. Stop the means of spread of the organism.
   - Patients and carriers should not be allowed to handle food for others.
   - Proper community disposal of all faeces and urine is essential.
   - Safe community water supply is essential.
   - Careful nursing of cases that are infectious is important. Staff must wash their hands carefully after caring for a patient.
3. Raise the resistance of susceptible persons.
   An oral, live typhoid vaccine (three or four doses 2 days apart but not if taking antibiotics or mefloquine) or injected Vi capsular polysacchroid typhoid vaccine (one dose) is far more effective than the old whole cell TAB vaccine subcutaneous injection. Immunisation will make it less likely for an immunised person to get typhoid. This is given, however, only to a person who has a particular risk of getting typhoid, such as travellers or occasionally household contacts of carriers or children in an endemic area or in an epidemic.

Brucellosis

Brucellosis is due to an infection with the *Brucella* bacteria. The infection is normally one of cattle, goats, sheep, camels and pigs and it can cause abortions in these animals. The bacteria can spread to people who live with or work with infected animals or who drink raw untreated (unpasteurised) milk or food made from milk which has come from infected animals.

The *Brucella* bacteria live mainly in the lymph tissues; but can affect joints and other parts of the body.

At first there can be a fever with severe pains and malaise which lasts for a few weeks. After this the patient usually slowly improves.

However, the fever may come back many times every week or every few weeks. The spleen sometimes becomes enlarged and sometimes very enlarged. Pain in a joint, especially the hip, is common. Chronic osteomyelitis of the spine or infections in almost any part of the body sometimes occur. Weight loss is common. Depression is common. Other parts of the body can be affected.

> Suspect brucellosis in a patient with a fever which comes and goes and who has difficulty walking.

In most people this prolonged infection is usually overcome by the body itself after a year or so; but in a few, the infection continues.

Diagnosis can be made only by special blood tests (serology) not possible in a health centre.

Treatment needs more than one antibiotic to stop relapses and may need to go on for 6–12 weeks and may need drugs used for tuberculosis (therefore, tuberculosis has to be excluded by X-ray and other tests). These things are not usually possible in a health centre.

Refer or *transfer* suspected cases to a Medical Officer for diagnosis and to rule out tuberculosis and for drug treatment.

Leishmaniasis

(a)

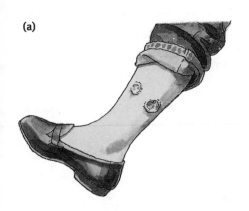

(b)

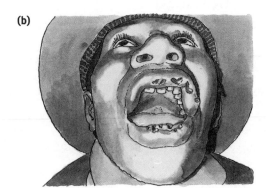

(c)

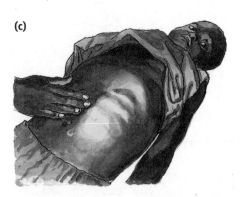

(d)

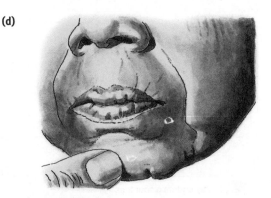

Figure 18.1 *Clinical signs of leishmaniasis. (a) A patient with cutaneous leishmaniasis. (b) A patient with mucosal leishmaniasis. (c) A patient with visceral leishmaniasis. (d) A patient with nodular post-kala azar dermal leishmaniasis (PKDL).*

Leishmaniasis is a group of diseases caused by an infection with one of the many species (types) of the protozoal organism called *Leishmania*. These live in macrophages (one of the defence cells from the blood which then go into most other organs) and then in some of these organs.

There are four main types of leishmaniasis.

1. Skin leishmaniasis (skin only) called 'cutaneous leishmaniasis' or dermal leishmaniasis.
2. Skin, but also mucous membrane leishmaniasis, which occurs only in South America and is called 'mucocutaneous leishmaniasis' or 'espundia'.
3. Skin, blood, bone marrow, spleen, liver and lymph node leishmaniasis called 'visceral leishmaniasis' (VL) ('visceral' means 'of the organs inside the body') or 'kala azar'.
4. 'Post–kala azar dermal leishmaniasis' (PKDL), when most of the organisms of visceral leishmaniasis have been killed by treatment for VL but some are still living in the skin (see Figure 18.1).

Skin leishmaniasis occurs in 82 countries; 1 million new cases occur each year; and 10 million are affected today (see Figure 18.2A).

Visceral leishmaniasis causes 500,000 new cases each year and 50,000 deaths each year (see Figure 18.2B).

The reservoir of infection includes not only infected people but also some infected dogs, rodents and many other animals.

The organisms are spread to man by the bite of many species (types) of sandfly which have been infected from an infected man or infected animal (see Figure 18.3).

Control and *prevention* of leishmaniasis follow the usual rules; but stopping the means of spread is usually the only practical method to use.

1. Kill the parasite in the original host or reservoir.
   (a) Find and treat patients with the disease; but this works only if man is the only host of that *Leishmania* in that area. Also, there are many cases without symptoms which are not found and treated. Also, treatment is either dangerous or expensive.
   (b) Find and kill any dogs or rodents or other animals with the disease; but first special tests are needed to prove that these animals do have the same *Leishmania* organism that is causing

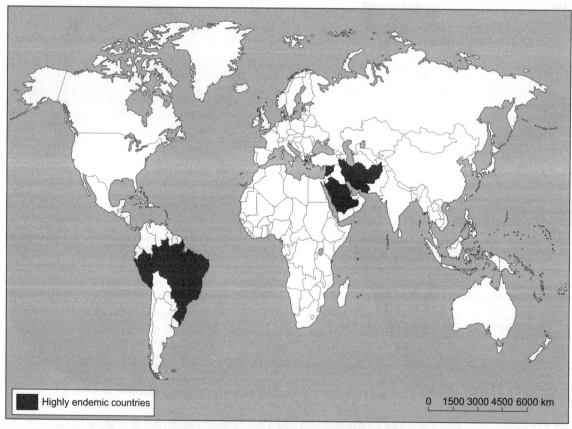

Highly endemic countries

0 1500 3000 4500 6000 km

Figure 18.2A *Distribution of cutaneous leishmaniasis. (Reproduced from Where does leishmaniasis occur in the world? www. who. int/leishmaniasis/leishmaniasis_maps/en/index2.html by permission of the WHO)*

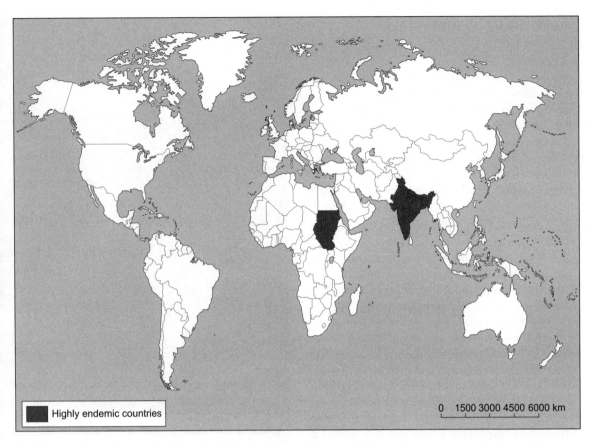

Figure 18.2B *Distribution of visceral leishmaniasis. (Reproduced from Where does leishmaniasis occur in the world? www. who. int/leishmaniasis/leishmaniasis_maps/en/index2.html by permission of the WHO)*

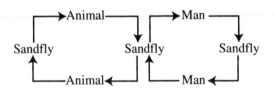

Figure 18.3 *Diagram to show the means of spread of leishmaniasis.*

the human disease and not another *Leishmania*, before all of these animals are killed. If foxes are affected they are difficult to find and kill. Dog collars containing deltamethrin greatly reduce infection of dogs and therefore people.

2. Stop the means of spread.
Sandflies breed in dark damp places like animal houses, rubbish dumps, anthills, crumbling stone-work, animal burrows and even pit latrines, etc. They do not usually fly more than a few hundred metres from where they breed. The following may therefore be effective:

(a) Move houses away from places where sandflies breed.
(b) Kill sandflies with regular spraying of residual insecticide where they breed.
(c) Protect people from sandflies by clothing, repellents and fine sleeping nets or door and window covers which are also treated with insecticide.

3. Raise the resistance of possible new hosts.
This can be done only for skin leishmaniasis. A sore used to be started by injecting aspirate from another person's sore into an area of the skin where a scar would not matter. This sometimes did stop sores starting in areas such as the face, where a scar would matter. It is, however, dangerous, as hepatitis or HIV infection may also be passed on.
Vaccines for immunisation are now available but only in some areas and they do have problems. Immunisation for visceral leishmaniasis is not yet possible.

4. Prophylactic treatment is not yet practicable (as safe effective cheap drugs for treatment of cases are not available).

Dermal (skin) leishmaniasis

Skin leishmaniasis occurs in many Old World countries; that is Africa, the Mediterranean, the Middle East and Asia, where it is called 'oriental sore'. It also occurs in the New World, that is Central and South America, where it is often more severe or widespread and can involve also the mucous membranes (see Figure 18.2A). It has been divided into types of increasing severity. At times, these differences are due to different strains of the organism, but more importantly the differences are due to different types of cellular immunity in the patient (similar to leprosy, see Chapter 15 pages 127–129).

1. *Single non-ulcerated or dry ulcerating lesions (e.g. 'oriental sore').* (See Figures 18.1 and 18.4.)

   Children are most often affected as most adults have been infected and have become immune.

   The incubation period is from weeks to months.

   At first, a small reddish itchy lump appears in the skin where the patient was bitten by the sandfly. A crust forms on top of the lump. The lesion gets bigger and usually becomes a rounded ulcer. The ulcer has thick raised edges and a discharge of blood and pus, which dries to form a dark crust (see Figure 18.4). Small new lumps may start around the edge of the ulcer. These lumps then get bigger and ulcerate. Eventually, as these join, a large ulcer up to 10 cm in diameter may be formed. Sometimes the lesion does not ulcerate and stays as a large lumpy mass. The ulcer is not painful. The ulcer usually lasts for months to a year and then heals leaving a thin scar.
2. *Multiple discharging lesions.*

   Sometimes there may be more than one lesion if the patient was bitten in several places. Sometimes new lesions form on the skin between the first lesion and the nearby lymph glands. Eventually all heal.
3. *Relapsing lesions.*

   These lesions heal or nearly heal only to get worse again, although eventually they do heal. If the condition goes on for a long time, severe scarring can result.
4. *Diffuse lesions.*

   If cellular immunity is poor, some organisms spread through all the skin producing nodules and loss of colour which can look like lepromatous leprosy. Ulcers form and do not heal (see Figure 18.6).

The *diagnosis* can be confirmed by aspirating some fluid through a fine needle from the edge of the ulcer and examination of this fluid under the microscope for the *Leishmania* organisms. (See Figure 18.4.)

Treatment includes the following:

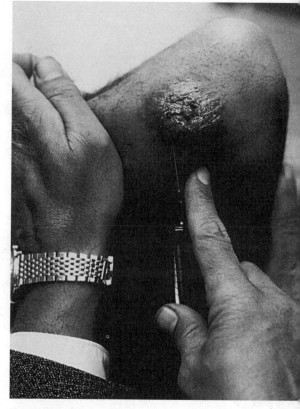

Figure 18.4 *A typical skin lesion of skin leishmaniasis. Diagnosis will be confirmed by aspirating some fluid, putting it on a slide and examining it under a microscope for* **Leishmania.**

1. Eusol (see page 524) dressings two or three times a day until the crust is gone and the ulcer is clean.
2. If there is a lot of secondary bacterial infection, give antibiotics such as penicillin or tetracycline; this is usually not needed.
3. Then keep the ulcer clean and dry under a dressing and it will probably heal in a few weeks.
4. Treat with paromomycin (aminosidine) 15% and urea 10% ointment for 4 (up to 12) weeks if available, as this usually halves the time to heal.
5. Transfer or refer to a Medical Officer for consideration for treatment with drugs injected into the lesion or as for kala azar if any of the following:
   • if the ulcer does not heal after the above treatment,
   • if the ulcer is on the face,
   • if there are a number of large ulcers (more than 4 ulcers) or very large ulcers,
   • if there are disseminated or diffuse lesions,
   • if there is mucous membrane as well as skin disease.

Epidemiology, control and *prevention* – see page 175.

Mucocutaneous (skin and mucous membrane) leishmaniasis.

This occurs in Central and South America. The worst kind is called 'espundia' in Brazil. In espundia the first lesion (see Dermal leishmaniasis) may be on the face, ears, elbows or knees. Either then, or months or years later, lesions appear in the mucous membrane of the nose and mouth. The nasal mucous membrane swells up and then ulcerates. The ulcer may slowly destroy all the tissues of the nose so that a terrible-looking hole is left in the centre of the face. The mouth, lips and throat may be affected (see Figure 18.1).

The patient does not have a fever or feel ill because of the infection. Diagnosis, treatment, prevention and control are as for dermal and visceral leishmaniasis.

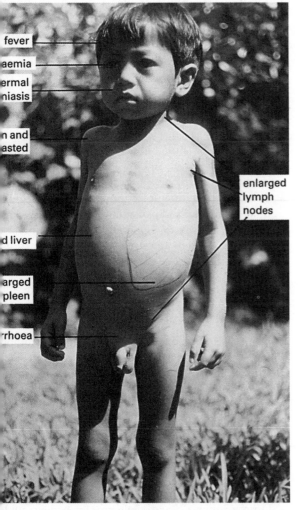

fever

aemia

ermal
niasis

n and
asted

enlarged
lymph
nodes

d liver

arged
pleen

rhoea

Figure 18.5 *A patient with visceral leishmaniasis. Note the features of the disease listed above.*

Visceral leishmaniasis (kala azar)

Visceral leishmaniasis occurs in many countries (see Figure 18.2B), but is particularly a problem in patients from India, Bangladesh, Nepal, Brazil, Ethiopia and especially Sudan.

A person is infected by the bite of an infected sandfly. The *Leishmania* organisms infect macrophages. They spread to the bone marrow where they damage the cells that make new blood. The organisms spread also to the lymph nodes, liver and spleen which are damaged and become larger than normal. Some patient's cellular immunity may, however, be good enough to control all signs of the infection.

In the Mediterranean region children and visitors are the ones mostly affected. In other areas, adults are affected too.

The illness starts with a fever. This is usually not severe at first and the patient continues his normal life. Sometimes, however, the fever comes with tiredness, weakness, loss of appetite and weight loss. The fever may be worse in the afternoon and again at night and occasionally is severe.

The spleen soon becomes enlarged, and often becomes very enlarged (see Figure 18.5).

The liver becomes enlarged but not very enlarged.

The lymph nodes may become enlarged (not often in India but often in Africa).

The patient becomes anaemic.

Bleeding may occur.

The patient may have repeated attacks of diarrhoea.

The patient becomes thin and wasted.

A darkening of the colour of the face, hands and feet used to occur in India, but now is not common.

Symptoms and signs of other infections (e.g. pneumonia, TB, gastroenteritis) may also develop especially as the patient's immunity gets less.

Dermal (skin) leishmaniasis may occur – often after treatment and when the patient is getting better (as the skin is then the place the organisms find it easiest to live). There are pale or reddish thickened areas of the skin on any part of the body. Lumps may form – especially on the face (see Figure 18.6).

Leishmaniasis may come back in a patient previously immune to or successfully treated for the disease if the patient's immunity decreases, especially if he develops HIV infection. Patients with HIV infection often get reactions to drugs used for treatment of VL. They also often do not get better with treatment.

The *diagnosis* can be best confirmed in the laboratory by finding the *Leishmania* organisms in a biopsy or aspi-

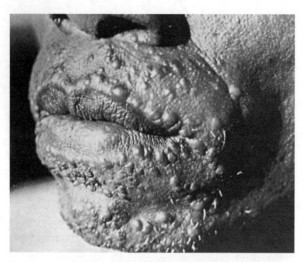

Figure 18.6 *A patient with dermal leishmaniasis. Do not confuse this condition with leprosy. (Source: W. Peters and H.M. Gilles, A Colour Atlas of Tropical Medicine and Parasitology, London, Wolfe Medical Publications 1981) (Dr D.M. Minter)*

rate (best from the spleen, although the biopsy can bleed, and spleen and liver biopsies therefore should not be done in the health centre). Aspirate from enlarged lymph nodes (see Chapter 14 page 110) or affected skin (see Figure 18.4) can be taken and sent to the laboratory.

Tests for antibodies against leishmaniasis are available. These tests, however, will be positive not only in patients with the disease but also infected persons whose cellular immunity is so good it does not let enough organisms grow to cause the disease, and also in patients who have had the disease but have been treated and apparently cured. These tests show only present or past infection but do not show that the patient's present illness is due to leishmaniasis. Sensitive laboratory tests exist but are not suitable for use in health centres. The direct agglutination test (DAT) is easier but needs a laboratory technician. The (rK39) immunochromatographic test strip is much easier to use (as it needs only blood from a finger prick put onto the strip) and quicker to get the result (20 minutes); but it still costs US$1 and is the only accurate method available for health centres. However, it is less often positive in Africa than in India in infected patients.

When no other tests are available, the formaldehyde gel test can be used. Put 1 ml of the patient's serum into a test tube. Add one drop of 40% (commercial) formaldehyde (formalin). If the patient has kala azar (but also other infections which cause a large increase in protein in the blood), the serum (1) becomes solid (so that if you tip the tube upside down the serum does not run

out) *and* (2) the serum does not stay clear (but goes a milky or dirty colour). Both (1) and (2) are needed for the test to be positive. The test is not positive until a few months after the patient has been infected, but other infections can also give a (false) positive result. It also may not be positive in more than half of the infected people.

Treatment is different in different parts of the world as the sensitivity of the organisms to drugs varies. Treatment is also by drugs with dangerous side effects. Unless you have been specially trained in the use of the best drugs for your area, transfer the patient for diagnosis and treatment to a Medical Officer.

Treatment also includes treatment of other serious conditions present such as malnutrition, malaria, other parasites, anaemia, etc. If these are not treated, side effects of the drugs for leishmaniasis are more common and more severe. Always immediately start treatment for these conditions.

Drugs to treat VL include (often in combination):

1. Pentavalent antimony injections – sodium stibogluconate or sodium antimony gluconate or meglumine antimonate; by IMI or IV infusion daily for 1 month; but severe (sometimes fatal) side effects occur, especially in the old or young or wasted patients, and also many organisms are now resistant.

2. Paromomycin (aminosidine) IMI is relatively cheap and reasonably safe and effective (and can be used with other drugs).

3. Aromatic diamidine injections – hydroxystilbamidine isethionate and pentamidine.

4. Amphotericin B, IV, especially for resistant organisms, is at present the most effective single treatment. The liposomal preparation is more effective and less toxic but expensive.

5. Oral treatment is now available using miltefasine 100 mg/kg daily for 4 weeks. It is usually very effective (even against organisms resistant to other drugs), has few side effects (but GI ones including vomiting well after drug administration and liver and kidney damage can occur).

It must not be given if pregnancy possible or if pregnant or during breastfeeding as it can cause severe damage to a baby. To stop resistance developing, every dose should be seen by the health worker to be swallowed (i.e. DOT like TB treatment) and it would be best used in combination with other drugs. It is still not cheap.

Drug treatment is not as effective for patients with HIV infection as for others. If the patient is also given nti-HIV treatment, this helps; but success is still less nd relapses more common than in non-HIV patients.

Epidemiology, control and *prevention* (see page 175).

African trypanosomiasis (sleeping sickness)

African trypanosomiasis occurs only in parts of West and Central Africa and of East and Southern Africa (see Figure 18.10).

African trypanosomiasis is an infection caused by a protozoal parasite called a trypanosome (*Trypanoma brucei*). There are two kinds of trypanosomes that affect man. If a trypanosome is in blood or other fresh fluids examined under the microscope, it can be seen to swim with its tail (see Figure 18.7).

Animals including pigs, cattle and large game are affected as well as man.

The trypanosomes are carried from infected animals or man by the tsetse fly (see Figures 18.8 and 18.9). There are at least two kinds of fly which carry the disease and they have different breeding, living and biting habits.

The trypanosomes cause a chronic disease which causes death. At first, a sore, called a chancre, may form where bitten. Then a fever occurs when the blood, lymph glands and other organs of the body are affected. Later, the nervous system is damaged and this damage is the usual cause of death. One type of trypanosome (*T. b. rhodesiense*) in East and Southern Africa may cause all of these things in a few months. The other type

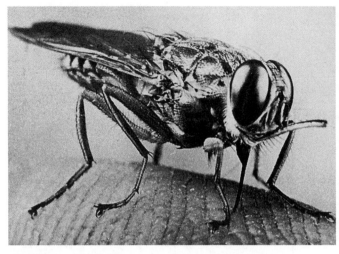

Figure 18.8 *The appearance of a tsetse fly. The actual size is about 15 mm in length.*

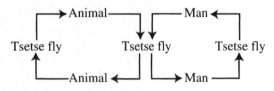

Figure 18.9 *Diagram to show how the trypanosomes can be spread.*

(*T. b. gambiense*) in West and Central Africa may take a year or more to cause death.

African trypanosomiasis occurs only in people who go into a tsetse fly infected area.

The first symptom is caused by the bite of a tsetse fly. It is painful, but the pain soon goes. However, if trypanosomes were injected by the fly, then 1–3 weeks later a reddish non-painful lump comes up at that place. It can form into an ulcer (chancre), especially if it is scratched. The lesion itself goes away in 2–3 weeks. Sometimes the person does not notice the lesion.

The trypanosomes, however, then pass into the blood and lymphatic system and cause any of the following. This is called Stage 1 or 'haemolymphatic' stage.

1. Fever with weakness, headache, etc. The fever may be there for a few days and then be gone for a few days over many months. However, the fever can be severe and present all the time. Everyone who has fever for no other obvious cause in an area where trypanosomiasis occurs must be investigated for trypanosomiasis. Wet and also stained thick blood films must be examined for trypanosomes before

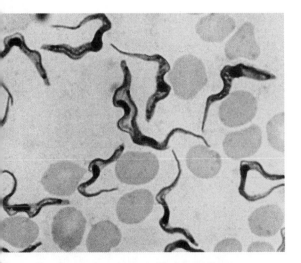

Figure 18.7 *A trypanosome magnified many times.*

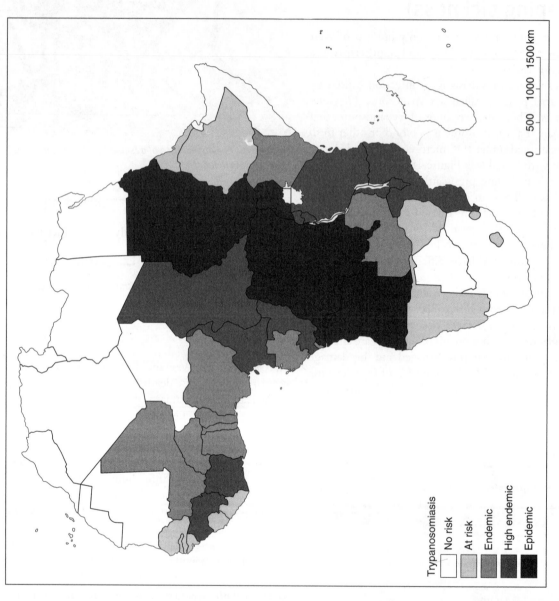

Figure 18.10 *The distribution of African trypanosomiasis.*
Reproduced from Control of Human African Trypanosomiasis: a Strategy for the African Region – Regional Committee

any other diagnosis is made. The examination should be repeated at least three times if the patient does not get better. The CIATT test (see below) is an easy quick test which may help diagnosis if available.

2. Lymph node enlargement. Any nodes may be enlarged but those at the back of the neck are the ones most commonly affected. The nodes are smooth, firm, painless and not stuck to the skin or other structures.

   If in an area where trypanosomiasis occurs, aspirate fluid from the node with a fine needle and have it examined for trypanosomes (see page 110).

3. Skin rashes or itchiness or oedema or thickening (especially of the face so that the patient's facial expression does not change much with emotional changes) may occur.

4. Enlargement of the spleen and liver.

5. Bone marrow damage with anaemia.

6. Heart damage with a fast pulse even when the fever is not present and later sometimes heart failure.

7. Kidney damage with proteinuria.

8. An autoimmune type disease with inflammation of many organs.

After some weeks in East African trypanosomiasis or months in West African trypanosomiasis the nervous system is infected. Signs of meningitis, encephalitis and organic psychosis then occur. (See Chapters 25 and 35.) The patient often has headache, abnormal behaviour, sleeps during the day but not at night, does not eat, shakes, becomes paralysed and passes into a coma and dies. Examination of the CSF shows an increase in the protein and in the cells. However, when there are no nervous system signs, a lumbar puncture should not be done just to see if the nervous system is involved. A lumbar puncture may cause infection of the nervous system from other parts of the body, if the nervous system was not yet infected, unless the patient is already on treatment.

If the patient is from or is in an area where trypanosomiasis occurs, then trypanosomiasis must be thought of and tests done for it in all cases of:

- fever without other obvious cause,
- lymph node enlargement,
- anaemia,
- wasting,
- sleepiness,
- meningitis,
- encephalitis,
- psychosis, and
- unconsciousness.

In any of these conditions, if another cause for the condition is not found and if the condition does not get better on the proper treatment for the diagnosis you made, then transfer the patient to a Medical Officer for the special tests to diagnose trypanosomiasis.

Tests

Special tests which show who has the infection (even if there are no symptoms and signs) are available. The card indirect agglutination test for trypanosomiasis (CIATT) is positive in almost all patients with symptoms and signs, and in infected people before symptoms and signs appear. It needs only blood from a finger prick. The card agglutination test for trypanosomiasis (CATT) is positive in only *T. b. gambiense* infections and has false positive and false negative results.

Other means of diagnosis need the trypanosomes to be seen under the microscope in body fluids, e.g.

- needle aspiration from the edge of the original sore,
- needle aspiration from enlarged lymph nodes,
- blood including wet films, thick films and use of special concentration methods,
- bone marrow aspiration,
- CSF obtained at lumbar puncture (which should not be done unless already on treatment).

Treatment

Treatment is more effective the earlier it is given. Early *gambiense* disease can be treated with IV pentamidine or suramin, but early *rhodesiense* disease can be treated only with IV suramin. These drugs kill only organisms in the body outside the brain. Once the brain has been infected, other drugs are also needed. Intravenous melarsoprol is the usual drug used for infection of the brain, but it has very serious side effects and in fact up to 15% of patients treated may die from these side effects, mainly encephalitis. Before the patient is fit for treatment with melarsoprol he will need treatment with suramin and/or pentamadine, as well as treatment of any anaemia, malnutrition, malaria, etc. Do not do a lumbar puncture before the patient is on treatment with suramin or pentamadine as, if the brain is not infected, the needle going into the CSF may spread the infection to the spinal cord and brain. A newer drug, eflornithine, is a much safer and more effective treatment than melarsoprol; but it is effective only for *gambiense* infections. A new oral drug (DB289) under trial may solve treatment problems. In view of the very serious side effects of most of these treatments and the expense of the other drugs, if you suspect or diagnose a case of trypanosomiasis, then transfer the patient to Medical Officer care at a

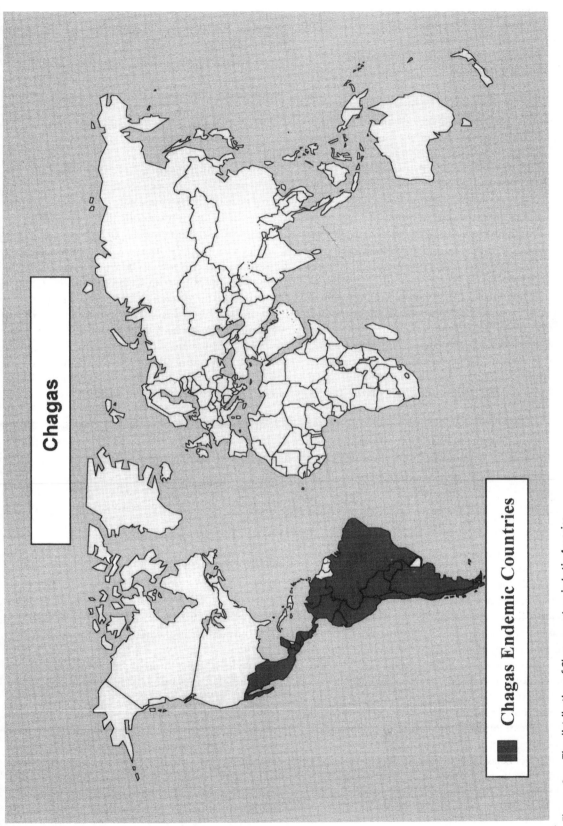

Chagas

Chagas Endemic Countries

Figure 18.11 *The distribution of Chagas vectors in Latin America.*
(Source: Pan-American Health Organization (PAHO/WHO) Program of Communicable Diseases, January 2003)

enter the heart and nervous system and cause both acute and chronic disease in these places.

Transfusion of blood or an organ transplant that contains the organisms will also cause infection. The infection can pass through the placenta from mother to child.

The acute disease affects children more often than adults but only one third of infected patients have this.

A lesion may appear where the organisms enter the body. This is usually on the face. If the organisms enter through the conjunctiva, there is swelling of the eyelids of the eye on that side of the face; the lids are firm and red and swollen enough to close the eye. If the organisms enter the skin at the site of a bite, there can be a painful red swelling with much hard oedema around it on the skin. The nearby lymph nodes are enlarged. The swelling and the enlarged lymph nodes stay for some weeks.

One to three weeks after the infection, the patient may develop a high fever and the liver, spleen and lymph nodes may be swollen. The pulse is often fast, even when the fever is not present, because by then the heart is also damaged. Meningitis and encephalitis can occur. The organisms can be found in the blood or the fluid aspirated from the swelling on the face or from an enlarged lymph gland, if it is examined under the microscope.

After 1–3 months the patient usually improves slowly; but the organisms stay in the body. They stay especially in the heart and in the nerves of the oesophagus and large intestine, which they slowly destroy.

After about 15 years of being well about 3% each year and eventually 30% of infected patients develop complications caused by this nerve and muscle damage. Eventually about one third of infected people develop complications. The patient may get heart failure or irregular pulse, or the patient may suddenly die because his heart stops. The muscles of the gastrointestinal tract may not contract properly and the patient may also develop difficulty in swallowing dry food and later any food or fluid; or aspirate (breathe in) food or drink, causing pneumonia. The patient may develop abdominal swelling and constipation. These things are due to the organisms causing chronic damage to the nerves and muscles of the heart; and the nerves and muscles of the oesophagus and end of the colon in the gastrointestinal tract.

If the patient has or gets HIV infection the acute trypanosomal infection may come back again or be more severe and the complications develop more quickly.

Diagnosis

Diagnosis can be made by seeing the trypanosomes in the blood only during the first illness but not afterwards. Special laboratory culture methods are interesting and accurate but too expensive for routine use. Serology tests including CFT and IFAT can be used to tell who has been infected; but other conditions can also cause a (false) positive test.

Treatment

Treatment is unsatisfactory. Previously nifurtimox, but now benznidazole, greatly reduce and in some patients get rid of all of the trypanosomes. The earlier treatment is given the better, as it will stop the acute disease, may cure the patient, and may delay or stop the late effects of the infection on the heart and gastrointestinal tract. Benznidazole seems now to be worth giving after the acute illness until the late stage of the disease; but in the last stage no drugs can cure the damage to the heart, gastrointestinal tract, etc. and treatment of the infection is too late to help the patient. Better drugs are needed which are more effective, have fewer side effects and do not need 2 months' treatment, usually in hospital, as at present. At the late stage of the disease only treatment of symptoms is possible.

If, therefore, you suspect the disease, especially if it is early before incurable heart or gastrointestinal tract damage, send the patient to a Medical Officer for diagnosis and treatment, unless you have been specially trained in the use of methods for these.

Treatment of heart failure is as usual; but if the patient has times when his heart beats irregularly or stops, or if the patient has gastrointestinal problems, special treatment by the Medical Officer will be needed.

Control and prevention

Control and prevention is as follows; but mostly by insecticides to kill the reduvid bug or by making better houses so there is nowhere for them to live.

1. Kill the parasite in the body of the original host or reservoir.
   Kill rodents, cats, chickens, etc. which live where people live, if these are known to be infected.
2. Stop the means of spread.
   The bug can be killed by various insecticides, including pyrethroids and gamma BHC applied to the house and places where domestic animals and birds live. This, however, is expensive and has to be repeated regularly until transmission of infection stops. After the initial insecticide treatment, use a special plaster which covers cracks between

bricks in the walls and itself will not later crack, and replace thatched roofs with galvanized iron to reduce the places where the bugs can live. Best of all, but usually not possible, is to rebuild houses with smooth walls and non-thatched roofs which have no hiding places for bugs. Sleeping under an insecticide-treated net will also help stop bugs biting the face. However, there are new ways of using insecticides, e.g. fenithrothion, which is put into paint which a family uses to paint inside the house; the use of traditional insecticides outside the house; and also the use of insecticide-treated bedclothes and nets, have proved effective.

All blood collected for transfusion should be tested for the parasite and not transfused if positive.

3. Raising the resistance of people is not yet possible.
4. Chemoprophylaxis is not yet possible (as the present drugs do not kill all the organisms in all treated people – even after 2 months of treatment).

Schistosomiasis (bilharziasis)

Definition and cause

Schistosomiasis is the disease caused by worms called schistosomes. These are small worms, like very short (1–2 cm) threads of cotton, which live in the veins of the pelvic organs for 3–5 years (sometimes longer). The female worm lays many eggs and these eggs damage the bladder, large intestine and liver and cause the disease.

Epidemiology

About three hundred million people are infected by schistosomiasis, many in the tropics, where there are collections of fresh water with snails living in them.

Three main types of schistosome affect people. Figure 18.13 shows the distribution of the different types.

1. *Schistosoma haematobium* and the less common *S. intercalatum* affect mainly the bladder of humans in Egypt, the Middle East and Africa only.
2. *S. mansoni* affects mainly the large bowel in people and baboons and rodents in Egypt, the Middle East, Africa, and South America.
3. *S. japonicum* (and the less common *S. mekongi*) affect the large and small bowel and other parts of people and many domestic and wild animals including horse and dog, in Japan in past times and now in China, Southeast Asia and the Philippines.

S. mansoni and *S. japonicum* live mainly in the pelvis in the veins which come from the bowel. The eggs

cause marked chronic inflammation of and ulceration of the wall of the bowel. This causes diarrhoea and dysentery. It also allows the eggs to enter the bowel and be passed in the faeces. *S. haematobium* lives mainly in the pelvis in the veins which come from the bladder and the genital tract. The eggs cause marked chronic inflammation and ulceration of the wall of the bladder. This causes blood in the last part of the urine passed. It also allows the eggs to enter the bladder and be passed in the urine. Inflammation around the eggs also damages the urethra, bladder, ureters and kidneys. It also damages the female genital tract and this leads to infertility, ulcers and tumours.

If the eggs in the urine or the stool get into water, the eggs release worm-like animals, now called miracidia. These miracidia swim around until they find certain snails in which they can grow. Then the worms leave the snail and are called cercariae. These cercariae swim in the water until they find a person or a person swallows the water they are in. They can go through the skin of a person or through the mucous membrane of the person's mouth. The worms then travel around the body of the person until they enter the pelvic veins, where they develop into adult schistosome worms (see Figure 18.14).

Some of the eggs laid by the female do not enter the bladder or intestine. Some are carried away in the blood in the veins from the bladder and intestine. These veins join to form the portal vein which runs to the liver (see Chapter 24 page 391). The eggs then damage the liver. Some eggs can be carried to other parts of the body as well as to the liver – especially the lungs and the spinal cord and brain – and damage these parts too.

The body may very slowly develop antibodies and cellular immunity. At first this causes severe inflammation around the eggs laid in the venules (little veins) with a lot of swelling around them. This swelling causes a lot of the symptoms. The inflammation lessens as better immunity

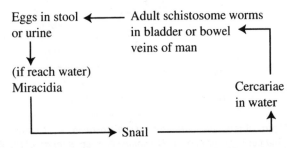

Figure 18.14 *Diagram to show the life cycle of schistosomes.*

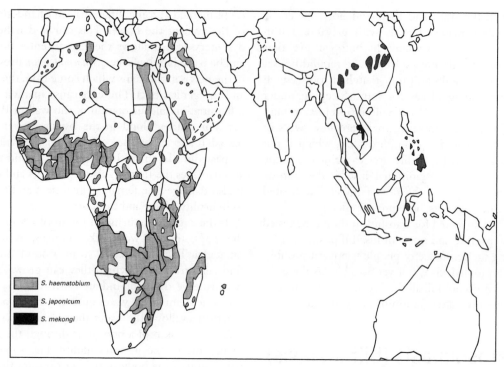

Figure 18.13A *The distribution of schistosomiasis (*Schistosoma haematobium, S. japonicum *and* S. mekongi*).*
(Source: The control of schistosomiasis: second report of the WHO Expert Committee. Geneva, WHO, 1993; WHO Technical Report Series No. 830.)

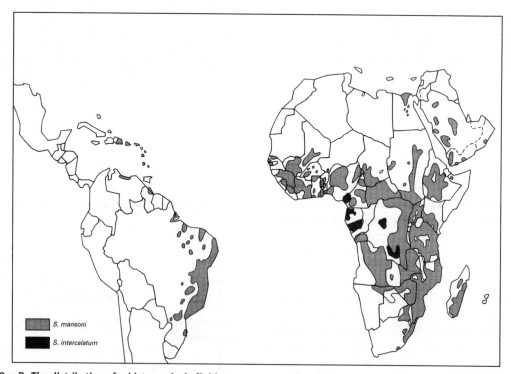

Figure 18.13B *The distribution of schistosomiasis (*Schistosoma mansoni *and* S. intercalatum*).*
(Source: The control of schistosomiasis: second report of the WHO Expert Committee. Geneva, WHO, 1993; WHO Technical Report Series No. 830.)

develops in most adults. Also, the better immunity stops a lot of new worms developing from reinfections.

Symptoms and signs

1. A mild skin itch and rash may come where and soon after the cercariae go through the skin.
2. Several weeks later there may be fever, malaise, cough, abdominal pain and allergic-type symptoms and signs. These are caused by the worms travelling around the body to the pelvic veins and starting to produce eggs. These symptoms last for 1–2 weeks. They are common only in *S. mansoni* and *S. japonicum* infections and only in the first infection.
3. Then the patient is quite well until either urinary (see 4 below) or intestinal (see 5 below) schistosomiasis develops. Either urinary or intestinal schistosomiasis may be followed by other complications (see 6 below).
4. Urinary schistosomiasis is caused by *S. haematobium* laying eggs in the veins of the wall of the bladder. Inflammation in these areas causes the bladder wall to be thick and ulcerated, and at times to bleed. Ulcers of the bladder wall cause blood in the urine. Usually the patient notices the blood in the urine when he has nearly finished passing urine. The patient also notices more blood after exercise. If there is a lot of blood in the urine, clots may form and there may be much pain (especially in boys). If there are not many worms the patient may slowly improve and have blood in the urine only sometimes. He may even get better. However, if there are many worms and especially if the patient gets new infections, then other problems develop. The bladder cannot stretch and the patient has to pass urine often (urinary frequency). Bacterial urinary tract infection may develop (see Chapter 26 page 443). After years, the ureter may become narrowed and cause chronic kidney failure (see Chapter 26 page 449). The urethra may become blocked and cause urinary retention (see Chapter 26 page 453). Cancer may start and grow in the damaged bladder. The female pelvic organs and the bowel can also be damaged. Ectopic pregnancy and infertility due to fallopian tube damage; ulcers and cancers of the cervix, vagina and vulva; and increased likelihood to get HIV infection if exposed to HIV all occur in infected women.
5. Intestinal schistosomiasis is caused by *S. mansoni* or *S. japonicum* laying eggs in the veins of the wall of the intestine. Inflammation in these areas causes the bowel wall to be thick and ulcerated and at times to bleed. This can cause abdominal pain, diarrhoea and dysentery (blood and pus in the faeces), but without any fever. If, however, salmonellae live in the worm, these can cause repeated attacks of bacillary dysentery, which will keep coming back until the worm is killed. If there are not many worms and no new infections, there may be no symptoms or the symptoms caused may go away. If there are many worms or if there are new infections, the symptoms may be severe. Infected lumps on the inside of the bowel may prolapse (come out) through the anus.
6. Complications can develop if the eggs are carried in the blood to the liver, lungs or nervous system.
   (a) The eggs can damage the blood vessels in the liver and cause portal hypertension (see Chapter 24 pages 395–398). The liver becomes large at first; but later small. The spleen becomes very large. The patient can become anaemic. Fluid can collect in the abdomen (ascites) and in the legs and back (oedema). The patient can vomit so much blood that he becomes shocked and dies.
   (b) The eggs damage the lung. The right side of the heart cannot pump the blood through the lungs and heart failure develops (see Chapter 27 page 461).
   (c) The eggs can damage the brain or spinal cord. The patient can develop paralysis or epilepsy or blindness or coma, etc. (see Chapter 25). This is more frequent in *S. japonicum* infections.

It is usually only those patients who have many schistosome worms in their body and repeated infections as the original worms die, who develop significant symptoms and signs of disease. Even those with marked disease may, however, greatly improve with treatment, as many of the symptoms are due to the acute inflammation around new eggs that are laid, and if no new eggs are laid and the inflammation slowly goes away, the patient will improve.

Tests

1. Urine test for blood if positive in known endemic area for *S. haematobium* almost always means infection.
2. Eggs may be seen through the microscope when the urine or stool is examined. Urine passed between 10 a.m. and 2 p.m. is the most likely to show the eggs. A concentration method and repeat examinations are needed to find eggs in the stool.
3. If laboratory tests are not available at the health centre, add boiled then cooled water to a sample of

urine or a sample of stool in a test-tube or bottle. Allow the urine to stand for 1 hour or the stool to stand for 1 night, then examine the tube through a magnifying glass against a dark background. Miracidia may be seen swimming in the tube if eggs were present.

Differential diagnosis

1. Fever.
   See Chapter 36 page 585.
2. Blood in the urine.
   In an area where schistosomiasis is common, almost all cases of blood in the urine are due to schistosomiasis.
   If there are
   • no eggs (or miracidia) in the urine, or
   • other urinary symptoms present, or
   • symptoms present in other systems, or
   • not cured by anti-schistosome treatment,
   then transfer the patient to the Medical Officer for diagnosis of other causes and treatment. See also Chapter 26 page 454.
3. Diarrhoea/dysentery
   Bacillary infections usually also cause fever. Amoebic infections and cancer of the intestine also cause dysentery or large intestinal symptoms and signs.
   If eggs or miracidia are not present in the stool and if the dysentery continues or keeps on coming back and does not improve after treatment with metronidazole and an anti-schistosome drug, then refer or transfer the patient to the Medical Officer for diagnosis of other causes and treatment. See also Chapter 23 pages 387–389.

Treatment

Do not spend a lot of time and money treating patients with mild infection and few symptoms of schistosomiasis if they are likely to become infected again soon. Give health education to these patients on how not to get more infections.

Also, many of the old drugs to treat schistosomiasis have serious side effects, which are more common if the patient has liver disease. Newer drugs are now available which are safer and easier to use but are expensive.

Also, the best drug for your area depends on which type of schistosome worm is the most common in your area.

Praziquantel is the usual treatment. It is effective against all schistosomes. The dose is 40 mg/kg once. For *S. japonicum* two doses of 30 mg/kg may be needed

– the second one 4–6 hours after the first, and given preferably after food in the evening. Tablets contain 600 mg or 150 mg. Side effects are mild – gastrointestinal upsets, dizziness, fever, skin rash. However, as mentioned, the drug is expensive. Not all worms may be killed with one dose.

Metriphonate 7.5–10 mg/kg body weight, given in three doses at intervals of 14 days, is effective treatment for *S. haematobium* only. It has very few side effects and is relatively cheap; but has the disadvantage of many people not taking the second and/or third doses.

Oxamniquine is given in doses that have to vary with the resistance of the schistosome worms in different areas. The doses vary from 15 mg/kg body weight as a single oral dose for adults and 10 mg/kg body weight for children with a second dose 4–6 hours later, up to 20 mg/ kg body weight for 3 days in a row. Oxamniquine has few side effects apart from occasional fitting and gastrointestinal symptoms, but is effective against only *S. japonicum*.

You must therefore find out the Health Department policy for:

• which patients you should treat,
• which drugs you should use,
• the doses, side effects and precautions you should take for these drugs.

Refer patients who have urinary problems or rectal problems or gynaecological problems, which are not helped by the drugs, to the next visiting Medical Officer. Surgery may help some of these patients.

Control and prevention

You can use most of the normal methods of control and prevention. However, experts need to study each area to find out which method is best. So again you must find out the Health Department policy for your area.

1. Kill the parasite in the bodies of the original host or reservoir.
   Patients with symptoms are treated.
   It is possible, after health education about methods of control of schistosomes, that the whole population will agree to co-operate in the programme. Only then can the community and health workers work out effective methods to distribute a drug (usually praziquantel) to all the population in the area.
2. Stop the means of spread of the parasite.
   (a) All people (including children) must use a toilet at all times. Proper toilets are needed for all people.

(b) Control or eradicate the vector (the snail).

Get rid of as many places where snails can live as possible (drain swamps, use landfill, etc.).

Niclosamide poisoning is the other method used. There are many ways of doing these things.

Specialists will advise what way is best for your area.

In many places it is not practicable to eradicate snails.

(c) Stop contact with water that has cercariae in it. Safe drinking water should be supplied. If water is left to stand in pots for 2–3 days before drinking, cercariae will die.

No one should swim or wash in infected water. Houses would be best built away from water and safe water piped to the houses. Ideally, safe swimming water should be supplied for children.

People should not work in infected water – this is almost impossible for many farmers or fishermen.

3. Raise the resistance of the people.

Immunisation is not yet possible but vaccines are at present being developed.

4. Prophylactic treatment.

This is used only in special circumstances.

19 Sexually Transmitted Diseases Including HIV Infection and AIDS

For an easy to understand and much more detailed guide to STD with syndromic diagnosis and treatment, see *Sexually Transmitted and other Reproductive Tract Infections* (WHO, 2005, or later edition). Modified tables and some other material have been reproduced in this book with permission of the World Health Organization (WHO). For details about this book and other information on HIV infection, see page 216.

Summary of STD diagnosis and management

Follow National Guidelines if they differ from this.

1. **Find out what syndrome the patient has.**
   (1) Urethral discharge ♂
   Gonorrhoea and chlamydia infections most likely.
   (2) Vaginal discharge ♀
   Without cervicitis
   Candida *and trichomonas and bacterial vaginosis most likely.*
   With cervicitis
   Cervicitis on examination, OR
   Partner symptomatic, OR
   Two or more of the following:
   - age < 21
   - single
   - > 1 partner
   - new partner in last 3/12
   Gonorrhoea and chlamydia infections most likely.
   (3) Sores or lumps in the genital mucous membrane or skin (♂+♀)
   Syphilis and chancroid most likely.
   (4) Swelling of the inguinal lymph nodes (♂+♀)
   With genital ulcer
   Syphilis and chancroid most likely.
   Without genital ulcer
   Lymphogranuloma venereum most likely.
   (5) Scrotal swelling (♂)
   Gonorrhoea and chlamydia most likely.
   (6) Lower abdominal pain (pelvic peritonitis) (♀)
   Gonorrhoea and chlamydia +/– ordinary and anaerobic bacteria most likely.
   AND as well as one or more of the above six
   (7) Risk of, or symptoms or signs of, HIV infection.
2. **Find out the patient's risk of getting and passing on this STD AND HIV infection.**
3. **Find out all of the patient's sexual partners who may be infected with this STD AND HIV infection.**

4. **Give treatment to the patient and all possibly infected persons for the most likely cause of the syndrome.**
   (1) Urethral discharge
   Gonorrhoea and chlamydia
   Ciprofloxacin 500 mg PO once OR*
   AND
   Doxycycline 100 mg PO for 7 days.
   (2) Vaginal discharge
   With cervicitis
   Gonorrhoea and chlamydia
   Ciprofloxacin 500 mg PO once or
   Ceftriaxone 250 mg IMI once if could be pregnant OR* AND
   Doxycycline 100 mg bd PO or
   Erythromycin 500 mg qid PO if could be pregnant for 7 days
   AND
   Treat as for bacterial vaginosis if this also present.
   Without cervicitis
   Candida and trichomonas and bacterial vaginosis
   Clotrimazole 500 mg intravaginally once
   AND
   Metronidazole 2 g PO once.
   (3) Sores or lumps in the genital mucous membrane and skin
   Syphilis and chancroid
   Benzathine penicillin 2.4 million units IMI once
   AND
   Doxycycline 100 mg PO bd or
   Erythromycin 500 mg qid PO if could be pregnant for 15 days.
   (4) Swelling of inguinal lymph nodes
   With genital ulcer
   Syphilis and chancroid
   Benzathine penicillin 2.4 million units IMI once

(continued on page 193)

AND

Doxycycline 100 mg PO bd or
Erythromycin 500 mg qid PO if could be pregnant
for 15 days.

Without genital ulcer
Lymphogranuloma venereum
Doxycycline 100 mg PO bd or
Erythromycin 500 mg qid if could be pregnant for
15 days.

(5) Scrotal swelling
Gonorrhoea and chlamydia
Ciprofloxacin 500 mg PO once OR*
AND
Doxycycline 100 mg PO for 7 days.

(6) Lower abdominal pain/pelvic peritonitis
Gonorrhoea and chlamydia +/– other bacterial
infection most likely
Ciprofloxacin 500 mg PO once or
Ceftriaxone 250 mg IMI once if could be pregnant
OR* AND
Doxycycline 100 mg PO or
Erythromycin 500 mg PO qid if could be pregnant
for 7 days

AND

Metronidazole 400 mg PO bd for 14 days
AND if does not improve,
Other antibiotics as for peritonitis.

(7) Give counselling and do test for HIV infection.

*If ciprofloxacin or ceftriaxone not available, then

- gentamicin 240 mg IMI once or
- SMX 4000 mg/TMP 800 mg orally once daily for
  1(–3) days; but only if proven effective in your area
  (see pages 56–57) or
- see Table 19.2 (pages 203–204).

**If patient not cured, look up and act on main reasons for this
including the following possibilities.**

(1) The patient (or partner) did not take all the treatment.
(2) The patient is still having sex with an untreated
    infected partner.
(3) Treatment for other possible causes of the syndrome
    needed.

Note:

1. If urethral or vaginal discharge, always find out if also genital or
   inguinal sore or lump; and treat this also if present.
2. If genital or inguinal sore or lump, always find out if urethral or
   vaginal discharge; and treat this also if present.
3. If any STD, always counsel and do test for HIV infection.

Anatomy

See Figures 19.1 and 19.2.

Pathology

Sexually transmitted diseases or infections (STD or
STI), also called venereal diseases (VD), are infections
usually spread by sexual intercourse but *sometimes* are

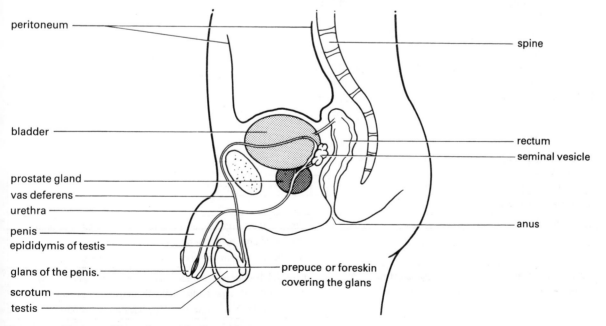

Figure 19.1 *Diagram of the male reproductive system.*

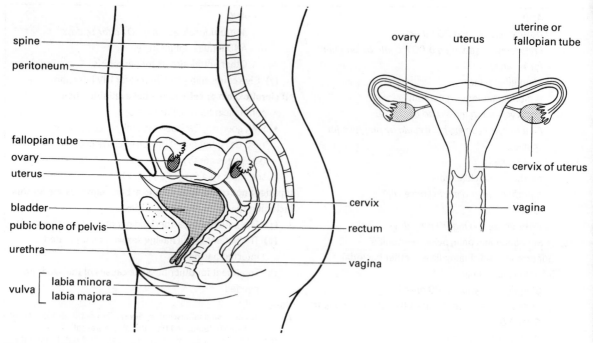

Figure 19.2 *Diagram of the female reproductive system.*

spread by non-sexual means. STD *usually* affect the genital tract but *sometimes* (especially HIV) do not affect the genital tract at first. Of course, *not all* genital tract diseases are STD (many are not).

The common STD and their causes are set out in Table 19.1 pages 194–195.

It is of great importance to realise that (except for HIV infection) STD usually show themselves in one of the following six ways called 'syndromes'. (A syndrome is a *group* of symptoms the patient complains about and clinical signs found during examination which may have a number of different causes.) The six syndromes include:

1. Urethral discharge or pain, especially on passing urine.
2. Vaginal discharge or pain, especially on passing urine.
3. Sores (ulcers) or lumps or pain in the mucous membrane or skin of the genitalia.
4. Swelling of the inguinal lymph nodes (called a bubo) near the genitalia with or without a genital ulcer.
5. Scrotal swelling of sudden onset in men.
6. Lower abdominal pain in women.

The details of the diseases which cause these syndromes are found on pages 205–216. A list of these diseases and a summary of the syndromes and other symptoms and signs the diseases cause follow in Table 19.1.

Table 19.1 Common sexually transmissible diseases.

Disease	Organism causing	Pathology and symptoms and signs
Bacterial infections:		
Gonorrhoea	*Neisseria gonorrhoeae*	Urethral discharge in males and females; cervicitis, vaginal discharge and lower abdominal pain in women; severe conjunctivitis in the newborn. May have no symptoms.
Chlamydial urethritis, cervicitis, etc.	*Chlamydia trachomatis* (certain types)	Urethral discharge in males and females; cervicitis vaginal discharge and lower abdominal pain in women; severe conjunctivitis in the newborn. May have no symptoms.

Table 19.1 (*continued*)

Disease	Organism causing	Pathology and symptoms and signs
Syphilis	*Treponema pallidum*	Anogenital ulcers (chancre); inguinal swelling; generalised skin rash; other severe problems later.
Chancroid	*Haemophilis ducreyi*	Genital ulcers with inguinal swelling (bubo) in the majority of cases.
Lymphogranuloma inguinale	*Chlamydia trachomatis* (certain types)	Little or no genital lesion. Enlarged inflamed inguinal lymph nodes.
Granuloma inguinale or Donovanosis	Calymmatobacterium or *Klebsiella granulomatis*	Nodular swellings and ulcerative lesions of the inguinal and anogenital areas.
Viral infections:		
Acquired immunodeficiency syndrome (AIDS)	Human immunodeficiency virus (HIV)	May be no symptoms; generalised lymph node swelling, persistent fever, skin rash, weight loss; many other serious infections, tumours, etc.
Herpes genitalis	Herpes simplex virus type 2 (HSV-2)	Anogenital vesicular lesions (blisters) and ulcerations.
Genital warts	Human papilloma virus (HPV)	Anogenital fleshy warts; cervical warts; years later cervical cancer (in women); penile cancer (in men).
Viral hepatitis	Hepatitis B virus (HBV)	Often no symptoms; nausea and malaise; enlargement of the liver; jaundice.
Cytomegalovirus infection	Cytomegalovirus (CMV)	Mild fever; diffuse lymph node swelling; liver disease, etc.
Molluscum contagiosum	*Molluscum contagiosum* virus (MCV)	Genital or generalised firm skin nodules with a depression in the centre.
Other:		
Trichomoniasis	*Trichomonas vaginalis* (protozoa)	Often no symptoms; a lot of frothy vaginal discharge.
Candidiasis	*Candida albicans* (fungus)	Thick curd-like vaginal discharge; vulval itching or burning.

Epidemiology

STD are very common all over the world. Hundreds of millions of new cases occur each year. In some places well over half of the population will have had at least one STD at some time in their life.

The infections usually live in the blood or body secretions (especially semen and vaginal fluid) of the infected person. These organisms then get into a new person when infected semen or vaginal fluid or blood gets through the mucous membranes of the genital tract or mouth or rectum of an uninfected person. The organism usually cannot get through the skin of an uninfected person unless the skin has a break (injury or ulcer, etc.) in it. Many organisms, however, can get through normal mucous membrane, even if the mucous membrane does not have a break. Penetrative sex (i.e. where the penis enters the vagina or rectum or mouth) and unprotected sex (where a male or female condom does not separate the mucous membranes of the people having sex) is the usual means of spread.

Some organisms, especially syphilis and HIV, can get through the placenta from a pregnant woman to her unborn baby. Organisms, especially HIV, could get into an uninfected person given an injection or tattoo or operation using instruments from which the blood and organisms from an infected person have not been removed. Of course HIV, HBV and syphilis can be transferred from an infected person to an uninfected person in a blood transfusion.

STD can be spread by the following ways.

1. Vaginal and even more easily anal intercourse:
   • All STD.
2. Oro (mouth to) genital contact:
   • Primary and secondary syphilis
   • Gonorrhoea
   • Herpes simplex virus
   • HIV virus.

3. Kissing:
- Herpes simplex virus
- Primary and secondary syphilis
- Hepatitis B.

4. Mother to child:
- Gonorrhoea
- Chlamydia
- Herpes simplex virus
- Hepatitis B virus
- HIV
- Streptococcal bacteria.

5. Blood transfusion:
- HIV
- Hepatitis B virus
- Syphilis.

6. Unsterile needles, syringes, other cutting or piercing instruments:
- HIV virus
- Hepatitis B virus.

How are STD usually transmitted?

By far the most common way is unprotected penetrative sexual intercourse (vaginal or anal or oral).

Other ways include:
- mother-to-child,
- during pregnancy (e.g. HIV and syphilis),
- at delivery (e.g. gonorrhoea, chlamydia, HSV-2 and HIV),
- after birth (e.g. HIV),
- through breast milk (e.g. HIV),
- unsafe (unsterile) use of needles or injections or cutting instruments or other contact with blood or blood products (e.g. syphilis, HIV and hepatitis),
- blood transfusions from infected people (e.g. HIV, HBV and syphilis).

Remember that the human immunodeficiency virus (HIV) is transmitted in the same ways as any other STI.

Not all acts of unprotected sexual intercourse cause infection. The following can increase the risk of infection:

1. Being female (with a large area of mucosal surface in the vagina);

2. Being young (the cervical mucosa in girls and young women has not fully developed and is more easily infected);

3. A culture where young women are married to older men (if the men are likely to have had previous intercourse and infection);

4. A culture where women are more likely to be raped or cannot easily refuse to have sex (men who are involved in these things are much more likely to have infections than other men);

5. Having HIV infection makes the likelihood of getting and developing complications of other STD greater;

6. Having other STD makes the likelihood of getting HIV infection greater;

7. Changing sexual partners frequently; having more than one partner; having casual sex or sex with sex workers or their clients; having sex with someone with a genital ulcer or urethral or vaginal discharge or HIV symptoms or signs or positive blood test; having sex with those who are injecting drug users; having sex with people who have had anal sex with other people;

8. Having sex when intoxicated from alcohol or drugs, and not thinking about the above precautions.

Symptoms and signs

The initial illness is an urethral or vaginal discharge, often with pain; or a genital sore; or inguinal swelling; but it can be more than one of these. Sometimes, however, these are mild and the newly infected person does not notice them. With HIV infection, there is usually no illness at the time of infection.

After the initial illness, especially in women, many patients have no symptoms or signs. The patient, however, is able to still pass the infection to others.

People who are infected often do not know they have the infection. It is not possible by looking at or talking to a person, to tell if he or she has an infection or not, unless the person is completely healthy with no symptoms or signs and also has never had sexual intercourse with anyone at all (or been infected from blood, etc.). Later on, infected patients (even those with no symptoms) can develop:
- epididymitis (swelling at back of the testis in the scrotum) (usually after an urethral discharge);
- pelvic peritonitis (lower abdominal pain) (usually after urethral or vaginal discharge with cervicitis);
- infertility (not able to have children) due to blockage of the fallopian tubes in women or the tubes from the testes in men (usually after cervicitis or urethral discharge);
- brain disease (usually years after infection with syphilis);
- heart disease (usually years after infection with syphilis);
- cancer of the cervix or penis (years after human papilloma virus infection);

blindness in the newborn baby (when the mother has gonorrhoea or chlamydia infection); stillbirth or severe organ damage in a baby (when the mother has syphilis or HIV);

all of the symptoms and signs of HIV infection and AIDS (see pages 222–234), but only if the patient has HIV infection.

It is important, therefore, to diagnose these diseases early when the patient has only one or two of the first four of the usual ways STD present (see these six syndromes on page 194); or at the latest when they have the fifth or sixth way STD usually present, and hopefully long before they develop any of the last seven of the complications above.

The aims of history and examination are as follows:

1. Find out which syndrome the patient has.
2. Find out the patient's risk of getting and passing on an STD.
3. Find out all the patient's sexual partners who may also be infected.

To do these properly, as the patient may be embarrassed or concerned:

1. Tell the patient that you need to ask personal questions to be able to help him or her and their partners; then ask them if you can do this.
2. Tell the patient that anything you find out will not be told to others (i.e. provide confidentiality).
3. Do the history and examination where others cannot hear or see (i.e. provide privacy).
4. Let the patient know you understand their problem and their worries and will not be critical of them. Be polite and respectful (i.e. develop rapport).
5. Use words and terms the patient understands and not medical terms which the patient would not understand.
6. Ask 'open' questions during the history of the present illness to find out all the patient's worries; and then 'closed' questions in the specific interrogation to find out the exact details of the illness and all the symptoms which may be present.
7. Make sure the patient knows exactly how to answer your questions (i.e. be specific).
8. Ask one question at a time.
9. Do not ask 'leading' questions that make the patient give the answer which he thinks you expect.
10. Keep your questions free of moral judgement or criticism, even if you do not agree with the ideas and behaviour of the patient.
11. Ask on several occasions, 'Is there anything else not so far talked about?'

Questions which often lead to helpful answers and allow you to ask for specific information are as follows:

1. To find out sexual orientation (that is, heterosexual or homosexual or bisexual) – 'Are you in a sexual relationship with a man or a woman?'
2. To find out about the risk of getting or passing on STD – 'Have you had any or many changes in sexual partners?'
3. To start the conversation or get it going again – 'Tell me about your sex life' or 'Tell me about what you do for sex?'

If the patient has an urethral discharge, find out if there is pain on passing urine (dysuria) or increased frequency of passing urine.

If the patient has an ulcer, find out if it came for no obvious reason or followed trauma; if it is single or if there is more than one; if there have been previous ulcer/s; if it is painful; what it looks like; if it is getting bigger; is there enlargement of lymph nodes; are there other symptoms.

If the patient has an inguinal bubo (enlarged inguinal lymph node), find out if there is a genital ulcer; is it painful; has the lump discharged; are there lumps elsewhere in the body?

If the patient has a vaginal discharge, is there any pain on passing urine (dysuria) or increased frequency of passing urine; what does the discharge look and smell like; how much discharge is there; is there an itch; is there pain on having intercourse; is there abdominal pain (and if so, related symptoms)?

If there is abdominal pain, is there vaginal discharge (if so, all its details); is there vaginal bleeding; has there been a missed or overdue period; is there painful or irregular menstruation; has there been painful or difficult childbirth or miscarriage?

If there is scrotal swelling or pain, has the patient had urethritis or a urinary tract infection or, if older, difficulty in passing urine (prostatic enlargement) or schistosomiasis; was the condition of sudden onset and very painful and the testis pulled up (twisting or torsion of the testis – a surgical emergency); has the condition come slowly (hydrocoele or cancer)?

The aim of the history and examination, however, is to make the diagnosis of the syndrome and not the actual disease the patient has. There are a number of reasons for this.

1. It is not usually possible to tell from history and examination what the exact cause of the infection is.
2. Tests to tell what the exact cause is are not usually available in the health centre.

3. Often the patient has more than one infection causing the syndrome.

The aim is firstly to find out what syndrome the patient has and then secondly to treat all the possible common serious causes of this syndrome. If the patient does not get better, then later on look for the unusual causes for this syndrome and treat them.

The syndromes are as follows:

1. Urethral discharge or pain.
2. Vaginal discharge with or without urethritis or cervicitis.
3. Sores or lumps or pain in the mucous membrane or skin of the genitalia.
4. Swelling of the inguinal lymph nodes both with and without a genital ulcer.
5. Scrotal swelling.
6. Lower abdominal pain.

Advantages of this 'syndrome case management' include:

1. The patient's symptoms are treated.
2. It does not miss mixed infections.
3. The patient gets treatment at the first visit.
4. Care of STD can be given by all health workers.
5. Flow charts have been made to help the health worker make correct decisions (see *Sexually Transmitted and other Reproductive Tract Infections,* WHO, 2005, or later edition).
6. More time is available for health education and counselling.

Urethral discharge or pain in the male

Urethral discharge which is caused by a sexually transmitted disease is usually caused by either:

1. *Neisseria gonorrhoeae,* also called the 'Gonococcus' which causes gonorrhoea, or
2. *Chlamydia trachomatis* infection.

Occasionally, other organisms are the cause. However, in up to 30% of patients there is more than one infection present. Treat urethral discharge, therefore, for both common infections. If symptoms do not go away other treatment can later be given.

Vaginal discharge or pain

Vaginal discharge due to STD is abnormal in colour, smell or amount. The patient may also have itchiness or swelling of the vagina or vulva, pain on passing urine or lower abdominal or back pain.

STD causes of vaginal discharge:

1. gonorrhoea causing cervicitis or urethritis;
2. *Chlamydia trachomatis* infection causing cervicitis;
3. *Trichomonas vaginalis* infection;
4. *Candida albicans* (*Monilia* or thrush) infection;
5. bacterial vaginosis when the normal organisms of the vagina are replaced with other bacterial organisms (especially *Gardnerella vaginalis* and anaerobes)
6. conditions which cause sores or lumps in the vagina including syphilis, herpes genitalis, condyloma accuminata, etc. (see below).

Always treat gonorrhoea and chlamydia. If the symptoms do not go away, give treatment for the other conditions.

Non-STD causes of vaginal discharge include neoplasms, polyps, foreign bodies, trauma, etc.

Non-pathological or normal vaginal discharge must not be considered abnormal and can occur after sexual intercourse, at the times of ovulation or just before menstrual periods, when oral contraceptives are taken and after the insertion of an intra-uterine contraceptive device (IUD).

Genital sores or lumps or pain

Sores or lumps or pain in the mucous membrane or skin of the genitalia or in the skin near the genitalia are usually caused by:

1. syphilis (usually single painless ulcer),
2. chancroid (also called 'soft sore') (usually many tender ulcers).

Other causes could be:

3. granuloma inguinale (also called granuloma venereum or Donovanosis) (at first a single painless ulcer which looks like cut meat),
4. lymphogranuloma venereum (also called lymphogranuloma inguinale) (often no genital ulcer but only inflamed inguinal nodes),
5. herpes genitalis (usually many painful small ulcers),
6. condyloma accuminatum (also called venereal warts) (wart like lesions),
7. amoebic ulcer (not always sexually transmitted),
8. pubic lice (not always sexually transmitted),
9. scabies (not always sexually transmitted), and
10. cancer (not itself sexually transmitted but can be a complication of human papilloma virus infection) (slow not sudden onset).

However, many cases are not typical; and definite diagnosis by examination without special tests is not possible.

In view of this, therefore, *the two common important causes, syphilis and chancroid, are always treated first*; and then if the patient is not cured, the diagnosis and treatment of others considered later.

Swelling in the inguinal lymph nodes near the genitalia (inguinal bubo)

If there is also an ulcer of the genitalia, then the causes are usually the same two important ones:

1. syphilis,
2. chancroid,
and other causes are also as listed above.

If there is swelling of the inguinal lymph nodes near the genitalia without a genital ulcer, the most important cause is:

• lymphogranuloma venereum.

In both of the above situations, many cases are not typical and the definite diagnosis by examination is not possible. *Always treat the most important causes as above.* If the patient does not improve, then consider the possibility that other causes are present and then treat these causes.

Scrotal swelling of sudden onset

Scrotal swelling caused by an STD is usually due to inflammation of the epididymis and is of sudden onset and painful. There is also urethritis, or it has been present recently. The common causes are:

1. gonorrhoea,
2. *Chlamydia trachomatis.*
Always treat for these two.

Other non-STD causes include:

1. acute torsion of the testis (twisting of the testis on its cord, which blocks the blood vessels and needs urgent surgery or the testis will die);
2. trauma;
3. mumps;
4. urinary tract infection, especially in older men with partial blockage of the urethra by the prostate;
5. TB (slow not sudden onset);
6. tumours of the testis (slow not sudden onset).

Lower abdominal pain in women due to 'pelvic inflammatory disease' (PID) i.e. inflammation of the uterus and/or fallopian tubes and/or ovaries and/or pelvic peritonitis.

The STD causes of PID are usually:

1. gonorrhoea,
2. *Chlamydia trachomatis.*
Always treat for these two.

Pelvic infections not due to STD can be due to:

1. post-partum or post-abortion infections;
2. intra-uterine contraceptive devices – especially in the first month after insertion;
3. bowel infections such as appendicitis and diverticulitis.

If pelvic inflammatory disease is not treated quickly, these infections can cause:

1. pelvic pain,
2. ectopic pregnancy,
3. infertility.

Non-sexually transmitted conditions of genitalia

These include:

• traumatic sores (i.e. injuries),
• foreign bodies,
• ordinary infection under foreskin (balanitis),
• cancer,
• amoebic ulcer,
• pubic lice,
• scabies, and
• many other skin conditions.

History, examination and tests

When you see a patient with either a genital sore or lump or an urethral or vaginal discharge or other condition which may be sexually transmitted, you should take a full history, do a full physical examination and do the necessary tests.

Remember:

1. One STD makes it more likely for the patient already to have other STD and HIV infection.
2. STD with ulcers or discharge make it more easy for the patient in future to be infected with HIV, or if the patient has HIV infection, more easy for them to pass HIV infection on to others.

Details about the main STD follow later in this chapter.

History (see Chapter 6 page 21 and page 197)

If for some reason you are not able to examine a patient, although not ideal, it would be better to treat the patient, and the contacts, for the syndrome the patient tells you in the history that he or she has, than not treat the patient and the contacts. Always try to do the examination, as you may well find the condition the patient has is quite different to what he says he has, or that the patient has other conditions as well as the one he told you about.

Physical examination (see Chapter 6 pages 23–25 and 'Symptoms and signs' pages 196–199)

Use the examination to make even more certain than just on the history which of the six syndromes the patient has.

Special things to note in the examination include:

All patients:

Make sure the consultation is private, i.e. others cannot see or hear. Explain what you need to do and why the examination is important. Ask the patient for permission to go ahead with the examination. Do not be impatient. Be confident but sensitive to the patient's needs. If the patient wants a relative or other person to be present, arrange this. Get the patient to lie down for the examination.

Wear disposable plastic gloves (which you throw away after seeing each patient), or reusable gloves (which you have sterilised before you use them again) to protect yourself.

Always ask yourself if there are any things to suggest HIV infection (see page 234).

At the end of the consultation you should be certain of the syndrome the patient has.

If you have no gloves you can still do almost all of the examination by looking and getting the patient to do the things you should do (e.g. pull back the foreskin, separate the labia, squeeze the urethra, etc.) and tell you what they feel (e.g. lump is hard or tender, etc.).

Male patients:

If you are a female, ask a male assistant to be present.

Look at the pubic hair for lice.

Examine the groin areas for ulcers or lymph gland enlargement.

Look at the penis for sores or ulcers. Feel if a sore is hard or soft and if it is tender. If the patient is not circumcised, pull back the foreskin so that you can examine the glans too. If you have no gloves, ask the patient to do this and the following procedure.

Squeeze the urethra gently to see if any discharge comes out of the urethra and if it is purulent or watery. If a laboratory is available, take a smear of any discharge.

Look at the scrotum for sores or ulcers. Gently feel each testis and epididymis for swelling, lumps or tenderness.

Put the patient onto his side and ask him to pull up his knees so that you can look at the perianal region for sores or discharge.

Only if you have been trained to do so, and know how to use the findings of the examination, do a pelvic examination through the rectum (PR) (see Chapter 26 page 444).

Female patients:

If you are a male, ask a female assistant to be present.

Look at the pubic hair for lice.

Examine the groin areas for ulcers or lymph gland enlargement.

Examine the abdomen.

Examine the perineum and genitalia. Cover the abdomen down to the knees with a sheet. Ask the patient to lie on her back and bend her knees until the heels touch the buttocks. Ask the patient to let her knees go apart. You then have a good view of the external genitalia.

Examine the vulva for any sores, ulcers, swelling or discharge.

Examine the perianal region.

Examine the internal surface of the labia after gently separating them. If you have no gloves, ask the patient to do this and the following procedure.

Feel if any sores are soft or hard and if they are tender.

If available, use a speculum to examine the vagina and cervix. If there is vaginal discharge use a swab on forceps to clean the cervix and then see if there is inflammation of the cervix or if pus is coming through the cervix.

If a laboratory is available, take a smear from the urethra and from inside the cervix.

Only if you have been trained to do so and know how to use the findings of this examination:

- Do a pelvic examination through the vagina (PV) (see Chapter 26 page 443), or if not possible, or if needed,
- Do a pelvic examination through the rectum (PR) (see Chapter 26 page 444).

Tests

Test the urine (see Chapter 26 page 445).

Do the following four tests only if a laboratory is available and your Health Department has told you to do them. You may be asked to also do other tests.

Tests other than urine are not usually done in the health centre.

1. Do the test for bacterial vaginosis.

2. Take 10 ml of blood and send the serum to the

laboratory with a request for the serological test for syphilis (VDRL or RPR; and if positive TPHA or FTA-Ab, which are more accurate, may be needed).

3. Make slides from swabs from the urethra and (in the female) inside the cervical canal for Gram stain and culture or put into a suitable culture material (e.g. Stuart's transport medium) to be sent to the laboratory for culture.

4. Take blood for testing for HIV infection, but only after counselling and consent.

Control and prevention

If after the history and examination and tests you think that the patient has a disease which may have been sexually transmitted, then you should use the usual means of control and prevention.

Kill the organism in the body of the original host or reservoir

Treatment can kill all the bacterial organisms. Treatment cannot kill all viral organisms, but drugs can control the growth of many of them so that they become few; but HIV infected people always are infectious.

All patients and all 'contacts' need to be found, investigated if possible and treated.

'Contacts' include the person who gave the patient the disease and anyone else the patient may have given the disease to, i.e. all persons the patient has had intercourse with up to 3 months before and also after the symptoms started, as well as the patient's husband/wife. This may at times include people of the patient's same gender or sex. Many of these 'contacts' will have no symptoms but still have infection and be likely to spread the infection to the patient again and to other people, and may themselves develop complications.

In most places you will not have enough money and staff to find contacts and offer them investigation and treatment, and there are disadvantages as well as advantages in this method of control. You will instead usually need to explain to the patient that he or she should:

1. bring contacts to you for treatment; or
2. give a 'contact card' (on which you write what treatment is needed and then give this to the patient); give enough to the patient to give one for each contact, so that the contact can then bring the card to the health centre and he or she will immediately get the correct treatment when this card is seen by the health worker;

3. at the very least, tell the contact that they may have the sexually transmitted disease and that they should come to the health centre to see you for treatment;
4. in only special cases be supplied with a course of treatment by you to give to the contact;
5. tell the contact not to have sexual intercourse until he or she has been treated.

If you have enough staff to do contact tracing and if this is the Health Department's policy, ask the patient for the names and addresses of contacts, as soon as an STD is diagnosed. Write all of the names in the STD register.

All contacts need:

1. treatment for the same disease the patient has,
2. treatment for any other STD diagnosed in the contact.

For every patient you treat:

1. Find out what the patient or contact who comes for treatment knows about STD and their treatment, and what questions and concerns they may have.
2. Tell them about any common side effects of the treatment.
3. Try to get them to take the full course of the treatment.
4. Try to get them not to have sexual intercourse again until the treatment is finished and they are cured.

Give health education to encourage all people who have the disease to come for treatment.

Health education should include:

1. how the diseases are spread;
2. the symptoms and signs of the diseases;
3. the serious results if no treatment is given, or if the person gets HIV infection; and
4. that the treatment is safe, and (except for HIV infection) effective, and free;
5. how not to get another infection, especially HIV infection (see pages 256–261), and how to use condoms, and what is and how to have safe sex;
6. a supply of condoms.

Stop the means of spread

Give health education so that people know that:

1. The means of spread is intercourse (with an infected person).
2. The only real safe sexual practice for an uninfected person is to have sexual intercourse with only one other uninfected 'faithful' (that is, one who does not have sexual intercourse with any one else) partner.

There is no way to tell from a person's appearance if they are infected or not. This can be done only by knowing the person and talking to the person about it and their not ever having had sexual intercourse with anyone ever; or if they have, having had treatment and now having no symptoms or signs and, if available, a negative blood test for HIV and syphilis (but see pages 233, 235, 210).

A person who has many sexual partners is at high risk of an STD. A person who has sexual intercourse with just one person, but that person has had many sexual partners, is at high risk of an STD. To reduce the risk of STD, people need to reduce the number of their sexual partners, although there will always be a risk until sexual intercourse occurs with only one uninfected faithful partner.

3. If a person has sexual relations with more than one person or with a possibly infected person, some things will reduce the risk of getting STD.

(a) Change sexual activities from high risk to low risk activities. High risk activities are when semen or vaginal fluid comes into contact with the partner's oral (mouth), genital or anal and rectal mucosa. Low risk practices are when these fluids come into contact only with skin which is not damaged (as most infections cannot enter through unbroken skin). This means that a low risk practice is when a man's penis does not enter the partner's vagina, anus or mouth.

(b) Use of a condom will greatly reduce the risk of infected semen or vaginal fluid getting into the other person. It is important that people not only know this, but are shown how to use condoms properly and do have condoms available, and do actually use condoms each and every time they have sexual intercourse. (See Appendix 1 pages 259–261.)

(c) Washing with soap and water after removing the condom will reduce the chance of infection. However, vaginal douching (washing inside the vagina) may make infections more likely.

It is most important that patients with STD are given the above information.

Health education about the above to groups at particular risk of STD, should be carried out whenever possible. These would include:
- sex workers,
- people who visit sex workers,
- STD patients,
- those who are away from their community and family and regular sexual partner, e.g. migrant workers, truck drivers, sailors, 'street' or homeless children and people, etc.

Health education of other special groups should be carried out whenever possible. These would include:
- school children, especially before they start having sex,
- young people, especially girls,
- groups of men,
- groups of women,
- those who can be reached by the mass media (radio, TV, newspapers).

If possible, some kind of measurement of the effects of these methods of health education should be carried out so that most effort can be put into those that are most effective in your area.

Giving people information and knowledge (health education), however, does not often make them change their behaviour. Counselling is also required.

Counselling includes:

1. Helping the patient to work out from what he knows and the information you give him, which of the unsafe sexual practices he was doing which led him to get this STD and put him at risk of getting another STD and especially HIV infection. Ask him to tell you these things.

2. Helping the patient to work out how to change his unsafe sexual practices into safe ones.

3. Helping the patient to work out how he can adopt these changes of sexual practice in his own daily life. If there are problems in doing this, help the patient to work out how to overcome these problems. Tell the patient how other people have solved the problem the patient has and what choices the person could make. If the patient has strengths and good ideas and practices, work out with him or her how these can be used to solve any problems the patient has. Help the patient make the best decisions.

4. At the end of all this, get the patient again to tell you what he or she is going to do. Help him feel motivated to want to do these things by praising the good intentions he has. This is to confirm the patient's decisions and motivate him to carry them out.

After education and counselling, the patient should know about:

1. STD and the treatment and importance of having all the treatment,

2. The need for sexual partners to also be treated,

3. What were/are the risks of STD and HIV the patient had/s,

4. The need to have only 'safe' sex,
5. Ways of solving any problems the patient has to change to having safe sex,
6. What he or she is going to do from now on and be motivated to do this.

Raise the resistance of susceptible people

Immunisation is not yet possible for most STD. It is available for hepatitis. Hopefully, it soon will become possible for HIV and possibly other STD.

Prophylactic treatment

Give prophylactic treatment with the proper treatment dose for the disease to a person who has had sexual intercourse with a person who is known to have a sexually transmissible disease, even if they do not have symptoms and signs of the disease.

Summary of management of a patient with an STD

What you should and can do for patients with suspected STD will depend on what part of the world you are in, what infections are common in your area, what antibiotics kill the organisms which cause STD in your area, etc. It will also depend on what things you have available to examine a patient (e.g. vaginal speculum or not), and if you have a good laboratory service (e.g. to do smears for gonococci, serological tests for syphilis, examinations for Donovan bodies, HIV serology, etc.). It will also depend on what antibiotics are available for you to treat the patients.

In view of these things, your Health Department will probably have drawn up a number of policies and probably flow charts for your area, to tell you what you are to do. You must follow the advice of your Health Department.

If such policies and flow charts are not available, the WHO flow charts should tell you what you should do if you choose the one which applies to your patient and the facilities you have. These flow charts and more details about STD and their treatment are found in the WHO book mentioned on page 192.

Drug treatment of the patient and contacts

Table 19.2 below shows treatment regimens for common STD.

Do not use ciprofloxacin or doxycycline or tetracycline in pregnancy.

Do not use doxycycline or tetracycline in childhood.

Table 19.2 Drug treatment of STD (based on WHO recommendations and publications).

| Vaginal discharge (without cervicitis) | Treat for vaginitis (candidiasis and *Trichomonas vaginalis*/bacterial vaginosis) Treat for cervicitis (in high gonorrhoea and chlamydia prevalence settings (see page 204) | Candidiasis
 nystatin 100,000 units tablet intravaginally once daily for 14 days, *or*
 miconazole or clotrimazole
 200 mg intravaginally once daily for 3 days, *or*
 clotrimazole 500 mg intravaginally as a single dose
Trichomonas vaginalis
 metronidazole 2 g orally as a single dose, *or*
 metronidazole 400–500 mg orally twice daily for 7 days
Bacterial vaginosis
 metronidazole 2 g orally as a single dose, *or*
 metronidazole 400–500 mg orally 2x twice daily for 7 days
<div align="right">(*continued on page 204*)</div> |

Table 19.2 *(continued)*

Urethral discharge Cervicitis	Treat for uncomplicated gonorrhoea and chlamydia	Gonorrhoea (uncomplicated)
		   ciprofloxacin 500 mg orally as a single dose, *or*
		   ceftriaxone 250 mg by IM injection as a single dose, *or*
		   cefixime 400 mg orally as a single dose, *or*
		   spectinomycin 2 g by IM injection as a single dose, *or*
		   TMP 800 mg / SMX 4000 mg (10 tablets) orally as a single dose, *or*
		   gentamicin 240 mg by IM injection as a single dose
		Chlamydia
		   doxycycline 100 mg orally twice daily for 7 days, *or*
		   tetracycline 500 mg orally 4 times daily for 7 days, *or*
		   erythromycin 500 mg orally 4 times daily for 7 days

Genital ulcers	Treat for syphilis and chancroid (and herpes in high HSV-2 prevalence settings)	Primary syphilis (chancre)
		   benzathine penicillin G 2.4 million IU IMI at a single session (often split into 2 doses at separate sites), *or*
		   procaine penicillin G 1.2 million IU by IMI daily for 10 consecutive days, OR (if allergic to penicillin)
		   tetracycline 500 mg orally 4 times daily for 15 days, *or*
		   doxycycline 100 mg orally twice daily for 15 days, *or*
		   erythromycin 500 mg orally 4 times daily for 15 days
		Chancroid
		   erythromycin 500 mg orally 3 times daily for 7 days, *or*
		   ciprofloxacin 500 mg orally twice daily for 3 days, *or*
		   ceftriaxone 250 mg by IMI as a single dose, *or*
		   azithromycin 1 g orally as a single dose, *or*
		   TMP 80 mg / SMX 400 mg tablets 2 orally twice daily for 7 days

Inguinal bubo with genital ulcer Inguinal bubo without ulcers on genitalia or legs, buttocks, etc.	Treat for syphilis and chancroid
	
	Treat for lymphogranuloma venereum
		Syphilis – see above
		Chancroid – see above
		Lymphogranuloma venereum
		   doxycycline 100 mg orally twice daily for 14 days, *or*
		   tetracycline 500 mg orally 4 times daily for 14 days, *or*
		   erythromycin 500 mg orally daily for 14 days, *or*
		   sulfadiazine 1 g orally 4 times daily for 14 days

Scrotal swelling	Treat for uncomplicated gonorrhoea and chlamydia If there is a strangulated hernia or torsion of the testis (testis very tender high and twisted) or acute injury – transfer for immediate surgery See page 199 for other causes	Gonorrhoea – see above Chlamydia – see above

Pelvic inflammatory disease	Treat for gonorrhoea and treat for chlamydia and also treat for ordinary and anaerobic bacteria
	If there is a pregnancy complication (late or missed period, bleeding from inside the cervix, miscarriage, abortion or birth in the last 6 weeks) (especially if abdominal pain and tenderness) remove any intra-uterine contraceptive device and provide condoms
		Gonorrhoea – see above
		Chlamydia – see above
		Ordinary and anaerobic bacteria
		   metronidazole 400 mg twice daily for 14 days, *but*
		   As for peritonitis if not improving (Chapter 23 page 349) and transfer

Remember:

1. Always treat the patient's contacts at the same time or as soon as possible after; and before the patient has intercourse with them again.
2. Give the patient condoms to use until cure and the partner is also treated.

Common sexually transmitted diseases

Gonorrhoea

Gonorrhoea is a bacterial infection which usually causes urethritis in men and urethritis and cervicitis in women, but can cause infections of the rectum or throat or eyes. It can also spread within the genital organs causing more severe infections of them and through the blood to other parts of the body, causing serious disease there or septicaemia.

Gonorrhoea is common.

The cause is the gonorrhoea bacterium (*Neisseria gonorrhoeae*).

The original host is an infected person. Some infected people have symptoms and signs, but some men and many women are carriers with no symptoms.

The means of spread is direct contact. In adults this is almost always by sexual intercourse. It can infect the eyes of a child if the mother's cervix or urethra is infected at the time of birth. It can infect the throat if infected genitalia are kissed.

Infection does not give any immunity.

Symptoms and signs, course and complications in the male

Symptoms and signs usually develop within a week; but they can take longer or never develop.

There is an urethral discharge (Figure 19.3). It is usually white or yellow (pus) and often a large amount. Dysuria and urinary frequency occur. The symptoms slowly improve over weeks or months, although a little white discharge may continue to be present each morning. But the infection does not go.

Complications include:
- abscess around urethra,
- inflammation of the epididymis and testis,
- sterility due to blocked epididymis and vas deferens,
- urethral stricture (i.e. narrowing of the urethra due to scarring where there was previous infection around the urethra) causing difficulty in passing urine and distended bladder,

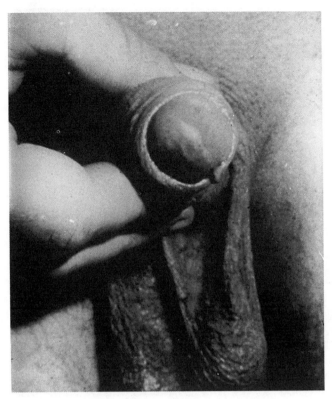

Figure 19.3 *Gonorrhoea in the male. The usual symptom and sign of gonorrhoea – urethral discharge.*

- severe conjunctivitis and iritis (spread by fingers from the genitalia),
- bacteraemia with pustular skin rash,
- acute infective arthritis or meningitis, etc.
- septicaemia.

These complications usually occur soon after infection. Sterility is a later complication. Urethral stricture occurs after many years.

Symptoms and signs, course and complications in the female

Symptoms and signs usually develop within a week; but they can take longer or never develop.

There is usually dysuria and urinary frequency and increase in vaginal discharge (Figure 19.4). This is often mistaken for a urinary tract infection. After treatment with a sulfonamide alone (which does not cure the infection), or after no treatment, the symptoms slowly improve over weeks or months. But the infection does not go. If the cervix is infected there may be pain during, and bleeding after, intercourse; tenderness if the lower abdomen is palpated; and on pelvic examination (PV) the cervix may have pus in the opening or be bleeding or be tender when moved.

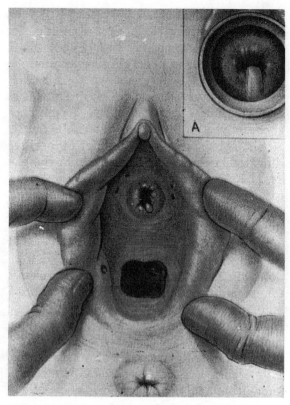

Figure 19.4 *Gonorrhoea in the female. Urethral discharge may be seen. On speculum examination of the cervix, discharge may be seen (inset A). However, the patient may not complain of these. She may have symptoms of urinary tract infection or of a vaginal discharge.*

Complications include:
- acute salpingitis,
- pelvic peritonitis,
- pelvic abscess,
- ectopic (tubal) pregnancies (due to blocked fallopian tubes),
- sterility (due to blocked fallopian tubes),
- severe acute conjunctivitis and iritis (spread by fingers),
- abscess in labia,
- bacteraemia with pustular skin rash,
- acute infective arthritis or meningitis, etc.
- septicaemia.

Tests (not usually possible)

Smear some discharge from the urethra and (in the female) from inside the cervix (Figure 19.5) onto a glass slide, fix it by heat and send it to the hospital laboratory for examination for gonorrhoea bacteria. If available, also collect a swab for culture, usually by putting it into a suitable transport medium such as Stuart's transport medium.

Send also the serum from 10 ml of blood with a request for serological tests for syphilis and HIV.

Diagnostic features

- Intercourse within previous week.
- Urinary pain and frequency.
- Urethral or vaginal discharge.
- Cervicitis.

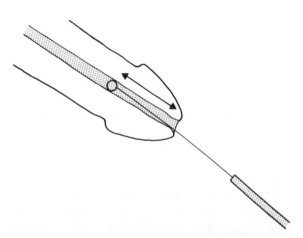

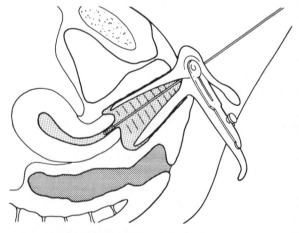

Figure 19.5 *Methods of collecting specimens for examination in the laboratory for gonococci. Use a sterile swab to collect pus from the urethra. If there is not enough pus to be collected on a swab then use a 100L sterile bacteriological wire loop but only if you have been trained how to use it. Use a sterile swab to collect secretions from the inside of the cervix. If you have Stuart's transport medium, collect specimens and put them in the transport medium and send them to the laboratory for culture and sensitivity testing. However, in a health centre all you can do yourself is to make a smear.*

Differential diagnosis

Females:

1. Pelvic inflammatory disease after childbirth or miscarriage.
   - Recent childbirth or miscarriage.
   - Discharge yellow pus.
   - Pelvic tenderness and/or masses.
   - Pus coming out of the cervix.
   - Pain when the cervix is moved during examination.
   - Possibly tenderness and guarding in lower abdomen.
   - Uterus enlarged and tender.
   - General symptoms and signs of infection.
2. Trichomonal infection.
   - Vulval and vaginal itchiness.
   - Discharge yellow and frothy and smelly.
3. Bacterial vaginosis.
   - Similar to trichomonal infection.
4. *Monilia* (*Candida* or thrush) infection.
   - Vulval and vaginal itchiness.
   - Discharge white, thick and lumpy.
5. *Chlamydia trachomatis* infections.
   - Symptoms or signs often mild or absent.
   - The symptoms and signs not diagnostic.
6. Other types of non-gonococcal infection not due to *Chlamydia trachomatis*.
7. Early pregnancy with increase in 'normal' vaginal discharge.
   - Period late or missed.
   - Uterus enlarged.
   - No pus or trichomonal or monilial discharge.
8. Others. See a gynaecology book.

Males:

1. *Chlamydia trachomatis* urethritis.
   - Discharge often less and more watery than gonorrhoea.
   - Discharge often has come after apparently successful treatment of gonorrhoea.
   - Common.
2. Trichomonal urethritis.
3. Other types of non-gonococcal urethritis which are not due to *Chlamydia trachomatis* either.

In all patients:
Note that 30% of patients will have both gonococcal and chlamydial infections.

Treatment

Give those drugs from the list in Table 19.2 page 204 your Health Department has told you to give.

Treat for gonorrhoea *ALL* clinical cases of gonorrhoea including:

1. All persons with urethral discharges.
2. All persons with 'urinary tract infections', especially young adults if there is a possibility of gonorrhoea.
3. All persons with vaginal infections if cervicitis or abdominal pain or tenderness present, and especially if the patient is a young woman and has had a recent change of sexual partner or if there is any other reason to suspect an STD.

Note that most cases of vaginitis in older women are not due to STD. If the above features are not present see a gynaecology textbook.

Treat for chlamydial infection *ALL* clinical cases of urethritis and cervicitis.

Note that 30% of patients will have both gonococcal and chlamydial infections. Treat all cases of urethritis and cervicitis for both gonococcal and chlamydial infections.

Find out if there is or was also a sore on the genitalia or anus. If so, treat for syphilis too. Treatment for gonorrhoea is not adequate treatment for syphilis (see page 210).

> Treatment for gonorrhoea needs a high concentration of the antibiotic but for only a short time. Treatment for syphilis needs only a low concentration of the antibiotic but for a long time.

If a patient with gonorrhoea (or cervicitis of other cause) gives birth to a baby before treatment, the baby may develop severe conjunctivitis and then blindness (ophthalmia neonatorum).

Treat such babies immediately with ceftriaxone 25–50 mg/kg IMI once (maximum dose 150 mg) AND oral erythromycin 50 mg/kg/day for 14 days AND also wash the pus out of the eyes with saline and then put in antibiotic ointment (e.g gentamicin) each 2–4 hours until settled. Povidone-iodine (aqueous not alcoholic) is used by some to treat all babies' eyes at birth to try to prevent any getting this condition.

Follow-up
Ask the patient to come back to be checked if not cured in 1 week.

If the patient is not cured, or if at first he or she seems to be cured but the condition comes back again, the three most likely possibilities are:

1. The 'contact' was not found and treated and the patient is still having intercourse with this infected person – this is the most likely.

2. The patient has gonococci resistant to the drugs used.
3. The patient has one of the other causes of urethritis (see 'Differential diagnosis' page 207).

Check the patient for all of these possibilities and take what action is needed.

Treat *Monilia* (*Candida* or thrush) vaginitis if present with nystatin (or other antifungal drug, e.g. clotrimazole in the recommended dose) vaginal tablets or pessaries 1–2 each night for 2 weeks. If these or other antifungal vaginal tablets are not available, all that can be done is paint inside the vagina daily with 0.5% crystal violet solution in water.

Treat trichomonal infection with metronidazole 2000 mg in one dose or with 200 mg three times a day for a week. Give to both the patient and the patient's sexual partner.

Treat non-specific vaginitis with metronidazole as above.

Do not give tetracycline or metronidazole to a patient who is pregnant – refer or non-urgently transfer the patient to the Medical Officer.

Refer or non-urgently transfer patients who may have drug resistant infections.

Refer/transfer

Refer or non-urgently transfer to the Medical Officer:

1. patients not cured by the above management (first make sure their sexual partner/s has/have been treated); and
2. patients who cannot be managed by the above scheme.

Control and prevention

See pages 201–203.

In gonorrhoea, all sexual contacts for 2 months before the patient developed symptoms should be found, examined if possible, but treated anyway (as not all infected people have symptoms).

Non-gonococcal infection including *Chlamydia trachomatis* urethritis, non-specific urethritis and cervicitis

Urethritis and cervicitis and their complications are often due to gonorrhoea. However, many other causes, especially *Chlamydia trachomatis,* do exist. Often these other causes do not produce as much urethral discharge as gonorrhoea, though most of the other complications of gonorrhoea can, and do, occur with these other infections. Pus may be seen in swabs taken of the urethral or other discharge, but gonococci are not seen.

In females, the cervix of the uterus (the opening into the vagina) as well as the urethra are commonly infected. Many infections cause no symptoms but there can be pain on intercourse, bleeding after intercourse or lower abdominal pain. Examination may show pus, tenderness on moving the cervix or signs of pelvic inflammatory disease. PID followed by infertility may occur.

About half of these cases are due to *Chlamydia trachomatis,* which is usually sensitive to the tetracycline group of drugs. Others of these cases are due to other organisms, some of which are successfully treated by tetracyclines and some of which are not.

Some organisms causing non-gonococcal urethritis cause other complications such as Reiter's syndrome (urethritis and conjunctivitis and arthritis) (see Chapter 29 page 488).

Treatment is the drug chosen by your Health Department from the list set out in Table 19.2 on pages 203–204.

Treatment of the sexual partners with the same drugs before the patient has intercourse with them again is essential.

Treatment of other contacts with the above drugs is also necessary.

Children born to women who have untreated *Chlamydia trachomatis* infections may develop severe conjunctivitis and blindness or pneumonia. As well as treating the mother, the baby should be treated immediately as on page 207. It is important to give erythromycin for 2 weeks.

Syphilis

Syphilis is a bacterial infection which causes a sore where the organism enters the body. This sore heals without treatment. However, the bacteria spread all through the body and cause serious subacute and chronic disease of many organs.

Epidemiology

Syphilis is common especially among young adults. The cause is the syphilis bacterium (*Treponema pallidum*). The only host is man.

The disease usually spreads from an infectious lesion (chancre, mucous patch or condyloma) during sexual intercourse. The organisms can enter a new person through broken skin or normal unbroken mucous membrane of the genitalia or mouth. Infection can also occur through infected blood which is transfused, or through the placenta to an unborn baby from an infected pregnant woman.

Previous infection with the similar yaws bacterium gives some immunity against syphilis.

Symptoms and signs, course and complications

Primary syphilis causes a chancre and enlarged lymph glands.

1. The chancre is the lesion at the site of infection (usually genitalia but can also be anus or mouth) (see Figures 19.6 and 19.7). First a painless lump develops. It soon ulcerates in the centre and clear fluid oozes from it. It is firm and hard, 'like a button' in the skin. It usually heals after 2–6 weeks, even without treatment. It may look different if secondary bacterial infection occurs.

   A female patient may not know she has a chancre if it occurs in the vagina or on the cervix

> Any ulcer of the genitalia is treated as syphilis no matter what it looks like.

2. The nearby lymph glands are usually hard but not tender.

   Secondary syphilis usually comes about 6 weeks after the primary sore heals. (But it can be earlier or much later.) There may be any or all of these common lesions:

1. A skin rash with bilateral (on both sides) round, red, non–itchy flat patches 5–10 mm in diameter.
2. A skin rash with bilateral red, non–itchy lumps which may become scaly or turn into pustules.

3. A skin rash called condylomata lata in warm moist areas such as the perineum, vulva (see Figure 19.8), scrotum, inner thighs, under breasts, etc. The above lumps here get bigger and the surface skin comes off to produce large painless raised moist grey areas. However, secondary infection may occur and change the appearance.
4. Mucous patches are painless, shallow grey ulcers with a narrow red margin (or edge). They occur on the lips or mouth, vulva, vagina, scrotum and penis.

> Any wet skin lesions in groin, perineum, axilla, etc. must be suspected of being syphilis (secondary syphilis).

5. Painless enlargement of all lymph nodes of the body.
6. General symptoms and signs of infection, e.g. malaise, fever, loss of appetite, loss of weight.

   Any of these symptoms of the secondary stage are present for 2–6 weeks and then go away, even without treatment. But they may return again many times.

   Tertiary syphilis occurs many years later, in one out of every two or three cases. 'Gumma', causing mostly non–inflamed ulcers on the skin as well as disease of the heart or disease of the brain, can occur. (In

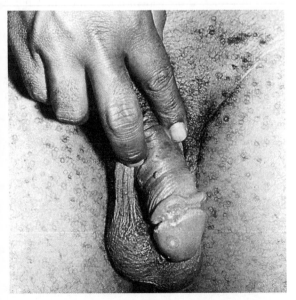

Figure 19.6 *Primary syphilis. A chancre on the penis. Note, however, that any ulcer on the genitalia is first treated as syphilis no matter what it looks like.*

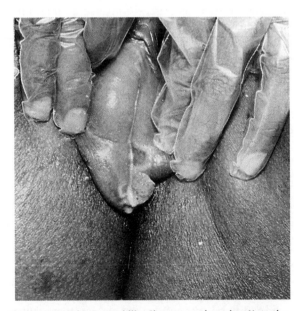

Figure 19.7 *Primary syphilis. Chancre on the vulva. Note the fairly typical appearance (see text). However, all ulcers in the genitalia are treated first for syphilis. Note also that in females the chancre may be in the vagina or on the cervix and not be noticed by the patient.*

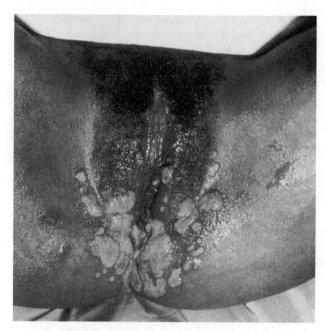

Figure 19.8 Secondary syphilis condylomata lata of vulva and perineum.

Diagnostic features

- Sexual contact about 3 weeks before.
- Hard, painless ulcerated sore on genitalia (or other area) with enlarged non-tender lymph nodes nearby. The sore heals after 2–6 weeks. However you should suspect syphilis in all ulcers on the genitalia.
- Two to six weeks later, skin rashes, condylomata lata, mucous patches, general symptoms and signs, and possibly disease of other organs can occur.

Treatment

1. Before giving treatment ask the patient about previous or present symptoms of urethral discharge. If discharge, give treatment for gonorrhoea and *Chlamydia trachomatis* (see page 204) as well as the treatment for syphilis (which will not cure gonorrhoea and chlamydia).

> Treatment for syphilis needs only a low concentration of the antibiotic but for a long time. Treatment for gonorrhoea needs a high concentration of the antibiotic but for only a short time.

2. Treat also for chancroid. See below.
3. See Table 19.2 page 204 for drug treatment. Use the drugs chosen by your Health Department.

Ask the patient to return for another clinical examination in a week. If the patient is not cured, investigate and treat for the other likely causes (see page 198).

Control and prevention

See 'Control and prevention' pages 201–203.

You should examine and test all groups of people who have a high risk of being infected, and treat them if necessary.

In areas where yaws is uncommon and syphilis occurs, do an STS on all pregnant women. Treat the woman, if the STS is positive, to stop possible congenital syphilis in her baby.

Chancroid (soft sore)

Chancroid is an infection caused by special bacteria (*Haemophilus ducreyi*). The main signs are one or many tender ulcers with ragged undermined edges on the genitalia and in half of the cases enlarged tender lymph nodes which can ulcerate. This infection seems to be becoming very frequent and in many areas is the most common cause of genital ulcer, especially in men and especially in HIV infected patients.

some tropical developing countries there have been only a few cases of tertiary syphilis. This is probably because syphilis has not been common for very long, as infection with yaws used to give some immunity to syphilis.)

Congenital syphilis. A child may be infected through the placenta, if his mother has syphilis. The child may be born dead or develop any of the signs of secondary or tertiary syphilis.

Tests

Send the serum of 10 ml of blood to the laboratory with a request for a serological test for syphilis (STS). A VDRL or RPR test is usually done. Occasionally, these tests are positive when the patient does not have syphilis. More accurate tests, e.g. TPHA or FTA-Ab may then be done.

The STS is positive in two out of three cases of primary syphilis but not until 3–4 weeks after the chancre comes.

The STS is positive in nearly all cases of secondary syphilis.

STS may remain positive for life. Re-treatment is needed only if a later test is about four times higher or more positive on titre testing than the original positive test; or the patient has further sexual intercourse with people with infectious syphilis.

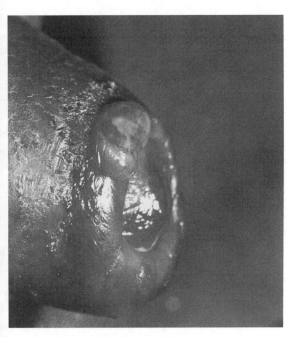

Figure 19.9 *Chancroid or soft sore ulcer.*

A small lump appears on the genitalia. The lump is on the surface of the skin or mucous membrane (different from syphilis, which is in the skin). The lump soon ulcerates. The edges are irregular and can be indeterminate. The edge of the ulcer is irregular and red, and it is covered with dirty pus (see Figure 19.9). The sore is very painful. Where the ulcer touches other parts of the body, new ulcers may appear. The ulcers are soft (again different from syphilis).

The lymph nodes in the groin on one or both sides become swollen, painful and tender in about half of the cases. These inflamed lymph nodes often form a fluid-filled (fluctuant) mass which bursts to leave a large ulcer (again different from syphilis).

However, it is not possible to tell, by examination alone, if the condition is definitely due to chancroid or syphilis or due to other infection.

Diagnosis is possible in a laboratory by examining the discharge from an ulcer under the microscope. Also, if this is done, send blood for STS and HIV serology.

Treatment – see Table 19.2 on page 204.

If lymph nodes look as if they will burst, then before this happens, aspirate (suck out) the pus through a needle put into the bubo through normal-looking nearby skin. Do not cut into the lump to let the pus out.

If the condition is not cured, consider both an antibiotic resistant organism, HIV infection or other conditions and refer to the Medical Officer.

Control and *prevention* – see pages 201–203.

Granuloma inguinale or Donovanosis

Donovanosis is caused by a bacterial infection (*Klebsiella* or *Calymmatobacterium* (or *Donovania*) *granulomatis*) but the organism is not very infectious. It is very common only in certain places including parts of the Pacific, Africa and India and South America. The main sign is a red ulcer on the genitalia without toxaemia. The lymph glands are usually affected only later and only in some cases.

The first lesion is usually a lump on one part of the genitalia. The lump soon develops into an ulcer. The ulcer is usually raised and irregular at its edges and bright red, because it is full of granulation tissue or like cut meat ('beefy red') and is not covered with a crust. The ulcer is not painful. The ulcer only slowly (over many weeks) gets bigger towards the groin areas or anus, usually in the folds of the skin (see Figure 19.10).

New lesions can appear on the genitalia; especially in places the first lesion touches.

Only if other infections are also present in the original ulcer do the lymph nodes in the groin areas become enlarged. However, the Donovanosis organism can spread to the lymph nodes and cause an ulcer, similar to the one on the genitalia, which slowly gets bigger. (This is why the disease is called also granuloma inguinale – see Figure 19.11.)

If not treated, the lesions all slowly get bigger and destroy a lot of tissue. Occasionally, the organism can spread to other parts of the body and start ulcers there

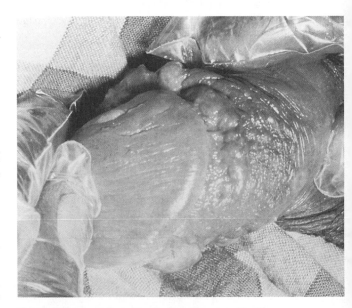

Figure 19.10 *Granuloma inguinale or Donovanosis. Ulcer on the penis filled with areas of granulation tissue.*

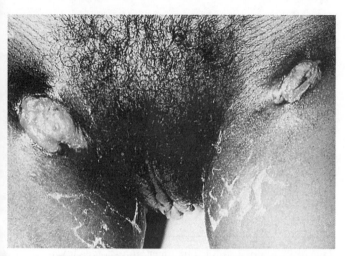

Figure 19.11 *Granuloma inguinale or Donovanosis. Vulval ulcer and granulations with spread of the disease to the lymph glands in the groin, which have ulcerated.*

too. After many years, if not treated, cancer can form in the edges of some lesions.

Diagnosis could be made by a simple test which can be sent to the laboratory. Clean the sore with saline. Local anaesthetic is not needed. Cut a *small thin* slice from the top of the edge of the sore with a sterile scalpel or razor blade. Smear the cut side on a glass slide or crush it between two glass slides. Fix it with alcohol. Send it to the laboratory with a request for examination for 'Donovan bodies'. This is often positive if the disease is Donovanosis. A proper biopsy would be diagnostic; but it is not usually needed.

For differential diagnosis and management see page 198.

Treatment – see Table 19.2 page 204.

Control and *prevention* – see pages 201–203. You need only trace and examine the regular sexual partner, as the disease is not very infectious.

Lymphogranuloma venereum (inguinal bubo)

Lymphogranuloma venereum is caused by a type of bacterial infection (*Chlamydia trachomatis*). It is also called lymphogranuloma inguinale. The usual signs are no ulcer on the genitalia but very enlarged inflamed inguinal lymph nodes with toxaemia and then ulceration of the inguinal lymph nodes.

One to three weeks after infection, a small blister or ulcer appears on the genitalia, and is usually not noticed. About 2–6 weeks later the lymph nodes in the groin become enlarged and inflamed. Pus forms in the lymph nodes, which then burst. As more nodes

are affected, many abscesses discharging whitish fluid develop. Abscesses can join to make large ulcers. The area affected increases. Sometimes abscesses and ulcers form in the anal region.

During this time the patient may have general symptoms and signs of infection such as malaise, fever, etc.

After some months the ulcers usually get better. But there is often a lot of deformity left. After years, there may be strictures (narrowing) of the rectum or urethra or vulva. There may also be chronic oedema of the genitalia.

Special tests for definite diagnosis are not usually done. Biopsy would be diagnostic.

Treatment – see Table 19.2 page 204.

Treat also for syphilis and chancroid if ulcer on genitalia at any time during this illness.

Aspirate any pus from lymph nodes before they burst, putting the needle through uninfected skin into the bubo and aspirating all the fluid before taking the needle out. Do not cut into the lump to let the pus out.

Control and *prevention* – see pages 201–203.

Venereal or anogenital warts (condyloma acuminatum)

Venereal warts are caused by one of the human papilloma viruses (HPV).

The warts are most common under the foreskin and on (and often around) the glans penis of the male. They are found on (and often around) the vulva and in the vagina and on the cervix of the female. They may also occur in the urethra and around the anus in both sexes.

The warts are soft pink fleshy growths like a cauliflower. There may be very many of them. They may grow very big (see Figures 19.12 and 19.13). Sometimes they look like warts on other parts of the body. They may get worse in pregnancy or if an HIV infection develops.

Infection with certain of the HPV organisms may, years later, cause carcinoma of the cervix of the uterus and possibly penile and other genital or anal carcinomas.

Always consider if the condition could be due to secondary syphilis or molluscum contagiosum. Always think of other STD and HIV being present.

Treatment is difficult. Small warts may just go away themselves. You should treat any other STD, especially any genital discharge (see page 203). Regular washing with soap and water will help. Paint the warts with

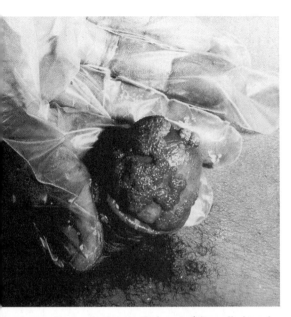

Figure 19.12 *Venereal or anogenital warts (also called condyloma acuminatum) of the penis.*

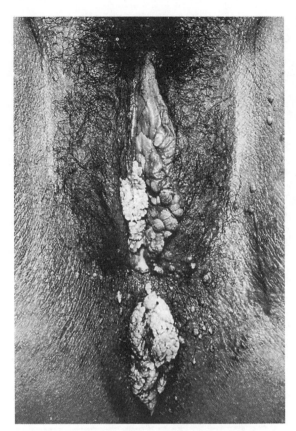

Figure 19.13 *Venereal or anogenital warts (also called condyloma acuminatum) of the vulva and anus.*

odophyllin 20% in tincture of benzoin, maximum ose 0.5 (1/2) ml; or touch them with a silver nitrate ick. Do not use podophyllin during pregnancy. Do ot put any podophyllin or silver nitrate on any normal art of the body. Wash off the podophyllin after 4 hours. .epeat the treatment each week until the warts are one. Podophyllotoxin 0.5% liquid applied twice daily or 3 days each 7 days is better but expensive, though atients may purchase this themselves. If the patient does ot get better or warts are in the urethra or cervix or the atient is pregnant, refer them to the Medical Officer.

A vaccine has just been developed by an Australian octor which will prevent most venereal warts and ne cancers (e.g. cervix) that may follow.

Control and *prevention* – see pages 201–203.

Herpes genitalis

Herpes genitalis is an infection with herpes simplex irus (usually HSV-2).

Infection with herpes genitalis virus causes a umber of small vesicles (blisters) to come up on the nucous membranes of the genitalia. The vesicles burst, nd shallow ulcers develop (see Figure 19.14). Some lcers join. The ulcers look like the 'cold sores' which nay appear on the lips during fever. The surface of ne ulcer is green-grey or white. Near the ulcer the nucous membrane is red. The ulcers are very painful, specially if urine touches them. The ulcers may look ifferent if they have secondary bacterial infection.

The lymph nodes in the groin are sometimes large, firm and tender.

During a first infection the patient may have the general symptoms and signs of infection – fever, malaise, etc.

The condition usually goes away after some weeks; but it may return many times for the rest of the patient's life. Tingling and other unusual feelings in the skin usually occur before another group of ulcers form. The patient is infectious any time ulcers are present, and should not have intercourse if the tingling or other feelings or ulcers are present.

Herpes genitalis comes back more often and spreads further and lasts longer and in general is worse if the patient develops an HIV infection.

If a pregnant woman has the infection with ulcers on the genitalia at the time of birth, the child may be infected at birth and get a severe infection and die. Caesarean section may be needed. Discuss delivery of pregnant women with herpes genitalis with the Medical Officer.

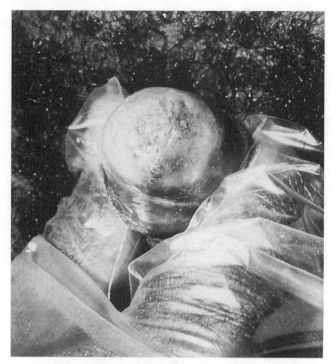

Figure 19.14 Herpes genitalis of the penis. Note the small vesicles on the glans. They soon burst to become ulcers and are very painful.

No *treatment* available in health centres cures the condition. Special antiviral drugs such as aciclovir 200 mg each 4 hours five times a day until healed makes the attack end more quickly, but they are very expensive and do not cure the patient and do not stop the infection coming back. Keep the affected area clean and dry. Treat as on page 226 or with methylrosanilinium 0.5% in water solution to put on the ulcers.

Control and *prevention* – see pages 201–203. As there is no curative treatment possible, it is not necessary to find contacts. The patient should not have sexual intercourse when infectious, i.e. when lesions or tingling, etc. present.

SIMPLIFIED TREATMENT OF SEXUALLY TRANSMITTED DISEASES

Urethral discharge

1. Ciprofloxacin 500 mg by mouth once on an empty stomach
   or
   Ceftriaxone 250 mg IMI once
   or
   Cefixime 400 mg orally once
   or

Spectinomycin 2 g IMI once
or
SMX 4000 mg and TMP 800 mg (co-trimoxazole) orally in 1 dose daily for 1(–3) day(s)
or
Gentamicin 240 mg IMI once
and

2. Doxycycline 100 mg orally twice daily for 7–10 days if not pregnant
   or
   Erythromycin 500 mg orally 4 times a day for 7–10 days if pregnant
   and

3. Treatment for genital sore if present.

Genital sore

1. Benzathine penicillin 2.4 million units IMI once
   and

2. Erythromycin 500 mg orally four times a day
   or
   TMP 160 mg and SMX 80 mg twice daily for 7 days if not pregnant
   and

3. Treatment of urethral discharge if present.

Other genital conditions

Balanitis

Balanitis is inflammation of the glans penis and the foreskin. It is more common in those who are uncircumcised, those who have phimosis, those who have diabetes and those who do not regularly wash under the foreskin. The inflammation can be caused by various types of organisms including bacteria, fungi and trichomonas.

The patient complains of a penile or urethral discharge; but on inspection the discharge is seen to come from under the foreskin and not the urethra. The glans penis is red, inflamed and sometimes ulcerated. The foreskin is inflamed and sometimes gangrenous.

Test the urine for sugar and refer or non-urgently transfer the patient for treatment, if he has diabetes.

Treatment includes benzathine penicillin 2,400,000 units (5 ml) IMI immediately in case it is syphilis; and if any urethral discharge see page 203.

The patient should wash the area regularly twice every day and apply gentian violet in water solution twice every day.

If the patient does not improve quickly give treatment with tetracycline and metronidazole (see page 215).

Prevention is by good personal hygiene.

Traumatic sores of penis or vulva

There are many causes for these, including small tears during intercourse.

Secondary bacterial infection can occur.

Give local treatment to the sore, e.g. 1% crystal violet in water solution twice daily after washing. As syphilis and chancroid cannot usually be excluded, give treatment for these (see page 204). Ask about previous or present symptoms of urethritis. Treat if there are symptoms (see page 204).

Amoebic ulceration of the genitalia

Amoebic ulcers are caused by a protozoal organism (*Entamoeba histolytica*) which normally lives in the bowel (see Chapter 23 pages 371–372).

The lesion starts on or near the genitalia because of direct spread of the organism from the anus; or anal intercourse; or intercourse with a person who has a genital amoebic ulcer.

The lesion is usually a fast growing (in days to weeks) painful ulcer which destroys much tissue. The ulcer is usually reddish in colour and covered with grey-white pus. If it is very acute, the discharge may be like watery blood. The lymph nodes nearby are usually enlarged and tender. (See Figure 19.15.)

Occasionally, the lesion may grow more slowly and look like a cancer of the penis, vulva or cervix.

Diagnosis can be made by immediate microscopic examination of discharge from the edge of the ulcer for *Entamoeba histolytica*; but this is not usually possible in a health centre. A biopsy would be diagnostic, but is not usually needed.

Treat with metronidazole 800 mg three times a day for 5–10 days. If nausea occurs, reduce the dose of metronidazole to 400 mg three times a day but continue for 10 days. Warn the patient not to drink alcohol while taking metronidazole. Give tetracycline together with the metronidazole if acute inflammation is present.

Cancer of the penis or vulva

You should suspect cancer in elderly patients who have had an ulcer for some weeks or months. The ulcer is often full of growing tissues with raised, turned out edges (see Figure 19.16). If it has spread to the lymph nodes, they will be very hard like stones.

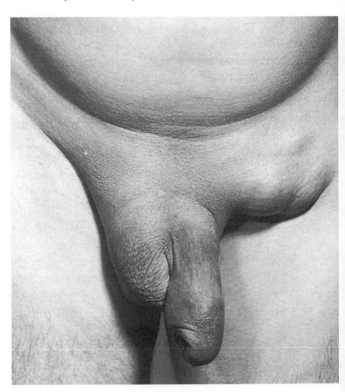

Figure 19.15 *A small amoebic ulcer of the penis. The ulcer did not improve after penicillin or after tetracycline. The patient was therefore treated with metronidazole and was cured. (A smear taken from the edge of the ulcer before metronidazole was given and immediately examined under the microscope showed amoebae.) Often amoebic ulcers are much larger than this ulcer.*

Figure 19.16 *Cancer of the penis. Note that any ulcer which has recently formed and does not get better after treatment with penicillin and then tetracycline and if necessary metronidazole, as well as any chronic ulcer, must be referred or transferred to the Medical Officer for a biopsy to see if it is a cancer.*

Any patient with a very suspicious ulcer should be transferred non-urgently for biopsy or biopsied and the biopsy sent for examination at the laboratory. While waiting for transfer or biopsy result, you should treat the patient for amoebic infection as on page 215. If the disease is cancer the only treatment is non-urgent transfer for surgery.

Scabies

See Chapter 32 pages 538–540.

Lice

See Chapter 32 page 540.

Human immunodeficiency virus (HIV) infection and acquired immunodeficiency syndrome (AIDS)

Dr Wendy Holmes and her collaborators at TALC have produced tape and slide sets on HIV infection from which most of the photographs for this section were generously supplied. Some parts of the text are based on ideas from these sets.

Other parts are based on the following excellent WHO publications:

- *TB/HIV: A Clinical Manual* by Drs Anthony Harries, Dermot Maher and Stephen Graham *et al.* (second edition, 2004);
- *Anti-retroviral Therapy for HIV Infection in Adults and Adolescents* (revised version, 2006);
- *Chronic HIV Care with ARV Therapy and Prevention* (2007);
- *Tuberculosis Care with TB-HIV Co-management* (2007).

All of these should be seen by health workers caring for HIV infected patients.

WHO regularly puts reports on their website with the latest information about diagnosis and treatment. Go to www.who.org and select 'Health topics' on the left upper corner, then select H (in the A–Z) and then select HIV. Reports from 2008 and later are of particular importance as these will have new information and should be seen and used.

Definition

Human immunodeficiency virus (HIV) infection slowly destroys the cellular immune system (see Chapter 10 page 41) of the body. This allows increasingly severe and frequent infections and also some tumours to grow.

Severely affected people are said to have Acquired Immunodeficiency Syndrome (AIDS). This, however, is what happens only many years after infection. At the time of infection there are no symptoms. A month or two later there may be a mild febrile illness. Then again for many years there may be no symptoms or signs or just a persistent generalised lymphadenopathy due to the virus in the lymph nodes. Then infections with common organisms occur more frequently than normal. The infections later become more frequent and more severe than usual because of the decreased immunity. The HIV itself can cause damage to some organs, especially the bowel and brain, and the virus itself can cause disease of organs. At the end there is so little resistance to infection that organisms which rarely cause infections in healthy people cause severe, often unusual and fatal infections or even cancers. Although there is now no cure for HIV infection, new genetic engineering techniques and new drugs may in future make cure possible. There are already anti-retroviral drugs which greatly slow the growth of the HIV infection and improve the patient's health. They are expensive, do have significant side effects and as yet are not everywhere available. The infections that HIV infection and loss of immunity allow to occur, however, can often be treated with drugs we already have. Counselling and support can greatly help patients and their family. Although there is no vaccine to prevent HIV infection, this may later become available. If practices that spread HIV are stopped, infection can already be avoided or prevented.

Epidemiology

HIV infection was first recognised in 1981. Tests on stored blood from people in Africa who died long before 1981 have now shown HIV to be present and to have caused their deaths. Even more recent investigations have suggested that about 100 years ago, the virus passed from monkeys, in which it does not cause a severe disease, to men, most probably when they butchered monkeys in the jungle for meat. There are in fact two different kinds of HIV – HIV-1 (the most common) and HIV-2 (mainly in West Africa). There are also different strains of these two viruses. The viruses are able to change and still do. It is of interest that there are other well known immunodeficiency viruses in other animals which are not infectious to man.

HIV is present in the body and especially the blood of infected people, who may be either apparently healthy carriers or be sick. The virus is also in some of the body secretions, mainly semen and vaginal secretions, but also discharges from wounds, milk and saliva. Infected blood, semen, vaginal secretions and possibly other infected secretions from a person infected with HIV may get into the body of another uninfected person by only a few special ways. By far the most common way for this to happen is through sexual intercourse (normal heterosexual intercourse and oral sex, but most easily by anal intercourse). Transmission may result from other close physical contact, but only if both the infected person and also the uninfected person have open wounds or sores and the blood or secretions from the infected person gets into the wounds or sores of the uninfected person. Transmission almost always occurs if infected blood is transfused. It is also likely if infected blood in needles or syringes is not properly cleaned out and sterilised after use and is then injected. This should never happen in health centres which use proper cleaning and sterilisation. However, it does happen when drug addicts share needles and syringes. It can happen in tattooing, traditional skin piercing, scarification and circumcision, when instruments are used but not cleaned and sterilised before being used on a further person. Infected pregnant women pass the infection to their unborn children in about 30% of cases either through the placenta or bleeding during birth. Up to 15% of babies uninfected at birth can later be infected, probably from the infected mother's milk (but without breastfeeding even more than this 15% would die of malnutrition, infections, etc.; and breastfeeding therefore should continue until 6 months).

It is not possible to be infected by caring for people infected by HIV (Figure 19.18) as long as their blood, semen or vaginal secretions, etc. do not enter the body of the carer by sexual intercourse, injection, needle stick injuries or through wounds or sores. It is safe, therefore, to eat, drink, talk and play with infected people. It is safe to hug and even kiss (safest without contacting saliva (although saliva has some HIV protective properties in it)) infected people. It would not be safe to use ungloved hands with cuts or sores on them to dress any open or bleeding wounds or sores of an infected person. It would not be safe to share razors, toothbrushes or tooth-cleaning sticks, which could go through the surface of the skin or mouth, etc. with an infected person. Any sexual intercourse, where the penis without a condom on it is placed in the vagina, anus or mouth, would be a danger to pass on infection. No symptom or sign occurs at the time of infection for a person to know they have been infected.

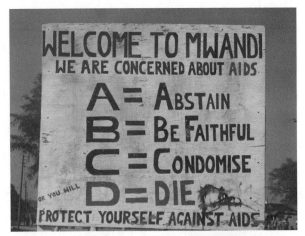

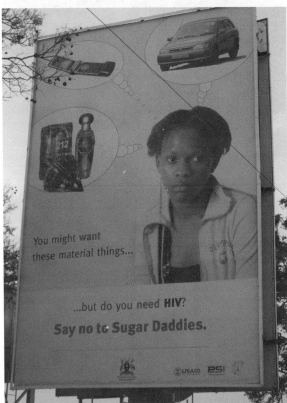

Figure 19.17 *Road signs in Africa warning how not to get HIV infection by the usual way it is spread, i.e. sexual intercourse.*

HIV infection is common. It quickly increased until 2005, but now control measures are slowly decreasing new cases. However, the amount of HIV infection varies greatly from country to country and area to area (Table 19.3 and Figure 19.19). It can vary far below 1% in some rural areas to up to 50% of some groups of adults in some cities. It is as common in women as in men. It is most common in young adults.

HIV DOES NOT SPREAD IN THESE WAYS:

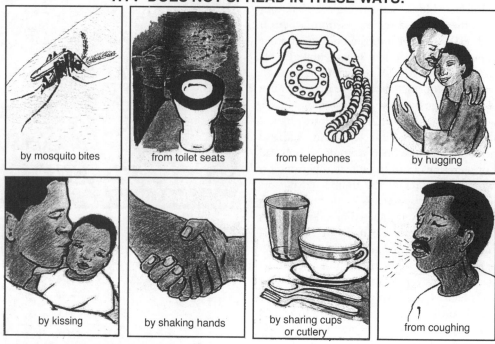

Figure 19.18 *HIV does not spread in these ways.*

HIV infection spreads
FROM the:
1. semen,
2. vaginal secretions,
3. blood,
4. milk,
5. discharges from sores or injuries

of an infected person
TO an uninfected person BY:

1. sexual intercourse through the mucous membranes of the vagina, urethra, penis, anus or mouth,
2. contact with skin, but only if the skin surface is broken, i.e. ulcers or injuries in the skin,
3. breast milk (occasionally),
4. blood transfusion,
5. instruments used for injections, surgery, tattooing, body piercing, cutting, etc. if not properly cleaned and sterilised.

About half the people in some hospitals are there because of HIV infection. The commonest cause of death in adults in some areas is HIV infection. (This is different from industrialised countries, where most HIV sufferers are either homosexual males or inject-ing drug addicts and they are given anti-HIV drug therapy to slow the growth of the virus and antibiotic treatment for most other infections and many patients live for many years.)

Table 19.3 WHO global estimates of the HIV/AIDS epidemic.

People newly infected with HIV in 2007	2,500,000
Number of people living with HIV/AIDS in 2007	33,200,000
AIDS deaths in 2007	2,100,000
Total number of AIDS deaths since the beginning of the epidemic until end of 2005	25,000,000

Data from *AIDS Epidemic Update, December 2007, UNAIDS/WHO.* http://whqlibdoc.who.int/unaids/2007/9789291736218_en.pdf by permission of the WHO.

Symptoms and signs

There are no symptoms or signs at the time of the infection.

After 2–4 weeks, but at times months after infec-tion, in about half of infected persons, a non-specific viral ('influenza'-like or 'glandular fever'-like) illness may occur. There may be fever, sweating, malaise, tiredness, loss of appetite, diarrhoea, pain in muscles or joints, headache, encephalitis, sore throat, enlargement

Regional HIV and AIDS statistics and features, 2008

	People living with HIV	New HIV infections 2008	AIDS-related deaths 2008	Adult HIV prevalence (%)
Sub-Saharan Africa	**22.4 million** [20.8–24.1 million]	**1.9 million** [1.6–2.2 million]	**1.4 million** [1.1–1.7 million]	**5.2%** [4.9%–5.4%]
South and South-East Asia	**3.8 million** [3.4–4.3 million]	280 000 [240 000–320 000]	270 000 [220 000–310 000]	0.3% [0.2%–0.3%]
East Asia	850 000 [700 000–1.0 million]	75 000 [58 000–88 000]	59 000 [46 000–71 000]	<0.1% [<0.1%]
Latin America	**2.0 million** [1.8–2.2 million]	170 000 [150 000–200 000]	77 000 [66 000–89 000]	0.6% [0.5%–0.6%]
North America	**1.4 million** [1.2–1.6 million]	55 000 [36 000–61 000]	25 000 [20 000–31 000]	0.4% [0.3%–0.5%]
Western & Central Europe	850 000 [710 000–970 000]	30 000 [23 000–35 000]	13 000 [10 000–15 000]	0.3% [0.2%–0.3%]
Eastern Europe & Central Asia	**1.5 million** [1.4–1.7 million]	110 000 [100 000–130 000]	87 000 [72 000–110 000]	0.7% [0.6%–0.8%]
Caribbean	240 000 [220 000–260 000]	20 000 [16 000–24 000]	12 000 [9300–14 000]	1.0% [0.9%–1.1%]
Middle East & North Africa	310 000 [250 000–380 000]	35 000 [24 000–46 000]	20 000 [15 000–25 000]	0.2% [<0.2%–0.3%]
Oceania	59 000 [51 000–68 000]	3900 [2900–5100]	2000 [1100–3100]	0.3% [<0.3%–0.4%]
TOTAL	**33.4 million** [31.1–35.8 million]	**2.7 million** [2.4–3.0 million]	2 million [1.7–2.4 million]	0.8% [<0.8%–0.8%]
December 2008	The ranges around the estimates in this table define the boundaries within which the actual numbers lie, based on the best available information.			

Approx. 74 000 new HIV infections a day in 2008

- About 1200 are in children under 15 years of age
- About 6300 are in adults aged 15 years and older of whom
  - almost 50% are among women
  - almost 40% are among young people (15–24)

Figure 19.19 *HIV and AIDS statistics and features, 2008. (Source: AIDS Epidemic Update December 2009, UNAIDS/WHO, November 2009)*

of all the lymph nodes in the body, a flat vague reddish rash on the trunk, etc. The virus by then has spread all over the body. It is called the 'acute seroconversion reaction' or 'primary HIV infection' as after it, the serum tests show antibodies to the HIV. There is no way, however, that this illness can be clinically recognised as (or diagnosed as) HIV infection in the health centre. The HIV blood test is still negative (although the virus protein (HIV DNA, etc.) tests would be positive, but are almost never available).

Serological tests usually available for HIV infection do not become positive until, at the earliest, 1–3 months after infection; but by 6 months 95% of infected people have a positive test.

Infants may not fully recover from the above illness and may 'fail to thrive' (not grow or gain weight), or within weeks or months they develop one or more of the complications below. However, most adults seem to recover from the seroconversion reaction and stay apparently well for months to up to 5–10 or even

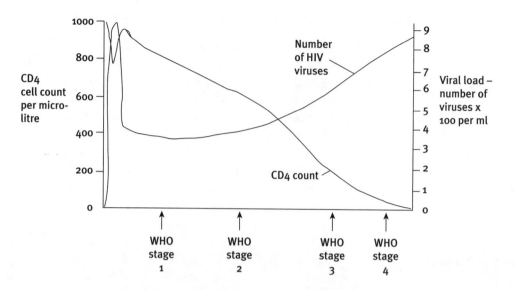

Figure 19.20 *Natural history of untreated HIV infection. WHO stage 1, no symptoms but may have persistent generalised lymphadenopathy (PGL); stage 2, minor symptoms and infections; stage 3, virulent infections, some opportunistic infections; stage 4, virulent infection and many opportunistic infections.*

many more years. Nevertheless, the virus is alive in the infected person's body and is able to infect others. The virus is also slowly damaging special parts of the body, most importantly the immune system; but also the nervous system and the bowel walls, skin, kidney, joints, etc. Most importantly, the lymphocytes (of the CD4 'helper' type), which are in the white blood cells and in lymph nodes, in the spleen and in other areas, are damaged and their numbers become fewer. These CD4 lymphocytes are responsible for cellular immunity (which protects against viral, mycobacterial, fungal and protozoal infections) and they also control B-lymphocyte cells so that they make antibodies in the correct amount. The patient's immunity, therefore, to infections and to some special cancers becomes less.

It may take some years (usually 5–10 years after infection and the seroconversion reaction, sometimes longer) for symptoms and signs to develop due to:

1. More infections and more severe infections than usual. These infections are caused by the usual organisms causing the common infections in the community (such as those organisms causing skin infections, mouth infections, bowel infections, sinusitis, pneumonia and TB). These more frequent and severe infections are caused or allowed by loss of immunity.

2. Unusual infections. These are allowed by severe loss of immunity. These infections are called 'oppor-

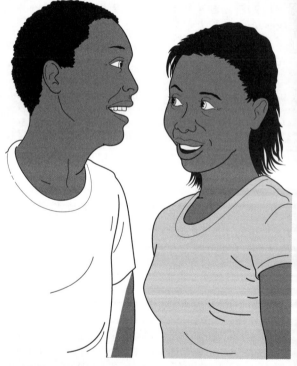

Figure 19.21 *These people have HIV infection stage 1. They still look happy and healthy and strong (but may not do so in 10 years unless treated). They will die young. It is not possible by looking at, or talking to, people to know if they are infected with HIV or not. HIV IS USUALLY SPREAD BY SEXUAL INTERCOURSE.*

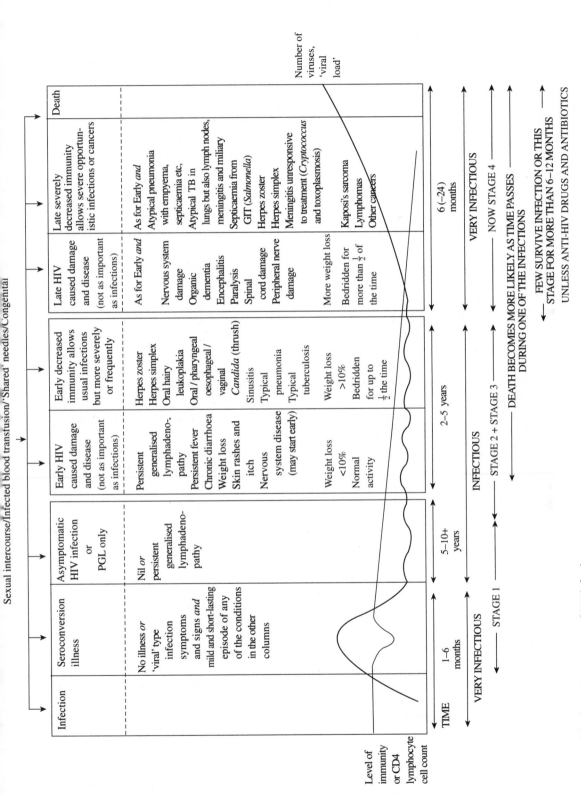

Figure 19.22 *This shows the progress of HIV infection.*

221

tunistic infections'. They are caused by organisms which normally do not grow in the healthy body and are normally killed or their growth mostly stopped by the healthy body's immunity. If, however, the body's defence or immunity is decreased, then they can take this 'opportunity' to grow in the body and cause an unusual infection, or a much worse infection than usual for that organism.

3. Unusual tumours, especially Kaposi's sarcoma or lymphoma, but others also. Many of these tumours may be due to virus infection and may be allowed by the loss of immunity.

4. Damage to some of the body's organs, especially the brain, lymph nodes, skin, bowel, kidney, joints, etc. These are caused by the virus itself.

Figure 19.22 (page 221) shows how HIV infection in a patient causes more and more loss of immunity as time goes by and what conditions are likely to be present at the different stages of loss of immunity.

The World Health Organization has put patients into the following groups or stages to help with diagnosis and management.

Clinical staging of HIV/AIDS for adults and adolescents

(Slightly simplified WHO Case Definitions 2007 for persons aged 15 years or more with positive HIV antibody test or other laboratory evidence of HIV infection.)

Primary HIV infection

- Asymptomatic (no symptoms)
- Acute retroviral syndrome (or seroconversion reaction)

Clinical stage 1 (no significant symptoms)

- Asymptomatic
- Persistent generalised lymphadenopathy (PGL)

Clinical stage 2 (mild symptoms)

- Moderate weight loss (< 10% of presumed or measured body weight), unexplained by other cause
- Recurrent bacterial respiratory tract infections (URTIs, sinusitis, bronchitis, otitis media, pharyngitis)
- Herpes zoster
- Angular cheilitis
- Recurrent oral ulcerations
- Papular (pimply) pruritic (itchy) eruptions (rashes)
- Seborrhoeic dermatitis
- Fungal nail infections of fingers

Clinical stage 3 (advanced symptoms)

Conditions where a presumptive (i.e. possible or provisional) diagnosis of HIV infection can be made on the basis of clinical signs or simple investigations

- Severe weight loss (> 10% of presumed or measured body weight), unexplained by other cause
- Chronic diarrhoea for longer than 1 month, unexplained by other cause
- Persistent fever (intermittent or constant for longer than 1 month), unexplained by other cause
- Oral candidiasis which persists or recurs
- Oral hairy leukoplakia
- Pulmonary TB at the time
- Severe presumed bacterial infections (e.g. pneumonia, empyema, pyomyositis, bone or joint infection, meningitis, bacteraemia)
- Acute necrotising ulcerative stomatitis, gingivitis or peridontitis (any very severe ulcers inside mouth)

Conditions where confirmatory diagnostic testing is necessary

- Unexplained anaemia (Hb < 8 g/dl), and/or low white cell count (< 500/mm^3) and/or low platelet count (< 50,000/mm^3) for more than 1 month

Clinical stage 4 (severe symptoms)

Conditions where a presumptive (i.e. probable or provisional) diagnosis of HIV infection can be made on the basis of clinical signs or simple investigations

- HIV wasting syndrome (even more weight loss with 1 month of either unexplained diarrhoea or unexplained fever or night sweats)
- Severe bacterial pneumonia which comes back
- Chronic herpes simplex infection (orolabial, genital or anorectal of more than 1 month's duration)
- Oesophageal candidiasis
- Extrapulmonary TB (i.e. TB in places other than lung)
- Kaposi's sarcoma

Conditions where confirmatory diagnostic testing is necessary (i.e. usually not able to be diagnosed or treated in a health centre)

- Pneumonia due to pneumocystis
- Central nervous system (CNS) toxoplasmosis
- Cryptococcal infection not just in the lungs, but also other organs including meningitis
- Disseminated non-TB mycobacterial infection
- Progressive multifocal leukoencephalopathy (PML) (a type of encephalitis)
- Candida infection of trachea, bronchi or lungs
- Diarrhoea, etc. due to cryptosporidiosis or isosporiasis
- Herpes simplex infection of organs (not just skin or mucous membranes)

- Cytomegalovirus (CMV) infection in retina of eye or other organ (not just the usual organs involved, i.e. liver, spleen or lymph nodes)
- Any fungal infection widely spread in the body (e.g. histoplasmosis, coccidioidomycosis, penicilliosis)
- Recurrent non-typhoid salmonella infection
- Lymphoma (cerebral or B cell non-Hodgkin's lymphoma)
- Invasive cervical carcinoma
- Visceral leishmaniasis (when not expected)
- HIV encephalopathy (encephalitis) or nephropathy (kidney failure) or cardiomyopathy (heart failure)

Clinical staging as above can be used to treat patients without CD4 or other laboratory testing. However, CD4 testing is very helpful, if available, to find out the severity of loss of immunity; and where CD4 facilities are available they should be used to make clinical decision-making more accurate. CD4 levels are not needed before starting anti-retroviral therapy (ART). They should be used only together with the clinical stage.

For clinical purposes, long-term prognosis has been shown to be related to the nadir (or lowest ever value) of CD4. It should be noted that the immunological staging of disease improves with successful ART.

CD4 levels in relation to the severity of immunosuppression:

Not significant immunosuppression $> 500/mm^3$
Mild immunosuppression $350–499/mm^3$
Advanced immunosuppression $200–349/mm^3$
Severe immunosuppression $< 200/mm^3$

HIV infection may at times show no symptoms or signs. It may at other times cause one or more or all of the following:

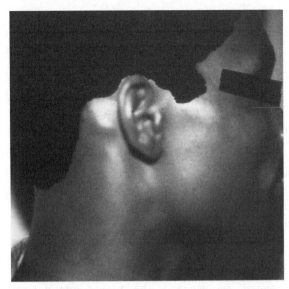

Figure 19.23 *Persistent generalised lymphadenopathy (PGL) in HIV infection.*

Notes on the symptoms, signs, diagnoses and management of conditions which occur in HIV infected people

Lymphatic system

1. *Persistent generalised lymphadenopathy* (PGL) due to HIV itself (Figure 19.23).
   There are enlarged lymph nodes without other symptoms in up to 30–50% of HIV infected people in stage 1. (These are not inguinal or groin nodes, which are often enlarged from chronic bacterial or filarial infections.)

The enlarged lymph nodes are:
- in more than one place and often symmetrical (the same on both sides),
- larger than 1 cm but usually smaller than 3 cm and do not continue to get larger,
- present for more than 3 months,
- have no other cause obvious (e.g. infection nearby, syphilis, TB, etc.) and are not tender.

Biopsy would be needed (as another diagnosis, especially TB, is more likely) if the lymph glands:
- are present in only one place,
- are large (4 cm or more in diameter) and continue to get larger,
- are tender or painful and there was no nearby infection,
- have local signs of chronic infection, e.g. are fluctuant or matted or have a sinus nearby,
- have other signs of infection including fever, night sweats, weight loss, etc.,
- are accompanied by a strongly positive tuberculin test.

See Chapter 14 pages 105, 110.

Respiratory system

1. *Recurrent acute respiratory infections of any sort.*
   These often occur early (i.e. stage 2) and are treated in the usual way (see Chapter 20).

2. *Sinusitis.*

   Causes face pain often on one side and tenderness and nasal discharge of pus and fever (see Chapter 20 page 282).

3. *Acute otitis media.*

   Causes ear pain, deafness, fever, swollen inflamed ear drum (see Chapter 20 page 280).

4. *Acute pharyngitis or tonsillitis.*

   Causes throat pain and fever (see Chapter 20 page 284).

5. *Acute bronchitis.*

   Causes cough and sputum but no signs of pneumonia (see Chapter 20 pages 286–287).

6. *Pneumonia.*

   This becomes more common as immunity decreases. Cough, sputum, chest pain, fever and chest signs occur as in non–HIV infected patients. *Streptococcus pneumoniae* is the most common cause. Treat as usual. Do not forget to give antibiotics to kill 'atypical' pneumonia organisms if penicillin is not quickly effective. However, look for complications such as empyema and lung abscess; and spread to other organs, causing such conditions as meningitis, acute septic arthritis and pyomyositis (see Chapter 20 pages 287–291).

7. *Unusual or opportunistic infections which can infect the lung (some infections only in certain areas).*

   (a) *Pneumocystis jeroveci (carinii).* An unusual fungus/protozoa with direct or airborne spread to the lungs of many people; but rarely causes disease unless the patient has immunosuppression. It can then cause pneumocystis pneumonia (PCP). The diagnosis is commonly made in industrialised countries by tests but rarely proven in developing countries; but it is still common. Suspect PCP in any HIV infected person if the patient has either (1) the typical features of PCP, i.e. slow onset of illness but later severe shortness of breath, cough, little or no sputum, fast pulse and breathing rate, often cyanosis, only an occasional crackle in the chest (and later death); or (2) pneumonia treated in the correct way (see Chapter 20 page 289) which gets worse. Diagnosis is by special examination in the laboratory of secretions collected from the lungs, not usually possible in a health centre. Treatment is by co-trimoxazole, i.e. sulfamethoxazole 1600 mg and trimethoprim 320 mg (4 single strength or 2 double strength tablets) each 8 hours for small adults and each 6 hours for large adults. If the patient is allergic to sulfonamides, give less

effective dapsone 100 mg once daily and trimethoprim 300 mg each 8 hours. Side effects to SMX/TMP are common including GI upsets (give metoclopramide), rash (give antihistamine), fever (give paracetamol), liver enzymes raised or hepatitis (stop if ALT is five or more times normal), low white cell count, etc. If reactions are severe, the treatment may need to be stopped; but transfer such problems to the Medical Officer. If the patient is very short of breath or cyanosed give oxygen, and also give prednisolone 50 mg daily to reduce after 5 days slowly as improves to none (but transfer such patients also to the Medical Officer as TB needs excluding and other treatment given). Prophylactic co-trimoxazole is needed after recovery for the rest of the patient's life unless the CD4 count rises with ART.

   (b) *Nocardia.* A soil bacterium which, if inhaled, can cause a subacute pneumonia (cough, sputum, fever, decreased weight, etc.); local invasion from the lung (and about one third of these develop empyema); dissemination (spread) to all parts of the body but especially to the brain, often with abscess formation; but sputum and CSF examination are often negative for nocardia. It is more common in HIV infected people. Treatment is with co-trimoxazole in the same dose as for pneumocystis.

   (c) *Melioidosis.* An infection by a bacterium (*Burkholderia pseudomallei*) which lives in soil and water in SE Asia and the Pacific, but also in other areas, and can enter the body through the skin or by inhalation. Skin infection may cause abscesses and the organism can spread through the body causing acute pneumonia, meningitis, etc. Inhalation of the organism can cause pneumonia, which is often chronic and looks like TB. Examination of the pus is usually diagnostic (see Chapter 17 page 161). Sometimes this responds to SMX/TMP but usually only to special antibiotics, e.g. third generation cephalosporins given for a long time.

   (d) *Cryptococcus.* A fungus which grows in warm soil, especially if there are pigeon droppings in it. Inhalation causes pneumonia, which is usually not a major problem and usually settles itself; but spread through the body often causes meningoencephalitis especially in immunosuppressed patients. Treatment requires intravenous antifungal treatment such as IV amphotericin B, followed by fluconazole and may need oral flu-conazole prophylaxis for life unless CD4 count rises with ART (see Chapter 25 page 414).

(e) *Penicilliosis marneffi*. A fungus most common in SE Asia which can cause lung infection and disease all over the body similar to miliary TB. Treatment requires IV amphoteracin B and then oral itraconazole for life unless the CD4 count rises with ART (see Chapter 20 pages 287–291).

8. *Tuberculosis* (see Chapter 14 page 111).

Always think of TB if chronic (more than 2–3 weeks) cough, especially if sputum, haemoptysis (coughing up blood even just once), shortness of breath, weight loss, fever, night sweats, fatigue and not cured by the usual antibiotics. Always send three sputum examinations for AFB from all such patients. TB is 5–10 times as likely if HIV infection is present than if it is not. About a third of HIV infected people in the world have also been infected with *M. tuberculosis*. Without HIV infection, only about 10% of *M. tuberculosis*-infected patients develop TB. About 50% of patients with both infections will develop TB disease. Up to half of the people seen with TB could also have HIV infection. In early HIV infection, where there is reasonable immunity, the symptoms and signs of TB will be the same as for other people (as above). However, later in the HIV infection, when there is little cellular immunity, TB may be unusual, e.g.:

• lower not upper parts of lungs affected;
• pleural effusions more common;
• sputum tests positive for AFB less commonly;
• the tuberculin test (Mantoux) usually negative;
• lymph node, bowel, meningeal and miliary TB more likely;
• unusual mycobacterial organisms (not *M.tuberculosis*), which do not cause infection in healthy people and could be resistant to the usual anti-TB drugs, can infect patients (but this occurs usually only late in the course of HIV infections);
• reactions to anti-TB drugs, especially thio-acetazone, are much more common and these reactions can be severe, causing loss of most of the skin and mucous membranes and death;
• interactions occur between some anti-TB drugs and some anti-HIV drugs. Some of these drugs (see page 244) should never be used together.

If these types of TB occur with HIV in your area, and sputum for AFB is negative, find out from your Medical Officer how you should send sputum for mycobacterial culture; if you should transfer the patient for X-rays and other tests; or if you should start anti-TB treatment in these patients.

If anti-TB drugs are started, they must be continued until the complete treatment is given, or resistant TB organisms will be produced (see Chapter 14 pages 112 and 123).

Patients with HIV infection who are started on anti-HIV drugs (ART) at the same time as anti-TB drugs often at first get worse on treatment. This is often due to immune reconstitution inflammatory syndrome (IRIS) (see page 248). This may be due to reactions of a patient to a drug, especially an NNRTI. If these are not the cause, it is most often because another infection such as pneumonia or malaria or meningitis, etc. has developed and needs diagnosis and treatment.

Patients with HIV infection and TB, who have been on treatment for TB without problems for some time, can then suddenly get worse. Although this could be due to the TB organisms becoming resistant to the anti-TB drugs, this is rare. It could be due to the patient having stopped the anti-TB drugs; so check for this. Most often it is due to another infection which needs diagnosis and treatment.

Always look for other infections, especially malaria, pneumonia and meningitis, which need treatment if a patient with both HIV and TB who is taking his treatment suddenly becomes seriously ill.

---

9. *Chronic cough from other causes.*

If the patient with a cough also has fever or continues to get worse on antibiotic treatment, even if the sputum tests for AFB are negative, in HIV infected patients, this is still often due to TB with unusual features (as above). It can, however, be due to another unusual infection (see 7 page 224). The patient needs transfer to the Medical Officer for chest X-ray and other special tests.

Think first, however, of all of the other causes of chronic cough and make sure that the patient does not have one which you can treat.

• Pneumonia not properly treated (see Chapter 20 page 287)
• Lung abscess
• Empyema (see Chapter 20 page 292)
• Bronchiectasis (see Chapter 20 page 299)
• Asthma (see Chapter 20 page 294)
• Chronic bronchitis and emphysema/chronic obstructive lung disease (see Chapter 20 page 297)

- Bronchial carcinoma (lung cancer) (see Chapter 20 page 300)
- Industrial lung disease (usually only if worked in factory or mine or cut stone or used asbestos) (see Chapter 20 page 301)
- Lung fluke – this worm can produce an illness with cough and red sputum which appears similar to TB (see Chapter 20 page 300)
- Unusual or opportunistic lung infections.

TREAT all apparent tuberculosis (but sputum for AFB negative) patients with:

1. further antibiotics – chloramphenicol if penicillin or other drug for usual pneumonia, and erythromycin or tetracycline for atypical pneumonia have not been effective; and
2. postural drainage and physiotherapy.

THEN if not effective:

1. transfer the patient to the Medical Officer; or if not possible,
2. give TMP 320 mg and SMX 1600 mg (co-trimoxazole) 4 of the 80/400 mg tablets three times a day for a small adult and four times a day for a large adult for 2 weeks, while waiting for the results of a second set of sputum examinations for AFB which you send.

THEN if not cured and if the second sputum tests for AFB negative (OR, if at any time before, the patient gets worse):

1. transfer to the Medical Officer for chest X-ray and further assessment; but if the patient looks as though he will die before transfer or if transfer not possible,
2. start anti-TB chemotherapy; but if started, the full course must be completed regardless of whether the diagnosis is confirmed or not.

Gastrointestinal problems

1. *Recurrent aphthous ulcers in the mouth.*
   Two or more episodes in 6 months of painful ulcers (yellow–grey base surrounded by inflammation).
   Treatment usually does not help as they are usually caused by a virus. Try hydrocortisone cream or ointment or a little powder from a crushed 5 mg prednisolone tablet put on to the ulcer 4 times a day. Try also the contents of a 250 mg tetracycline capsule in 10 ml of water held in the mouth for 5 minutes daily for 3 days.
2. *Chronic herpes simplex virus infection around mouth (usually HSV-1) or genitalia or anus (usually HSV-2).*
   These are painful small blisters which burst to leave an ulcer with a grey base surrounded by a red inflamed

area. They are very common in normal people, but become increasingly severe as immunity decreases (Figure 19.27 page 230). Keep the area clean and dry. Give antibiotics for secondary bacterial infection only if this occurs. A mixture made from nystatin (5 ml of solution or a crushed lozenge, tablet or pessary) and metronidazole (two 200 mg tablets crushed up or 5 ml of oral solution) and, if available, aciclovir (a crushed tablet or the contents of a capsule or the powder for one injection) to make 10–20 ml of solution and then painted onto the ulcers 3–4 times a day, may help. Aciclovir tablets orally help but do not cure; and are not usually available (see also page 214).

3. *Oral hairy leukoplakia.*
   Oral hairy leukoplakia (Figure 19.24) is probably caused by the Epstein–Barr virus (EBV). It causes patches of white material along the sides of the tongue. This white material is often in ridges or a series of lines. The material is stuck on and cannot be pushed off with a tongue depressor or spatula. It usually causes no symptoms and usually needs no treatment. Its main importance is that when you see it, you should immediately ask yourself if this patient could have HIV infection.
4. *Candidiasis or moniliasis.*
   'Thrush' infection in the mouth, throat and oesophagus, and in women in the vagina, is due to infection with the usual *Candida* or *Monilia* fungal organisms.
   Candida is a fungus which normally lives in all normal mouths and vaginas. An overgrowth of *Candida* occurs if other organisms in these areas are killed by antibiotics or if there is more than the usual amount of sugar present (i.e. diabetes mellitus), or if the patient is inhaling steroid drugs for asthma, and at times in the vagina of pregnant women and in the mouths of normal babies.

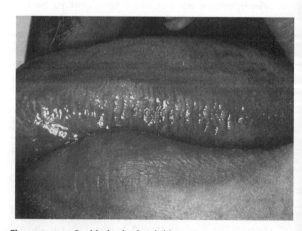

Figure 19.24 *Oral hairy leukoplakia.*

If none of the above apply, it is likely the patient who has *Candida* infection has HIV infection.

The growth of *Candida* in the mouth makes white patches which, if scraped off, leave a red inflamed mucosa. At times, there is just the very red inflamed swollen mucosa. There may be inflamed cracks in the corners of the lips (angular cheilitis) if the lips are affected. Pain, worse on eating or drinking if the mouth is affected, occurs. Pain in the front of the chest, worse on swallowing if the oesophagus is affected, occurs. Vaginal discharge and vulval itching, if the vagina is affected, occurs. These candida infections are very suggestive of HIV infection (see Figure 19.25).

Treat gastrointestinal tract candida infection with anti-candida drugs such as nystatin, natamycin, clotrimazole, fluconazole or amphotericin mixtures or lozenges, or if these are not available, methyl rosanilinium (crystal or gentian violet) 0.5% water solution, held in the mouth for as long as possible, then swallowed, three times a day after eating and before sleeping.

Treat genital candida with nystatin or clotrimazole cream or pessaries (see page 203).

Treatment of *Candida* anywhere can be with very effective oral drugs such as itraconazole or fluconazole 100–200 mg daily, but these are very expensive, can cause hepatitis and are not usually available.

5. *Angular cheilitis.*
This is diagnosed if there are inflamed cracks or splits in the corner of the mouth.

This occurs in candida infections which can be caused by HIV infection. It can, however, also occur if the teeth or dentures are worn down, the corners

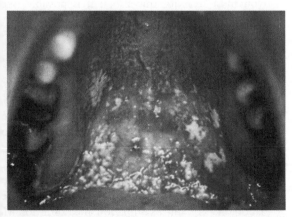

Figure 19.25 *This appearance of* Candida *in the mouth should make you think of HIV infection if other conditions do not exist.*

of the mouth are always wet and also if there is vitamin B deficiency and also iron deficiency (usually with anaemia).

6. *Acute severe ulceration of the gums or infection around teeth* ('acute necrotising ulcerative gingivitis/ periodontitis').
There is severe pain, ulcers of the gums around the teeth, infection around the teeth which become painful and loose, bad smell, etc. Treat with penicillin and metronidazole, mouth wash with salty water and methylrosanilinium (gentian violet) 0.5% aqueous solution, after each meal and at night.

7. *Difficulty or pain when swallowing.*
Candida (thrush) infection in the oesophagus is the usual cause (see page 226). Treat with nystatin or natamycin or amphotericin lozenges or drops or crushed up antifungal tablets or vaginal pessaries, three times a day after meals and at night. All of these must be dissolved as slowly as possible in the mouth. The patient should not eat or drink until 1 hour afterwards. If nothing else is available, methylrosanilinium (gentian violet) 0.5% aqueous (water, not tincture) could be tried. Oral fluconazole 100–200 mg or itraconazole 100–200 mg would be the best treatment but both are very expensive, may have side effects and interactions with other drugs (including some ART) and are not usually available.

8. *Chronic diarrhoea and/or progressive weight loss and/or 'slim disease'.*
Diarrhoea is often severe but can come and go. The bowel motions are often just watery without blood or mucus and the patient may have some colic around the umbilicus but it is usually mild and often absent. Weight loss keeps on occurring and is often severe, often more than 10 kg and up to 20% loss of the previous body weight (Figure 19.26).

The cause of this may be one of the usual infections but especially salmonella (see Chapter 23 pages 372–373). It could be due to a TB infection of the bowel wall. It could be due to special opportunistic infections which immunosuppressed patients are likely to get. Cancers including Kaposi's sarcoma and lymphoma also occur in the bowel and cause diarrhoea and weight loss. If none of these are present, it is probably due to the HIV infection itself damaging the bowel wall and stopping food being absorbed; or the drugs used in treating HIV doing a similar thing.

If possible, send stool tests for AFB as well as for ordinary infections and for cysts, parasites and amoeba.

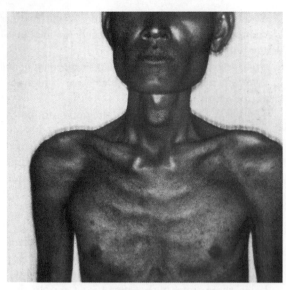

Figure 19.26 *In parts of Africa this is called 'Slim Disease'.*

Treat with oral rehydration fluids. If the diarrhoea is chronic despite rehydration and treatment of possible infections, give anti-diarrhoeal drugs (e.g. codeine phosphate 30 mg 4–6 hourly if needed).

For management of bowel infections see Chapter 23 page 388. Always try treatment with SMX 800 mg/TMP 160 mg twice daily for 10 days (for *Salmonella, Shigella* and *Isospora belli*); then chloramphenicol 500 mg 1 g four times a day (for resistant *Salmonella*, etc.); then metronidazole 400 mg three times daily for 10–14 days (for *Clostridium difficile* and *Microsporidia*) if not improving on the chloramphenicol for 5 days (but continue the chloramphenicol for 5 more days); then, if still not settled, possibly try erythromycin 500 mg qid for 10 days (for *Campylobacter*). However, do not continue giving any one of these drugs for more than 10 days for each. If not given before, always give at some stage albendazole 400 mg daily for 3 days (for intestinal worms and *Microsporidia*).

Special drugs such as ciprofloxacin and other quinolones or fourth generation cephalosporins for particular bacterial infections, or albendazole for parasitic infestations such as *Microsporidia* and strongyloides may be started in a hospital by the Medical Officer if blood and stool tests and cultures showed that they would be effective. However, they are very expensive; they do not always work; if they do work they often need to be continued as prophylactic treatment or the condition returns; and they are not usually available. Most patients know

the cause of the illness and that it will cause death soon and prefer to stay at home on treatment of symptoms only.

If chronic diarrhoea and weight loss, always try:

1. Rehydration fluids; and
2. Trimethoprim 160 mg and sulfamethoxazole 800 mg twice daily for 7–10 days; and if still present,
3. Chloramphenicol 500–1000 mg qid for 7–10 days (or other drug if you are told to use instead); and if not gone by 5 days, add also
4. Metronidazole 400 mg tid for 7–14 days; and at some time, also,
5. Albendazole 400 mg daily for 3 days.

But always send stool for tests including for AFB as a very common cause for weight loss is bowel TB.

See also chronic diarrhoea (Chapter 23 page 387).

Nervous system disease

1. *Acute meningitis* (see Chapter 25 page 409).
   Streptococcus pneumoniae (the pneumococcus), which has spread to the brain through the blood from the respiratory tract, is the most common cause in HIV infection. Other bacteria can also cause meningitis. Viruses such as herpes simplex and cytomegalovirus can cause encephalitis which may look like acute meningitis. Do a lumbar puncture with the precautions needed to avoid HIV infection. Give chloramphenicol 2 g by IVI or IMI immediately and then see Chapter 25 pages 411–412 about other meningitis treatment which is essential. Do not forget the possibility of cerebral malaria and you must treat for this also if it is possible (see Chapter 13 page 82).
2. *Subacute and chronic meningitis* (see Chapter 25 pages 414–415).
   Mycobacterium tuberculosis is the most likely cause. Fungus infections, most commonly *Cryptococcus*, are the next most likely cause. (Other infections, especially *Toxoplasma* and *Nocardia*, which are more likely to cause intracranial masses, and also syphilis, are possible causes.) Transfer such patients to the Medical Officer.

   If transfer is not possible, do a lumbar puncture and examine the CSF, and if possible send it to the laboratory for full examination including for *M. tuberculosis* and *Cryptococcus*. Treat the patient with anti-TB drugs, although pyrizinamide is essential and streptomycin may help (but not if pregnant), i.e. 2(HRZE)S/1(HRZE)/5(HR)E or 5(HR)3E3. The full course must be given once it is started. Treat the patient also with sulfadoxine 500 mg and pyrimethamine 25 mg, two tablets twice daily for 6 weeks (but not if in the first 14 weeks of pregnancy; and folinic acid should be added) (treatment for *Toxoplasma* but also *Nocardia*); or if not available or the patient is pregnant, treat with sulfamethoxazole and trimethoprim in the dose for *Nocardia* on page 224 (as this drug has an effect against *Toxoplasma* also). If the patient recovers, it is not certain whether it was the anti-TB or the anti-protozoal treatment which worked. Anti-TB treatment must be completed and SMX 800 mg/TMP 160 mg daily prophylactic treatment should be continued for life or until the CD4 count is above 200 if given ART.

Of course, if *Cryptococcus* is present, the patient will get worse and die unless given amphotericin B, etc. (see Chapter 25 page 414).

3. *Cerebral tumour or inflammatory intracranial mass* (see Chapter 25 page 421).

Cancers including lymphomas, Kaposi's sarcoma, secondary carcinoma, etc. are common – no curative treatment is possible and the patient will soon die.

Inflammatory intracranial masses due to pyogenic abscesses, *Toxoplasma* and *Nocardia* and occasionally due to TB, *Cryptococcus*, viruses, (and even schistosomiasis and cysticercosis, etc.) can occur and may be curable.

Transfer the patient to the Medical Officer for a brain scan and other tests to see if a trial of treatment is worthwhile.

If transfer not possible, do not do a lumbar puncture, but give chloramphenicol 1 g qid (± metronidazole) (for pyogenic abscess), sulfadoxine and pyrimethamine or SMX/TMP (as above) (for *Toxoplasma* and *Nocardia*), 2(HRZE)S/1(HRZE)/5(HR)E or 5(HR)3E3 (as above) (for TB); and see Chapter 25 pages 421–422 for other possible drugs.

If possible, give also dexamethasone 12 mg daily or prednisolone 50 mg daily; then slowly reduce the dose to zero over 1 month.

4. *Encephalitis* (see Chapter 25 page 415).

HIV and also herpes and CMV are well-known causes of encephalitis, especially late in the disease.

5. *Headache.*

Always think of the above four conditions and see Chapter 25 page 427.

Never forget:
- local causes – do examination for dental abscess, otitis media, sinusitis, etc.;
- infections, especially malaria, syphilis, trypanosomiasis – send blood for tests for these;
- meningitis, especially chronic meningitis – see above;
- encephalitis – see above;
- cerebral tumours or abscesses or inflammatory masses – see above;
- drugs which can cause headache.

Refer the patient to the Medical Officer. If this is not possible, consider treatment with chloramphenicol; sulfadoxine and pyrimethamine or SMX/TMP; TB drugs; dexamethasone, etc. (see left and Chapter 25); but this will not improve tumours (except for a short while), fungal infections, virus infections, etc.

6. *Confusion or delirium (acute organic psychosis)* (see Chapter 35 pages 568–569, 572).

Think especially of:
- malaria, pneumonia, meningitis, septicaemia;
- low oxygen from anaemia, heart failure, pneumonia, pneumothorax;
- dehydration;
- drug reaction;
- acute liver failure, especially from reaction to drugs;
- syphilis – send blood test and treat;
- meningitis, encephalitis, cerebral tumours and inflammatory intracranial masses, etc.;
- trypanosomias – do a blood test (but not a lumbar puncture if trypanosomiasis is possible).

7. *Dementia (chronic organic psychosis)* (see Chapter 35 pages 568–569, 573).

HIV itself can cause 'progressive multifocal encephalopathy' and other reasons for dementia. Always, however, think of all the conditions which can affect the brain, especially the first four conditions in this nervous system section; but also conditions affecting the blood going to the brain (see Chapter 35 page 568).

8. *Difficulty walking* (see Chapter 25 page 426).

This is usually due to something pressing on the spinal cord or disease of the spinal cord or peripheral nerves.

- Spinal TB or spinal bacterial abscess. Examine for signs of these (see Chapter 14 page 105) and refer urgently to the Medical Officer for X-ray if any suspicious signs. If transfer not possible, immediately give chloramphenicol for 2 weeks and TB drugs (see left).

- Syphilis – send blood for serological test for syphilis.
- Schistosomiasis – if in an area where schistosomiasis occurs, give praziquantel 30 mg/kg one dose and a further dose 6 hours later and refer to the Medical Officer.
- Vitamin B_{12} and folate deficiency – send blood for examination for macrocytosis.
- Side effects of isoniazid given without pyridoxine – give pyridoxine 50(–100) mg daily.
- Damage to the vertebrae or discs from injury.
- Tumour pressing on the cord.
- Peripheral neuritis (see below).
- HIV infection itself can cause damage to the cord (transverse myelitis) and peripheral neuritis.

Refer almost all of these patients to the Medical Officer for investigation.

9. *Sight getting worse.*
   - If on ethambutol, stop ethambutol (which can cause blindness) and replace with streptomycin.
   - CMV infection of retina of eye.
   - Toxoplasmosis of retina of eye.
   - All usual causes of loss of vision also (see Chapter 31 page 520).

   Transfer all cases to the Medical Officer urgently.

10. *Peripheral neuropathy or neuritis.*
    Pain or burning in the feet is the usual complaint. This is often due to the virus itself. However, all the causes and especially drug causes and including isoniazid if not given with pyridoxine and anti-HIV drugs (ART), must be thought of (see Chapter 25 page 420).
    - If on anti-TB treatment, give pyridoxine 100 mg daily and, if available, also vitamin B compound.

    In other cases give:
    - vitamin B compound if available,
    - amitriptyline 25 mg at night (to help symptoms) or *if this is ineffective,*
    - try an anti-convulsant such as phenytoin 100–300 mg at night or carbamazepine 100–200 mg twice daily.

    Treatment of CNS conditions by the Medical Officer may include dexamethasone or prednisolone at first in large doses if there is a chronic inflammatory condition or a mass affecting the CNS (and appropriate accompanying prophylactic treatment for TB, malaria, etc.).

Skin and mucous membrane disorders

Skin itching and rashes can be due to the HIV itself or to other infections. Also, many of the non-infective skin conditions such as seborrhoeic dermatitis or psoriasis are worse during HIV infections. Kaposi's sarcoma also occurs. Skin reactions due to drugs including those for HIV and opportunistic infections are common.

1. *A chronic itchy maculopapular rash which may later become nodular and darkly pigmented.*
   This is very common.
   It is usually worse on the back of the hands and arms and top of the feet. Scratch marks are seen as it is very itchy. This may be due to the HIV itself. It may be called 'papular folliculitis'. An antihistamine (e.g. promethazine 25 mg at night or chlorpheniramine 4 mg three or four times a day) and calamine lotion may help the itch of the HIV rash. Corticosteroid creams such as hydrocortisone 1% could be tried, but continue these only if they greatly help.

2. *Herpes simplex infection.*
   Herpes simplex viruses can cause small but painful vesicles which burst to form ulcers with a grey base surrounded by inflamed red mucosa or skin. Usually, HSV-1 occur on the lips or nose during fevers ('cold sores') and HSV-2 on the genitalia (herpes genitalis). In HIV infection they also appear in other places, spread further, last longer and come back more frequently.

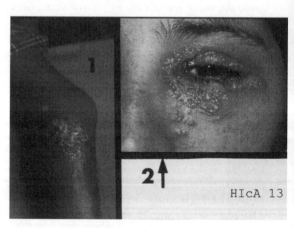

Figure 19.27 *Photograph 1 shows an inflamed ulcerated area with a discharge of pus and blood. Some areas have healed. This patient had a chronic bacterial skin infection which improved with treatment but then came back. This was because of decreased body defence due to HIV infection. The treatment is more antibiotic and more dressings until it is fully healed.*
Photograph 2 shows a patient with herpes simplex infection around the eye. Herpes in such an unusual place with so many vesicles should make you think of decreased immunity and HIV infection.

Keep the area clean and dry. Give pain relief if needed. Give antibiotics only if secondary bacterial infection. See page 226 for a skin paint to use. Aciclovir 200 mg each 4 hours 5 times a day would help, but not cure; and is expensive and not usually available.

See page 226.

3. *Herpes zoster* (see Chapter 16 page 153).
This is due to infection with the usual chickenpox virus.

This is normally a condition of older adults. It is uncommon in young people unless they have HIV infection. If herpes zoster occurs in patients under 50 years of age, or if more than one nerve is affected, or if repeated attacks occur, always think of HIV infection.

Keep area clean and dry. Treat any secondary bacterial infection with antibiotics. Give pain relief; powerful drugs may be needed. If eye affected, pad and transfer urgently to Medical Officer. Aciclovir, if available, would help – the dose is 800 mg 4 hourly, five times daily, for 1 week.

See Chapter 16 page 153.

4. *Molluscum congagiosum* (see Chapter 32 page 546).
Molluscum contagiosum is normally a condition affecting children. If an adult is affected, especially if severe or widespread, this is very suggestive of HIV infection.

5. *Candidiasis* (see pages 226–227).

6. *Tinea* (see Chapter 32 pages 527–531).
One special kind of fungus infection causes inflammation around the hairs.

7. *Impetigo/furuncles* (see Chapter 32 page 532).
Care with all of the many details of treatment for this condition is needed.

8. *Syphilis.*
A rash due to secondary syphilis must always be thought of (see pages 209–210).

9. *Minor skin injuries and infections may become quickly severe and at times cause septicaemia.*
These are usually due to infection with usual skin organisms such as staphylococci. Always think of HIV infection as well as diabetes mellitus in such patients. Give an anti-staphylococcal antibiotic and see Chapter 32 page 532 and Chapter 12 for management.

10. *Scabies* (see Chapter 32 pages 538–540).

11. *Seborrhoeic dermatitis* (see Chapter 32 page 548).

12. *Psoriasis* (see Chapter 32 page 549).

13. *Kaposi's sarcoma* (see page 232).

14. *Drug eruptions or skin reactions to drugs.*

In patients who have HIV and a skin rash, always think of the possibility that the rash is due to drugs.

Especially important are:
• anti-HIV drugs, especially nevirapine (NVP),
• anti-TB drugs,
• co-trimoxazole,
• but any drug the patient is taking.

High fever (PUO)

Fevers or night sweats are usually due to infection with the usual infectious organisms including *M. tuberculosis* and at times the unusual or 'opportunistic' organisms which can cause infections.

See Chapter 36 pages 585–587 for diagnosis and management.

Treatment will probably include antimalarials and antibiotics (including chloramphenicol) for septicaemia (often for organisms from the bowel such as salmonellae) and transfer for tests if the patient is not cured. If at any time the patient gets worse or there is no diagnosis after special tests at the hospital, anti-TB drugs (which must be continued until the full course is completed) may be necessary.

Leishmaniasis and other protozoal tropical diseases

These are due to infection with the usual organism.

Patients who were previously infected with leishmaniasis organisms but had immunity so good that no signs developed and patients who had leishmaniasis previously and were successfully treated, may develop clinical leishmaniasis after they become infected with HIV. Drug addicts who inject when they are in, or have been, in areas where visceral leishmaniasis occurs may be infected with leishmaniasis and/or HIV from infected blood in needles. Blood tests for leishmaniasis are much less often positive in patients with HIV even though they have leishmaniasis. In patients infected with HIV, visceral leishmaniasis may not respond as well as expected to treatment. The patient may develop more rashes and other side effects to treatment than expected.

See Chapter 18 pages 175–180.

Leishmaniasis, malaria, American trypanosomiasis (Chagas' disease) (but not African trypanosomiasis (sleeping sickness)), toxoplasmosis, the common bowel protozoa, *Giardia lamblia* and the unusual bowel protozoa *Cryptosporidium* and *Cyclospora* (although not *Entamoeba histolytica*) have been shown to become worse after HIV infection develops. It would be expected that this is true for other infections but has not yet been proven.

A

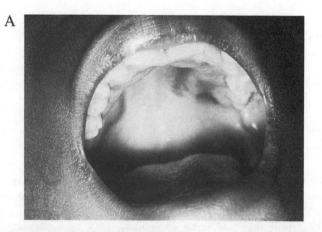

B

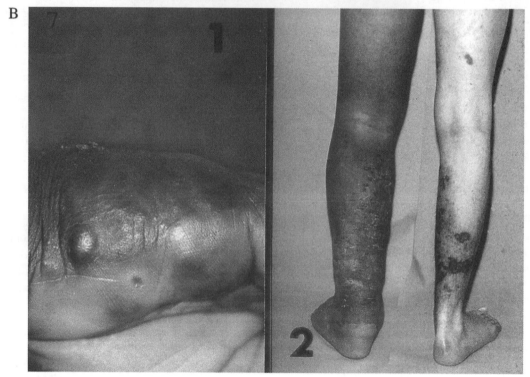

Figure 19.28 *Kaposi's sarcoma of (A) mouth, (B) hand and legs.*

Kaposi's sarcoma

Kaposi's sarcoma is a cancer or tumour which is due to overgrowth of the lining cells of a blood vessel. It is probably caused by a special herpes virus (KSAV or HHV8). Slow-growing Kaposi's tumours on the hands and feet in patients who are otherwise well have been present in Africa for years. However, in people who lose normal immunity, especially from HIV infection, the lesions of Kaposi's sarcoma grow more quickly and more and more keep coming. They especially affect the roof of the mouth, tip of the nose,

lower eyelid, penis and groin; but they can spread all over the body (Figure 19.28) and inside the body also. They can look like a plaque or nodule. They can be red but become black. They can ulcerate. There is surrounding oedema. Lymph nodes, lungs, bowel and other organs can also be involved.

Cancer chemotherapy drugs usually do help but are expensive and may not be available. Radiotherapy may help but is usually not available. Sometimes one of the newer non-steroidal anti-inflammatory drugs (e.g. ibuprofen) may help a little. No other specific treatment is possible. Kaposi's sarcoma, however, may greatly decrease if the patient is started on anti-retroviral treatment. Always give symptomatic treatment.

Lymphomas

See Chapter 22 page 339.

These are probably due to Epstein–Barr virus.

Anaemia

See Chapter 21 pages 314–319.

Think also of the possibility that the anaemia is due to side effects of any drugs being given.

Kidney disease

See Chapter 26.

Note that HIV itself can cause a type of glomerulo-nephritis and/or kidney failure (pages 446, 449).

Cardiovascular system problems

HIV infection itself can cause heart failure.

Treat heart failure. See Chapter 27 page 464.

Opportunistic infections may destroy adrenal glands causing shock and need hydrocortisone (Chapter 30 page 504) as well as shock treatment (Chapter 27 page 461).

Eye problems

See Chapter 31 pages 519–520.

Arthritis

See Chapter 29.

Bacterial arthritis is common. Treat in the usual way with aspiration and antibiotics.

Gout, if on any TB treatment with pyrazinamide, could be a side effect of pyrazinamide.

For all cases give acetylsalicylic acid, or, if ineffective, consider an NSAID, e.g. ibuprofen.

Table 19.4 Symptoms and signs which suggest HIV infection is possible.

Think of HIV infection if you note the following:	
Past history	• sexually transmitted infection (STI) • herpes zoster (shingles) which often leaves a scar • recent or recurrent pneumonia • severe other bacterial infections (sinusitis, meningitis, pyomyositis, septicaemia, etc.) • recently treated TB
Symptoms	• weight loss (> 10 kg or 10% of original weight) • diarrhoea (> 1 month) • mouth pain or ulcers • retrosternal pain on swallowing (oesophageal candidiasis) • burning sensation of feet (peripheral neuropathy) • chronic cough or any symptom suggesting TB • any STI • symmetrical generalised lymphadenopathy
Signs	• herpes zoster or scar of herpes zoster • any STI • symmetrical generalised lymphadenopathy • itchy papular skin rash • Kaposi's sarcoma of HIV type • chronic meningitis or unexplained neurological condition or organic psychosis • oral candidiasis • angular cheilitis • oral hairy leukoplakia • ulceration of gums • large ulcers inside mouth • persistent herpes simplex ulcers around mouth or genitalia • fever of unknown cause • sinusitis, pneumonia, meningitis, pyomyositis, gastroenteritis • wasting/weight loss

> Always look in the mouth of any patient. Many mouth lesions are highly suggestive of HIV infection, and others are almost diagnostic.

Tests

Tests to diagnose HIV infection

Tests on serum or plasma from blood are available to diagnose HIV before severe disease develops. Without a test there is no way to be absolutely certain in a health centre that a patient definitely has HIV infection until perhaps stage 4 HIV disease.

Blood tests can diagnose HIV infection by showing antibodies to HIV. These tests are of two main types. EIA (previously called ELISA) tests for HIV antibodies need a laboratory and trained laboratory staff and

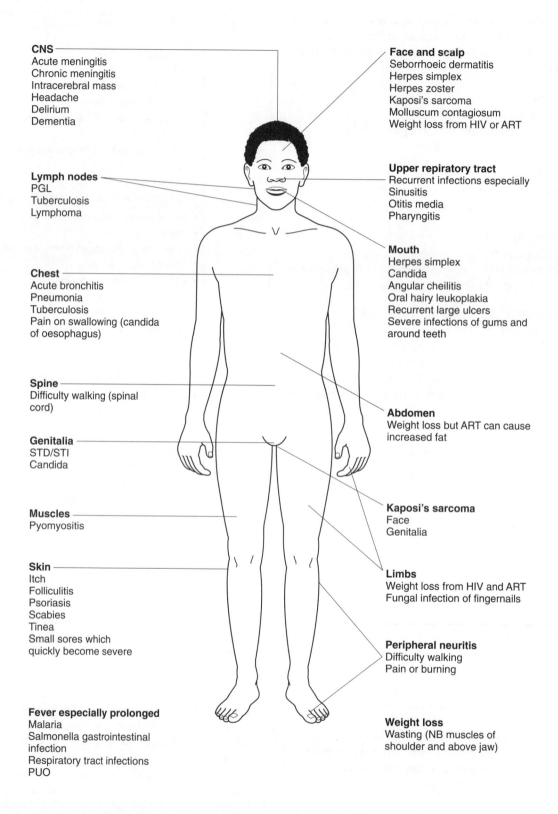

CNS
Acute meningitis
Chronic meningitis
Intracerebral mass
Headache
Delirium
Dementia

Lymph nodes
PGL
Tuberculosis
Lymphoma

Chest
Acute bronchitis
Pneumonia
Tuberculosis
Pain on swallowing (candida of oesophagus)

Spine
Difficulty walking (spinal cord)

Genitalia
STD/STI
Candida

Muscles
Pyomyositis

Skin
Itch
Folliculitis
Psoriasis
Scabies
Tinea
Small sores which quickly become severe

Fever especially prolonged
Malaria
Salmonella gastrointestinal infection
Respiratory tract infections
PUO

Face and scalp
Seborrhoeic dermatitis
Herpes simplex
Herpes zoster
Kaposi's sarcoma
Molluscum contagiosum
Weight loss from HIV or ART

Upper repiratory tract
Recurrent infections especially
Sinusitis
Otitis media
Pharyngitis

Mouth
Herpes simplex
Candida
Angular cheilitis
Oral hairy leukoplakia
Recurrent large ulcers
Severe infections of gums and around teeth

Abdomen
Weight loss but ART can cause increased fat

Kaposi's sarcoma
Face
Genitalia

Limbs
Weight loss from HIV and ART
Fungal infection of fingernails

Peripheral neuritis
Difficulty walking
Pain or burning

Weight loss
Wasting (NB muscles of shoulder and above jaw)

Figure 19.29 *Symptoms and signs which suggest that HIV infection is possible.*

are used for testing 90–100 or more blood samples at one time, when they are fairly cheap to use. Simple or rapid tests for HIV antibodies are used to test just one patient at a time and do not need a laboratory or trained staff. They are more expensive, but more suitable to use in a health centre.

Blood tests exist which can show the HIV itself, e.g. HIV RNA, HIV DNA and HIV p24 antigen. These tests are expensive and not usually available in a health centre. They may be used for (1) diagnosis (but usually only in infants who may not have HIV infection but who have HIV antibodies from their mother), or (2) determining the severity of the HIV infection ('viral load'), or (3) determining the response to HIV drug treatment (if successful, the viral load falls a lot in the first 4–6 weeks and may seem to be zero by 4–6 months), or (4) to find out if drug resistant HIV is present.

Tests not using blood (e.g. urine or saliva), although available and used in some epidemiological studies, are not reliable or accurate enough for diagnosing HIV in any one particular patient.

A blood test for HIV is needed only if it will change the management of the patient. In some places, if not enough medical staff or drugs are available to give proper treatment, diagnosing HIV disease earlier by the blood test will not change much that can be done for the patient.

The blood test for HIV can, however, greatly help the patient and the health worker caring for the patient (see below).

The blood test for HIV is also essential in any hospital or health centre which gives blood transfusions; and the HIV serology test must be done and be negative on any blood before it is transfused.

It may take 3 and occasionally up to 6 (or more) months after infection before the antibody test becomes positive. A negative blood test does not make it certain that the patient does not have HIV infection.

Pre-test counselling is needed before an HIV blood test is taken, to help the patient decide to have the test or not and to be prepared for the result.

The advantages of having the test include (if positive):
- no continuing worry about having or not having HIV infection,
- able to make better decisions for the future, e.g. getting pregnant,
- what to do to prevent infection, especially TB (including drug prophylaxis),
- knowing to get early treatment of any infection,
- being considered for anti-retroviral therapy,

- avoidance of drugs with a high risk of side effects to HIV patients,
- knowing what to do to stop HIV being passed on to others, including use of condoms and never donating blood,
- having any HIV services available offered to the patient.

The disadvantages of getting the test include (if positive):
- unable to get life insurance,
- unable sometimes to get visas to travel overseas,
- risk of loss of job,
- risk of loss of family support,
- risk of discrimination from the community.

Counselling should prepare patients for a positive result as, when told a positive result, patients do not often recall what is then said to them. Counselling should also prepare them for a negative result so that they can use the relief that comes from this to reinforce preventive measures against possible future exposure to AIDS infection.

If a patient may have HIV infection:

1. Give information and counselling about a test for HIV.
2. Strongly recommend the patient has the test.
3. Do the test unless the patient does not agree to it.

Laboratory tests which you need to be able to get done if you have been trained how to give anti-retroviral drugs (ART) and are going to give these in your health centre

1. HIV diagnostic testing.
2. CD4 count:
    - on diagnosis to tell if patient needs ART (< 350),
    - each 6 months if patient did not need treatment, to tell when does need ART (< 350),
    - if patient does need ART, to judge effectiveness of ART or if need to switch ART because of HIV resistance to first line drugs or need to stop ART because of HIV resistance to second line drugs,
    - any other time needed.
3. Sputum for AFB if possibility of TB needing treatment (preferably before ART).
4. Blood tests for malaria.
5. Pregnancy testing in women before start EFV.
6. Hb before and then 4, 8 and 12 weeks after starting AZT.

7. ALT (or AST) and possibly other tests of liver function before and then 2, 4, 8 and 12 weeks after starting NVP in women with CD4 counts between 200 and 350; or other people with hepatitis or liver problems.
8. Urea and creatinine and electrolytes (kidney function tests) before and each 6 months if started on TDF.

These tests are not all available at a health centre.

You should, however, be able to send blood, sputum or other specimens to the laboratory for these tests if you are giving ART. If you are not able to get the results of blood tests, see if you can send the patient for care to someone who can do and get the results of these tests. See box on page 241.

Differential diagnosis

The two conditions most likely to be confused with HIV infection are TB without HIV infection (see Chapter 14 pages 101–126) and depression (see Chapter 35 pages 575–577). Of course, it is possible for patients with HIV infection to develop both of these conditions.

HIV infection can be diagnosed with certainty only by a positive blood test in a patient who may have HIV infection, especially if there are consistent symptoms or signs.

HIV, later in its course, is probable if there are conditions present which occur in stage 3 or stage 4 of the disease.

Suspect HIV infection in a patient who has an infection which:

1. does not respond as usual to treatment, or
2. comes back unexpectedly after treatment appeared to cure it,
3. is an unusual infection,
4. is in a person who is from one of the risk groups for HIV infection, i.e.
   • sex worker,
   • patient with an STD,
   • someone who has had many sexual partners or whose present sexual partner has had many sexual partners,
   • someone who has spent a long time away from his family and community (e.g. immigrant worker or truck driver or sailor),
   • male homosexual,
   • drug addict.
5. has another of the other common HIV conditions, especially continuing weight loss or diarrhoea.

Definition of AIDS

Acquired Immunodeficiency Syndrome, i.e. AIDS, has in the past been used to describe different conditions by different people. WHO recommends that the term AIDS be used:

1. for epidemiological surveillance (see Chapter 5),
2. for any clinical stage 3 or 4 HIV disease,
3. where CD4 testing is available when CD4 count is less than 350/mm³ in any stage of the disease.

Management

There is, at the time of writing, no cure for HIV infection.

A great deal of help, however, can be given to people with HIV infection, including the following:

1. Give correct information and suitable things to read:
   • Counselling (see below);
   • Choosing and preparing a personal treatment supporter for the patient.
2. Prophylactic drug therapy to prevent some of the most likely infections to occur. Give, at present, co-trimoxazole to almost all patients. See also page 258 about isoniazid and other drugs.
3. Treatment to cure or control infections and other conditions which have occurred because of loss of normal immunity (see pages 223–233).
4. Start on or refer suitable patients for treatment with drugs to decrease the number of HIV in the body to allow immunity to (at least partly) come back, i.e. anti-retroviral therapy (ART) (see pages 240–242).
5. In all cases, treat the symptoms caused by conditions due to the loss of immunity and those caused by the HIV itself.
6. Follow up the patients and carry out the administrative procedures needed to ensure good patient management and best possible disease control.
7. Use each patient with HIV infection as an opportunity to give health education about how HIV infection can be avoided or prevented.

1. Counselling and choosing a personal treatment supporter

Giving correct information and suitable things to read

WHO has prepared a 'Patient Self-Management Booklet', a 'Caregiver Booklet', a 'Patient Education Flipchart' and other aids to help the health worker in giving correct information and literature. Your own Health Department will probably have supplied you with such things which are most suitable for people in your area. Use these aids for health education and give literature to the patient and care givers. Every patient will have different needs for information and you must use your skill in deciding what information and literature is needed at each consultation.

Counselling is the most important part of managing HIV infection. Counselling is not for the health worker to tell people what they should do (especially as this may make them decide to just continue to do exactly what they are already doing). Counselling is to make it clear to people all the different options (or things they can do) in this situation, and to help them to make their own decision to choose the best of these options.

Listen to what the patient says after encouraging them to talk about themselves, their circumstances, their problems and their feelings. Show them that you understand them and feel the same feelings that they feel. Give correct information about all the important things above, to help them make correct decisions. Help them to actually come to a decision, and if possible, a good one. Try to not let them just stay as they are without a plan. Support them, and try to give them confidence in what they decide to do, and help them to do it.

Counselling needs privacy so that people can say and act how they really think and feel. Counselling needs to be done by people who are accepted and trusted by the patient and have the knowledge and the time to do the counselling properly. It is likely that it is best for a special couple of health workers, or if these are not available, religious or community or other leaders to be found, who can be given the knowledge and have the time to spend doing this counselling, as it cannot all be done by the officer in charge of the health centre.

Counselling will occur at many different times.

Preventive counselling

This is done every time the subjects of sexual relations, drug addiction, etc. come up. Give advice as to how to prevent the transfer of HIV infection.

Pre-test counselling

Do this before the HIV test (see page 235).

Post-test counselling if the HIV test is positive

This takes time and privacy. Tell the patient only when both of these are available. See Figure 19.30.

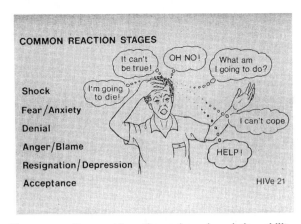

COMMON REACTION STAGES

Shock
Fear/Anxiety
Denial
Anger/Blame
Resignation/Depression
Acceptance

It can't be true! OH NO! What am I going to do?
I'm going to die!
I can't cope
HELP!

HIVe 21

Figure 19.30 *You must have time, privacy, knowledge, ability to help and you must show the patient you understand and care if you are going to properly counsel a patient who has a positive HIV test.*

Some patients cry. They need to be allowed to do so. Some patients are so shocked that they understand nothing of what is said to them. They need to be made to talk and engage in conversation. Some patients become angry. It is important that the health worker also does not become angry. Some patients become agitated. It is important that the health worker should stay calm.

Supply information on HIV infection according to what the patient can understand. Give appropriate literature for them to take home and read.

Ask what the particular worries are going to be straight away and help them try to deal with these first. Discuss how the patient will tell his partner.

Discuss which family members will help and how to get their help. Discuss what support groups are available and how to get their help.

Discuss 'safe sex' and the precautions that should be taken and supply condoms (see Appendix 1 pages 259–261). *Discuss avoidance of pregnancy* and supply contraceptives.

Discuss the place of drug therapy (see page 240).

Help the patient decide to follow a healthy lifestyle. The following are important:
- good nutrition with calories, protein and vitamins, i.e. cereals, vegetables, fruit and if possible meat or chicken or fish or eggs to improve his resistance,
- physical exercise,
- good relationships with family, friends, etc.,
- keeping productive in the family and community and if possible still at work.

Tell the patient how to try to avoid the organisms which cause opportunistic infections in HIV infected patients.

- Drink only safe water, preferably boiled or filtered and treated with chlorine.
- Eat meat only if it is well cooked.
- Use safe water to wash fruit and vegetables if eaten raw, before eating.
- Protect food from insects and animals.
- Wash hands well after contact with cats, dogs and other animals, raw meat, soil, faeces (including babies).
- If working in a health centre or hospital, wear gloves.
- Avoid contact with human and animal faeces.
- Do not swim in water contaminated by human or animal faeces.
- Avoid injury, scratches or bites from animals.
- Avoid dust when gardening, but especially from bird faeces.
- Avoid people who have (untreated) TB, but also herpes zoster with sores or crusts (but not if just scars or pain after an attack) or any other infectious disease.
- Avoid unprotected sex.
- Avoid injecting drugs for 'recreation'.
- Avoid needle stick and other injuries.
- Avoid cats (which carry toxoplasmosis) and young dogs.

Tell the patient about prophylactic treatment. This will almost always be co-trimoxazole and, in some if indicated, isoniazid and other drugs (see page 258).

Make sure the patient knows what symptoms mean he should come quickly for early diagnosis and treatment of any infection which could occur (especially TB).

Tell the patient that treatment for symptoms caused by infections or the HIV infection itself is available and will be given to him by you.

Tell the patient you can give to him or refer him at the proper time for anti-retroviral treatment (ART); then help the patient take ART regularly and correctly; and know what problems mean he should be sent for specialist advice (see pages 240–242).

Tell the patient he can live normally and yet not infect others if he follows the rules.

- Safe sex only; especially important is the use of condoms if any sex.
- Avoid getting blood or body secretions on others.
- Do not donate blood for transfusion.

Discuss how care can be carried out at home (see page 258).

Crisis counselling

This is given when a problem gets too much for the patient to cope with and they become distressed or agitated. This counselling is to help them get back in control of the situation again.

Counselling about anti-HIV drugs (ART) if the patient may be helped by them (see page 240)

Only some patients may be helped by these drugs. Even if the patient is one who could be helped, counselling is needed to:

1. Inform him of the many problems with ART. The patient must understand these and decide he will really continue on ART when problems do occur, i.e. he must convince the counsellor he is motivated to get ART.
2. Inform him that all doses of all of the drugs once or twice each day have to be taken (as if less than 95% are taken, the treatment is not effective). The patient must understand this and convince the counsellor that he will take all these drugs every day, i.e. he has potential for adherence.

Only when the patient wants to and will take the treatment should the treatment be started.

Counselling about adherence to ART
(see above and page 247)

At times, even after the patient has improved on ART, the symptoms and signs may come back again. There are other causes; but the most common cause is that the patient is not taking all of the doses of the drugs every day. Counselling is then needed to find out why this has happened and help the patient overcome these problems so that from then on he will adhere to treatment (as otherwise there is no point in trying to continue).

Choosing and preparing a personal treatment supporter

This person needs to be someone who can learn all the patient needs to know about HIV infection and its care and prevention of spread and help the patient carry out all these difficult things.

This person, e.g. partner, parent, child, sibling, friend, HIV support group member, religious leader, etc. needs to be trusted by, and chosen by, the patient; accept the patient's condition and keep it confidential; learn about HIV and its management; and be with the patient twice each day at the time of drug therapy to make sure the drugs are taken, etc.

This supporter will need education and support himself from the health worker and should be present

t any consultations before, as well as after, treatment
s begun.

Post-test counselling if the HIV test is negative

Explain that the HIV test takes 3 months (but occasionally longer, rarely up to 3 years) to become positive after infection and this must be taken into account. Use the patient's happiness at the test's results to try to make sure that in future he lives and behaves in such a way that there will never be further worries about another HIV infection in that patient.

2. Give what prophylactic drugs are available to try to stop infections occurring because of loss of immunity

At present, most patients should be started on co-trimoxazole

Co-trimoxazole (see Chapter 11 page 56) is a combination of sulfamethoxazole (SMX) and trimethoprim (TMP) which may be able to stop the growth of, or kill, the organisms that cause some cases of:

Pneumonia   *Pneumococcus* (bacterium)
             Pneumocystis jiroveci (fungus/protozoa)
Diarrhoea   Non-typhoid *Salmonella*
                (NTS) (bacterium)
             Isospora (protozoa)
             Cyclospora (protozoa)
Meningitis ⎫ *Toxoplasma* (protozoa)
Encephalitis⎭ *Nocardia* (bacterium)
Malaria   *Plasmodium falciparum* (protozoa)

Patients with decreased immunity from HIV infection do get more of the above infections and often die from them. If they are given co-trimoxazole, many trials have shown that they have fewer of these infections and a greatly decreased (up to 50%) death rate. (This is not fully understood as some of the above organisms have developed resistance to co-trimoxazole; but co-trimoxazole as yet does work.)

All HIV infected patients with significantly decreased immunity should therefore routinely be given co-trimoxazole. These would include the following:

	If no CD4 testing possible	If CD4 testing possible
WHO clinical stage		1 if CD4 < 350
	2	2 if CD4 < 350
	3	3 regardless of CD4 count
	4	4 regardless of CD4 count

The dose is 160 mg trimethoprim + 800 mg sulfamethoxazole (one double strength or 2 single strength tablets) every day.

All HIV infected pregnant women at any stage of pregnancy should be treated from the time of diagnosis (but would then not need sulfadoxine/pyrimethamine intermittent treatment for malaria).

All children who themselves have HIV, and all children who had a mother with HIV, should be treated from the age of 4–6 weeks until it is shown the child has no HIV infection and is not at risk of getting it (i.e. has stopped breastfeeding, preferably by 6 months and at the latest by the age of 1).

If the patient is allergic to co-trimoxazole but does not have a severe allergy with, e.g. Stevens–Johnson syndrome (see Chapter 14 page 117), the patient may be able to continue the co-trimoxazole with the help of an antihistamine; but if the condition gets worse, the patient may be able to be desensitised by stopping the drug until the rash is gone and then giving one sixth of the usual dose of the drug on Day 1, and then adding another one sixth of a dose daily until the usual dose is reached. If this does not work, dapsone 100 mg daily could be used instead (but is not as efficient).

Stop the co-trimoxazole if:

1. Child who has had exposure but has not been infected with HIV after the risk of infection less, i.e. after has finished breastfeeding.
2. Adult on ART.
   If CD4 count available:
       after count > 200; probably best > 350 if in an area where malaria; *and*
       at least 6 months treatment completed.
   If CD4 count not available:
       after WHO stage improves and is better than 2 *and*
       after at least 1 year of treatment.

Other prophylactic drugs (isoniazid and others)
See pages 258–259.

3. Treatment to cure or control infections and other conditions occurring because of loss of immunity
See pages 223–233.

The methods, including drugs needed for treatment of most of the chest, bowel and other problems caused by the loss of immunity or the HIV itself, are available in health centres. Other drugs which may be tried and which you may read about in other books, are very expensive and often have severe side effects and need to be given in hospitals. However, many are not available even in many hospitals. As well as this, the condition often returns soon after the drugs stop. In most health centres, the most important treatment as outlined in the sections of this book, is all the treatment that is possible. As well as this, many patients may prefer to stay at home for their treatment and collect drugs for symptoms as needed, attending the health centre only for treatment of any severe infections, etc. that occur.

Patients are usually treated in a normal health centre ward. However, all the precautions to prevent spread of HIV as outlined on page 257 and as for hepatitis B (see Chapter 24 page 394) and universal precautions (see Chapter 11 pages 61–63) are carried out. Also, do not put patients who have HIV infection together with patients who have or may have TB and have not been on proper anti-TB treatment for at least 2 weeks, as the HIV patients can easily be infected by TB organisms.

There are patients you need to refer to the Medical Officer if they could be helped by anti-HIV drugs (see below).

4. Give anti-retroviral drugs (ARD) anti-retroviral therapy (ART) if needed and if available

Anti-retroviral therapy (ART) is the giving of anti–retroviral drugs (ARD) to a patient infected with HIV to try to stop the HIV (a retrovirus) from continuing to replicate (i.e. multiply or increase in numbers). Then, as older viruses die, the total number of viruses will fall. Then the CD4 T lymphocyte cells will recover and increase in number. Opportunistic and other infections will then become fewer and damage done by the HIV virus will decrease. The patient will feel and look much better.

In all populations of HIV, however, some viruses are a little different to most of the other viruses. Some will naturally not be stopped from multiplying by (i.e. will not be sensitive to) any one particular anti-HIV drug given; even if most of the other viruses are sensitive to this drug. These few resistant viruses, however, may well be sensitive to other anti-HIV drugs. If only one anti-HIV drug is given, most of the viruses will be stopped from multiplying and the patient will improve. The few resistant viruses, however, will continue to multiply and later on become very many and the patient will then again become worse. As well as this, the viruses in the patient will be resistant to that

drug already given, although most but not all of the viruses are probably sensitive to another anti-HIV drug. If only one new anti-HIV drug is then given, the patient will again improve but later get worse again and the virus will be resistant to the second drug as well. **Therefore, one anti-HIV drug alone should never be given.** The only exception to this is the very short course of treatment given at birth to try to stop the newborn baby of an HIV positive mother becoming infected. If, however, at least three anti-HIV drugs, which act in different ways, are given from the start of treatment, the multiplication of the virus is greatly reduced and it takes much longer for resistant viruses to develop and the patient stays well much longer. The use of at least three anti-HIV drugs (i.e. anti-retroviral therapy or ART) together, is called Highly Active Anti-Retroviral Therapy or HAART.

HAART usually starts to improve the patient within a couple of weeks.

Problems with anti-HIV treatment include:

1. ART and even HAART is NOT a CURE for HIV infection.

   The patient will look better, feel better, have fewer infections, and live longer. Opportunistic infections which have already occurred may go away and not return. The infections expected for that stage of the disease may not occur. Eventually, however, resistant viruses will appear and the disease returns. In the meantime, the PATIENT IS STILL INFECTIOUS to others and must still use a condom if he or she has sex, not allow their blood or body secretions to get into other people, not donate blood for transfusion, etc.

2. The treatment is for all of the patient's life. If ART is stopped, the virus will soon grow again and the patient will become ill.

3. All of the prescribed drugs in the correct dose at the correct times of the day must be taken every day. No doses of the drugs should be missed, even when more than one dose daily is needed. Unless 95% or more of all prescribed doses are taken, the virus will soon grow in the patient and be resistant to the drugs.

4. Anti-retroviral treatment is not the most important part of treatment of the HIV infected patient. Do not forget the essential things discussed under the other headings.

5. Side effects of the drugs can occur. If these do happen, the patient must not just stop the drugs. The patient should immediately see the health worker to have the drug causing the problem

changed or switched to another (or if not able to do so immediately, refer or transfer the patient to another health worker or the hospital where this can be done).

Most side effects occur in the first few weeks of treatment. However, the patient needs regular monitoring or checking, e.g. each month, about side effects of drugs, as well as for infections, weight, etc.

6. The drugs are expensive.
7. You may not have been trained how to use these drugs and follow up and monitor people on these drugs. You must be able to do or get the results of the pathology tests needed to give these drugs safely. Not all health workers can be trained in this. If you have not been trained and/or cannot get the pathology test results, if there is any problem with the patients not taking all doses regularly or drug side effects or clinical problems with the patient, immediately arrange for a health worker trained in these things to see the patient, or immediately refer or transfer the patient to the Medical Officer or hospital.
8. Do not start ART immediately. Counselling is needed. The patient must have enough damage done to his immune system or to his body by the HIV infection itself, that infections or other problems are starting to occur or will soon occur. These mean that the patient will spend a lot of time sick and may die. The problems caused by the HIV infection must be far more than the side effects caused by the anti–HIV treatment. Also, only when the patient wants (is motivated) to take the drugs and is certain he will take all doses (has the potential for adherence) should the ART be started.

Anti-retroviral drugs used for anti-retroviral therapy (ART)

If anti-retroviral drugs are not being used in your area, it is not important for you to know about them.

If ARDs are being used, you may not need to know all about them. You do, however, need to know at least:

1. When to send patients to *start ART* (see pages 241–242).
2. What drugs are being used in your area.
3. What side effects these drugs can cause.
4. Where to immediately send patients if side effects occur to *substitute* a new drug for the toxic drug (as you must not just stop the drugs and do nothing else).
5. What drugs to immediately (within hours) give to a person who has possibly just been infected with HIV, especially:

- health worker with needle stick or other injury or otherwise contaminated with infectious body fluids,
- person who has been raped,
- baby being born to an HIV infected woman.

6. What suggests the ART is no longer effective and the patient needs to be sent to *switch* to different ART.
7. What suggests that the second line ART is no longer effective and the patient needs to be sent to find out if the ART should be *stopped*.

Anti-retroviral drugs belong to two main classes:

1. reverse transcriptase inhibitors (RTIs)
2. protease inhibitors (PIs).

Reverse transcriptase inhibitors (RTIs) are further divided into two groups:

1. nucleoside and nucleotide reverse transcriptase inhibitors (NRTIs)
2. non–nucleoside reverse transcriptase inhibitors (NNRTIs).

At present, the anti-retroviral drugs (abbreviations in brackets) approved for inclusion in WHO's 'Model List of Essential Drugs (EDL)' are as follows:

NRTIs	NNRTIs	PIs
Zidovudine (AZT, ZDV)	Nevirapine (NVP)	Ritonavir (RTV) as 'pharmaco-enhancer'
Didanosine (ddl)	Efavirenz (EFV/EFZ)	Saquinavir (SQV)
Stavudine (d4T)		Indinavir (IDV)
Lamivudine (3TC)		Nelfinavir (NFV)
Abacavir (ABC)		Lopinavir/ ritonavir (LPV/r)
Tenofovir diso-proxil fumerate (TDF)		
Emtricitabine (FTC)		

Indications for use of ART

At present, most countries start a patient on ART if the patient is in one of the following groups.

1. HIV infected patient IF:
   - stage 4,
   - stage 3,
   - stage 2 if no CD4 count available but total lymphocyte cell count less than 1200/mm³,
   - stage 1 and 2 (as well as 3 and 4) if CD4 lymphocyte count available and near 200/mm³ (or less), although less than 350 if severe infection or TB or pregnant.

However, the above may change and you must follow the guidelines for your country.

ART is *not* normally given if the patient has:
- severe kidney disease (renal failure),
- severe liver disease (hepatic failure),
- another incurable disease likely to lead to death soon.

2. A person who has possibly been infected by an HIV infected person (to try to stop the infection developing).
3. A woman who is or may have HIV infection and who is pregnant or delivering a baby (to try to stop the baby being infected).
4. A baby before, during and after birth if the mother is HIV positive.

WHO clinical staging	CD4 testing not available	CD4 testing available
1	Do not give ART	Start ART if CD4 count is below 200 cells/mm³
2	Do not give ART	Start ART if CD4 count is below 200 cells/mm³
3	Start ART	Consider ART if CD4 count is below 350 cells/mm³
		Start ART if pregnant or severe infection or TB
		Start ART in others before CD4 count drops below 200 cells/mm³
4	Start ART	Start ART no matter what CD4 cell count

Do not give ART if:

1. The diagnosis of HIV is not confirmed.
2. The patient does not meet (the above) criteria for ART.
3. The patient has certain other conditions (see below).

Do not give ART in the health centre without Medical Officer help (refer the patient to the Medical Officer in hospital) if:

1. The patient has a clinical stage 4 condition (other than thrush or herpes simplex) or severe illness or prolonged fever not helped by proper treatment (see Chapter 36 pages 585–587) which needs special treatment in a hospital.
2. The patient is already on anti-TB drugs, as ART may cause a drug reaction (see page 244) or immune reconstitution inflammatory syndrome (IRIS) (see page 248) needing hospital treatment.
3. There is already severe anaemia (Hb < 8g%) or peripheral neuritis, as ART may make these worse.

4. The patient has known significant liver disease or jaundice, as ART often affects the liver.
5. Some chronic illnesses such as heart disease, kidney disease or diabetes mellitus, as ART may cause problems and not help a lot.
6. The patient has had previous ART, as HIV drug resistance may be a problem.
7. The patient is a drug addict, especially one who uses IVI drugs, as liver and other disease may also be present and patient may not take ART reliably.

Choice of ART regimen

Follow the guidelines of your Health Department, if different from the following.

If the patient is female, do not give certain drugs if pregnant and advise her that oral contraceptives may not work (use condoms or other means for contraception).

Always use the drugs in co-formulations or blister packs if these are available.

IF a patient needs ART,
START treatment, usually with AZT + 3CT + NVP; but

IF a patient needs ART but also:
- HIV-2 infection or
- problem with NVP or EFV (i.e NNRTIs) (possibly), or
- hepatitis infection with also liver function abnormality (possibly), or
- rifampicin treatment for TB (possibly), or
- pregnant woman with CD count well above 200 cells/mm³ (possibly),

START instead AZT + 3TC + ABC,
i.e. leave out the NNRTI and add another NRTI.

IF toxicity from one of the drugs,
SUBSTITUTE a different drug in the same group (or if NNRTI, change it to an NRTI).

IF failure of above ART (i.e. if HIV becomes resistant),
SWITCH to second line therapy with:
    ritonavir boosted PI and
    two NRTIs not used before,
    usually LPV/r + ddl + ABC.

IF failure of second line therapy,
STOP ART if dying and treatment of cause not possible; but OTHERWISE CONTINUE.

Follow the guidelines in your country.
At the time of writing, the WHO guidelines

...re that the best first line or standard treatment is with two NRTI drugs and one NNRTI drug, i.e.:

One of the following two NRTIs – lamivudine (3TC)[1] or emtricitabine (FTC)[2], AND

One of the two NNRTIs – nevirapine (NVP)[3] or efavirenz (EFV)[4], AND

One of the other NRTIs – zidovudine (AZT)[5] or tenofovir (TDF)[6] or abacavir (ABC)[7] or stavudine (d4T)[8].

$$\left.\begin{array}{c} \text{AZT (or d4T)} \\ \text{or} \\ \text{TDF (or ABC)} \end{array}\right\} \text{AND 3TC or FTC AND} \left\{\begin{array}{c} \text{NVP} \\ \text{or} \\ \text{EFV} \end{array}\right.$$

The usual regime is AZT + 3TC + NVP.

Notes about ARD which may alter the choice of these drugs

Because of the following notes about the above drugs (1–8) and other problems with ART drugs, if the patient is:

• TB infected (page 244),
• a woman in childbearing years (page 245),
• a child being born to an infected HIV mother (page 246),
• exposed to HIV and needs prophylaxis (page 246),
• a hepatitis sufferer (page 247).

1. Lamivudine (3TC)
   • An effective safe cheap drug almost always used.
2. Emtricitabine (FTC)
   • Similar action to 3TC but more expensive (do not use as well as 3TC).
3. Nevirapine (NVP)
   • Not if HIV-2 infection as HIV-2 is resistant (use 3 NRTI drugs).
   • Rashes including Stevens–Johnson syndrome can occur. Start low dose and if rash, do not increase until rash goes. Do not start at same time as cotrimoxazole (which also can cause these rashes).
   • Hepatitis occasionally. Do not start at same time as other liver damaging drug; or if already hepatitis with ALT raised × 5; or if CD4 count well above 200 unless do ALT tests for hepatitis after start,
   • EFV better than NVP if rifampicin also given.
   • Can be used if is, or may get, pregnant (EFV best not in early pregnancy).
4. Efavirenz (EFV)
   • Not if HIV-2 infection as HIV-2 is resistant (use 3 NRTI drugs).
   • Rashes and hepatitis less than for NVP.
   • CNS problems can occur; use carefully if psychiatric or neurological problems.

• Possible fetal abnormalities if used in first 3-4 months of pregnancy.
• Better than NVP if used together with rifampicin.
• If pregnant woman with CD4 count well above 200, may cause hepatitis and may have to use three NRTI drugs.

5. Zidovudine (AZT) or (ZDV)
   • Can cause headache or nausea.
   • Can cause anaemia, especially in area where malaria, and low white cell count. Needs regular Hb checks.
   • Can cause lipodystrophy or lactic acidosis.
   • Do not use with d4T.
6. Tenofovir (TDF)
   • Effective safe drug.
   • Reduce dose if kidney not working well.
   • May cause fetal bone damage; best not to give if pregnant.
   • Can cause gastrointestinal symptoms.
7. Abacavir (ABC)
   • Has less lipodystrophy, lactic acidosis, peripheral neuritis, etc.
   • But 5% of patients get severe allergic type reaction.
8. Stavudine (d4T)
   • Effective, cheap and no tests needed.
   • But significant lipodystrophy, lactic acidosis, peripheral neuritis, etc.
   • Now not used much.
   • Do not use if isoniazid given for TB.

A less effective but satisfactory alternative first line regime would be three NRTI drugs, e.g.:

Lamivudine (3TC) + zidovudine (AZT) + abacavir (ABC) OR tenofovir (TDF)
This could be considered IF:

1. HIV resistant to NNRTI:
   • HIV-2 is always resistant
   • infection from known HIV-1 resistant patient.
2. Known or likely toxicity for NNRTI, e.g.:
   • Rash, e.g. starting also SMX/TMP,
   • Hepatitis already with some signs of liver failure, e.g. ALT × 5 or more normal,
   • Pregnant woman with CD4 count well above 200 cells/mm³,
   • Rifampicin needed for TB.

The second line or reserve treatment with a P1 and two NRTIs would only rarely be given first, e.g. if the above problems but the three NRTIs not possible.

DO NOT GIVE for first line treatment of HIV infection:

1. Only one or even only two ART drugs, as HIV resistance will soon develop.
2. Protease inhibitor (PI), as this is kept for people with HIV resistant to first line drugs.
3. Didanosine (ddI), as this should be kept for use with PIs for people with resistant HIV.

DO NOT GIVE the following combinations of ART:

1. Zidovudine (AZT) and stavudine (d4T), as the effect of one stops the effect of the other.
2. Stavudine (d4T) and didanosine (ddI), as both have similar side effects.
3. Lamivudine (3TC) and emtricitabine (FTC), as both have similar effects and two are not better than one.
4. Tenofovir (TDF) and didanosine (ddI) and any NNRTI, as HIV resistance soon occurs.
5. Tenofovir (TDF) and lamivudine (3TC) and abacavir (ABC), as HIV resistance soon occurs.
6. Tenofovir (TDF) and lamivudine (3TC) and didanosine (ddI), as HIV resistance soon occurs.

Interactions between ARD and drugs used to prevent or treat opportunistic infections

There are many such interactions or bad effects from using drugs together. These include:

- co-trimoxazole when given with zidovudine (AZT) can cause damage to the bone marrow and blood, especially anaemia and low white cell count;
- antifungal drugs such as ketoconazole and fluconazole may stop the body getting rid of PIs and NVP, and vice versa; this may result in increased serum levels of PI and increased toxicity;
- rifampicin reduces the blood levels of many ARTs; and can cause hepatitis with protease inhibitors and NVP.

ART for patients with TB

ART is needed by all patients with TB who:

1. have extrapulmonary TB (which makes them stage 4 HIV disease) (except just lymph node TB),
2. have stage 4 by other criteria,
3. have stage 3 and the CD4 count is < 350 mm^3,
4. have any stage and the CD4 count is < 200 mm^3.

The diagnosis of TB is often the first indication that a patient may have decreased immunity and therefore HIV infection. Patients with known HIV infection in areas where PTB is common often develop TB. TB in patients with HIV infection is often unusual (see page 225) with sputum negative for AFB, involvement of lower rather than upper parts of the lungs, often extrapulmonary TB, and often infection with unusual *Mycobacteria* (not *M. tuberculosis*) causing the disease.

The first thing to do is immediately confirm the diagnosis of TB and immediately get the patient started on routine TB drug treatment. See Chapter 14 pages 112–122. This will stop the patient infecting others and start him on the road to recovery.

The next thing to do, if the patient is not known to have HIV infection, is to find out if the patient has HIV infection by counselling and doing an HIV antibody test; and then find out how badly his immunity is damaged by doing WHO clinical staging (see page 222) and sending blood for CD4 lymphocyte count.

If the patient has severe immunodeficiency (CD4 count < 200), the patient needs urgent ART; but if the patient improves on the anti-TB treatment and ART can be delayed at least 2 or if possible 8 weeks – this is better. If the patient is not very severely immunosuppressed, delay ART until after the intensive phase of anti-TB drug treatment using rifampicin is over. Reasons for delaying ART include (1) there are reactions between rifampicin and some ART drugs and (2) the risk of immune reconstitution inflammatory syndrome (IRIS). If the patient is WHO stage 1 or 2 or 3 and the CD4 count is above 350, delay the TB treatment until after 8 weeks, or if doing well until the end of TB treatment.

If the patient has to be given ART as soon as anti-TB drugs are started, it may be best to use three NRTIs. If two NRTIs and one NNRTI are used, as long as the patient is not pregnant, use efavirenz (EFV) rather than nevirapine (NVP) and contraception.

The recommended ART regime for an HIV patient with TB started 2–8 weeks after anti-TB treatment has been started is the two usual NRTIs and one NNRTI (see page 243).

1. Efavirenz (EFV) is preferred to nevirapine (NVP) as it has less interaction with rifampicin.
2. Efavirenz (EFV) cannot be used in early pregnancy and nevirapine (NVP) is used.
3. Nevirapine (NVP) and possibly efavirenz (EFV) may be best not used if pregnant with CD4 count near 350, as there is a greater risk of liver and other problems the higher the CD count is above 200 – use three-drug NRTI regime instead (see page 243).
4. Efavirenz (EFV) and nevirapine (NVP) cannot be used if HIV-2, as they are then not effective. A three-drug NRTI regime (see page 243) would be used instead.

If the patient develops TB whilst on ART, the question arises if the HIV could be resistant to the ART. Although ART reduces the incidence of TB in HIV infected patients by 80%, 20% of patients can develop it. Refer all patients who develop TB while on ART to your Medical Officer. It is very unlikely, if TB develops in the first 6 months of ART, that the HIV is resistant. It may be if the patient develops atypical TB after the first 6 months of ART that the HIV is resistant (whereas not so if the TB is typical or just a lymph node). Careful evaluation of the TB, HIV, CD4 count, viral load, ART and other things are needed; and treatment with a PI which will need boosting and problems with rifampicin or rifabutin use, etc. all need Medical Officer care.

ART in women who are of childbearing age (i.e. may become pregnant)

ARTs do affect the hormones used for oral contraceptives and they then may not prevent pregnancy. IM hormonal contraceptives may be still effective. The use of condoms, however, is recommended for all women on ART who:

1. do not want to become pregnant (which would be the best decision), or who
2. want to avoid other STDs, or who
3. are taking efavirenz (EFV) or tenofovir (TDF) in their ART; as EFV, if taken in early pregnancy, can cause fetal CNS abnormalities and TDF may also cause fetal abnormalities.

The main concern with ART in women who could become pregnant (or who are pregnant) is the possibility that one or more of the ART will damage the fetus.

1. Efavirenz (EFV) may cause fetal CNS abnormalities if taken in the first 12–16 weeks of pregnancy. This drug should not be given unless it is certain the patient will use barrier contraception (usually condoms) to stop pregnancy, or is pregnant after 16 weeks and it is certain she will use barrier contraception after the baby is born so that she cannot become pregnant again while on EFV. The risk of fetal abnormalities is, however, not so high that if EFV is taken in early pregnancy abortion should be considered. If the patient is on EFV and becomes pregnant, it could be changed to NVP if she was less than 12–16 weeks pregnant.
2. Tenofovir (TDF) may cause some abnormalities if given during pregnancy and should be used in the same way as EFV (above).

If a pregnancy test is not available, if a woman answers 'yes' to any one of the following questions, it is unlikely that she is pregnant.

1. Has your last menstrual period started within the last 7 days?
2. Have you had NO sexual intercourse since your last normal period?
3. Have you been using a reliable contraceptive properly and always?
4. Have you given birth in the last 4 weeks?
5. Have you had a miscarriage or abortion in the last 7 days?
6. Have you given birth less than 6 months ago AND had no menstrual period AND are now fully or almost fully breastfeeding?

ART for women who are pregnant

HIV counselling and testing should be given to all pregnant women in places where HIV is common. Diagnosis of HIV will allow co-trimoxazole and ART to keep the woman in better health and stop the transmission of HIV to the child. If the HIV test is positive, also do a blood test for syphilis or give penicillin treatment for syphilis to prevent possible fetal damage.

A pregnant woman with HIV infection should have both her WHO clinical stage assessed (although weight loss is difficult to determine), and her CD4 count done, to determine if she herself needs treatment, screening for TB, prophylaxis with SMX/TMP, and advice about avoiding malaria, etc.

ART for the pregnant woman is given as for all other adults; except that also women with WHO clinical stage 3 and a CD4 count of less than 350 would be treated.

WHO clinical stage	CD4 testing not available	CD4 testing available
1	Do not give ART	Treat only if CD4 count < 200
2	Do not give ART	Treat only if CD4 count < 200
3	Give ART	Give ART if CD4 count < 350
4	Give ART	Give ART no matter what CD4 count

ART should be started as soon as possible in the pregnancy if the woman has indications for it.

ART usually consists of AZT + 3TC + NVP twice daily.

Women who become pregnant while taking ART should continue treatment, but if in the first 16 weeks of pregnancy and on EFV, change EFV to NVP (as this is safer for the baby in the first 16 weeks).

TDF may cause fetal damage and 3TC is preferred.

NVP is effective for the woman and effective in stopping spread of the HIV to the baby. However, in a woman with a CD4 count much higher than 200 and near 350 there is an increased risk of hepatitis. The woman needs to know to come back quickly if symptoms of hepatitis (yellow eyes, skin rash, fever, abdominal pain, etc.) for review and probably switching away from NVP. It is also best that the ALT pathology liver test is done at 2, 3, 8 and 12 weeks after starting treatment. The NVP should be stopped if there are symptoms and signs of hepatitis, and the ALT rises to 5 or more times the normal level. A third NRTI would be given in the place of NVP. If the patient is more than 16 weeks pregnant when first seen and it is certain that her contraception will be used so well that no pregnancy will occur after this birth, then EFV would be started instead of NVP, as it is less likely to cause hepatitis. Otherwise, a three-drug NRTI could be used from the start. If the patient has HIV-2, then again a three-drug NRTI is needed, e.g. AZT + 3TC + ABC.

Women with HIV infection with indications for ART who present late in pregnancy or labour, should still be started on ART and the ART continued during and after labour.

Women with HIV infection but who do not have indications for treatment for themselves, should, however, still have some drug treatment to try to stop infection of their baby. At the least this will be (but may later be increased):

> AZT starting at 28 weeks of pregnancy or as soon as possible after this, AND
>
> NVP single dose + AZT + 3TC during labour, AND
>
> AZT + 3TC for 7 days after birth.

After birth, the woman who needs ART should continue ART while breastfeeding.

ART for infants born to women who have HIV infection

All infants born to mothers infected with HIV should be given anti-retroviral therapy. If the mother has had ART for more than a month before delivery, then the infant should have AZT for 7 days after birth. If the mother has had less than 4 weeks ART before delivery, the infant should have 4 weeks AZT. If the mother has had no ART then the infant should be given a single dose of NVP (2 mg/kg orally) and 4 weeks of AZT (4 mg/kg twice daily). The sooner the treatment is given to the infant after birth, the more effective it is.

ART after possible HIV infection by exposure to the blood or bodily secretions of an HIV infected person

'First aid' where a person is exposed by possibly HIV infected body fluids includes, IMMEDIATELY:

1. Spit out any fluids in the mouth or wash off any fluids elsewhere.
2. Make any punctured wound bleed by holding it under running water; but do not squeeze.
3. Do not squeeze or rub or suck any site.
4. Wash the area immediately with a lot of water and soap but do not use soap in the eyes or mouth.
5. Do not rub or scrub the area or use strong solutions such as alcohol, bleach or iodine.
6. Do not put a dressing on the area.

Collect blood for HIV testing from both persons involved.

Persons who need prophylactic ART include:

1. Health workers who have had:
   * needle stick injury or injury with a sharp instrument used on the patient,
   * the mucous membrane of the eyes or mouth splashed with blood or other body fluids of the patient,
   * skin with injury or ulcer, etc. if exposed to blood or secretions from the patient,
   * normal skin which is exposed to large amounts of blood or secretions from the patient.
2. Persons who have been raped.
3. Persons possibly given HIV infected blood (when 80–90% chance will be infected).

Zidovudine (AZT/ZDV) 1000 mg daily (a higher dose than is now used) for 4 weeks has been shown to reduce the risk of developing HIV infection by 80%.

A two-drug regime for 4 weeks is probably more effective, e.g.:

1. Zidovudine (AZT/ZDV) 300 mg bd and lamivudine (3TC) 150 mg or emtricitabine (FTC) 200 mg once daily (instead of 3TC), or
2. Tenofovir (TDF) 300 mg daily and emtricitabine (FTC) 200 mg once daily or lamivudine (3TC) 300 mg once daily in place of FTC.

A three-drug regime may be more effective; but if it causes more side effects and is taken for less than 4 weeks, it would be less effective than a two-drug regime taken for 4 weeks. It may be indicated if resistant HIV, especially resistant HIV-1, is suspected. A protease inhibitor would be the best drug to add, e.g. lopinavir/ritonavir (LPV/r) 400 mg/100 mg bd with food; but would not be likely to be available. Efavirenz (EFV/EFZ) could be considered as long as not early pregnancy or HIV-2 infection, or if it is possible the person already has HIV infection, in preference to nevirapine (NVP); or a third NRTI added.

It is most important to start treatment as soon as possible; if possible in 1–2 hours. The earlier the treatment, the more effective it is. After 2–3 days it is unlikely to be effective.

Do not continue prophylactic ART if it is later shown that either;

- the person getting the prophylaxis is already HIV positive and does not need prophylaxis (or needs triple therapy), or
- the person suspected of passing on HIV is not HIV positive unless he has stage 4 disease (when he is so immunosuppressed that the HIV test may be negative), or there is a reason to believe he may have been infected in the previous 3 months (before the HIV test becomes positive).

The person getting the prophylaxis should use condoms if they have sex until a blood test 3 months later is negative.

Hepatitis B is an even greater risk to the person getting the prophylaxis than HIV infection; and active and passive immunisation for hepatitis B should be given as needed (see Chapter 24 page 395).

ART in a patient with a hepatitis virus infection

HBV infection affects up to 400 million and HCV up to 180 million people. Many of these people also have HIV infection. These can occur together very commonly in areas where there are unsafe injecting practices and blood use.

HIV makes HBV and HCV infections develop more quickly into chronic liver disease (cirrhosis). The effect of HBV infection on HIV infection is not known.

Some drugs which treat HIV infection are also treatment for hepatitis virus infection. Lamivudine (3TC) and emtricitabine (FTC) (although as these two have the same action, they should not be used together) are effective against HBV. If, however, one is used alone, the HBV does develop resistance to it. Tenofovir (TDF) treats both HIV and HBV infections, and if used together with 3TC or FTC will help prevent resistance of HBV to 3TC and FTC. Nevirapine (NVP) is also effective for treatment of HIV and HBV but can itself cause liver damage. Do not start NVP if ALT 5 or more times the normal level; and if NVP is used and ALT rises to, or above, 5 times the normal level, stop the NVP. Efavirenz (EFV), which has fewer liver side effects, is therefore preferable to NVP.

If a patient for HIV treatment has also HBV infection, then treat both HIV and HBV with:

3TC
or   and TDF and EFV.
FTC

If a patient is on ART drugs for both HIV and HBV infection and then gets hepatitis, this may be because of:

1. Immune reconstitution inflammatory syndrome (IRIS) (see pages 248 and 252), or
2. Side effects of drugs causing hepatitis.

Refer such patients to the Medical Officer about:

1. Continuing ART and treatment of IRIS (preferable, if possible), or
2. Cessation of ART until settles and then use of alternative drugs, preferably still with 3TC.

Hepatitis (sometimes fatal) can occur if ART, active against HBV, is suddenly stopped. When such a patient is re-started on new ART, it is best if at least 3TC is included.

Monitoring the efficacy of ART

Good effects or failure of ART are judged by:

1. clinical improvement:
   - gain in body weight,
   - decrease in occurrence and severity of HIV-related diseases (infections and malignancies),
   - change back to a better WHO clinical stage.
2. increase in total lymphocyte count (but not helpful in showing how much improvement);
3. improvement in CD4 + T lymphocyte counts;
4. plasma viral load level improves or seems to disappear (not usually available).

The response is better and quicker if the patient is not in stage 4 and the CD4 count is not very low.

The patient may seem sometimes to get worse when treatment first started, as:

1. it takes time for the HIV viral load to fall if CD4 count very low, or
2. immune reconstitution inflammatory syndrome (IRIS) may occur, especially if anti-TB treatment is started (see pages 248, 252),
3. drug toxicity may occur (see pages 248–253).

Early AVR toxicity

(In first few weeks) includes:

1. hypersensitivity (allergic type) reaction to NNRIs, especially skin rashes, abnormal liver function tests (ALT) or jaundice and hepatitis, etc.,
2. anaemia and low white cell count from AZT,
3. IRIS (see opposite).

Immune reconstitution inflammatory syndrome (IRIS)

After 2–12 weeks of ART in 10–25% of patients with another infection (especially TB and cryptococcus, especially if treatment of infection has only just started), and especially if the CD4 count is very low.

Table 19.5 Anti-retroviral drugs (ARD), doses, side effects and other information.

Drug	Formulations	Dose and dose frequency	Unwanted side effects	Other
Nucleoside/nucleotide reverse transcriptase inhibitors (NRTIs)				
Zidovudine (AZT or ZVD)	Oral Liquid 50 mg/5 ml Capsules: 100 mg; 250 mg Tablet 300 mg Solution for IV infusion 10 mg/ml in 20 ml vial	180 mg/m² twice daily Maximum dose: 300 mg twice daily	Nausea, diarrhoea and other GI upsets Headache Tiredness and weakness Anaemia Loss of white blood cells with infections and mouth ulcers, etc. Do regular FBC for 4 months Lipodystrophy and lactic acidosis Blue/black nails	Stored at room temperature but best in glass jars out of light. Can give with food. Doses of 600 mg/m² twice daily have been given for HIV encephalopathy. Do not use with d4T (each stops the effect of the other). Cheap. Effective. Safe.
Lamivudine (3TC)	Oral solution 50 mg/ml Tablet 150 mg	4 mg/kg twice daily Maximum dose: 150 mg twice daily, or 300 mg once daily	Nausea Headache Tiredness and weakness Muscle pain and weakness Anaemia Loss of white blood cells and infections and mouth ulcers, etc.	Well tolerated. Can give with food. Store solution at room temperature (use within 1 month of opening). Tablet can be washed, mixed with a small amount of food and taken immediately.
Emtricitabine (FTC)	Capsule 200 mg Oral liquid 10 mg/ml	200 mg once daily	Similar to 3TC but more costly	Store at room temperature.
Didanosine (ddl) (dideoxyinosine)	Powder (buffered) for oral liquid 100 mg 167 mg 250 mg packets Buffered chewable tablets 25 mg 50 mg 100 mg 150 mg 200 mg Enteric-coated unbuffered capsules 125 mg 200 mg 250 mg 400 mg	> 60 kg 400 mg once daily < 60 kg 250 mg once daily	Nausea Diarrhoea Neuropathy or peripheral neuritis Pancreatitis (upper abdominal pain and tenderness and vomiting) and can cause death	Suspension – if refrigerated will keep for 30 days – must shake well. Others stored at room temperature. Should be taken on an empty stomach at least 30 minutes before or 2 hours after eating. Enteric-coated beadlets in capsules can be opened and sprinkled on small amount of food.

Table 19.5 (*continued*)

Drug	Formulations	Dose and dose frequency	Unwanted side effects	Other
Stavudine (d4T)	Powder for oral liquid 5 mg/ml Capsules 15 mg 20 mg 30 mg 40 mg	< 30 kg 1 mg/kg twice daily > 30 kg 30 mg twice daily (maximum dose 30 mg twice daily)	Neuropathy or peripheral neuritis Lactic acidosis Lipodystrophy syndrome Pancreatitis (see above) These stop this cheap effective drug being used much	Large volume of solution. If refrigerated can keep for 30 days – must shake well. Needs to be stored in glass bottles. Capsules opened up and mixed with small amount of food are well tolerated (stable in solution for 24 hours if kept refrigerated). Do not use with AZT (each stops effect of other).
Abacavir (ABC)	Oral solution 20 mg/ml Tablet 300 mg	< 16 years or < 37.5 kg: 8 mg/kg twice daily > 16 years or > 37.5 kg: Maximum dose 300 mg twice daily or 600 mg once daily	Nausea Diarrhoea Tiredness and weakness Not able to sleep normally Severe hypersensitivity or 'allergic' type reactions in 5% Stop permanently if occur Lipodystrophy, lactic acidosis, neuritis, etc.	Syrup well tolerated or can crush tablet. Can give with food. **Must warn about hypersensitivity reaction.** Stop permanently if hypersensivity reaction (fever, short of breath, rash, GI symptoms, etc.)
Tenofovir (disoproxyl furomate) (TDF)	Tablet 300 mg (equivalent to 240 mg tenofovir disoproxyl)	300 mg once daily	If kidney problems (failure) reduce dose Best not if pregnant, as possible fetal brain damage Nausea Diarrhoea. Headache Occasional pancreatitis and lactic acidosis	Effective. Safe.
Non-nucleoside reverse transcriptase inhibitors (NNRTIs)				
Nevirapine (NVP)	Oral liquid 50 mg/ 5 ml Tablet 200 mg	120 mg/m² once daily for 2 weeks, then 120–200 mg/m² twice daily Maximum dose > 13 years 200 mg once daily for first 2 weeks, then 200 mg twice daily	Skin rash which can be severe or life-threatening (Stevens–Johnson syndrome) Jaundice, hepatitis Nausea Diarrhoea	If rifampicin co-administration, use with care (EFV fewer interactions). Store suspension at room temperature. Shake well. Can give with food. **Warn about rash.** Do not increase first dose if rash occurs (if mild/moderate rash, stop drug; when rash cleared, restart dosing from beginning dose; if severe rash, do not restart NVP). Drug interactions. HIV-2 is resistant.

Table 19.5 (*continued*)

Drug	Formulations	Dose and dose frequency	Unwanted side effects	Other
Efavirenz (EFV or EFZ)	Oral liquid 150 mg/5 ml (note: syrup requires higher doses than capsules, see dosing chart) Capsules 50 mg 100 mg 200 mg Tablets 600 mg	15–20 kg: 250 mg (300 mg = 10 ml) once daily 20–25 kg: 300 mg (360 mg = 12 ml) once daily 25–30 kg: 350 mg (450 mg = 15 ml) once daily 33–40 kg: 400 mg (510 mg = 17 ml) once daily Maximum dose: 40 kg and above 600 mg once daily	Mental and psychiatric disturbances including dreaming, sleeplessness, depression and suicide Encephalitis Damage to fetus if given in first 1/3 of pregnancy is possible Hepatitis and skin rashes less often than NVP Nausea, diarrhoea	Store at room temperature. Capsules may be opened and added to food but very peppery taste; however, can mix with jam or sweet foods. Can give with food (but avoid after high fat meals which increase absorption by 50%). Best at bedtime, especially first 2 weeks to reduce CNS side effects. Drug interactions. HIV-2 is resistant
Protease inhibitors (PIs)				
Lopinavir/ ritonavir (LPV/r)	Oral solution: 400 mg lopinavir + 100 mg ritonavir/ 5 ml Capsules: 133.3 mg lopinavir + 33.3 mg ritonavir Tablets: heat stable: 200 mg lopinavir + 50 mg ritonavir	6 months to 13 years: 225 mg/m² LPV + 57.5 mg/m² ritonavir twice daily Or weight-based dosing: 7–15 kg: 12 mg/kg LPV + 3 mg/kg ritonavir twice daily 15–40 kg: 10 mg/kg LPV + 2.5 mg/kg ritonavir twice daily Max. dose: > 40 kg: 400 mg LPV + 100 mg ritonavir (2 tablets or 3 capsules or 5 ml twice daily) Dose may be increased in long-term patients to 3 tablets twice daily with EVF or NVP.	Nausea Vomiting Abdominal pain Diarrhoea Pancreatitis Tiredness and weakness Headache	Preferably oral solution and capsules should be refrigerated; however, can store at room temperature up to 25°C (77°F) for 1 month. Liquid formulation has low volume but bitter taste. Capsules large. Tablets best preparation. Should be taken with food. See drug interactions.

Table 19.5 (*continued*)

Drug	Formulations	Dose and dose frequency	Unwanted side effects	Other
Indinavir (IDV)	Capsules 200 mg; 333 mg; 400 mg Also co-formulations with ritonavir	Maximum 800 mg tid with fluid Dose with ritonavir (IDV/r) 800 mg + 100 mg twice daily	GI upset Headache Kidney stones Hepatitis Raised blood glucose Blood disorders Lipodystrophy	Give with ritonavir but **check for latest dose (reduction).** See drug interactions.
Saquinavir (SQV)	Capsule 200 mg Also co-formulations with ritonavir	1000 mg bd after food SQV/r 1000 mg + 100 mg twice daily but **check for latest dose (reduction)**	GI upsets Nausea Headache Lipodystrophy Hepatitis Raised blood sugar	Give with ritonavir but **check for latest dose (reduction).** See drug interactions.
Nelfinavir (NFV)	Powder for oral suspension (mix with liquid): 200 mg per level 5 ml teaspoon (50 mg per 1.25 ml scoop) Tablet: 250 mg (tablets can be halved, can be crushed and added to food or dissolved in water)	55 to 65 mg/kg twice daily Maximum dose: > 13 years 1250 mg twice daily	Nausea Diarrhoea Skin rash Changes in body fat and blood glucose	Powder is sweet, faintly bitter, but gritty and hard to dissolve; must be made up only just before being given in water, milk, formula, pudding, etc. – do not use acidic food or juice (increases bitter taste). Because of difficulties with use of powder, crushed tablets preferred (even for infants) if appropriate dose can be given. Powder and tablets can be stored at room temperature. Take with food. Note drug interactions (less than ritonavir-containing protease inhibitors). Can give with ritonavir but **check for latest dose (reduction).**
Ritonavir (r)	Oral liquid 400 mg/5 ml Oral solid dosage form 100 mg (usually soft capsules)	100–200 mg bd	Nausea Diarrhoea Abdominal pain Pancreatitis Allergy Tiredness	Not used alone as treatment; but to increase the effect of other protease inhibitors taken with it. Note drug interactions.

IRIS occurs. There is an increase of the symptoms of the infection and also fever, and other symptoms of inflammation in the body caused by the improved immunity attacking the infection.

All other possible causes of the fever, etc. (especially other infections) need to be looked for, and if found, treated.

Treatment includes, if possible, continuing the ART; treatment of the other infection; use of anti-inflammatory drugs (including prednisolone 0.5 mg/kg/day until settled and then slowly reduced and ceased) (and usual drug prophylaxis when giving prednisolone).

Always, if possible, transfer patients with IRIS for Medical Officer assessment.

Later AVR toxicity

Set out in Table 19.6 (below) but also Table 19.5 (pages 248–251).

If a patient has a significant reaction to an anti-retroviral drug, it may or may not need stopping. If it does need stopping, do not just continue the other two drugs. You must substitute another drug not likely to have this same side effect. This would mean changing someone from one NRTI to another NRTI; or from NVP to EVF or NVP to an NRTI.

See Table 19.6 below for details.

Table 19.6 ART side effects, the drug/s most likely to cause these side effects and what action to take (including substituting another drug).

Problem	Probable cause	Management
Acute pancreatitis (upper abdominal pain and tenderness and vomiting, etc. See Chapter 24 page 400)	d4T and ddI	Stop ART. Give pancreatitis treatment. When settled start ART with, instead, an NRTI with low pancreatic toxicity risk. AZT, ABC, TDF and 3TC are less likely to cause this type of toxicity.
Diarrhoea	ddI (buffered formulation) NVF, LPV/r and SQV/r	Usually goes away by itself without need to stop ART. Symptomatic treatment should be given.
Skin rashes (mild to severe, including Stevens–Johnson syndrome or toxic epidermal necrolysis) – see Chapter 14 page 117	NVP, EFV (rarely)	In very mild cases give antihistamines and watch carefully as it may go without need to change ART. If mild/moderate rash, non-progressing and without mucosal involvement or systemic signs, consider a single NNRTI substitution (i.e. from NVP to EFV). In moderate and severe cases, stop ART and give supportive treatment. After settles, resume ART with three NRTIs (or two NRTIs + PI).
High blood sugar and fats	PIs	Consider replacing the suspected PI by PI drug with less risk of metabolic toxicity (e.g. ?NFV) or other drug. Diet suitable for diabetes and physical exercise, etc. are needed.
GI intolerance, with taste changes, nausea, vomiting, abdominal pain and diarrhoea	All ARDs (less frequent with d4T, 3TC, FTC and ABC)	Usually goes away by itself without need to stop ART. Symptomatic treatment should be given.
Blood abnormality, especially anaemia and low white cell count	AZT	If severe (Hb < 6.5 g%) and/or neutrophil count < 500 cells/mm³, replace by an ARD with minimal or no blood toxicity (e.g. d4T, ABC or TDF) and consider blood transfusion.
Hepatitis (loss of appetite, nausea, abdominal pain, dark urine, ALT more than 5 times normal – see Chapter 24 pages 393–395)	All ARDs (particularly with NVP and ritonavir-boosted PIs)	Increase in ALT by more than 5 times can be due to NVP; however, changes can occur with all ARDs. If ALT is at more than 5 times normal level stop ART and watch. After it becomes normal, replace the drug most likely to have caused the condition.

Table 19.6 (*continued*)

Problem	Probable cause	Management
High bilirubin without hepatitis	ATV (a PI used by some HIV specialists)	Generally asymptomatic but can cause jaundice (without ALT elevations). Replace ATV with other PI.
Hypersensitivity (allergic) reaction with respiratory symptoms, fever and without mucosal involvement	ABC	Stop ABC and **do not restart**. Symptomatic treatment. Giving ABC again may lead to a severe and life-threatening reaction. Give other NRTI.
Lactic acidosis (shortness of breath, weakness, nausea, vomiting, abdominal pain), which may come over weeks or months; and needs blood lactic acid test to diagnose. See Chapter 13 page 74.	All NRTIs (particularly d4T and ddl)	Stop ART and give symptomatic treatment. After settles, re-start ART, replacing the offending NRTI. ABC, TDF and 3TC are less likely to cause this type of toxicity.
Lipoatrophy, when fat at edge of body (face, limbs) is lost. Fat accumulation with fat at centre of body (abdomen, breasts, back of neck) increases. Can be called 'lipodystrophy'	d4T or AZT PIs But any NRTI also	Early replacement of the suspected ARD (e.g. d4T by TDF or ABC). Physical exercise may help.
Neurological (CNS) changes or psychiatric changes (sleep disturbances; depression; behaviour and personality changes)	EFV	Usually goes away by itself without need to stop ART. Symptomatic treatment if required. If a previous psychiatric disturbance has occurred there is a higher risk of a more severe reaction. Effects may be made worse by alcohol or drugs.
Renal stones (kidney stones with ureteric colic. See Chapter 26 page 450 and Chapter 36 page 593)	IDV	If using IDV, stop it and give fluids, pain relief and other symptomatic treatment (50% recurrence rate). Replace IDV with another PI.
Renal toxicity (kidney failure – serum creatinine high. See pages 449 and 453)	TDF	Stop TDF and give fluids and symptomatic treatment. After settled, start ART using another drug.
Peripheral neuropathy or neuritis (with pain or weakness of limbs) See Chapter 25 page 420	d4T and ddl	Consider replacement by an NRTI with minimal or no neurotoxicity (AZT, TDF or ABC). Give symptomatic treatment and see Chapter 26 pages 420–421

Note: 'Mitochondrial dysfunction' means the body cells are stopped from working properly and is the name given to lactic acidosis and/or hepatitis, and/or pancreatitis, and/or peripheral neuropathy, and/or lipodystrophy, and/or myopathy, etc. which then happens. It is usually due to NRTIs.

Switching ART because of drug failure/HIV drug resistance

This should normally be done by the Medical Officer. This should be done only if it is certain that the first line drugs are not working, i.e.:

1. at least 6–12 months treatment with the first line ART (it may take that long for the ART to improve the patient);
2. no doses were missed; if 3 doses, i.e. 1½ days in a month or 5% of all doses (or more) missed, then treatment is not effective; explain and help the patient take all doses regularly for 6–12 months;
3. other infections have been diagnosed and treated (especially TB);
4. IRIS is not present or has been treated;
5. the prophylactic treatment needed (e.g. co-trimoxazole) is being taken regularly.

If all of these have been considered, things which are used to diagnose the need to change ART drugs include:

1. Clinical failure:
   • WHO stage 4 (or perhaps stage 3) has come for the first time; or has come back after going away for 6–12 months on ART.

Table 19.7 Switching ART because of drug failure/HIV drug resistance.

Treatment failure criteria	WHO stage 1	WHO stage 2	WHO stage 3	WHO stage 4
CD4 failure < count before treatment or < 50% of highest count or < 100 **Viral load testing** not usually available	Do not switch regimen. Follow patient for development of clinical signs or symptoms. Repeat CD4 cell count in three months.	Do not switch regimen. Follow patient for evidence of further clinical progression. Repeat CD4 cell count in three months.	Consider switch to second line regimen (but not if CD4 count > 200).	Switch to second line regimen.
CD4 failure and **Viral load failure** (<10,000)	Consider switch to second line regimen.	Consider switch to second line regimen.	Switch to second line regimen.	Switch to second line regimen.

- If the stage change is diagnosed because an infection (especially TB) has occurred, give proper treatment of the infection. If treatment successful – ART failure less likely. If treatment fails – ART failure more likely.
- Make sure the clinical state is not just IRIS.
2. CD4 cell failure:
   - Fall of CD4 count to the level when started ART (or less).
   - Fall to half of the highest CD4 count when on ART (or less).
   - CD4 levels below 100 on repeated tests.
3. Virological failure:
   - Plasma viral load of above 10,000 copies/ml (test rarely available).

The CD4 count is the best guide if done:
1. *before* start ART; but after treatment of any other condition is completed,
2. *after* each 6 months of treatment,
3. *again* if doubt about ART failure; *but only after* any infection, etc. treated.

Send blood for CD4 count where possible before considering changing treatment.

Drugs used if first line ART fails/HIV drug resistance occurs ('switching treatment')

This will need three more drugs which have never been given to the patient before.
1. A protease inhibitor (PI) is the basis of the new treatment.
   - It should be boosted (or made more effective) by giving ritonavir (r) (not by itself a treatment) together with the PI.
   - Any PI is probably effective. However, at present lopinovir (LPV) is the only PI which is available with ritonavir (r), which is not damaged if the drugs get hot; and at present LPV/r is the drug usually used.

2. The second drug is usually didanosine (ddl), especially if the enteric-coated (EC) preparation is available (to reduce GI side effects), as this is usually not used as a first line drug.
3. A third drug often helpful is abacavir (ABC) (with the ddl).
4. An alternative combination to ddl and ABC is tenofovir disopropyl furanate (TDF) and abacavir (ABC).
5. If the patient had only three NRTIs as first line therapy, then there is the possibility of
   - a boosted PI, and
   - an NRTI, e.g. ddl and
   - an NNRTI.

LPV/r + ddl (or TDF) + ABC, OR
LPV/r + NNRTI (e.g. NPV) + an NRTI (e.g. ddl)
(as long as the patient has not had an NNRTI).

Table 19.8 WHO suggestions for switching treatment if first line ART drugs fail/HIV drug resistance occurs.

	First line regimen	Second line regimen
Standard strategy	AZT or d4T + 3TC + NVP or EFV	ddl + ABC + LPV/r TDF + ABC + LPV/r TDF + 3TC (± AZT) + LPV/r
	TDF + 3TC + NVP or EFV	ddl + ABC + LPV/r ddl + 3TC (± AZT) + LPV/r
	ABC + 3TC + NVP or EFV	ddl + 3TC (± AZT) + LPV/r TDF + 3TC (± AZT) + LPV/r
Alternative strategy	AZT or d4T + 3TC + TDF or ABC	EFV or NVP + ddl + LPV/r

Always use the drugs in one co-formulation or blister pack (if possible) so that there is no possibility that one of the drugs can be accidentally or purposely not taken.

When to stop ART (failure of second line treatment)

When newer drugs become available, it may be possible to give further different drug treatment if the HIV becomes resistant to second line treatment. At present, however, if the criteria which indicate failure of first line ART occur when the patient is on second line ART, no further more effective ART is available.

Normally, however, even if the second line ART is not controlling the HIV, the ART is usually continued, as it is still probably slowing the progress of the HIV. If it is stopped, the patient often becomes quickly worse and dies.

The ART, however, would be stopped if:

1. the ART is causing side effects which worry the patient, or
2. the patient is obviously dying and no other treatment is possible.

The main aim of the treatment then would be to keep the patient without pain and as comfortable as possible with treatment of all symptoms until he died.

5. Treat symptoms

Symptom treatment – see pages 223–233, 236–239.

6. Follow-up and administrative procedures

Follow-up and administrative procedures – follow the guidelines for your country.

Patients and the personal treatment supporter need to be seen regularly, be supplied with drugs regularly and have all the forms and registers, etc. filled in at these times and sent as needed to the Health Department.

Make arrangements for the supply of ART drugs, usually monthly. At this time, not only should questions be kindly asked about the regularity of tablet taking; a tablet count should be done to make sure the patient is taking at least 95% of his doses. (*Only 3 missed doses a month may make the treatment not work.*) If the patient is not taking all the drugs, the health worker must find ways of helping the patient and the treatment supporter to solve this problem.

- Patients with clinical stages 1 and 2 will usually need to be seen at least each 6 months.
- Patients with clinical stages 3 and 4 will usually need to be seen each month.
- Patients in any stage who develop any new problem need to be seen immediately.
- Patients who are started on ART will usually need to be seen each 2 weeks for 2 months and then each month.

When you see the patient, ask not only how he has been and if any problems have developed, but also ask about the major symptoms in all body systems, in case a problem is developing that the patient does not mention. Check the basic observations and examine any part of the body the symptoms suggest is affected; but particularly the skin, mucous membrane, lymph nodes, colour for anaemia or jaundice and if any evidence of TB or of injuries from violence. If needed, do a psychiatric examination. If possible, check the eyesight. Make sure you find out about and solve any family, work and social problems as well as physical and psychological problems.

Ask also about any problems the treatment supporter has and solve these.

If the patient is on ART with AZT, blood tests at least for Hb are needed at 0, 4, 6 and 12 weeks. If the patient is on NVP, especially if a high CD4 count or if pregnant or if a previous liver problem, then an ALT is needed each 2 weeks for 3 months.

Each 6 months the patient should have a full clinical staging done and recorded (with a 'T' for treatment before it) and, if possible, a CD4 count.

Refer any patient with problems you cannot solve to the Medical Officer and make sure the consultation takes place and the problems are really solved – further action is needed if they are not.

Control and prevention

1. Kill the organism in the body of the original host or reservoir

This is as yet not possible. ART at present does greatly reduce the number of HIV in the body but never gets rid of them all. It is just possible that in the future a drug that does this will be found. Another possibility is that a genetic engineering method of taking and altering the HIV protein and then giving this to the patient may get rid of the HIV (which does the damage) from the body. At present, however, although ART greatly reduces the number of HIV particles in the body temporarily, there is no cure and no way of making the infected person completely or permanently non-infectious to others.

2. Stop the means of spread

This is most important. See below.

3. Increase the resistance of possible new hosts

This is not yet possible. It is hoped, however, that one of the many vaccines being tested or more likely a vaccine not yet made may be able to immunise against HIV infection. Keeping the genital tract healthy makes it less likely to be infected if exposed to HIV. Avoiding and correctly treating STDs will therefore help.

4. Prophylactic treatment

Curative drugs, effective preventive vaccine, etc. for HIV infection are not yet available. Prophylactic treatment is therefore not usually possible. However, any health worker or other person possibly infected by needle stick or other such injury likely to cause infection, any person who has been raped, any person who has incorrectly been given possibly HIV infected blood and other people in other situations where infection is possible, should immediately start on 4 weeks' treatment with at least two anti-HIV drugs. Doing this greatly reduces their chance of infection (see page 246). Babies born to mothers with HIV infection should be treated at birth and for 1–4 weeks afterwards. This greatly decreases their risk of infection (see page 246).

Prophylactic treatment is, however, possible for some of the bacterial, protozoal and other infections more likely in people with HIV infection. Co-trimoxazole and at times isoniazid and other drugs (see pages 239 and 258) may be used.

Ways to stop HIV spread

Stop the spread by unsafe sexual practices

Encourage all people to get their HIV test done.
If it is positive, encourage them to practise only safe sex and not to infect anyone else. If the test is negative, encourage these people from then on to have only safe sex and not become infected.

Ensure information about safe sexual practices is available to everyone.
The only really safe sexual practice for an uninfected person is to have sexual intercourse with only one other uninfected 'faithful' partner (that is, one who has not had and will not have sexual intercourse with anyone else). There is no way to tell from a person's appearance, or by what they say, if they are infected or not. This can be done only by knowing for certain the person has never had sex with anyone else and has not otherwise been likely to have been infected and is also well. If the person has a negative HIV blood test at least 3–6 months after the last time they had intercourse and is well, it is unlikely they are infected.

A person who has many sexual partners is at high risk of HIV infection. A person who has sexual intercourse with just one person, but that person has had many sexual partners, is also at high risk for HIV infection. To reduce the risk of HIV infection, people need to reduce the number of their sexual partners, although there will always be a risk until sexual intercourse occurs with only one uninfected faithful partner.

If a person has sexual relations with more than one person or with a possibly infected person, the following will reduce the risk of getting HIV infection.

1. Change sexual activities from high risk to low risk activities. High risk activities are when semen or vaginal fluid come into contact with the partner's oral (mouth), genital or anal/rectal mucosa. Low risk practices are when these fluids come into contact only with skin which is not damaged (as unbroken skin is not able to be entered by the virus). This means that a low risk practice is when a man's penis does not enter the partner's vagina, anus or mouth; or a woman's vaginal fluid does not enter the partner's urethra, anus or mouth.

2. Use a condom. A condom will greatly reduce the risk of infected semen or vaginal fluid getting into the other person to almost none; but not to absolutely none. It is important that people not only know this, but are shown how to use condoms properly and do have condoms available and do actually use condoms each and every time they have sexual intercourse. See Appendix 1 page 259.

3. 'Microbicides' are chemicals which can kill microorganisms. There are some (including a cheap fruit) that are now under test that will hopefully kill HIV in the vagina. They are likely to be much less than 100% effective. Even if they have some effect, however, they would still be very helpful for women whose only other protection is the female condom if the male does not use a male condom. As yet, none have been proven to be effective.

4. Trials are being done to see if intravaginal hormones will make the vaginal mucosa more resistant to infection.

5. Male circumcision reduces the risk for men of being infected from an HIV infected partner by about 60%, i.e. it is only partly effective. It offers no protection for the partner. It would help but would be carried out only as part of the HIV prevention programme. It has health risks and must be done as a surgical procedure by trained operators after counselling and without forcing the patient. It must be done confidentially. 'Female circumcision' (female genital mutilation) does not help and may make infection more likely.

6. Washing the penis immediately after intercourse reduces the risk to the male.

It is most important that patients with HIV infection are given the above information.

Health education.
Health education about safe sex to groups at particular risk of HIV infection should be carried out whenever possible. These would include:
- sex workers,
- people who visit sex workers,
- STD patients,
- those who are away from their community and family, e.g. migrant workers, truck drivers, sailors, etc.

Health education of special groups should be carried out whenever possible. These would include:
- school children, preferably before they are likely to have sexual intercourse for the first time,
- young people,
- groups of men,
- groups of women,
- those who can be reached by the mass media (radio, TV and newspapers).

If possible, some kind of measurement of the effects of these methods of health education should be carried out so that most effort can be put into those types of health education which are most effective.

Stop the spread of infection by transfusion of infected blood

1. Do not transfuse anyone unless blood is really needed.
2. Do not transfuse blood unless the HIV test on that blood is negative before the blood is transfused.
3. Do not collect blood for transfusion from anyone who has any risk factors for HIV in the previous 3–6 months, as they still could be infected but the HIV test not yet be positive.

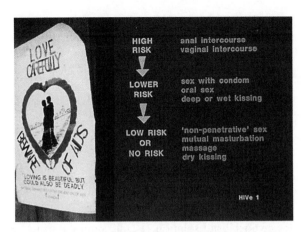

Figure 19.31 *Posters and literature which are understood by the people in your area are needed to get them to understand how HIV infection is spread and how not to get the infection.*

4. Tell patients who have HIV infection they must not donate blood.

Stop the spread of infection in the health centre

1. Do not allow health workers to get blood on them from patients in case the patient's blood is infected. Wear gloves and an apron or gown when doing dressings, etc. and use a 'no touch' technique. Use a mask which is waterproof and glasses or goggles if health workers are doing something which splashes droplets of blood or body fluid near the face including surgery and at childbirth and lumbar puncture. Do not do 'mouth to mouth resuscitation'. Instead, use a barrier method (face shield or mask) (see Chapter 37 page 611). If blood does get on to a health worker, gently but completely wash off all this blood with soap and water. Then see page 246.
2. Make sure health workers do not accidentally get injuries from needles and other sharp instruments. Do not put caps back on needles after the needle has been used. If possible, use disposable needles which, together with other sharp disposable contaminated objects, are dropped into a strong 'sharps' plastic or cardboard container which, when full, is burned, then buried. If a needle stick injury occurs or a person gets blood or other body fluids onto or into them, see page 246 for first aid and if needed prophylactic ART. First aid must be carried out immediately. If exposure is onto only unbroken healthy skin, the risk is minimal.
3. Give prophylactic ART (see page 246 for details) if exposure is through the skin or onto mucous

membrane. It should be started within the first hour. Then take blood for HIV serology from the exposed person (and also from the suspected HIV infected person if they have not already had a positive test) (see pages 246–247).

4. Sterilise instruments, etc. correctly. See Chapter 11 pages 61–63 for more details.
   - Soak for 30 minutes in disinfectant; then clean them carefully, wearing gloves, mask and eye protection; then sterilise by autoclaving or by steam or by boiling for 20 minutes or by dry heat at 170°C.
   - Suitable antiseptics include chlorine as in sodium hypochlorite solution (10,000 ppm chlorine) or household bleach diluted 1 in 10; gluteraldehyde 2% solution freshly prepared; formalin 4% solution; povidone-iodide 2.5% (Betadine); hydrogen peroxide 6%. Note that chloroxylenol (e.g. 'Dettol') and phenolic antiseptics and alcohol are not adequate.
5. Ensure all wounds, etc. are covered.
6. If a health worker is HIV positive, that health worker should not do any surgery or any procedure where the health worker's blood could get onto or into any patient.
7. Have laundry washed at high temperatures or with disinfectants.

Stop the spread of HIV in the home

1. See also page 117 and pages 236–238.
2. For the washing of plates, spoons, clothing, etc. use ordinary soap or detergent and water. If possible, use hot water or dry them in the sun.
3. Clothing, bedclothes, floors, etc. soiled with body fluids should be covered with household bleach diluted 1 in 10 for half an hour and then cleaned as usual.
4. The HIV patient must be told how he must not get his blood or body fluids into anyone else's body. This will include safe sexual practices, including never having sex unless a condom is used, not sharing sharp items such as razors, toothbrushes or tooth cleaning sticks, etc.

Stop the spread of HIV by drug addicts

1. Discourage people from becoming drug addicts.
2. Discourage drug addicts from using injected drugs.
3. If drug addicts do inject themselves, either get them to use a clean needle and syringe for each injection by using disposable needles and syringes, or tell them how to clean the needles and syringes and sterilise them with a 1 in 10 solution of household bleach for half an hour.

Stop the spread of HIV to unborn and newborn children from infected mothers

1. Advise any HIV patient against any pregnancy.
2. Supply contraceptive advice and condoms.
3. Try to make the birth of any child as free of blood as possible, e.g. no artificial rupture of the membranes, no episiotomy unless essential and try to get none of the mother's blood on the baby, especially when cutting the cord or at the birth of the placenta.
4. Give prophylactic ART to the mother and the child (see pages 245–246).
5. Do not stop HIV infected mothers breastfeeding their own child for the first 6 months, especially if the mother is on ART. The risk of this child contracting HIV from his mother's milk is less than the risk of the child dying from malnutriton or gastro-enteritis, etc. if not breastfed. See page 217. Present evidence suggests it may be safest for breastfeeding to stop at 6 months if the child is still not infected.

Chemoprophylaxis of some of the infections more likely in patients with HIV infection and decreased immunity is possible (see 2 page 239)

1. Co-trimoxazole, i.e. SMX 800 mg and TMP 160 mg daily. See page 239 for details.
2. Other drugs, if available, if the patient was started on them by the Medical Officer after treatment of the following infections. (Many of the following diagnoses are not usually able to be made in the health centre and many of the following drugs are not usually available in the health centre.)
   - (a) Co-trimoxazole SMX 800 mg/TMP 160 mg daily, if:
     - pneumocystis, or
     - toxoplasma, or
     - diarrhoea which settled on this drug.
   - (b) Fluconazole 200 mg once daily for cryptococcus infection.
   - (c) Itraconazole 200 mg twice daily for histoplasma infection.
   - (d) Ganciclovir 5 mg/kg daily for CMV infection.
   - (e) Ciprofloxacin 500 mg twice daily for 6–8 months for salmonella (NTS) infection in blood.
   - (f) Isoniazid 300 mg/day for 6 months or longer for patients infected with TB (positive Mantoux test) but no evidence of tuberculous disease:

- if cough, sputum negative for AFB AND satisfactory chest X-ray AND
- no evidence of TB elsewhere;
- but only in areas where TB uncommon; as long as the patient is otherwise well and does not have liver disease and does not drink much alcohol, when side effects of isoniazid are common.

At the time of writing, the situation with HIV is different in different areas. What action the health worker should take will depend on how common HIV infection is in his area, how it is spread in that area and what facilities for diagnosis and treatment exist. What should be done will be set out in the country's health policy about HIV infection. These

things can always be discussed with the supervising Medical Officer. The action to be taken will depend on the above and should be written down under the headings in this book. Remember, however, that the situation and the correct thing to do will change as time goes by as the epidemiology of the disease and its treatment changes.

Appendix 1   Condoms

Male condoms

Condoms prevent pregnancy, although they are not 100% effective. However, pregnancies reported with

How to use a condom

1. Check the expiry date and the manufacture date.

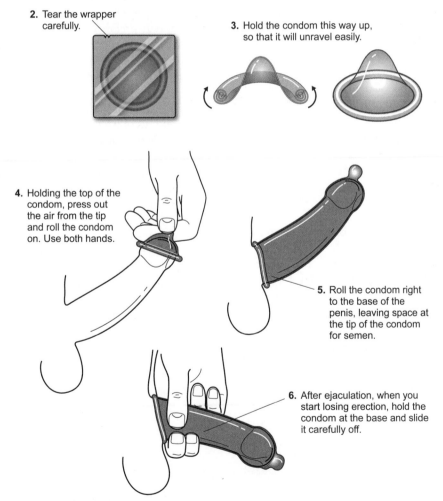

2. Tear the wrapper carefully.

3. Hold the condom this way up, so that it will unravel easily.

4. Holding the top of the condom, press out the air from the tip and roll the condom on. Use both hands.

5. Roll the condom right to the base of the penis, leaving space at the tip of the condom for semen.

6. After ejaculation, when you start losing erection, hold the condom at the base and slide it carefully off.

Source: World Health Organization.

condom use are often due to user failure rather than product failure.

Condoms are a key part of HIV prevention, as is abstinence and being faithful to one's partner. All these three strategies make up the 'ABC' of HIV/AIDS prevention. With consistent and correct use of condoms, there is a near zero risk of HIV. Studies of couples where one partner is infected show that with consistent condom use, HIV infection rates for the uninfected partner are below 1% per year.

Condoms are also effective barriers against other diseases such as herpes simplex, hepatitis B, chlamydia and gonorrhoea.

High rates of condom use have resulted in dramatic drops in the numbers of sexually transmitted infections (STI). After condom use rates rose among Thai sex workers from 14% in 1989 to 94% five years later, STI dropped from 400,000 to 30,000 per year. Condom use in Thailand and Cambodia has resulted in drops of HIV rates of more than 80% since the peak of the epidemics.

There are many things said about condom use **which are all wrong** (including all of the following):

- Condoms can get lost inside the woman.
- Condoms cannot be carried in a pocket or wallet or purse whenever there is the possibility you may have sexual intercourse.
- Condoms do not protect against STI, including HIV.
- It is OK to use glycerine or water-based lubricants with condoms.
- Pull the condom tight over the head of the penis to ensure a snug fit.
- Squeeze the air out of the top of the condom as you put it on.
- Condoms should be stored in a cool, dark, dry place.
- Condoms cannot be kept in a pocket or wallet indefinitely.

Condoms **can** provide a number of possible advantages.

- They help women to avoid pregnancy.
- They prevent transmission of STI, including HIV.

- Condoms reduce the risk of transmission of an STI if a patient does not wait for the STI to be cured before having sex but, ideally, the health care provider would encourage him to wait.
- Women feel dryer inside.
- The patient will feel safer, with fewer worries.
- Many men can prolong intercourse if they wear a condom.
- Bed linen needs washing less often.

Female condoms

Female condoms are becoming more widely available and have the advantage for women that their use is more in their control than use of male condoms. One type of female condom is currently on the market, under various names. It is made of polyurethane plastic, which is sturdier than latex. Only one size is made and fitting by a health care provider is not required. Unlike latex male condoms, which are weakened by oil-based lubricants, the female condom may be used with any type of lubricant without its strength being affected. It is prelubricated, but users may add more lubricant.

Female condoms may offer a similar level of protection as male condoms, but they are more expensive. Some studies have shown that the female condom is acceptable to both women and their male partners.

Despite its advantages, the female condom has some problems. The device protrudes from the vagina and thus requires the acceptance of the male partner. Also, it cannot be used at the same time as the male condom, which means it cannot provide back-up protection if the male condom breaks or slips.

Research into other female-controlled methods is underway. Microbicides (chemicals that kill STI organisms) are being tested for their safety and effectiveness in protecting against STI and HIV, as are other barrier methods such as the diaphragm. None of these methods has yet been shown to provide protection, however, equal to the male condom.

Instructions for use of a female condom

The female condom is a soft, loose-fitting sheath with a flexible polyurethane ring at each end. The inner ring at the closed end is inserted into the vagina. The outer ring at the open end remains outside the vagina during intercourse and covers outer genitalia.

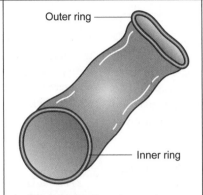

Outer ring

Inner ring

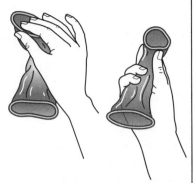

1. Remove the female condom from the package, and rub it between two fingers to be sure the lubricant is evenly spread. If you need more lubrication, squeeze two drops of the extra lubricant included in the package into the condom sheath.

2. The closed end of the female condom will go inside your vagina. Squeeze the inner ring (enclosed end) between your thumb and middle finger. Insert the ring into your vagina.

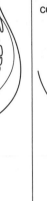

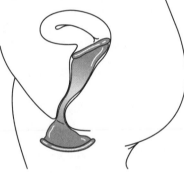

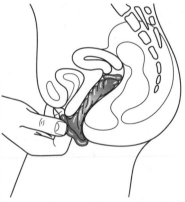

3. Using your index finger, push the sheath all the way into your vagina as far as it will go. It is in the right place when you cannot feel it.

Do not worry, it cannot go too far.

4. The ring at the open end of the female condom should stay outside your vagina and rest against your labia (the outer lip of the vagina). Be sure the condom is not twisted. Once you begin to engage in intercourse, you may have to guide the penis into the female condom. If you do not, be aware that the penis could enter the vagina outside of the condom's sheath. If this happens, you will not be protected.

5. After intercourse you can safely remove the female condom at any time. If you are lying down, remove the condom before you stand to avoid spillage. Before removing the condom from the vagina, make sure you twist it to prevent semen from spilling.

Dispose of the female condom safely (where it cannot cause any hazard). Do not reuse it.

Source: World Health Organization.

20 Disorders of the Respiratory System

Anatomy and physiology

All the cells of the body need oxygen to be brought to them, not only to do their work but just to stay alive. The cells make carbon dioxide while they live and work, and if the carbon dioxide is not taken away, it will poison the cells.

Air is about 20% oxygen, 80% nitrogen and much less than 1% carbon dioxide. The body cells take oxygen from the air and excrete carbon dioxide into the air (where it is used by plants which make it into oxygen again).

The oxygen and carbon dioxide are taken to and from the body cells in the blood. The respiratory system is where the body takes the oxygen from the air and puts it into the blood, and the carbon dioxide from the blood and puts it into the air. Taking air in and out of the respiratory system is called ventilation. Exchanging the oxygen and carbon dioxide is called respiration.

The respiratory system is in two parts – the upper respiratory tract and the lower respiratory tract (see Figure 20.1).

The upper respiratory tract is above the lowest part of the larynx or voice box. The work of the upper respiratory tract includes taking air to and from the lower respiratory tract, and warming, moistening, filtering and purifying the air; also speech, hearing and other things. The upper respiratory tract is often called the 'URT' or the ear, nose and throat 'ENT'. Figures 20.2, 20.3, 20.4 and 20.5 show the parts of the upper respiratory tract.

The lower respiratory tract consists of the trachea, bronchi and lungs (see Figure 20.1).

Air is taken to the lungs by air passages. Air enters the mouth or nose, goes through the larynx then down the trachea, which divides into two main bronchi. Each main bronchus divides into smaller and smaller bronchi (see Figures 20.1 and 20.6). The smallest bronchi end in little air bags or sacs known as alveoli. If the lungs are taken from a dead person, scissors can be used to cut along the bronchi, tracing each one, until they finally become so small that they cannot be seen. The appearance is something like the branches of a tree and the system of bronchi is often referred to as the bronchial tree. The smallest bronchi, called bronchioles, divide and lead into air sacs or alveoli (see Figure 20.11).

The lungs (see Figures 20.1, 20.7, 20.8) are inside the chest – one on each side. They are separated by the heart and the other structures of the mediastinum. The right lung consists of three smaller separate parts or lobes (upper, middle and lower lobes) and the left lung of two smaller separate parts or lobes (upper and lower lobes, although a part of the left upper lobe is called the lingular lobe). Each lobe has one bronchus bringing air to and from it.

Each lung is surrounded by a thin but strong airtight membrane called the pleural membrane or the pleura. The pleura surrounding and fastened to each lung is in turn surrounded by another layer of pleura which is on the inside of and fastened to the chest wall and the mediastinum. The two layers of pleura are not fastened to each other and so can easily move over each other. There is normally nothing between the two layers of pleura, except a thin layer of slippery fluid. (See Figure 20.9.)

Breathing is done by the muscles of the chest wall and the diaphragm (see Figure 20.10). During breathing in, the muscles pull the rib cage outwards

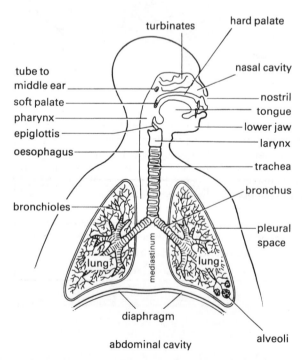

Figure 20.1 *Anatomy of the upper and lower respiratory tracts.*

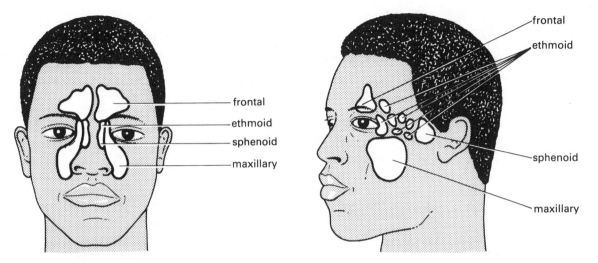

Figure 20.2 *Diagrams to show the position of the paranasal sinuses.*

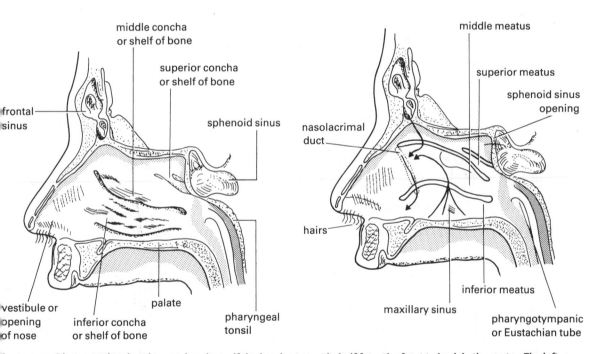

Figure 20.3 *Diagrams showing the nasal cavity as if the head were cut in half from the front to back in the centre. The left diagram shows structures of the lateral (side) wall. In the right diagram parts of the conchae are removed to show the way the paranasal sinuses and naso-lacrimal duct (see Figure 31.1) drain into the nasal cavity.*

nd upwards and the diaphragm downwards. When the chest wall (with the outer layer of pleura) moves away, the lungs (with their inner layer of pleura) follow, and the lungs expand. The lungs expand because negative pressure (or vacuum) is developed between the pleura lining the inside of the chest wall and the pleura lining the outside of the lungs when the chest and diaphragm start to move away from the lungs. During breathing out, the muscles relax and the lungs, which are somewhat elastic and stretched, contract and pull the chest wall and diaphragm with them – again because of the negative pressure between the pleura of the lungs and the pleura of the chest wall. The weight of the chest wall helps.

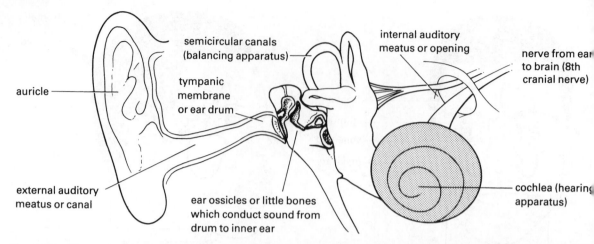

Figure 20.4 *Diagram to show the ear especially its subdivisions into outer, middle and inner ear and its anatomy. The middle ear is connected to the nasopharynx (back of the nose and throat) by means of the Eustachian or pharyngotympanic tube or canal. The ear drum or tympanic membrane does not allow air or fluid to go from the outer ear to the middle ear and middle ear to outer ear.*

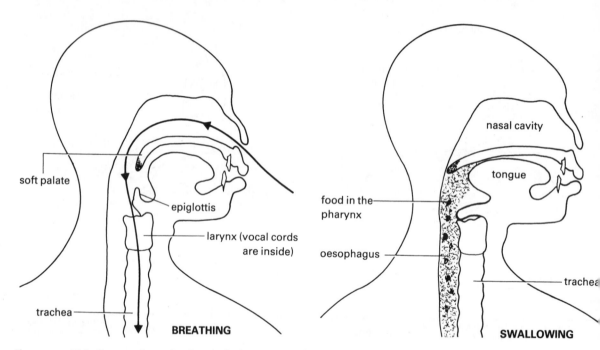

Figure 20.5 *This diagram shows the changes in the upper respiratory tract during breathing and swallowing. Note the positions during swallowing of the soft palate (to stop food going into the nose) and of the epiglottis (to stop food going into the larynx and trachea, bronchi and lungs). This does not occur when the patient is deeply unconscious.*

A system of blood vessels (called the pulmonary circulation) goes through the lungs. The pulmonary artery takes blood pumped by the right side of the heart. This blood is rather blue and is low in oxygen and high in carbon dioxide. The blood vessels divide into smaller and smaller vessels. When they are very small capillaries, exchange of oxygen and carbon dioxide occurs between their blood and the air in the alveoli. (See Figure 20.11.) The capillaries then join up to form veins. The blood in them is taken back to the left side of the heart by the pulmonary veins.

The blood in the pulmonary vein is more red, and it has a high content of oxygen and a low content of carbon dioxide.

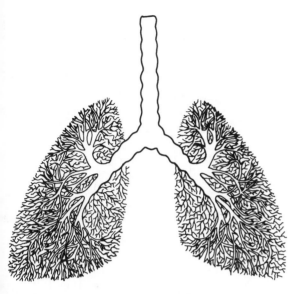

Figure 20.6 *Diagram to show how the bronchi divide to form smaller and smaller bronchi (like branches of a tree). The smallest air passages lead into air sacs or alveoli (see Figure 20.11).*

The left–over air with high carbon dioxide content and low oxygen content is breathed out of the lungs through the bronchi, etc. and fresh air with high oxygen and low carbon dioxide content is breathed into the alveoli.

Pathology of the respiratory tract

Most diseases of the respiratory tract are caused by infection. These infections are usually caused by viral, bacterial or tuberculosis organisms; but there are others. HIV infection decreases immunity and allows respiratory infections to become much more common and severe. Tobacco smoke irritates and destroys the lungs. Diseases caused by smoking (especially chronic obstructive lung disease (COLD) and lung cancer) will become more common as so many young people in developing countries have started to smoke tobacco. Some diseases are caused by allergy. Some are caused by dust and fumes in mines and factories. A few are caused by other things known and unknown.

Symptoms and signs of diseases of the respiratory tract

Symptoms of diseases of the upper respiratory tract

Ear

• pain in ear
• discharge from ear
• deafness

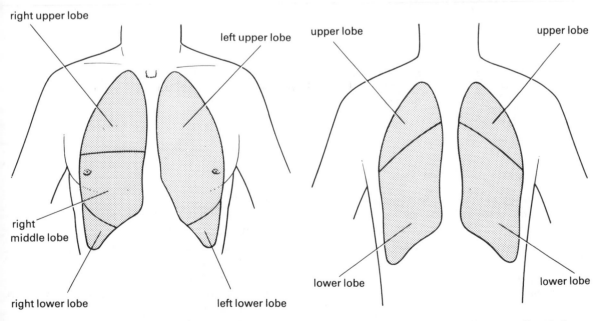

Figure 20.7 *Diagrams to show the position of the lungs in the chest and to show which lobes of the lungs are affected when abnormal signs are found during examination of the front and back of the chest.*

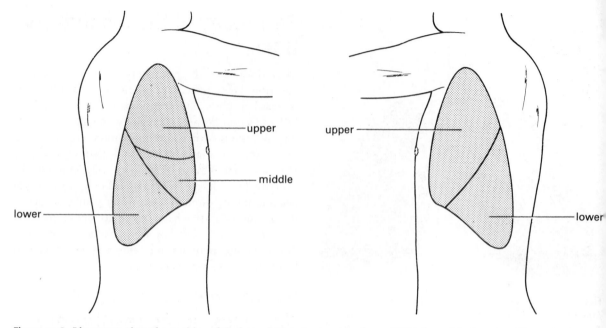

Figure 20.8 *Diagram to show the position of the lungs in the chest and to show which lobes of the lung are affected when abnormal signs are found during examination of the lateral (side of the) chest.*

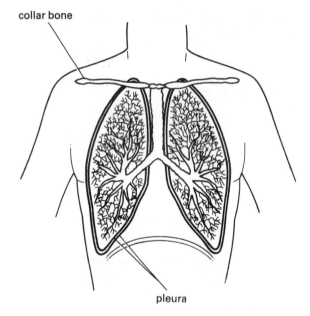

Figure 20.9 *This diagram shows the relationship of the two layers of pleura to each other. (See also Figure 20.1.) There is normally no air and only a little fluid in each pleural space or cavity.*

Nose

• nasal discharge
  – clear fluid
  – pus
  – blood
• pain in face or forehead (over paranasal sinuses)

Throat

• sore throat
• hoarse voice or loss of voice

All

• cough

For causes and management of these symptoms, see pages 302–307 onwards.

Signs of diseases of the upper respiratory tract

Ear

• external canal
  – discharge (clear fluid, pus, blood)
  – foreign body
  – injury
  – dermatitis
  – inflammation of the whole canal
  – furuncle (pimple or boil)
• drum
  – retraction (pulled in)
  – bulging (pushed out)
  – inflammation (dilated vessels, dull or red or yellow, loss of light reflex)
  – perforation (hole)
• hearing – all degrees of deafness

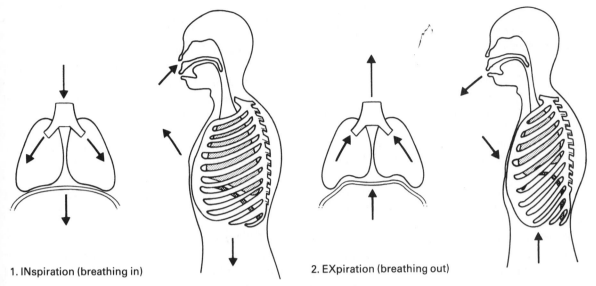

1. INspiration (breathing in)   2. EXpiration (breathing out)

Figure 20.10 *Diagram showing how the ribs and diaphragm are used to ventilate the lungs.*

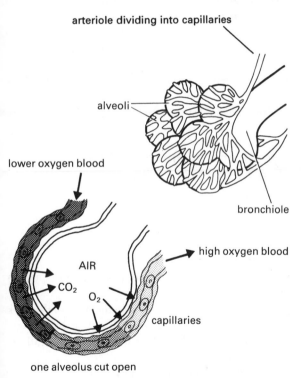

arteriole dividing into capillaries

alveoli

lower oxygen blood

bronchiole

high oxygen blood

AIR

CO_2

O_2

capillaries

one alveolus cut open

Figure 20.11 *Diagrams showing anatomy and physiology of the small air sacs and blood vessels.*

Nose

• discharge
 – watery fluid
 – pus
 – blood

• mucous membrane
 – inflammation
 – thickened blue-pink 'allergic' appearance

Mouth and throat

• inflammation of all or a part (especially tonsils)
• pus over a part (especially tonsils)
• post-nasal discharge

All

• cough

Use the auriscope to inspect the external ear canal and the ear drum like this:

Hold the auriscope in your right hand. Pull the pinna (outside ear) upwards and backwards with the finger and thumb of the left hand to straighten the external ear canal. Rest your right hand on the side of the patient's face. Then, if the patient suddenly moves, your hand will also move, and the auriscope cannot push into his ear and damage it. Use the largest speculum possible to push into the ear without hurting the patient much.

It may hurt the patient a little to push the speculum of the auriscope into the canal. There may be wax in the canal. Both of these things are normal.

Pain on moving the ear, swelling and redness of the skin lining the canal (either in one area or involving the whole canal), or pus in the canal itself, all suggest inflammation of the external canal (external ear inflammation).

The ear drum is normally white. It also reflects the light, in its lower part, as a bright white triangle called the 'light reflex' (Figure 20.12).

The ear drum may be retracted (pulled back) if the Eustachian tube is blocked and the air is absorbed into and taken away by the blood.

The ear drum may be pink or red, small dilated blood vessels may be seen running in from the edge, the light reflex may not be present and fluid levels may be seen behind the drum in early acute inflammation of the middle ear.

A little later in acute middle ear inflammation tissue fluid goes into the passages and pushes the ear drum outwards (i.e. it bulges). As it cannot bulge where it is held in the centre by a little bone, the drum then looks like the buttocks of a baby at a breech birth.

The drum may be perforated (broken) and pus may come out of the hole and even fill the ear canal in late acute middle ear inflammation.

If you cannot see the eardrum clearly because of wax or pus in the canal, gently clean the canal with a swab (or by syringing) until you can see the drum clearly (see page 281).

To test the hearing of an ear

Block the other ear of the patient with one of your fingers which you keep moving in his ear (to make a noise so that he can hear nothing else with that ear); do not let him see your mouth; ask in a quiet voice questions which need answers that are more than just 'yes' or 'no'.

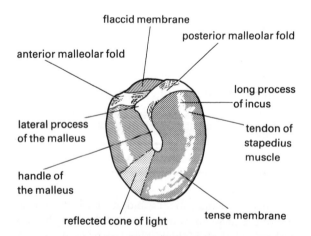

Figure 20.12 *Diagram to show the normal left ear drum, also called tympanic membrane. The names of the parts of the membrane and of the small bones (see Figure 20.4) are not important. It is important to look at the ear drums of many normal as well as sick patients, so that you can recognise a normal ear drum.*

Examination of the nose using a torch or auriscope

Put the patient's head back and press gently on the end of his nose. This will open the nostrils and allow you to look in. If you have a large speculum for the auriscope, use this to look inside the nose – you will be able to see much better.

Red, swollen mucous membrane will be seen in acute rhinitis. If the infection is viral, you may see watery discharge on the mucous membrane. If the infection is bacterial, you may see pus on the mucous membrane.

A blue or pale, swollen, watery-looking mucous membrane suggests an allergic rhinitis or hay fever.

Tenderness of sinuses

Tenderness can be tested for by pressing firmly or tapping the bones containing the sinuses (above and below the eyes).

Examination of the mouth and throat, using a torch and tongue depressor

Examine the inside of the mouth, the tongue, the soft palate, the tonsils and the back of the throat for redness and swelling and pus from acute inflammation. You may need to press the tongue down and ask the patient to say 'Ah' to see the back of the throat wall. You may see pus from the nose running down the back of the throat (called post-nasal discharge or drip).

Symptoms of disease of the lower respiratory tract (lung)

- Cough
- Sputum
  - white (mucus)
  - yellow or green or brown (pus)
  - jellylike (mucus)
- Haemoptysis (blood coughed up or blood in sputum)
- Pain in chest
  - tracheal (tearing or burning in the front of the neck or centre of the chest present only on coughing)
  - pleural (at the side of the chest, worse on breathing or coughing)
  - central dull continuous ache
- Shortness of breath
  - on doing exercise (what?) or on walking (how far?) or on climbing stairs (how many?)
  - at rest in the day sitting down
  - at rest in the night in bed
- Wheezing

For causes and management of these symptoms, see pages 302–307 onwards.

Table 20.1 Summary of the symptoms and signs of the common lung diseases.

	Pneumothorax	Fluid in pleural cavity	Lobar pneumonia	Broncho-pneumonia	Acute bronchitis	Asthma	Chronic bronchitis, emphysema†	Bronchiectasis	Laryngeal or tracheal obstruction
Temperature	varies	varies	*raised	often raised	*often raised	*normal NOT raised	*normal	sometimes raised	varies
Sputum	varies	varies	*pus	pus	*pus sometimes	*thick mucus NOT pus	*mucus	*pus or mucus	varies
Respiration rate	sometimes fast	sometimes fast	*fast	often fast	sometimes fast	slow	usually normal	normal	slow
Respiration type	sometimes shallow	sometimes shallow	*shallow	often shallow	normal	deep	usually normal	normal	*deep stridor
Movement	*decreased	*decreased	*decreased	normal	normal	decreased	decreased	normal	normal or decreased
Percussion	very resonant	*very dull 'stony' dull	*dull	normal	normal	normal or more resonant	normal or more resonant	normal	normal
Breath sounds	*reduced or absent	*reduced or absent	*reduced	normal	normal	normal or reduced	normal or reduced	normal reduced	normal or reduced
Type of breath sounds	varies or absent	varies or absent	*bronchial	normal	normal	normal	normal	normal	normal
Wheezes or rhonchi	none	none	none	none	usually present	*present	present	none	*stridor
Crackles or crepitations	none	none	*present	*present	usually absent	usually absent	usually absent	*present	none

* These are the important signs for this condition.
† Also called chronic obstructive lung disease (COLD) or chronic obstructive airways disease (COAD) or chronic obstructive pulmonary disease (COPD).

Table 20.1 summarises the symptoms and signs of the common lung diseases.

Signs of disease of the lower respiratory tract (LRT)

Look for

- Rate of breathing (16–20 breaths/minute normal; above 20 abnormal; above 30 very abnormal)
- Type of breathing (deep or shallow, use of extra muscles, insuction, grunting, prolonged expiration, etc.)
- Deformity of chest or spine

Palpate or feel for

- Decreased movement of (1) all of chest, (2) part or parts of chest

Percuss or tap for

- Dullness or abnormal resonance of (1) all of chest or (2) part or parts of chest

Auscultate or listen for

- Amount of breath sounds (normal or decreased)
- Breath sounds (bronchial instead of normal)
- Crackles (or crepitations)
- Wheezes (or rhonchi)
- Rubs

in { all of chest or parts or parts of chest }

Ask the patient to cough. *Listen* to type of cough. *Look at* any sputum. (Is it pus, mucus or blood?)

Examination of the rate and type of breathing or ventilation (but often called incorrectly 'respiration')

The normal rate is 16–20 breaths/minute. The type of breathing is often more important than the rate.

Is the patient distressed or not? Is the patient taking rapid shallow breaths which suggest pneumonia, or deep wheezing breaths which suggest asthma? Is there any indrawing of the soft tissues above and below the clavicle and between and below the ribs ('insuction') and dilation of the nostrils on breathing in? Is there grunting during breathing out? Insuction, dilation of the nose and grunting mean that the patient is having to do much extra work in order to breathe. This is common in pneumonia (especially in children), and in asthma and chronic respiratory disease (especially in the old).

Wheezing is when you hear the whistling noises of the air moving through the air passages without the stethoscope. The causes are the same as for wheezes or rhonchi heard with a stethoscope (see page 273).

Stridor is when you hear a loud whistling or crowing noise during breathing *in*. (Noisy breathing *out* is not as important.) It is caused by obstruction of the larynx or trachea. Stridor is always dangerous. Stridor is very dangerous if there is also insuction, rib recession (lower ribs moving *in* not *out* during breathing in), and the neck and abdominal muscles are being used for breathing.

Ask the patient to take a deep breath and look at the chest movement once again. Stand back from the patient when looking for these signs. See how well the chest moves. If he has great difficulty in moving both sides of the chest wall, it is said the chest wall is 'fixed' – usually a sign of over- or hyper-inflation. Is one side moving and the other not moving? *The side which does not move is the side with the disease in it.*

Palpation of the chest (Figure 20.13)

Palpate the chest to find out if there is decreased movement of (1) all of the chest, or (2) part or parts of the chest.

You must find out from examining many normal people how much chest movement is normal – it is usually more than 1 cm on each side.

Disease affecting all of the lungs will cause decreased movement of all of the chest and the same amount of decrease on both sides. This decreased movement of all the chest is caused by chronic obstructive lung disease and acute asthma.

Disease of one part of the lung causes decreased movement of the chest on the same side. This decreased movement of one part of the chest is caused by lobar pneumonia, tuberculous pneumonia, pleural fluid, lung cancer, pneumothorax and others.

> The side of the chest which moves less is the abnormal side.

Percussion of the chest

Press the middle finger of the left hand firmly over the area you are percussing. Place the finger in the same line or direction as the ribs in that area and between the ribs (over the muscles between the ribs). Percuss or hit the middle of this finger in a light and loose fashion with the bent middle finger of the right hand.

Percuss the chest wall in a systematic fashion. Percuss the sides front and back of the chest wall (see Figure 20.14).

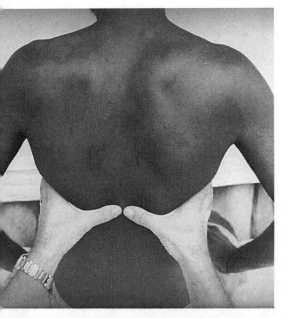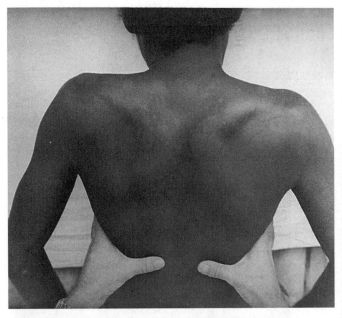

Figure 20.13 *Photographs to show method of palpation of the chest for movement. Press your finger-tips firmly into the lateral chest wall so that they stay in the same place between the ribs. Put your finger-tips in such a position that when the patient breathes right out, then the ends of your thumbs just meet in the midline of the spine. (See left photograph.) Then get the patient to take slow deep breath in (and out). Let the palms of your hands and your thumbs slide over the skin; but do not let your finger-tips move. The movement of each side of the chest is shown by how far the ends of your thumbs move away from the spine in the midline. (See right photograph.)*

Percuss the *same* part of *each* side of the chest and decide if the percussion note is normal or not and equal or not on both sides before percussing another part.

Feel *and* listen for the type of percussion note. The percussion note may be either dull or resonant (hollow sounding).

Normally the chest over the lungs is resonant, but it may be a little dull if the person is very muscular or fat. The area of resonance moves down 2–5 cm during breathing in as the diaphragm moves down and the lungs expand.

Percussion over the heart, liver and large muscle masses in the shoulders will give a dull note.

Percussion over the air in the stomach will give a very resonant note (see Figure 20.15).

The percussion note will be dull if anything more solid than lung filled with air is underneath.

The percussion note will be dull over an area of pneumonia because there is a lot of fluid in the alveoli. The percussion note will be very dull when there is pleural fluid as no air is under the chest wall there.

In patients who are acutely ill with breathlessness and fever, see if the percussion causes pain. Pain on per-cussion is a sign of pleurisy usually due to pneumonia.

The percussion note will be very hollow if only air and not air and lung are underneath the chest wall, e.g. pneumothorax.

Auscultation of the chest

Listen in all areas including the axillae using a stethoscope (see Figure 20.14).

Listen in one place and then in the same place on the opposite side of the chest next. Decide if the breath sounds are present or not (air entry is normal or not), if they are normal or not, and if crackles or wheezes are present or not in the *same* places on *both* sides, before you listen to another place on the chest.

It is better to use the bell of the stethoscope when you listen to the breath sounds. Do not press hard when you use the bell.

Listen for three things when you auscultate:

1. *The quantity of the breath sounds* (amount of air entry).

   Compare both sides of the chest and see if breath sounds are the same. The breath sounds may be loud, or soft, or absent. Breath sounds are softer or absent, if less air is entering that part of the lung under the

271

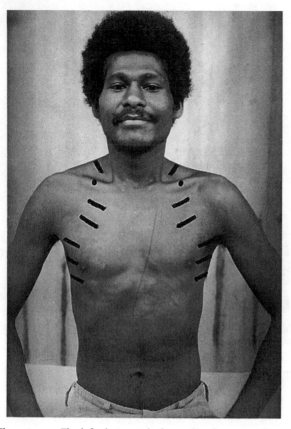 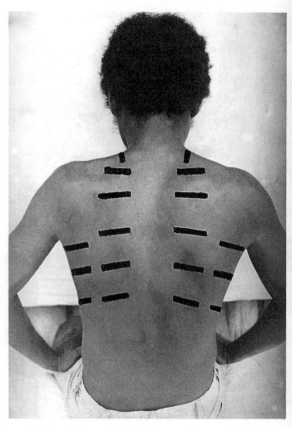

Figure 20.14 *The left photograph shows sites for percussion and auscultation of the posterior and lateral chest wall. The right photograph shows sites for percussion and auscultation of the posterior and lateral chest wall.*

stethoscope. Breath sounds may be softer (or less) over an area of pneumonia and may be softer or even absent over a collection of pleural fluid. Breath sounds may be soft in all areas if not much air is entering any part of the lung, e.g. severe chronic obstructive lung disease or very severe asthma.

2. *Quality of the breath sounds* (type of breath sounds). The breath sounds normally have a quality which is a bit like the sound of rubbing the hands together or the rustling of leaves in a tree. These types of breath sounds are called 'vesicular'.

Over the trachea the normal breath sounds you hear are louder, and sound something like blowing air over the top of a bottle. These types of breath sounds are called 'bronchial'. You hear bronchial breath sounds or bronchial breathing at the chest wall only if something solid *in the lung* (not in the pleura) conducts these breath sounds from the trachea to the chest wall.

You hear bronchial breathing only over large areas of pneumonia or tumours (and very occasion-

ally over very large tuberculous cavities with thick fibrous tissues around them, or at the upper level of plural fluid which squashes the lung into a solid mass). You do not often hear bronchial breathing in diseases other than pneumonia. Bronchial breath sounds are not always easy to hear; but are very helpful if they are heard.

3. *Added sounds.*

Added sounds are sounds which are not normally present. There are three kinds of added sounds which you may hear – 'crackles' which used to be called 'crepitations' (crackling or bubbling sounds), 'wheezes' which used to be called 'rhonchi' (whistling sounds) and a 'pleural rub' (a rubbing or scraping sound).

Crackles or *crepitations* are the crackling noises made by alveoli or bronchi which are closed but snap open and vibrate, and by air bubbling through fluid in bronchi. Causes include:

(a) acute infections of the alveoli (lobar pneumonia, bronchopneumonia);

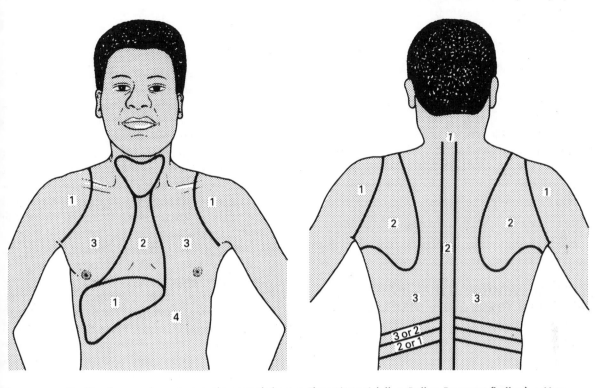

Figure 20.15 *Quality of percussion note over the normal chest. 1. Flat or 'stony' dull. 2. Dull. 3. Resonant (hollow). 4. Very resonant (very hollow).*

(b) chronic infections of the alveoli (tuberculosis);

(c) chronic damage to the bronchi with fluid in the bronchi (bronchiectasis);

(d) oedema of the lungs (left heart failure); and

(e) some cases of chronic obstructive lung disease, and after some attacks of asthma.

Wheezes, which used to be called *rhonchi*, are whistling sounds made by air going through narrowed bronchi. (These sounds are also called wheezing, when you do not need a stethoscope to hear them.) They are often louder during breathing out. Causes include:

(a) asthma,

(b) acute bronchitis,

(c) chronic obstructive lung disease.

(d) foreign body or tumour in a large airway if heard on only one side or part.

A *pleural rub* is a creaking, grating or rubbing noise usually heard in breathing in and out over one area. It is not changed by coughing (wheezes often are), but may be changed by pressing hard on the chest and thereby changing the position of the pleura. It is caused by pleural inflammation.

The important conditions that produce abnormal chest signs

1. Obstruction of the trachea or larynx, e.g.
   - infections, e.g. croup, acute bacterial epiglottitis, laryngotracheobronchitis, diphtheria,
   - allergy (angio-oedema),
   - foreign body inhaled,
   - tumour.
2. Obstruction of the bronchi, e.g.
   - pus, e.g. acute bronchitis,
   - mucus, e.g. chronic obstructive lung disease,
   - spasm of the muscles, e.g. asthma,
   - foreign body,
   - tumour.
3. Fluid in the alveoli, e.g.
   - heart failure (left heart),
   - pneumonia (all types).
4. Solid lung (consolidation), e.g.
   - lobar pneumonia.
5. Fluid in the pleural cavity, e.g.
   - watery – effusion,
   - pus – empyema,
   - blood – haemothorax.

6. Air in the pleural cavity
- pneumothorax.

Positions of lung lesions (see Figure 20.7)

Upper lobes or parts

- suspect TB

Lower lobes or parts

- suspect bacterial pneumonia
- suspect TB in patient with HIV infection if it does not get better on treatment for pneumonia
- suspect inhaled food, vomit, etc.

Right middle lobe or lower front right side of chest

- suspect TB and inhaled foreign body, food or vomit as well as ordinary bacterial pneumonia

General symptoms that may be caused by respiratory disease

1. Fever
2. Weight loss
3. Malaise

General signs that may be caused by respiratory disease

1. The temperature may rise in any infection.
2. The pulse rate may increase in any infection, or any disease of the lungs that does not put enough oxygen into the blood.
3. The breathing rate and type of breathing may be abnormal (see page 270).
4. Cyanosis is the blue colour of the blood caused by low oxygen concentration in the haemoglobin of the blood.

It is easiest to see cyanosis where blood is close to the surface of the body, and there is little or no pigment (e.g. the mucous membranes of the tongue and inside the mouth, conjunctivae, and under the fingernails and toenails). Cyanosis is caused by haemoglobin that does not have oxygen. (Haemoglobin with oxygen is red. Haemoglobin without oxygen is blue.)

There must be 1.5–5 g of haemoglobin without oxygen in each dl (100 ml) of blood to make the blood look blue. In a very severely anaemic person (with a haemoglobin of less than 5 g/dl) you may not see cyanosis, even if their haemoglobin does not have much oxygen. They may not have the necessary amount of haemoglobin without oxygen to show the blueness of cyanosis.

If the blood in all parts of the body is blue, i.e. there is cyanosis of the tongue *and* the fingernails and toenails, this may be caused by:

(a) the patient not breathing enough (for any reason);
(b) some diseases of the lungs, especially pneumonia;
(c) some diseases of the heart;
(d) some poisons in the blood which stop the haemoglobin combining with oxygen (e.g. sodium nitrite in 'anti-rust' tablets).

If only part of the body is cyanosed and blue but the tongue is a normal pink, then the lungs, heart and blood must be normal, the blood must be circulating slowly through just the cyanosed area, and most of the oxygen is being taken out before the blood leaves that area.

Be careful not to mistake the blue colour in the pigment or normal colouring of some people's mouths and lips for cyanosis.

5. Clubbing of the nails. Clubbing is said to be present, when on looking at the back of the finger from the side, the normal angle between the nail and the finger is lost. Later on, the end of the finger may become swollen, and look like the head of a drumstick (see Figure 20.16).

Clubbing is usually caused by chronic respiratory diseases, but usually only those caused by chronic infection or cancer. It sometimes occurs in heart disease (some infective and congenital), chronic liver and bowel disease and other conditions. Very occasionally it is inherited.

Do not call curved finger nails (which are not important), clubbing. With curved nails there is still a normal angle between the base (or back or top) of the nail and the back of the finger.

Clubbing does not occur with usual chest infections (but sometimes does with tuberculosis) or with chronic obstructive lung disease or with asthma. If clubbing is present, look for a serious chronic disease, especially chronic infection in the chest or lung cancer.

Symptoms and signs of HIV infection in patients with respiratory disease

Persons who have decreased immunity from HIV infection are very likely to get respiratory diseases, especially acute bacterial sinusitis and pneumonia, pulmonary tuberculosis and unusual lung infections. In fact, a respiratory infection may be the first illness a patient with HIV infection gets.

Always check people with respiratory disease for the common signs of HIV infection, e.g. itchy papular skin rash, herpes simplex, herpes zoster (shingles) scars, oral thrush, angular cheilitis, gingivitis, mouth

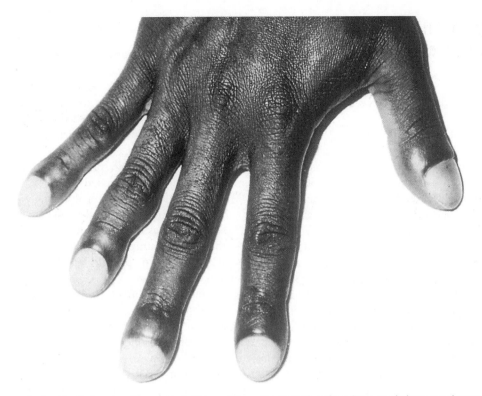

Figure 20.16 *A patient's hands with severe clubbing of the nails. Note that there is no angle between the proximal (body) end of the thumb nail and the back of the thumb. In this severe clubbing the whole of the end of the finger is swollen. The fingernail does not seem to be firmly attached and seems to be floating (or be fluctuant) on top of the tissues at the end of the finger.*

ulcers, oral hairy leukoplakia, symmetrical generalised lymphadenopathy, etc. (See Chapter 19 pages 222–234.)

Send blood for HIV test after counselling if HIV possible.

> Always think of HIV infection in every patient with respiratory disease, but especially:
>
> 1. acute sinusitis
> 2. pneumonia
> 3. tuberculosis
> 4. unusual lung infections.

Tests in respiratory disorders

Chest X-ray

A chest X-ray is not usually possible in a health centre. It also takes a lot of training to be able to understand and use an X-ray properly. Fortunately, most conditions can be accurately diagnosed and treated without the use of an X-ray.

Sputum examination

1. For AFB (see Chapter 14 pages 108–109).
2. For other bacteria and parasites.

   Gram stain for pus cells and the types of bacteria and culture of these bacteria, to test to what antibiotics they are sensitive, needs sputum to be kept at body temperature and arrive at the hospital laboratory within a few hours after being spat up. A Gram stain is possible if the sputum is put on a slide, smeared, fixed and sent. Examination for parasites, e.g. lung fluke, strongyloides, etc. is also possible under the microscope.

Blood test for HIV infection

See Chapter 19 pages 233–235.

Tests of lung function

1. Peak expiratory flow rate (see pages 310–311).
2. Spirometry is much more helpful but rarely available.

Summary of methods of treatment of respiratory diseases

1. Treat infections with antibiotics; or, if TB, anti–TB drugs.

   Use penicillin first. It is usually effective. In some places where penicillin is not freely available, or where the common organism such as pneumococci may have developed high resistance to penicillin or where injections are if possible not given because of the risk of HIV infection, other drugs such as sulfamethoxazole/trimethoprim (SMX + TMP or co-trimoxazole) are used first. One of the disadvantages of such oral SMX + TMP is that all of the drugs may not be taken for the full course by the patient. Another disadvantage is that in some communities, there are a lot of reactions, especially of the skin, to sulfamethoxazole. Another problem is that many organisms have become resistant to SMX + TMP, especially if SMX + TMP is being used for HIV patients in your area. You need to find out from your Health Department what you should do and change the book as needed. Amoxicillin or ampicillin, especially if given together with clavulanic acid (co-amoxyclav), is very good treatment but is more expensive and has the above problem of not all being taken if given orally. Give chloramphenicol instead of penicillin if the infection is severe and may cause death. Ceftriaxone or other third generation cephalosporin by IMI or IVI is sometimes given in hospitals instead of chloramphenicol. Use tetracycline or doxycycline if penicillin or SMX + TMP does not work and the patient is not likely to die soon from the infection, and especially if he may need repeated courses of antibiotics. Do not give tetracycline to a pregnant woman or a child; use amoxicillin or ampicillin or erythromycin instead (or, even better, amoxicillin and erythromycin). If available, amoxicillin + clavulanic acid (co-amoxyclav) and erythromycin would be the best treatment for all non-pregnant patients if penicillin or SMX + TMP did not work. Give chloramphenicol if penicillin and then tetracycline or amoxicillin and erythromycin do not work; but look first for other reasons why the antibiotics are not working. See Chapter 11 pages 56–61.

   Give streptomycin *only* for tuberculosis. Do not use it for any other respiratory infection. Give at least two anti-TB drugs to all cases of TB for every dose of the planned treatment. See Chapter 14 page 112.

2. Treat bronchial narrowing (causing wheezing and/or rhonchi) like this:
   (a) Treat the cause if possible (antibiotics in infection; stopping smoking if COLD, etc.)
   (b) Give epinephrine/adrenaline injection or salbutamol (or alternative) to inhale (breathe in) or to take orally; and if needed
   (c) Ipratropium bromide (or alternative) to inhale and if needed
   (d) Adrenocorticosteroid preferably to inhale or taken orally; and if needed
   (e) Aminophylline or theophylline orally or injection or suppository; but does not help more if the patient has asthma and has already had all of the above treatment in proper doses.

3. Remove sputum or pus (if present) from the airways like this:
   (a) Encourage a patient to breathe deeply and cough sputum up.
   (b) Suck out the pharynx using a mechanised sucker if the patient cannot cough.
   (c) Physiotherapy (see page 299).
   (d) Postural drainage.
   (e) Postural sleeping (with head of bed down).
   But do not continue with any of these methods if the treatment produces less than 15 ml of sputum.

4. Treat a cough like this:
   (a) Treat the cause.
   (b) Remove sputum from airways (See 3 above).
   (c) Do *not* give an effective anti-cough drug if the patient has sputum, as any sputum present should be coughed out. Codeine phosphate (and morphine) are effective in stopping coughing.
   (d) 'Cough medicine' does not help. Give it only if the patient wants medicine very much, and does not need effective drugs.

5. The patient, if a smoker, should stop smoking.
   All the lung conditions are made worse by smoking tobacco or marijuana, etc.
   Smoking causes chronic obstructive lung disease and lung cancer (and blood vessel and other diseases).
   It is very important that the patient does not start smoking again.

6. Treat low oxygen in the blood, which has caused cyanosis of the whole body including the tongue, with intranasal oxygen 1–4 litres/minute (see Chapter 7 page 34). Do not give more than 1–2 litres/minute if patient has COLD as it could stop the patient breathing.

7. Treat swelling of the nasal mucous membrane with:

(a) Ephedrine or other vasoconstrictor nasal drops, which narrow the blood vessels and make the swelling of the mucous membrane less; but do not give for more than 7–10 days.

(b) Oral antihistamines (e.g. chlorphenamine or promethazine) if allergy.

8. Analgesics if pain. If the pain stops the patient coughing up sputum, give analgesics, but you *must* then *make* the patient cough up the sputum (see 3 above), otherwise the infection will get worse.

9. Rest and nursing are important for acute severe diseases.

Prevention of respiratory disease

1. You can do one thing which is more effective than anything else to prevent respiratory disease. That is to *prevent children from starting to smoke tobacco and help people who do smoke tobacco stop smoking.* Smoking tobacco is the most common preventable cause of disease and death in the world today.

The World Health Organization has estimated that there are about 1100 million tobacco smokers in the world and about 75% of these are now in developing countries. It is predicted that by the year 2025 tobacco smoking will cause 10 million deaths each year and 7 million of these deaths will be in developing countries. During this century it is expected that half a billion deaths will be caused by smoking tobacco. Most of these people suffer years of terrible disease with shortness of breath, pain and other discomforts before they die.

Although the tobacco companies and others claim that smoking does not cause disease and death, this is untrue. Scientific studies have proved that tobacco causes disease and death, including:

• chronic bronchitis and emphysema (or chronic obstructive lung disease),
• lung cancer,
• many other cancers including of the lips, mouth, oesophagus, kidney, bladder and others,
• heart attacks,
• strokes,
• many other cardiovascular diseases including peripheral vascular disease,
• pregnancy complications, lower birthweight babies and more likely death of the newborn of a smoking mother,
• lung disease in the children of parents who smoke.

Most of these diseases only come 20 or more years after the person starts to smoke and many people who smoke do not think they will be the ones affected. However, one in every three smokers dies earlier than might be expected due to smoking. Younger people may be more influenced by the studies which show smoking does cause wrinkles and loss of 'good looks', a decrease in athletic and sports performance, decrease in sexual performance and enjoyment, and decreased fertility.

Once smokers give up tobacco their health starts to improve almost immediately. They also have more money to spend on more worthwhile things.

It is therefore our duty to:

(a) Help educate the population, especially children before they start smoking, about the dangers of smoking and the benefits of not smoking. We should support all health education programmes and do what we can to help in our own community. For example, if we can get a well known local sporting hero to support the programme (as long as he or she is a committed non-smoker), this could be a big help.

(b) Advise smokers to stop and encourage children not to start smoking whenever we see patients as part of routine health education.

(c) Give literature with facts about smoking and how to stop smoking to patients.

(d) Try to organise and help 'support groups' for people trying to stop smoking.

(e) Advise people that for about the same cost as cigarettes, they can buy 'nicotine replacement therapy'. Nicotine is the addictive chemical in tobacco (although it is not the chemical in smoke which does most of the damage). If a smoker uses nicotine therapy instead of smoking, it is much safer. More importantly, as it produces less pleasure than smoking, most people can then after a couple of months slowly reduce the nicotine and eventually stop it (more easily than they can reduce and then stop smoking tobacco). Nicotine replacement therapy comes in the form of:
• chewing gum or tablets,
• transdermal patches,
• powder to inhale.
The most effective treatment is to use a patch or gum throughout the day, together with powder to inhale when there is a craving for a cigarette. It is important that patients use the therapy correctly, according to the instructions on the packet.

(f) If smokers want to stop but really are not able to, refer them to the Medical Officer to see if they would be suitable for a trial of a drug such as bupropion or varenicline. This drug, which they would have to buy, together with the above things, gives people a very good chance of stopping smoking.

(g) Of course, it is essential that you and all health workers set a good example by never smoking tobacco.

If all of the above things are done (and (f) is not usually needed) many smokers can stop smoking, prolong their lives and save themselves years of suffering.

2. *Prevention of measles and whooping cough* by vaccination will stop many people having damage done to their lungs and upper respiratory tract when they are infants. Their lungs will then be less likely to have diseases such as bronchiectasis when they become adults. Otitis media and sinusitis will be less likely in childhood or adulthood.

3. *Early and proper treatment of respiratory infections* will cure them and not let them go on to cause chronic infections such as bronchiectasis and chronic sinusitis.

4. Tuberculosis is a very common cause of lung disease. BCG vaccination may reduce the chance of miliary and meningeal tuberculosis. *Early diagnosis by sputum tests for AFB and proper treatment with DOTS* will stop the infection destroying a lot of lung tissue. This is important as the patient cannot, of course, grow new lungs to replace damaged or destroyed lung tissue.

Diseases of the respiratory system

The common cold

The common cold is an acute viral infection of the upper respiratory tract. It can be caused by one of many viruses.

Symptoms may include sneezing, watery nasal discharge, sore throat, cough, watery eyes, mild fever and malaise.

On examination, there may be mild fever and red swollen watery mucous membranes of the upper respiratory tract.

There are no abnormal signs in the chest and the sputum has no pus in it. There are no general signs of severe disease.

Complications can occur, including acute otitis media, acute sinusitis, tonsillitis, acute bronchitis and pneumonia caused by bacteria. These complications may need treatment with antibiotics.

Treatment

Examine all the respiratory tract to see if there is a complication which needs treatment (especially otitis media).

Treat as an outpatient.

Tell the patient to come back if a complication develops (especially pain in the ear or deafness; or shortness of breath or pus in the sputum).

There are no anti-viral drugs to help. You can only treat the symptoms:

1. Rest may be needed.
2. Give paracetamol 0.5–1 g or acetylsalicylic acid 300–600 mg each 6 hours if needed for headache or aches and pains.
3. Give ephedrine or other vasoconstrictor nasal drops (which narrow the blood vessels), if the nose is blocked.
4. Cough mixture does not help. Give it only if the patient wants medicine.
5. Give antimalarials if malaria is possible. (See Chapter 13 pages 79, 80.)

Influenza

Influenza is an acute viral infection of *all the respiratory tract*. It is caused by one of the influenza viruses (Type A, B or C).

It is very contagious from 1 day before symptoms for 7–10 days. It is transmitted by inhaling droplets or airborne droplet nuclei from infected sneezing or coughing persons; and also by direct contact for 2 hours with things touched or sneezed or coughed on by infected persons.

Usually it is an epidemic disease. Type A is the most likely cause of an epidemic.

Severe general symptoms and signs of infection occur:
• sudden start of the symptoms,
• fever,
• pains all over the body,
• loss of appetite, and
• feeling too sick to walk around.

But only mild respiratory tract infection symptoms and signs occur:
• cough (but little or no sputum),
• sore throat,

• tracheal pain, and

• slight redness of the upper respiratory mucous membranes.

There is improvement after a few days; but the patient may not get better for two weeks and may feel tired or depressed for many weeks.

If influenza virus pneumonia develops, without first improving, the patient gets worse and worse with cough, haemoptysis, shortness of breath, cyanosis and often death.

If a secondary bacterial pneumonia develops, usually after first improving, the patient gets suddenly worse (see page 288) and the cause is usually a pneumococcus or staphylococcus. (Staphylococci are often resistant to ordinary penicillin.)

Viral pneumonia can occur in all ages including healthy young adults, who may die. Secondary bacterial pneumonia is more common in old people, or patients with chronic and lung diseases. Pneumonia is the usual cause of death in influenza epidemics.

Examine all the respiratory tract, and look at any sputum. Find out if there is a complication (especially pneumonia) which needs treatment.

Treat uncomplicated cases as an outpatient.

Tell the patient to come back if any complication develops (especially bad cough, shortness of breath or pus in sputum).

Treat the symptoms as for a common cold (see page 278) – rest, paracetamol or acetylsalicylic acid and possibly antimalarial drugs.

Admit for inpatient treatment if any serious complications, especially pneumonia, develop and treat as usual. If improvement in pneumonia is not rapid, change to chloramphenicol (see page 289). (Di)cloxacillin may be needed for some staphylococci.

Notify (page 36) the Medical Officer if an epidemic occurs (e.g. more than 20 cases in 1 month), or if any deaths, especially from a viral type pneumonia (see above) and in a previously healthy person, occur.

Control and prevention Immunisation is effective but expensive, difficult to organise and usually not possible in developing countries. Patients should cover their noses and mouths when sneezing and coughing; not spit; and stay at home for 7–10 days. Others should keep 2 m from infected patients; avoid crowds; and (as hands may have got viruses on them) wash hands often and try not to touch the face, nose or mouth.

H1N1 2009 influenza A ('swine flu')

See Appendix 4 page 310.

H5N1 (avian) influenza A ('bird flu')

There is a Type A influenza virus with H5N1 glycoprotein in its outside coat which at present is causing an epidemic of influenza with many deaths (i.e. it is virulent) in birds – but it is not very infectious to humans. It is called 'avian influenza' or 'bird flu' (avian means belonging to a bird). There is a big worry that a person or a pig, both of which *can* be infected by both human and avian influenza, will get an infection with *both* human and avian influenza virus *at the same time,* when it is *possible* that the two viruses will combine to form a new virus. This new virus may be (1) very infectious (like the present human influenza) and (2) very virulent and cause many deaths (like the present avian influenza). As well, no people (*nobody*), even those previously infected or immunised against human influenza, would have immunity to this new virus. Were this to happen, as well as the usual influenza symptoms and signs, viral pneumonia, gastroenteritis, encephalitis, conjunctivitis, bleeding and likely death would occur even in previously healthy people. In addition, a huge epidemic or even pandemic (epidemic affecting the whole world) could occur. Such 'new' viruses were formed at least three times in the last century. The influenza pandemic which occurred in 1918–1919 caused more than 50 million deaths – more deaths than the whole of World War I from 1914–1918 caused.

If this new influenza virus forms and spreads, you will be given instructions from your Health Department about what you should do. This may include:

1. Immunisation of all with a vaccine (if it can be developed) to give immunity to the new virus.
2. Rapid diagnostic testing (if it can be developed) of possibly infected people.
3. Isolation of patients and contacts, including stopping all people from travelling.
4. Education of the public about ways of stopping transmission, including covering the mouth and nose when coughing or sneezing, not spitting, etc. (The wearing of masks is more important for the patient than the uninfected public.)
5. Education of health workers as to how to barrier nurse patients to prevent more infections.
6. Treatment of patients and possibly contacts with antiviral drugs such as the M2 ion channel blockers (e.g. amantadine and rimantadine) or more likely neuraminidase inhibitors (e.g. oseltamivir and zanamivir) or newer drugs.

Prevention includes keeping wild birds away from people's domestic birds, killing and safely burying or burn-

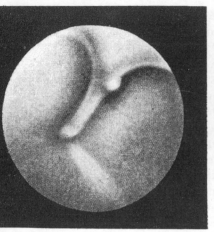 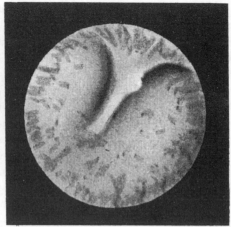 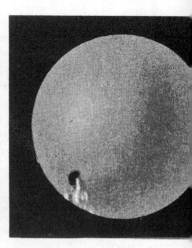

Figure 20.17 *Left: normal ear drum. Middle: acute otitis media. Right: otitis media with perforated drum.*

ing infected birds, keeping pigs and people separate from birds and when available, immunisation of all people.

Severe acute respiratory syndrome (SARS)

This is a new (since 2003) infection caused by a virus (coronavirus) previously infecting only bats and civet cats. It spreads by inhalation of droplets or droplet nuclei or by direct contact or on things which have been in contact with the virus – all from the infected animal or patient. The incubation period is up to 10 days. At first, there is a fever with or without some gastroenteritis or respiratory symptoms. Then 3–7 days later, the patient gets a cough and gets more and more short of breath, then cyanosed, then dies. There is no known treatment. A vaccine is under test. Prevention is by strict isolation of the patient and strict barrier nursing. This stopped what may have been a huge epidemic or pandemic occurring, and at the time of writing there are no known cases in the world. But the infection could return. Notify (page 36) any suspected cases (similar to influenza viral pneumonia, see page 279) immediately to your Medical Officer and immediately start isolation precautions (see Chapter 11 page 61).

Acute middle ear inflammation (acute otitis media)

Acute middle ear inflammation is a common acute infectious inflammation of the middle ear. It is often caused by a virus, and fluid not pus often forms in the middle ear. Acute middle ear infection due to bacteria also occurs and often develops with or after a viral or bacterial upper respiratory tract infection, especially if these block the Eustachian tube and pus forms in the middle ear.

Symptoms include:

- pain and a feeling of fullness in the ear,
- deafness,
- discharge from the ear, if the drum bursts, and
- general symptoms of infection sometimes, e.g. fever, malaise, gastroenteritis.

Signs (see Figure 20.17) can include:

- inflammation of the ear drum (the drum may be pink or red, there may be small blood vessels seen running in from the edge and the normal white colour and light reflex are not seen),
- fluid or pus seen behind the ear drum,
- bulging of the ear drum,
- rupture of the ear drum, with a hole in the drum and pus in the external canal,
- deafness, and
- general signs of infection including raised temperature and pulse rate.

Many cases get better without treatment. Some cases develop complications. These include:

- 'glue ear' with partial deafness (the acute infection settles but thick fluid is left filling the middle ear),
- chronic otitis media (continuing infection causes the ear drum to burst) and pus comes out of the ear,
- acute mastoiditis (a tender swelling of the bone (not just the lymph node) behind the ear),
- meningitis,
- acute tonsillitis.

Treatment

Treat as an outpatient. Admit for inpatient treatment if there is discharge of pus from the ear.

1. Give paracetamol or acetylsalicylic acid 0.5–1 g with, if needed, codeine 30 mg every 6 hours if pain.
2. Tell the patient to blow his nose often (to try to open up the Eustachian tube).
3. Give ephedrine or other vasoconstrictor nasal drops if available four times a day.
4. Give an antimalarial drug if malaria likely (see Chapter 13 pages 79, 80).
5. If a viral infection, with this (or no) treatment it will probably get better in a couple of days.
6. If it does not get better or if the patient has general symptoms and signs of infection when seen give procaine benzylpenicillin 1 g or 1,000,000 units daily or SMX 800 mg/TMP 160 mg orally twice daily until cured (6–10 days).

   If the above are not successful, give tetracycline or doxycycline or even better, amoxicillin 500 mg + clavulanic acid 125 mg about 8 hourly but, if pregnant, amoxicillin alone.
7. Do ear toilet and put in ear drops (see below) *if* the ear is discharging. Do this daily or more often if there is a lot of discharge. Continue the ear toilet and ear drops until the discharge stops.
8. After the ear toilet put 5 drops of boric acid 3% or acetic acid 1% or salicylic acid 1% in alcohol ear drops into the ear.

Method for ear toilet

Cut the end off a clean size 8 feeding tube (or cut the needle off a scalp vein set) so that the tube is about 5 cm (2 inches) long. Put this onto a clean 5 ml or 10 ml syringe.

Draw up 2 ml of normal saline made with $2\frac{1}{2}$ ml ($\frac{1}{2}$ teaspoonful) of salt in 200 ml (1 cup) of clean water (better than just water).

Put the cut end of the feeding tube *gently* into the ear. *Do not put the tube deep into the ear or you may damage the ear.*

Inject the saline *slowly* into the ear. Then suck out the saline and pus from the ear into the syringe. Throw away this dirty saline. Fill the syringe with clean saline again. Repeat the treatment until no more pus comes out.

Dry the ear like this (called 'wicking') – roll up a small piece of soft absorbent tissue or toilet paper into a spear shape, put it into the ear, leave it there for 1 minute, then take it out.

Look with an auriscope at the canal and drum. If there is still pus, etc., repeat the cleaning with the syringe and the drying with paper. Continue until the drum is seen and the drum and canal are clean and dry.

After use, clean the syringe and feeding tube very well. Then soak them in antiseptic solution.

This method is very effective and not dangerous.

Another method of doing ear toilet

Clean inside the canal with a *small* piece of cotton wool wrapped around the end of a *very thin* swab stick. Do not push it into the drum. Use a new piece of cotton wool when the cotton wool on the stick becomes dirty or wet. Continue until you can see the canal and drum are clean and dry (through the auriscope). This method is harder for most health workers in health centres to do, and is also less effective.

Transfer

Transfer to Medical Officer care if:

1. acute mastoiditis develops (urgent),
2. the ear drum does not return to normal or the patient is deaf in that ear after 3 weeks of treatment (non-urgent).

Chronic middle ear inflammation (chronic otitis media)

Chronic middle ear infection is a chronic infection of the middle ear by bacteria.

It can be a complication of untreated or badly treated acute middle ear inflammation or due to anatomical abnormalities in the upper respiratory tract (URT) (including enlarged adenoids) or decreased immunity. It is likely, however, that in many patients specific organisms infect the URT and continue to live there (called 'colonisers') despite antibiotic treatment and cause repeated or chronic infection.

There are symptoms and signs of discharge of pus from the ear from time to time. The ear drum is perforated (has a hole in it) and does not heal. The patient is partly deaf.

Treatment

Treat as an outpatient. Admit for inpatient treatment, if necessary for ear toilet.

Ear toilet and drops daily as for acute middle ear inflammation (see above), until the discharge stops. If there is a lot of discharge, the ear toilet (or at least with paper spears) followed by drops may be needed 2–4 times daily.

Treat as for acute middle ear inflammation (see above) if there has been evidence of acute otitis media in the last 6 weeks, or if the ear suddenly gets worse or if there is no improvement on the above treatment for 1 week. Antibiotics, however, will not help unless there has been a recent acute infection and most organisms by then are resistant to ordinary antibiotics; and antibiotics will not heal the ear drum.

Tell the patient that he must try to keep inside his ear dry (no swimming, care with washing, dry carefully if water does get inside, etc.).

Refer (do not normally transfer) the patient to the next visiting Medical Officer as some cases can be helped by an operation.

Prevention is by having good nutrition, good general health, having all possible immunisations and by early proper treatment of acute rhinitis or sinusitis or chronic sinusitis.

External ear inflammation (otitis externa)

External ear inflammation is an acute or a chronic inflammation of the skin of the external canal of the ear. The inflammation is usually caused by an infection with bacteria and occasionally with fungi. This infection often complicates an injury or a chronic non-infective dermatitis (see Chapter 32 page 548) of the skin inside the ear. There may be inflammation of all of the skin of the canal, often with pus formation. At other times there is a furuncle (pimple or boil) (see Chapter 32 page 532) in one area.

Treatment

Treat as an outpatient.

1. Ear toilet and ear drops daily, or if needed 2–4 times a day (see page 281).
2. Use boric acid 3% in alcohol or acetic acid 1% or salicylic acid in alcohol ear drops, 3–5 drops after the ear toilet. If this does not work, try crystal violet (methylrosanilinium chloride) 0.5–1% in alcohol solution 3–5 drops after the ear toilet.
3. If the condition is severe, insert glycerine and ichthammol 10% on a gauze wick deep into the ear canal daily, until the condition is cured or improved enough to use ear drops.
4. Tell the patient to keep the ear dry (no swimming, care with washing) and to dry the inside of the ear carefully if water does get in.
5. Give paracetamol 0.5–1 g or acetylsalicylic acid 0.5–1 g if needed every 6 hours for pain.
6. Antibiotics are not usually needed and most organisms are resistant to ordinary antibiotics.

If the external ear inflammation returns many times:

1. tell the patient to always keep the inside of the ear dry (no swimming, care during washing, dry carefully if water does get inside, etc.);
2. use boric acid 3% (or acetic acid or salicylic acid) in alcohol ear drops or even just alcohol ethanol or methylated spirits as ear drops once or twice every week even when the ear seems to be well; or if not successful
3. use hydrocortisone 1% cream (as well as 1 and 2 above) in the ear daily until it improves, then 2–3 times a week.

Foreign body in the ear

A foreign body in the ear may cause pain or discharge or no symptoms.

If the foreign body is an insect, put cooking oil (not hot) into the ear; when the insect is dead, syringe the ear. You can syringe many other foreign bodies out of the ear. However, do not put water into the ear if the foreign body is a vegetable (e.g. dry bean) which may swell. Instead, try sucking on it with the end of a small tube attached to a strong sucker. Do not use forceps as you can easily push the foreign body further into the ear and damage the ear drum. Try using a paper clip straightened out with one end squashed to make a narrow loop like this:

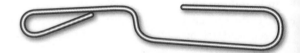

Lie the patient on his side. Get someone to hold the head still. Pull the ear backwards and upwards. Put the loop in gently from the side until you see it past the foreign body. Gently hook it behind and pull the foreign body out. If the patient is unco-operative or has a lot of pain, he may need a general anaesthetic.

Sinusitis

Acute sinusitis is an acute viral or bacterial infection of one or more of the paranasal sinuses (see Figures 20.2 and 20.3). It is much more common in patients with HIV infection. It may become chronic.

There are often general symptoms and signs of infection – fever, etc.

Local symptoms and signs of inflammation are almost always present as follows:

- Pain over the affected sinus. Sometimes there is also a general headache or pain in the nearby teeth or eye.
- Tenderness over the affected sinus.
- There is often nasal mucous membrane swelling, and, if a bacterial infection, pus in the nose and throat.

Always look for other signs suggesting HIV infection and consider counselling and sending blood for HIV test.

Treatment

1. Paracetamol 0.5–1 g or acetylsalicylic acid 0.5–1 g with, if needed, codeine 30 mg if required for pain.
2. Antimalarial drug (see Chapter 13 pages 79, 80) if malaria possible.
3. Ephedrine or other vasoconstrictor nasal drops, 2–3 drops into each nostril four times a day.
4. Tell the patient how to wash out the nose with saline once or twice daily (see page 303). This is very important.
5. Procaine benzylpenicillin 1 g or 1,000,000 units IMI daily or SMX 800 mg/TMP 160 mg bd.
6. Add an antihistamine only if there is evidence of allergic rhinitis.
7. If it does not get better change penicillin to tetracycline or doxycycline with metronidazole or, if available, amoxicillin and clavulanic acid or, if pregnant, amoxicillin alone.

Foreign body in the nose

The most common symptom caused by a foreign body in the nose is a discharge of pus from one side of the nose.

> If a patient has discharge of pus from one side of the nose always look for a foreign body in the nose.

If you can see the foreign body remove it with a paper clip (see 'Foreign body in the ear' page 282) rather than forceps. If you cannot see the foreign body or if the foreign body is hard or round and you cannot easily get it out, then try to remove it with a probe. Gently push a thin round-ended metal probe along the floor of the nose (i.e. almost straight in; but pointed a little downwards as well as backwards) until it touches the back of the throat. Then press the end you are holding downwards until the end in the patient's throat hits the top of the back of the nose. The foreign body will then be on top of and in front of the probe. Slide the probe out, keeping your end gently pressed down as far as possible. The foreign body often comes out in front of the probe. Sometimes a general anaesthetic is needed to see and remove the foreign body.

Bleeding nose (epistaxis)

Causes of a bleeding nose include:

1. a cause not found (common),
2. a small crusted area on septum (in the middle just inside the nose) which has cracked (common),
3. trauma,
4. strong nose blowing or sneezing,
5. others – snakebite, rare blood diseases, diphtheria, etc.

Treatment

1. Treat any underlying cause found.
2. Sit the patient up.
   - Pinch his nose tightly together between finger and thumb. Do not release the pressure for 10 minutes.
   - Let the blood run out of his mouth into a dish.
   - Do these things for 10 minutes by the clock. Do not stop before 10 minutes are over.
   - Release the pressure but do not blow the nose or pull any clots of blood out. See 6 below.
   If this does not stop the bleeding, then:
3. Put in anterior nasal pack. Soak a long strip of narrow gauze bandage in 1 in 10,000 solution of epinephrine/adrenaline (mix 9 ml of saline with 1 ml of the 1 in 1000 epinephrine/adrenaline solution used for injection). Use long narrow forceps to pack the gauze in layers into the nose. Start off by putting the first layer as far back as possible. (See a reference book for details.) If this does not stop the bleeding, remove this anterior nasal pack, put in a posterior nasal pack (see below) and then another anterior nasal pack, starting off as far back as possible and pressing it onto the posterior nasal pack.
4. A posterior nasal pack can be made with a Foley's urethral self-retaining balloon catheter. Push the catheter through the bleeding side of the nose until the tip can be seen at the back of the throat when the patient opens his mouth. Make sure the balloon is not behind or below the tongue. Inflate the balloon of the catheter with 4–10 ml of air or saline. Then pull the catheter forward as far as it will go until the balloon is stuck in the back of the nose. Fasten the catheter to the face with sticking plaster to keep the catheter pulled firmly forward so that it will press on any bleeding site at the back of the nose. Then put in an anterior nasal pack.
5. Treat for shock or anaemia if necessary. (See Chapter 27 page 468 and Chapter 21 page 316.)
6. When the bleeding has stopped, gently put antibiotic compound ointment or white soft paraffin into the nose, three times a day for a few days, to soften and heal any hard cracked area.

7. If unable to stop the bleeding, transfer the patient as an emergency to the Medical Officer, making sure an IV drip is running.

Allergic rhinitis (hay fever)

An allergic reaction of the mucous membrane of the nose is called allergic rhinitis or 'hay fever'. The allergic reaction often affects the eyes too (allergic conjunctivitis) and the throat.

The allergy is usually to something breathed in – often house dust or a plant pollen.

The nose (and often eyes and throat) become itchy, watery and sore. The patient often sneezes a lot and rubs his nose and eyes. He may feel as if he has a fever.

On examination the mucous membrane is thickened, bluish-pink and has watery material covering it. There is no pus in the nose. The temperature is normal.

The condition may continue for hours or days or weeks or months.

Try to discover what is causing the reaction. The patient must try to avoid this. But this is not often possible.

Treat with an antihistamine, e.g. chlorphenamine 4 mg 2–4 times daily or promethazine 10–25 mg at night; and if needed, but for no longer than 1 week, ephedrine or other vasoconstrictor nasal drops each 4 hours. If the patient wishes to buy and use every day mometasone or budesonide or fluticasone or beclomethasone nasal spray according to the directions, these are much more effective.

Acute tonsillitis and diphtheria

Acute tonsillitis is an acute bacterial or viral infection of the tonsils and surrounding area of the throat. This causes acute inflammation and usually pus formation in the throat and the general symptoms and signs of infection.

The patient complains of a sore throat worse on swallowing or turning the head, and headache and fever.

The patient may be quite sick with a high temperature and fast pulse. The tonsils and inside the throat are red and swollen and usually there are spots of white or yellow pus on the tonsils. The lymph glands in the neck are often swollen and tender.

Complications can occur, including an abscess behind the tonsil or at the back of the throat or under the chin. Any of these can block the airway. After

1–3 weeks rheumatic fever (see Chapter 29 page 486) or acute glomerulonephritis (see Chapter 26 page 446) can occur.

Diphtheria is a special kind of upper respiratory tract infection. It is a bacterial infection caused by *Corynebacterium diphtheriae*. It usually causes respiratory infections ('diphtheria'), but it can cause skin infections (usually ulcers, e.g. 'desert sore'). It also puts toxins into the blood which can stop the heart or peripheral nerves working properly. It spreads by droplets or direct spead. It is more common in children than adults. It usually causes tonsillitis, often with neck swelling, but can cause infection of the larynx (voice box) or nose. The diagnostic feature is a greyish covering or membrane over the affected area, usually the tonsils, which is firmly stuck on and cannot be pushed off with a tongue depressor as pus can be. Around the edge of the grey covering is an area of inflammation which sometimes bleeds. The illness can vary from mild to severe. In severe cases, within the first couple of weeks shock or complete blockage of the larynx can cause death. In the next couple of weeks heart failure can occur. Some weeks later damage to motor nerves (which control muscles) can result in things swallowed coming back up the nose, difficulty seeing and even weakness of the arms and legs.

Treatment

1. Procaine benzylpenicillin 1 g or 1,000,000 units IMI daily is preferable to SMX 800 mg/TMP 160 mg twice daily. Amoxicillin 500 mg (but not if glandular fever) +/- clavulanic acid 125 mg (but not if pregnant) three times a day is effective.

2. Paracetamol 0.5–1 g or acetylsalicylic acid 0.5–1 g four times a day if needed for pain.

3. Antimalarials if malaria possible (see Chapter 13 pages 79, 80).

If the patient has an acute very severe infection, give benzyl (crystalline) penicillin.

If an abscess starts to block the airway, see below.

If you think the patient has diphtheria, treat with benzylpenicillin but immediately contact the Medical Officer about the use of diphtheria antitoxin (10,000–100,000 units) and examination and antibiotic treatment and immunisation with toxoid of contacts. If there is difficulty in breathing or if stridor occurs, arrange urgent transfer, as tracheostomy may be urgently needed. If the airway does become completely blocked, do an urgent laryngostomy (see Chapter 37 page 613). Diphtheria can be prevented by immunisation, especially DPT or triple antigen given during childhood. (See Chapter 10 page 46.)

Acute infections which block the airway

Acute bacterial infections in the throat, epiglottis, larynx or trachea can cause death by blocking the airway. This block may be caused by an abscess or infective swelling or membrane or secretion which can be seen; but sometimes one of these things is so far inside the throat or in the larynx or trachea that it cannot be seen.

Suspect possible blockage of the airway if:

1. You can see a swelling which could block the airway; or
2. The patient has difficulty in breathing. Stridor means death may be close; and especially if
3. The patient looks very 'sick'.

If a blockage of the airway is possible, *treat* like this:

1. Immediately give antibiotics as for septicaemia (IVI chloramphenicol 2 g, see Chapter 12 page 64).
2. Nurse carefully (suck out when needed; give oxygen when needed; etc.). Observe carefully every 15 minutes.
3. Give epinephrine/adrenaline and antihistamines if allergy is possible (see Chapter 10 page 44).
4. Transfer patient if he does not quickly improve.
5. If there is any swelling that will block the airway and cause death before transfer is possible, cut the skin or mucous membrane only; then push closed artery forceps into the pus and open them up to let the pus drain out.
6. Do an emergency laryngostomy if incision is not possible. See Chapter 37 page 613.

Obstructive sleep apnoea syndrome

This syndrome (OSAS) exists when the patient has:

1. snoring, usually loud,
2. times when his snoring and breathing stop during sleep (the patient will not know; only others who see him or hear him sleep will know),
3. daytime sleepiness (or irritability or depression or other symptoms).

Snoring and breathing stop as the patient has relaxed his throat muscles so much when asleep that he has sucked the sides of his throat together when breathing in and this blocks his airway. Low oxygen in the blood when the patient stopped breathing will have woken him up. Waking up will have tightened up all his muscles and pulled the insides of his throat apart, and this starts him breathing again. The patient will not know any of this has happened as he usually goes back to sleep again within seconds. The repeated waking during sleep to breathe, even if there is enough length of sleep, causes sleepiness the next day.

This condition is more common in

- people who are overweight or obese,
- men; or women after the menopause,
- the middle-aged and elderly,
- people who drink alcohol or take sleeping tablets before sleeping,

but anyone can be affected.

The patient is usually seen as

- the husband or wife is worried by the snoring or the stopping of breathing,
- the patient is tired all the time.

Special tests to diagnose it and special treatment (continuous positive airway pressure or CPAP, or a mandibular advancement splint) are possible but are expensive and usually not available even in hospitals.

If you suspect a patient has this condition, talk to the Medical Officer about it, but the following things may help the patient and would do no harm.

1. If overweight, the patient should exercise and diet to get back to the normal weight for his height. This is in fact the most important part of the treatment.
2. The patient should never sleep on his back. The patient should put something very uncomfortable on his back, either in his sleeping clothes or in a belt worn around the chest, etc. so that any time he rolls onto his back he is so uncomfortable he has to roll on to his side or front.
3. If the nose is blocked, treat the nose so that he can breathe through his nose.
4. Try the effect of a chin strap or bandage which goes from under the chin to over the top of the head to hold the lower jaw forward and keep the mouth closed during sleep.
5. Get the patient to push his lower jaw forward as far as it would be comfortable for him to keep it all night (about 2 mm less than as far forward as it will go). Get him to bite onto a 'boil and bite' footballer's mouth-guard in this position. Wear this mouth-guard to bed each night (the chin strap should hold his teeth in the mouth-guard). This will hold not only his lower jaw but also his tongue forward and will help keep his airway open.
6. Try sleeping propped up a little or with the head of the bed raised.
7. Do not have alcohol or sleeping tablets before sleeping.

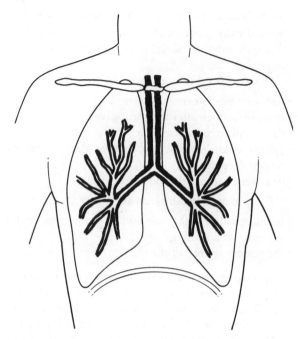

Figure 20.18 *Diagram showing the changes in acute tracheitis and bronchitis. The mucous membrane lining all the air passages is inflamed and swollen and sometimes covered with pus. These things cause narrowing of all the airways to all parts of the lung. The alveoli themselves are normal.*

Acute laryngitis, tracheitis and bronchitis

Acute bronchitis is a common acute inflammation of the mucous membrane lining the inside of the bronchi (see Figure 20.18). If the trachea is inflamed, acute tracheitis is also present. If the voice is hoarse or lost, the larynx is inflamed.

Acute bronchitis is usually caused by an infection with viruses or bacteria; but chemicals and smoke can also cause the inflammation.

General symptoms and signs of infection may be present, including:

• malaise and
• fever.

Symptoms of a chest infection may be present, including:

• cough, which can last for 3 weeks (even with treatment),
• tracheal pain (pain in the front and middle of the neck and upper chest during coughing),
• sputum made of pus if bacterial infection, and
• shortness of breath and wheezing.

Signs of bronchial obstruction (wheezes) are usually present but there are no signs of pneumonia:

• chest movement unchanged,
• percussion note unchanged,
• breath sounds unchanged to all areas, but
• wheezes (and occasionally coarse crackles) in all areas.

Treatment

Treat as an outpatient.

Tell the patient to return if shortness of breath gets worse (pneumonia or asthma).

1. If pus in sputum or 'sick', procaine benzylpenicillin 1 g or 1,000,000 units IMI daily or SMX 800 mg/TMP 160 mg twice daily until cured (usually 5–7 days). Tetracycline or doxycycline or amoxicillin +/- clavulanic acid or amoxicillin alone if pregnant are alternatives.
2. Paracetamol 0.5–1 g or acetylsalicylic acid 0.5–1 g every 6 hours if required for pain.
3. A 'bronchodilator', e.g. salbutamol metered aerosol 100 mcg (μg) 2 puffs or tablet 4 mg or alternative drug each 4–6 hours *if* wheezing and shortness of breath present.
4. Inhalation (the breathing in) of steam (from a cup or tin of boiling water), for 5 minutes three or four times a day.
5. An antimalarial drug if malaria possible (see Chapter 13 pages 79, 80).

Bronchopneumonia

Bronchopneumonia is an acute infection of groups of alveoli in the lungs (see Figure 20.19).

Bronchopneumonia is usually caused by bacteria.

Bronchopneumonia usually develops as a complication of another condition which has either:

1. stopped the patient moving around and breathing deeply and/or
2. has allowed bacteria to come into the lungs from the upper respiratory tract, e.g.
   • after anaesthetics, operations, accidents,
   • old or sick people lying in bed, or
   • measles or whooping cough.

There are the general symptoms and signs of infection:

• the patient has another condition but is not as well as he or she should be or is getting worse,
• fever (but not always),
• fast pulse, etc.

Symptoms of a chest infection are usually present (but not always):

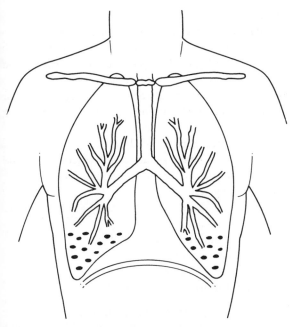

Figure 20.19 *Diagram showing the changes in bronchopneumonia (in this case of both lower lobes – the most common places affected). Scattered groups of alveoli are involved. Bronchi are usually normal. However, disease of the bronchi can also be present.*

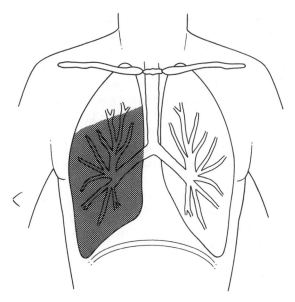

Figure 20.20 *Diagram showing the changes in lobar pneumonia (in this case the right lower lobe). One whole lobe (or section) of lung is solid (bronchi and alveoli filled with organisms, fluid and blood cells). The solid lung extends from large central airways to the edge of the chest wall.*

• cough,
• sputum (made of pus), and
• shortness of breath.

Signs of the chest infection include:

• sputum made of pus,
• respiratory rate usually fast and shallow,
• normal movement, normal percussion note and normal breath sounds, but scattered crackles throughout the lungs, often mostly low down at the back.

Treatment

1. Antibiotics – procaine benzylpenicillin 1 g or 1,000,000 units IMI daily or SMX 800 mg/TMP 160 mg twice daily or amoxicillin 500 mg (without clavulanic acid 125 mg if pregnant), until cured. (See page 289 for details about other antibiotics.)
2. Physiotherapy twice daily (see Chapter 20 page 299).
3. Tell the patient to take 10 deep breaths and cough each hour when awake.
4. Tell the patient to move around in bed and, if he is able, make him get out of bed and walk around.
5. Antimalarials if malaria possible (see Chapter 13 pages 79, 80).
6. Treat any underlying condition.

Prevention of bronchopneumonia is by encouraging activity in old, ill or postoperative patients.

Lobar pneumonia

Lobar pneumonia is a very common cause of sickness and death in the tropical and developing world.

Lobar pneumonia is an acute inflammation of all the alveoli in one lobe or one part of the lung. (See Figure 20.20.) The affected part of the lung becomes filled with organisms, plasma and blood cells and becomes 'solid' (often called 'consolidation').

The cause is usually the bacterial organism *Streptococcus pneumoniae* (the pneumococcus). Other bacteria (especially *Staphylococcus aureus, Haemophilus influenzae*), 'atypical' bacteria (e.g. *Legionella, Mycoplasma*, Q fever and *Chlamydia*), *Mycobacterium tuberculosis*, rickettsia, as well as viral, fungal and other organisms can cause pneumonia. If pneumonia does not improve on treatment as it should, always think of it possibly being due to atypical bacteria or TB.

Inhaled chemicals (e.g. kerosene) or acid if gastro-oesophageal reflux or smoke from a large fire, etc. are often causes of non-infective bronchitis and pneumonia; often followed by infective pneumonia.

Pneumonia is very common in patients with decreased defences against infections. The most common of these decreased defences is HIV infection.

In all patients with pneumonia (especially if severe or repeated attacks), ask yourself if there is anything in the history or examination to suggest HIV infection. In some places half of the patients who have pneumonia have HIV infection (see Chapter 19 page 224).

Pneumonia due to organisms which normally cannot grow in the lungs but take the opportunity to do so if there is decreased immunity in HIV infection (opportunistic infections) are common in HIV infected patients, e.g. pneumocystis, nocardia, cryptococcus, etc. (see Chapter 19 pages 224–225).

Pneumonia is common with diseases which have damaged the defences in the lungs, e.g. COLD and bronchiectasis.

Pneumonia is common if acid from reflux (page 351) or organisms from sinusitis or decayed teeth repeatedly get into the lungs during sleep.

Pneumonia is most likely to cause death in those who are young or old, or who have HIV infection or have no spleen (including from sickle cell anaemia), or who have any chronic medical condition such as diabetes mellitus, heart condition, anaemia, etc., or if they have something else wrong with their lungs, especially COLD or bronchiectasis.

'Atypical' pneumonia is due to 'atypical' or unusual organisms (*Legionella, Mycoplasma Chlamydia* and Q fever). The pneumonia behaves in an 'atypical' (unusual) way, often with a severe disease but few chest signs. These organisms are uncommon but not rare and can be quite common in some areas. The organisms do not die if given penicillin, but do die if given erythromycin or tetracycline/doxycycline.

Symptoms

- The start of the infection is usually sudden; but sometimes there has been an upper respiratory tract infection before.
- A rigor at first is common; or just fever.
- Cough is almost always present.
- Sputum usually – rusty looking (from blood) or made of pus.
- Pleuritic chest pain (pain at the side of the chest but occasionally in the shoulder or in the upper abdomen, worse when the chest moves, e.g. on deep breathing or coughing and relieved by keeping the chest still, e.g. by holding or lying on the painful side).
- Shortness of breath

Signs

- High temperature.
- Fast pulse rate.

- Sometimes cyanosis.
- *Breathing fast and usually shallow, sometimes irregular due to pain. Breathing rate and type* are *the most important signs to show pneumonia is present (when there is a chest infection) and to show how severe it is (if pneumonia is present).*
- Respiratory distress if severe – insuction and/or dilated nostrils on breathing in; grunting on breathing out. (See page 270.)
- In the affected area of the chest:
  - patient can often point to the place where the pleuritic pain is over area of pneumonia,
  - movement less,
  - percussion note dull (percussion often causes pain),
  - breath sounds or air entry less,
  - bronchial breathing,
  - crackles (or crepitations),
  - pleural rub sometimes.

The rate and type of breathing is a very good sign for the presence and severity of pneumonia. It is difficult for the chest muscles to stretch a 'solid' lung. And chest movement often causes pleuritic pain. So the patient often takes shallow breaths which do not exchange as much oxygen and carbon dioxide as normal respiration with normal lungs. So breathing usually has to be fast when it is shallow.

If the pneumonia is more severe (and the patient has to do much extra work to breathe and his lungs do not exchange oxygen and carbon dioxide well and the body needs more oxygen than when it is not fighting an infection) there are signs of respiratory distress:

1. indrawing of the soft tissues between the ribs and below and above the clavicles when the patient breathes in (called 'insuction');
2. use of neck and shoulder muscles when he breathes in;
3. dilation of the nostrils when he breathes in; and
4. grunting when he breathes out;
5. as well as fast respiratory rate.

The earliest signs in the chest are usually increase in the respiratory rate, decreased movement of the affected side and decreased breath sounds. Percussion at this stage often causes pain. At first there may be no, or only a few, crackles or crepitations. It is often a day or two before many crackles are heard. Not all the signs do develop in every case. If you give antibiotic treatment early fewer signs develop. Sometimes you can hear a pleural rub if inflammation of the pleura (pleurisy) has developed.

Complications

- Heart failure (see Chapter 27 page 461).
- Septicaemia sometimes with shock (see Chapter 12 page 64).
- Jaundice (see Chapter 24 page 401).
- Pleural effusion (see page 292).
- Empyema (see page 292).
- Pneumothorax (see page 293).
- Lung abscess.
- Infections in other organs especially meningitis (see Chapter 25 page 409) and arthritis (see Chapter 29 page 485).
- Others.

Tests

Tests are not usually needed. But, if the pneumonia is severe or unusual, or does not get better when it should, do tests for HIV and send sputum for AFB (see Chapter 14 page 108).

Treatment

Without treatment 20–40% of severe cases die.

Management includes:

1. Antibiotics until cured.
   - Procaine benzylpenicillin or alternative if it is a mild case.
   - Benzyl (crystalline) penicillin, if it is a moderate case.
   - If benzylpenicillin is not improving the patient, but it is not a severe case, amoxicillin with (if not pregnant) clavulanic acid and add erythromycin; or change to tetracycline or doxycline (if not pregnant).
   - Chloramphenicol, if the above do not cure or if severe case at diagnosis.
2. Antimalarial drugs as indicated.
3. Treatment of symptoms, especially pain.
4. Oxygen, if needed.
5. Physiotherapy, if very much sputum.
6. Look for and treat complications, especially
   - heart failure,
   - septicaemia/shock,
   - infections in other parts, especially meningitis; but also arthritis,
   - pleural fluid, and
   - pneumothorax.
7. Look for and treat other important conditions (e.g. severe anaemia).
8. Consider counselling, then HIV testing in all patients.

---

9. If the pneumonia is unusual or is not improving on all of the above treatment, look for TB and think of unusual and 'atypical' and opportunistic infections. Treat these if needed.
10. Transfer the patient if necessary.

Treat according to severity.

Mild
- no respiratory distress[1] and breathing RR < 30 and PR < 100 and
- no cyanosis and
- no complications[2]
See below.

Moderate
- respiratory distress[1] but not severe and breathing RR < 40 and PR < 120 and/or
- cyanosis if present but not marked and
- no complications[2] except, if there is COLD, the patient may have heart failure.
See below.

Severe
- respiratory distress[1] and breathing RR > 40 and PR > 120 and/or
- cyanosis and/or
- complications[2]
See below.

Mild case
Treat as an outpatient.

1. Procaine benzylpenicillin 1 g or 1,000,000 units IMI; *or* (if effective in your area) SMX 800 mg/ TMP 160 mg orally twice daily; or amoxicillin 500 mg with, if not pregnant, clavulanic acid 125 mg about each 8 hours; give until 2 days after fever and symptoms have gone (usually 5–7 days).
2. Antimalarial drugs if indicated (see Chapter 13 pages 79, 80)
3. Paracetamol 0.5–1 g or acetylsalicylic acid 0.5–1 g every 6 hours if necessary for pain.

If the patient is not much improved after 5 days, or if he gets worse, look for a complication, especially a pleural effusion. If no complication that needs special treatment is found, then treat as a moderately severe case.

---

1   Respiratory distress is (1) indrawing of soft tissues between the ribs and below and above the clavicles when the patient breathes in (insuction); (2) use of neck and shoulder muscles when he breathes in; (3) dilation of the nose muscles when he breathes in; (4) grunting when he breathes out. It is not distress from pain during breathing.

2   Complications include: (1) heart failure, (2) shock/septicaemia, (3) infections in other organs, (4) pleural fluid, and (5) pneumothorax.

Moderate case

Admit for inpatient treatment.

1. Benzylpenicillin 600 mg or 1,000,000 units IMI every 6 hours until improved, then procaine benzyl-penicillin 1 g or 1,000,000 units IMI daily; or better treatment, if available, would be amoxicillin 500 mg with, if not pregnant, clavulanic acid 125 mg each 8 hours. Give until 4 days after all fever has gone.
2. Antimalarial drugs if indicated (Chapter 13 pages 79, 80).
3. Paracetamol or acetylsalicylic acid 0.5–1 g every 6 hours if necessary if pain. Add codeine 30 mg if needed.

If the patient is not much improved after 2–5 days, but is not severely sick, then:

1. Add erythromycin 500–1000 mg every 6 hours; or change penicillin or amoxicillin to tetracycline 500 mg every 6 hours, or doxycycline 100 mg twice daily, but if pregnant only add erythromycin. This is also treatment for most 'atypical' pneumonias.
2. Send sputum for AFB and blood for HIV test.

If the patient gets worse at any time treat as a severe case with chloramphenicol (see below).

Severe case

Use this treatment for severe cases (the patient will die soon if the treatment is not successful) and moderate cases not cured by treatment.

1. Chloramphenicol 2 g immediately, then 1 g every 6 hours until much improved, then 750 mg every 6 hours. Give chloramphenicol for 10 days or until cured – whichever is longer. If the patient has shock or is *very* sick or cannot swallow or is vomiting, give IV or IM chloramphenicol (if shock, IV needed) until he can take oral chloramphenicol. In other cases give oral chloramphenicol. In hospitals, ceftriaxone (or one of the other third generation cephalosporins or a quinolone which are also very effective), may be used.
2. If the patient does not quickly improve and has or could possibly have HIV infection, **add** treatment for pneumocystis with SMX 1600 mg and TMP 320 mg each 8 hours for a small, and each 6 hours for a large adult and also prednisolone 50 mg daily. He may get worse at first but should be improved in 3–5 days.

   Transfer the patient as soon as possible for tests and possible prophylatic SMX/TMP and ART (see Chapter 19 page 224).

3. Antimalarial drugs if indicated (see Chapter 13 pages 79, 80). You should give IV or IM artesunate or IM artemether or quinine and a companion drug to *very* sick patients (see Chapter 13 page 80).
4. Oxygen at 2 litres per minute by intranasal prongs, if the patient is cyanosed or very short of breath.
5. Paracetamol or acetylsalicylic acid 0.5–1 g every 6 hours for pain. Add codeine 30 mg if needed.
6. Look for complications (page 289) and other conditions (especially severe anaemia) that need treatment.
7. If no better in 3–5 days, looks as if will die, and transfer not possible, start TB drugs and finish the course (see Chapter 14 page 115).

Look for infection elsewhere in all cases of pneumonia

Look in all other places in the respiratory tract but also in other organs.

Look very carefully for meningitis. Do lumbar puncture if indicated.

Treat with chloramphenicol if meningitis or severe infection elsewhere.

Think of HIV infection in all cases of pneumonia

Ask for contacts and past history and look for signs which could suggest HIV infection (see Chapter 19 pages 222–233).

Do necessary counselling and send blood for HIV test (see Chapter 19 pages 233–235).

Think of opportunistic infections if the patient has HIV infection

Think of:

1. TB with unusual clinical features for TB (see page 225);
2. *Pneumocystis jeroveci* (see page 224);
3. nocardia (see page 224);
4. melioidosis – in Asia and the Pacific (see page 161);
5. cryptococcus (see page 224);
6. other fungal infections – in some parts of the world.

Look for tuberculosis in almost all cases of pneumonia

Send sputum for AFB *if*:

1. Previous chronic cough (ask *all* patients if they had a chronic cough before the present illness).

2. Pneumonia is in an upper lobe or in the (right) middle lobe.
3. Patient not as acutely sick as you would expect when he has marked chest signs.
4. Past or family history of TB, or other history that suggests TB.
5. Wasting or lymphadenopathy or other sign that suggests TB.
6. Patient does not get better as quickly as expected, or patient not cured after 2 weeks of proper treatment.
7. Patient does, or may have, HIV infection.

Send sputum for AFB (three smears) from these patients. If the smear is negative and you still suspect TB, send three more smears for AFB after 1–2 weeks of treatment with antibiotics.

Think of 'atypical' pneumonia

See page 228.

If a patient on treatment for pneumonia is getting worse, think of atypical pneumonia and if he needs treatment with erythromycin or doxycycline.

Think of special infections in special areas

Some infections are common only in some areas (e.g melioidosis in SE Asia or fungal infestations in SE Asia and America) and need special drugs for treatment. If you are in one of these areas where these infections occur, always think of these diseases being possible and treat or transfer such cases as you have been told.

Pneumonia which does not resolve (get better)

Think of the following:

1. Decreased immunity – HIV infection, etc.
2. Underlying disease of the lungs – TB, lung fluke, bronchiectasis, COPD, lung cancer, Kaposi's sarcoma, inhaled foreign body, industrial lung disease, asthma, etc.
3. Repeated aspiration (breathing in) of food, fluid or stomach material *especially* if gastro-oesophageal reflux or oesophageal disease or neurological disease (e.g. stroke or not fully conscious) or an alcoholic or a nasogastric tube being used;
4. Unusual organism causing the pneumonia, e.g.
   • *M. tuberculosis*
   • pneumocystis or nocardia (see Chapter 19 pages 224–225), if HIV needing SMX and TMP in large doses;
   • *Staphylococcus aureus* if following influenza needing dicloxacillin or alternative;

• 'atypical' pneumonia caused by *Legionella* or *Chlamydia* or *Mycoplasma* or Q fever needing tetracycline or erythromycin;
   • melioidosis needing special antibiotics from the Medical Officer, etc.
   • fungal infections needing special antifungal antibody from the Medical Officer.
5. Complication of pneumonia, e.g. pleural effusion; empyema; lung abscess; blockage of a large airway by a plug of pus, foreign body, tumour; etc.
6. Does the patient really have pneumonia; or could it be another condition?

Transfer

Transfer these cases to Medical Officer care:

1. severe cases which do not improve, or get worse after 2 days chloramphenicol (urgent);
2. cases not cured after 2 weeks chloramphenicol (non-urgent);
3. those with complications that you cannot treat at the health centre (urgent).

Prevention

Pneumococcal vaccine, polyvalent, 0.5 ml injection gives good protection for about 5 years against pneumococci, which cause many cases of pneumonia. Ask if it is available for those in your population who are most at risk of dying from pneumonia – the young; the elderly; those with splenectomy or severe sickle cell disease; HIV infection; chronic obstructive lung disease; or any chronic medical condition such as heart condition, diabetes mellitus, etc. Sometimes it is given to all children.

Pleural fluid

There are often no symptoms of fluid in the pleural cavity, but there may be shortness of breath and/or pleuritic pain. (See Figure 20.21.)

Signs of fluid in the pleural cavity include (on the affected side):

• movement less,
• percussion note very dull ('stony dull'),
• breath sounds or air entry less (usually none), and
• no crackles or wheezes but occasionally a pleural rub.

There may *also* be symptoms and signs of the cause of the pleural fluid.

When you diagnose fluid in the pleural cavity:

1. *Always do a diagnostic pleural aspiration* to find out what kind of fluid it is.
   Draw up 5 ml of 1% lidocaine local anaesthetic into a 20 ml syringe. Clean the skin with antiseptic

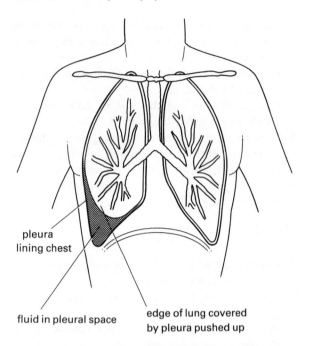

pleura
lining chest

fluid in pleural space

edge of lung covered
by pleura pushed up

Figure 20.21 *Diagram showing the changes with pleural fluid on the right side in the standing position. The fluid in the pleural space pushes the lung up. The fluid can fill almost all the chest and squash (collapse) almost all of the lung so that no ventilation is possible.*

at the top (not at the bottom) of where the pleural fluid is (the highest place where it is dull to percussion). Do not put the needle into the lower part of the chest where the liver or spleen are.

Without touching the skin or needle inject some lidocaine into the skin, muscle and onto the bone at the top of the rib (not at the bottom of a rib where the blood vessels are). Then while slowly injecting some more lidocaine, slide the needle over the top of the rib into the pleural cavity to a depth of about 2 cm. If you are in the pleural cavity, when you pull the plunger of the needle back fluid comes out. If you are in the lung, air comes out and you should take the needle out, sucking as you go (in case you get into the pleural fluid outside the lung).

Look at the fluid. Is it clear or blood or pus?

(a) Clear (usually yellow) fluid ('effusion'). This can either be a transudate which is just watery fluid (like oedema) or an exudate which has a lot of protein in it (and is often due to an infection).

- Stand a sample of fluid in a clear glass bottle for half an hour. If a web forms in it or it clots and part become solid, it is likely to be an exudate.

- Get a solution of 2.3 g of copper sulfate dried crystals ($CuSO_4$ $5H_2O$) dissolved in distilled water made up to 100 ml and keep in a small capped bottle. Put 1 drop of pleural fluid into this bottle. The drop will float if it is a transudate and will sink if it is an exudate.
- Use a urine dip stick to test for protein and sugar. If the protein is high (> 30 g/l) it is an exudate, but if low (< 30 g/l) it is a transudate. If the sugar is normal it is not likely there is infection in the fluid, but if the sugar is low there may be infection.
- If possible, send a sample of the fluid to the laboratory with some in a bottle used for a blood count (which has anticoagulant in it) and some in a clear sterile bottle and ask for Gram and AFB stains, cell count, protein, sugar and specific gravity (SG) and an explanation of the results.

(b) Pus ('empyema').

(c) Blood ('haemothorax')

You must transfer all patients with pus or blood to a Medical Officer immediately for drainage of all the fluid and other treatment.

2. *Always find out the cause*

If the patient does not have
- clear fluid which is a transudate and pneumonia or heart failure, or
- clear fluid which is a transudate or exudate and sputum positive for AFB

THEN you must transfer the patient to a Medical Officer for diagnosis and treatment (even if the effusion goes away – early TB often causes an effusion which goes away without treatment but the TB infection stays and gets worse).

(a) Pneumonia can cause an effusion (clear yellow fluid). If this is a transudate, it will usually go away itself with treatment of the pneumonia. If it is an exudate or an empyema, it all should be drained urgently and the patient needs urgent transfer to a Medical Officer.

(b) Tuberculosis can cause an effusion (clear yellow fluid). This can be a transudate or an exudate, but usually does not have AFBs in it. If the patient is put on anti-TB treatment, this will almost always clear itself.

(c) Heart failure, which will cause only an effusion (clear yellow fluid). This will be a transudate and go away with treatment of the heart failure.

(d) Many other conditions can cause fluid, pus or blood in the pleural cavity, all of which need transfer to the Medical Officer for diagnosis and/or treatment.

Pneumothorax

A pneumothorax is when there is air in the pleural cavity (see Figure 20.22).

Symptoms include shortness of breath and at times pleuritic pain.

Signs may include (on the affected side):

- movement less,
- percussion note very resonant or hollow (difficult to be sure of this but compare with the other side), and
- breath sounds or air entry less.

There may also be symptoms and signs of the cause of the pneumothorax (NB tuberculosis).

Contact your Medical Officer urgently about management of any case you diagnose.

Transfer all cases urgently.

If there is severe shortness of breath, put a plastic cannula, or a needle only if no cannula available, into the pleural cavity immediately. The best place is in the mid-clavicular line in the second intercostal space (i.e. 2–3 cm below the middle of the clavicle), pushing the cannula in just at the top of the rib (not at the bottom of a rib where the blood vessels are). Make a valve for the cannula or needle before you put it into the chest with part of a surgical rubber glove, like this:

1. Take a rubber surgical glove or, if unavailable, a plastic glove and cut a small 1 cm slit at the top of one of the glove fingers.
2. Then cut that glove finger from the glove, where it joins the palm of the glove.
3. Put the glove finger, where it joined the glove palm, around the hub of the cannula which is to go in the chest (i.e. where the cannula can join onto a syringe).
4. Tightly tie the glove finger onto the cannula or needle with suture material or cotton around the hub of the cannula.

This will allow air to go out of the chest, through the cannula and the slit in the glove, but it will not allow air to go back into the chest as the glove will be pushed into the end of the cannula by the air and stop the air going in.

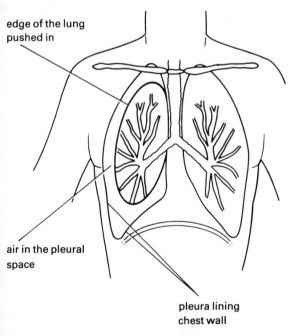

edge of the lung pushed in

air in the pleural space

pleura lining chest wall

Figure 20.22 *Diagram showing the changes in a pneumothorax. The air in the pleural space pushes the lung towards the trachea. The air can fill almost all the chest and completely collapse (squash) the lung so that no ventilation of that lung is possible.*

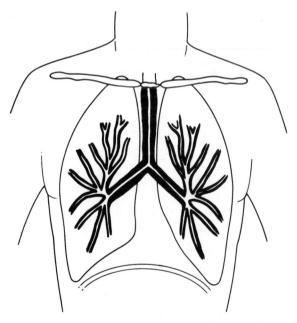

Figure 20.23 *Diagram showing changes during an attack of asthma. All the bronchi going to all parts of the lung are narrowed by a thick layer of thick mucus, swelling of the mucous membrane, and contraction of the bronchial muscles. Between attacks the bronchi return to normal.*

Asthma

Asthma is a condition of non-infectious inflammation of the bronchi. This causes times when all of the bronchi are narrowed (see Figure 20.23), causing episodes of shortness of breath and wheezing called attacks of asthma. Between attacks, the bronchi may not be narrowed and there may be no symptoms or just a cough.

You often cannot find the cause of a patient's asthma in a health centre. There may be a family history of asthma or allergies. There may be a history of attacks of shortness of breath or cough; or of allergies (see Chapter 10 page 44) to things breathed in, or swallowed (including drugs), or touched. Often asthma is caused by allergy to dust (especially house dust) or pollens. Sometimes it is caused by reaction to organisms that have caused respiratory infection or worms in the body. It can be caused by gastro-oesophageal reflux. Make sure the asthma is not caused by the patient taking acetylsalicylic acid tablets.

The bronchi have bronchial muscle spasm, swelling of the bronchial mucous membrane, and a thick layer of jelly-like mucus on the bronchial walls. There is shortness of breath, cough and sputum.

Symptoms include:

• sudden shortness of breath, most common at night or when the patient starts sudden exertion or if he goes into cold air,
• a feeling of tightness in the chest,
• wheezing,
• often repeated little coughs, and
• usually a history of previous attacks and being well in between attacks or having only a cough.

Signs include:

• temperature normal (no fever),
• breathing slow and deep with wheezing and sometimes coughing,
• pulse rate fast if a severe attack,
• white or jelly-like sputum (not pus),
• chest – wheezes or rhonchi in all areas especially when the patient breathes out.

There are two very important exceptions to the above:

1. In some patients the asthma does not ever go away completely (especially people who do not have the allergic type of asthma and whose asthma started when they were in middle or late adult life). These patients do have acute attacks of asthma. But between acute attacks they may have chronic shortness of breath and wheezes may be heard on examination of the chest. Some just have cough. This is called 'chronic asthma'.

2. Some patients have very severe attacks when almost no breath sounds on breathing in can be heard. In this case the patient is very anxious, has respiratory distress (see page 270), has a very fast pulse rate, is cyanosed, has decreased breath sounds or air entry and few wheezes or rhonchi can therefore be heard. This patient is near death.

Treatment

Asthma can be treated properly only if the lung function can be measured. Symptoms and signs are not very accurate. Ask if you can be supplied with measuring equipment – even a 'peak flow meter' which is very cheap (see Appendix 3 page 310). The aim of treatment is to have lung function always 80% of predicted or above. If it is less than 50% of predicted consider the asthma as severe and life threatening until it gets above 50%. Measure the patient's lung function each time you see him and any time he has an attack.

Educate the patient and relatives:

1. There is no cure for asthma.
2. Drugs can control chronic asthma but must be taken regularly in the correct dose at the correct time of the day.
3. Acute asthma is very dangerous and can kill the patient. If he gets an acute attack and is very short of breath he should use the treatment he is told to use and come to the health centre immediately.
4. If the patient is given prednisolone he must not at any time himself just stop the drug; he must not take more than he has been told to take; but he must take the larger dose he has been ordered if he has an acute attack and immediately come to the health centre. He must also take his regular isoniazid and antimalarials if the medical officer has ordered these. He must have regular check-ups.

For a list of asthma drugs see Appendix 1 page 308.

For details about a 'large volume spacer' see Appendix 2 pages 309–310.

Treatment of chronic asthma

1. Give salbutamol 100–400 mcg of metered aerosol through a large volume spacer or salbutamol 4 mg tablet or ephedrine 30 mg tablet when needed up to four times a day and at night. Reduce the dose if side effects occur (shaking, nervousness, sweating, giddiness or palpitations).

Increase the dose slowly if no side effects but still asthma. Do not give more than 400 mcg metered aerosol or 2 tablets four times a day. If treatment is needed daily, add regular beclomethasone and if this is not available ipratropium and if this is not helpful aminophylline until the patient has no symptoms; and then give the salbutamol only if needed.

2. Add beclomethasone metered aerosol.

Start with 100 mcg in one dose regularly in the morning every morning.

Use a large volume spacer.

Tell the patient to have a mouthful of water then gargle then spit out after the drug.

Increase the dose if needed each month up to 500 mcg daily; but no more. (Medical Officers may use up to 1200 mcg only in special circumstances.) Do not give more than needed.

When well for 1 month, try reducing the daily dose by 1 puff each month to find the lowest dose which will keep the patient well.

Use salbutamol only if needed.

3. Add ipratropium metered aerosol 20 mcg/puff through a large volume spacer if asthma control still not good or if beclomethasone not available.

Give 1 puff after the beta 2 agonist four times a day and if needed at night.

Increase up to 4 puffs four times a day if needed.

If it does not help the patient, stop ipratropium.

4. Add aminophylline or theophylline if necessary if the patient is taking more than two or more doses of the salbutamol daily and if beclomethasone or ipratropium not available or does not control the symptoms.

Increase the dose until:
• the asthma is controlled, or
• there is nausea, or other side effects (then reduce dose a little), or
• you are giving 400 mg four times a day (do not give more).

5. Find and avoid or treat the cause if possible.

Remember always to check that acetylsalicylic acid, other NSAID or beta-blocker or other drug or food which can be avoided, is not the cause.

6. Refer all cases to the Medical Officer for the review of the diagnosis and treatment.

7. The present best treatment where available would be a combination of a long acting beta 2 agonist (e.g. eformoterol or salmeterol) twice daily and an inhaled adrenocorticosteroid (e.g. beclomethasone or budesonide or fluticasone or ciclesonide) once (or twice) daily; using preferably dry powder preparations but otherwise metered aerosols through a large volume spacer.

8. Treat any acute attacks which occur (see below).

Treatment of acute attack asthma

1. Give intranasal oxygen 2–4 litres/minute for a moderate or a severe attack.

2. Give salbutamol 400–800 mcg 4–8 puffs over 8 minutes through a large volume spacer or 2.5–5 mg nebulised or (4 mg orally but only if no inhaled drugs available) if it is a mild or moderate attack and repeat if needed in 1 hour and then each 2–4 hours. If it is a severe attack give also epinephrine/adrenaline tart. 1:1000 solution 0.5 ml ($\frac{1}{2}$ ml) subcutaneous injection.

> DO NOT give both salbutamol (or similar drug) and epinephrine/adrenaline at the same time or either within 4 hours of the other unless severe attack.

3. If the attack is moderate or severe and the patient has been taking prednisone, prednisolone or other cortisone-like drug, urgently consult the Medical Officer. If the patient does not quickly improve, give 50–60 mg (12 of the 5 mg tablets or 2 of the 25 mg tablets) of his prednisolone (or 6–12 times his usual total daily dose of other cortisone-like drug) immediately and daily until you get further advice from the Medical Officer. If no prednisolone is available, give hydrocortisone 200–300 mg IVI immediately and daily.

4. Find and avoid or treat the cause, if possible. Do not give acetylsalicylic acid (give paracetamol instead) unless you know acetylsalicylic acid does not cause an attack of asthma in this patient. If a respiratory infection treat with antibiotic.

5. Do *not* give morphine, pethidine or sleeping tablet. Instead, if mentally abnormal, treat as a severe attack; also look for other causes of mental abnormality (see Chapter 35 pages 571–572).

> IF the symptoms and signs go and the peak flow is above 65% of predicted within 2 hours,
> THEN discharge on salbutamol 400 µg/mcg 4 puffs of metered aerosol or 5 mg (1 tab) four times a day for 5 days; then only if necessary up to four times a day; and beclomethasone 400 µg/mcg daily.
>
> IF symptoms and signs do not all go in 2 hours,
> *or*
> IF the peak flow is less than 65%,
> *or*
> IF it is a severe attack from the start,
> THEN immediately treat as follows (as well as 1–5).

6. If the attack is still moderate or severe and the peak flow less than 65% after 1 and 2, or if the patient takes prednisolone or other cortisone-like drug regularly, then the patient really needs a large dose of oral prednisolone 50 mg or hydrocortisone 200–300 mg IV. Contact the Medical Officer about what you should do. If this large dose is given, it needs to be reduced a little each day to be back to zero in the next 7–10 days. If this cannot be done because the asthma comes back and the patient needs to stay on some prednisolone, the Medical Officer must tell you and the patient what dose he should take and what needs to be done about prophylactic isoniazid and antimalarials and follow-up. Do not just give the patient prednisone without arranging the above as this will probably cause the patient to die.

7. If needed add ipratropium 4 puffs (80 mcg) through a large volume spacer four times a day.

8. Give salbutamol each 4 hours. If asthma very severe give epinephrine/adrenaline 0.5 mg SCI every 4 hours.

9. If prednisolone or hydrocortisone not available and the patient not improving, give aminophylline or theophylline. (If prednisolone, salbutamol or epinephrine/adrenaline and ipratropium have been given, aminophylline or theophylline will not be of any more help; so do not give them.)

Do NOT give any injection of aminophylline if the patient has been taking aminophylline or theophylline tablets or has had an aminophylline injection in the last 12 hours; as an overdose can cause death.

Give aminophylline or theophylline orally or aminophylline IV for a moderate attack or IV for a severe attack. *Give IV slowly* – take 10 minutes by the clock.
- Small adult (< 50 kg) 300 mg orally *or* 250 mg IV
- Large adult (> 50 kg) 400 mg orally *or* 375 mg IV.

Do not give this large dose of aminophylline or theophylline if the patient has taken regular oral aminophylline or theophyllline or had a large oral dose in the last 12 hours. In these cases, start an aminophylline drip (see below),

---

Start an aminophylline drip.
Add aminophylline solution:
- 150 mg for a small adult (< 50 kg) *or*
- 225 mg for a large adult (> 50 kg)
to 0.5–1 litre of 4.3% dextrose in 0.18% sodium chloride.

Use only half of these doses of aminophylline if the patient has heart failure or liver disease or if a macrolide antibiotic, e.g. erythromycin or roxithromycin (which increases blood theophylline levels) is being given.

Give the above every 8 hours. Continue until the attack has completely gone.

If the patient is a smoker *and* if the asthma does not improve *and* if there are no toxic effects, you can double the dose of aminophylline.

If there is continuous nausea or any vomiting or headache that does not go away, or anything to suggest an epileptic fit, then stop the aminophylline drip for 8 hours; and after this, restart it at half of the previous rate, or (better) reduce the dose of aminophylline in each flask to half the previous dose and continue to run the drip at the same rate.

10. If there is any suggestion of an acute bacterial infection (temperature raised, pus in sputum, signs in chest, etc.) give antibiotics.

11. When the patient improves:
    (a) Stop oxygen.
    (b) Change epinephrine/adrenaline injections or salbutamol nebulised to salbutamol metered aerosol 4 puffs or one (or two) 4 mg tablets four times a day.
    (c) If given, change aminophylline drip to aminophylline or theophylline tablets four times a day. Start 100 mg four times a day. Increase the dose if necessary.
    (d) Continue ipratropium.
    (e) Continue the prednisolone, reducing to zero by 7–10 days.

When the patient is better he can go home with a supply of his drugs, and return for review each week. If well and peak flow 80% or more when seen on the first week, stop prednisone; the next week stop ipratropium; the next week make salbutamol just prn; and then each *month* try reducing the beclomethasone by 1 puff. If at any time the asthma comes back, increase the treatment until it settles and then continue on one dose above the dose where the asthma returned.

The patient should return for review regularly to see if:
(a) lung function is 80% of predicted, in which case the dose of treatment may be able to be reduced;
(b) lung function is not 80% of predicted, in which case the dose of treatment should be increased.

If any patient is on prednisolone all the time, the Medical Officer must see him; decide about isoniazid and malaria prophylaxis and order what dose of prednisolone (usually 50 mg) the patient should take immediately if an acute severe attack when he comes to the health centre for continuing treatment.

Transfer to Medical Officer care if there is:

1. Very severe asthma which does not improve, or is worse, after 8 hours of proper treatment for a severe case, i.e. if:
   - PR 120 or more,
   - severe shortness of breath and breathing distress, or
   - cyanosis
   (urgent – emergency);
2. Severe asthma after 2 days of full treatment (urgent);
3. Repeated acute attacks needing repeated inpatient care during several months (non-urgent).

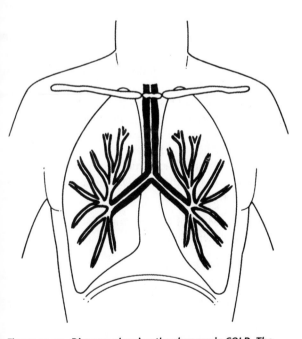

Figure 20.24 *Diagram showing the changes in COLD. The bronchi going to all parts of the lung are narrowed by (1) a thick layer of mucus on the surface of the mucous membrane, (2) the mucous membrane itself is thickened and (3) the irregular size of many damaged bronchi, many of which collapse when the patient breathes out, thus trapping air in the lungs.*

Chronic obstructive lung disease

Chronic obstructive lung disease (COLD) (also called chronic obstructive pulmonary or airways disease (COPD or COAD) or chronic bronchitis and emphysema) is a common chronic non-infective disease of the bronchi and lungs.

The mucous membrane lining the bronchi is thickened and covered by a layer of mucus. This narrows the bronchi and causes shortness of breath, cough and sputum. The walls of the bronchi, because of years of irritation and inflammation, are of irregular size and are weak. When the patient breathes out, many of the bronchi collapse before the air from the alveoli can go through them. This traps air inside the lung. This causes shortness of breath. Alveoli have been irritated and inflamed and many are destroyed. This also causes shortness of breath. Because of all these, not enough oxygen is put into the blood and often not enough carbon dioxide got out of the blood. (See Figure 20.24.)

COLD is caused by smoking tobacco or other leaves or chemicals; smoke from fires in homes without proper chimneys; some smoke or special dusts at places of work; or repeated attacks of lung infections. These things irritate, inflame and destroy the lungs.

Symptoms
- Chronic cough (on most days for at least 3 months of the year for at least 2 years).
- Sputum which is white or mucus (except if there is also acute chest infection, when pus).
- Shortness of breath – at first during exercise or respiratory infection, but later all the time.
- Wheezing at times.

Signs
- Middle-aged or old person who usually has been a smoker or had repeated chest infections, etc. (as above).
- Normal temperature.
- Normal pulse.
- Increased breathing rate (if severe).
- Wasting (if severe).
- Chest – hyperinflation, i.e. looks as if the patient is holding his breath in all of the time; abnormal use of neck and shoulder and abdominal muscles for breathing; and indrawing of the skin and soft tissues above and below the clavicles and over the upper and lower chest during breathing in ('insuction') (if severe).
- Only a little but equal movement on both sides (the chest is almost fully expanded *all* the time).

- The percussion note often more resonant (hollow) than normal but on both sides.
- Breath sounds – air entry often decreased equally on both sides.
- Wheezes (or rhonchi) and sometimes crackles (or crepitations) – heard equally on both sides and more often low down in the chest.
- Peak flows usually but not always low (peak flow readings measure severity of asthma but not COPD well).

Complications

- Acute bronchitis (see page 286) and pneumonia (see page 287) which occurs more and more often.
- Asthma (see page 294) is very common.
- Heart failure (see Chapter 27 page 461).

The patient usually gets worse slowly over years, and dies because of one of these complications.

Tests

Always send three sputum smears to the laboratory for examination for AFB. See Chapter 14 page 108.

Do not diagnose COLD until smears have been negative for AFB.

Treatment

Treat as an outpatient.

Admit for inpatient treatment only if a complication (pneumonia, moderate or severe asthma or heart failure) develops.

1. Tell the patient he has to stop smoking to have any chance of improving. (See page 277 to help him stop.)
2. If there is wheezing or rhonchi then supply:
   (a) ipratropium bromide metered aerosol 20 µg/mcg/puff, 2 puffs through a large volume spacer four times a day regularly which often helps a lot.
   (b) salbutamol metered aerosol 200–400 mcg (2–4 puffs) through a spacer or 4 mg orally four times a day if necessary for attacks of shortness of breath (as well as (a)).
   If an attack of asthma see page 294.
   (c) aminophylline or theophylline tablets regularly (see page 295) if there is shortness of breath all the time; or as required (see page 295) if there are only attacks of shortness of breath, could be tried.
3. The inflammation in the airways in COPD is different to the inflammation in asthma. Asthma inflammation responds well to corticosteroids, whereas COPD inflammation usually does not.

The Medical Officer may at times try corticosteroids and continue them if they are effective. New drugs are being tried for COPD inflammation but are not yet generally available.

4. *Show* the patient how to look for pus in his sputum (yellow or green colour).
   Tell the patient to look every day and to come for antibiotics immediately if he sees pus.
   Treat any chest infection immediately, until there is no pus in the sputum (it is white again).
   Treat as follows: procaine benzylpenicillin 1 g or 1,000,000 units IMI daily *or* SMX 800 mg/TMP 160 mg twice daily for 5–10 days. If this fails give: tetracycline 250–500 mg four times a day or doxycycline 100 mg daily *or* amoxicillin 500 mg with, if not pregnant, clavulanic acid 125 mg three times a day.
   Use chloramphenicol only for infections which threaten life.
5. Look for heart failure. If it is found start hydrochlorothiazide 25–50 mg daily and only if needed, add furosemide/frusemide 40–80 mg daily, and see 'Heart failure' (Chapter 27 page 461).
6. Do not give oxygen unless there is a complication (e.g. pneumonia). Do not give oxygen faster than 2 litres/minute intranasally as too much oxygen may make the COLD patient unconscious and cause death. If the patient's blood is measured and shown to be low in oxygen all the time $PaO_2 < 50$ mmHg or 6.7 kPa, oxygen 2 l/minute by nasal prongs as long as it is for more than 15 hours a day may stop heart failure. This is not possible because of the expense. Short treatments with oxygen when there is no complication are of no help at all – useless and waste of oxygen and money.
7. Never give morphine, pethidine or phenobarbitone (as these may stop the COLD patient breathing and cause death).

Transfer to Medical Officer care is not necessary as no more treatment is possible at a hospital.

Control and prevention

1. Treat chest infections quickly and properly.
2. Do everything you can to stop people smoking tobacco (see page 277).

Lung diseases caused by worms

A number of lung diseases can be caused by worms.

Bronchitis and pneumonia can be caused by the larvae of worms (e.g. hookworm or roundworm) as they travel through the lung.

Asthma and other chest pains and other symptoms can be caused by worm larvae (e.g. roundworm or hookworm) as they travel through the body, or by some of the filarial worms.

Chronic lung disease with heart failure can be caused by schistosomiasis, but usually there are signs of portal hypertension also.

Haemoptysis, pneumonia or chronic lung disease or a condition like TB can be caused by lung flukes (see page 300).

None of these conditions can be diagnosed without the help of a laboratory. Do not worry. If one of these conditions is very common in your area, you will be taught how to diagnose and treat it. Otherwise, the condition will be diagnosed when you refer or transfer the patient to a Medical Officer (usually when the patient does not get better with your treatment).

Bronchiectasis

Bronchiectasis is a condition when there is permanent damage to the bronchi of part of the lung. The bronchi are permanently dilated (widened) and cannot (as normal bronchi can) push fluid or anything else in

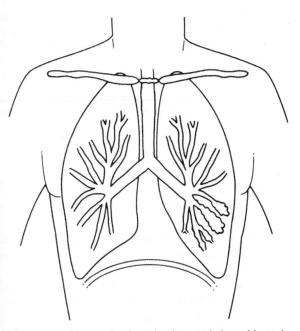

Figure 20.25 *Diagram to show the changes in bronchiectasis affecting some of the bronchi of the left lower lobe. The bronchial walls have been weakened or destroyed. The bronchi therefore became irregular in size and shape. The bronchial mucous membrane has been destroyed. The bronchi therefore cannot move secretions out through the bronchial tree. The bronchi therefore become filled with secretions. The bronchial secretions often become infected and form pus.*

them upwards against gravity to get rid of them from the lung. The bronchi become infected. They finally become just like tubes or bags full of pus (see Figure 20.25).

Bronchiectasis is caused by obstruction and infection (at the same time) of bronchi which are not treated and cured quickly. This infection and obstruction may be caused by TB or pneumonia or bronchitis (especially attacks complicating measles or whooping cough) which are not treated quickly or properly.

Symptoms include:

- Chronic cough that is present every day and worse after waking in the morning or after exercise.
- Sputum in large amounts (e.g. 20–200 ml or more daily) which is often made of pus (e.g. green or yellow or brown and often smells bad).
- Sometimes blood in the sputum.
- Shortness of breath; but only late in the disease.

Signs of bronchiectasis are few until late in the disease. At first there is only one sign – crackles (or crepitations) in the affected part of the lung which stay there after deep breathing and coughing and are always there in the same place every time the patient is examined.

Signs which come later include: wasting, anaemia, and clubbing of the fingers.

Attacks of acute bronchitis and pneumonia are common.

Try to diagnose bronchiectasis when there is only cough, sputum and crackles in one area.

Send sputum for AFB to check the patient does not have TB.

Treatment includes:

1. Postural drainage and physiotherapy for 15–30 minutes once or twice *every* day of the patient's life is the only treatment which really helps. Most patients will not do this; but without this, any other treatment is of no real help. Show the patient how to raise the foot of a straight bed by using blocks of something about 0.25–0.5 m high; lie on this with the head at the low end of the bed and the affected part of his lung (i.e. where the crackles are heard) upwards (i.e. on the roof side); then take deep breaths and cough up the sputum as he (or someone else) hits the affected part of the lung with the palm of the hand. Even better, someone should use both hands to squeeze the patient's chest as he breathes out and coughs, and at the same time shake or vibrate the chest. Tell the patient to do this for 15–30 minutes each morning, and also if

possible each evening. Also tell the patient to sleep on a straight bed if possible; even better, sleep with the foot of the bed raised.

2. Antibiotics as for pneumonia if there is an acute bacterial infection (but do not continue the antibiotic if it does not cure the infection). Antibiotics will not work if the patient does not also have the postural drainage and physiotherapy.

3. Salbutamol or other asthma treatment drugs if there is shortness of breath or wheezing which is improved by the asthma drugs.

4. Surgery to cut out the whole part of the lung which has bronchiectasis in it can help only very occasionally.

Discuss treatment of the patient with the next visiting Medical Officer.

Pulmonary tuberculosis

See Chapter 14 page 101.

Lung flukes

Paragonimus westermani and some other small worms about 10 mm long normally live in the lungs of dogs, cats, pigs and other animals in Asia, parts of the Pacific and West Africa. Their eggs are coughed up or passed in the stool and if they reach fresh water, develop in crayfish and crabs, ending up in their muscles. When animals eat these crabs, etc. the worms travel from the bowel to the lung, where they live by destroying part of the lung and making little 'nests' about 1 cm in diameter. These cause cough, sputum, haemoptysis, chest pain, fever, etc.

Man can become infected by eating uncooked freshwater crayfish and crabs. The symptoms in man are the same as for animals and very similar to those of TB. Diagnosis can be made by finding the eggs in the sputum or stool.

The main problem is making the diagnosis. If a patient appears to have TB and repeated tests do not demonstrate AFB in the sputum, it is worthwhile requesting sputum and stool examination for eggs of *Paragonimus* if this parasite is known to occur in the area.

Treatment is with praziquantel 25 mg/kg three times a day for 2–3 days.

Prevention is of course not eating uncooked crabs or crayfish, even if they are pickled.

Lung cancer (carcinoma of bronchus)

This cancer is common only in populations where smoking has been common for 20 or more years (and chronic bronchitis and emphysema is therefore usually also common). Unfortunately, although previously rare, smoking tobacco has now become more and more common in developing countries.

The cancer grows in areas of the bronchi irritated by tobacco smoke breathed in for many years. This growing cancer can cause cough, sputum and if it bleeds, haemoptysis. Initially, it often looks like TB but the sputum for AFB is negative. Later, as the tumour grows, it can block up the whole bronchus in which it is growing and cause shortness of breath and the part of the lung supplied with air by it to collapse or get infected. Infection will look like a pneumonia but it will not get better with antibiotics, or if it does, soon come back again. If the cancer spreads to the pleura at the edge of the lung, this can cause a pleural effusion (as pneumonia also can). If it presses on nerves in the centre of the chest, this can paralyse the diaphragm (causing shortness of breath and chest signs like pleural fluid) or paralyse the vocal cords (causing hoarseness). It often causes a constant severe ache or pain in the chest. It can spread not only inside the chest but through the lymph vessels or blood to the lymph glands above the clavicle (causing a hard, lumpy swelling), to the liver (which becomes hard and lumpy and the patient may become jaundiced), to the bones (which can ache or give severe pain and at times break) or the brain (where it can cause epilepsy or paralysis or loss of consciousness, etc.) or in fact to any part of the body (and there produce symptoms and signs). It can cause severe malaise and loss of weight. It is a common cause of finger clubbing. Symptoms can be severe.

The best treatment is to cut the tumour and the surrounding lung out while the tumour is still small and before it has spread anywhere else. Some types (small cell carcinomas) are best treated with (very expensive) chemotherapy. Even with the best treatment, 85–90% of patients will still die of this cancer before 5 years are up; and without treatment usually all within 2 years, although with small cell lung cancer within 12 weeks. In most cases, the most important part of the treatment will be to relieve the terrible pain and symptoms that lung cancer causes as it will not be possible to cure the patient.

Diagnosis is difficult and includes sputum examination for cancer cells or bronchoscopy (that is, looking inside the airways of the lungs with a special instrument and taking a biopsy of any cancer seen) and these are not possible not only in health centres but also in many hospitals. Treatment, as mentioned, is difficult, expensive and often does not cure the patient.

Remember, therefore, that lung cancer exists mainly in smokers, although unfortunately also in those who live or work with smokers and breathe in the smoker's smoke. Diagnosing and treating it, however, is not anywhere near as important as correctly diagnosing and treating pneumonia, TB, HIV infection, etc. as these conditions can be cured or helped; and correct management not only helps the patient but also stops the condition spreading to others.

Lung cancer is just another of the reasons why you should do all you can to stop children from starting to smoke and help smokers give up smoking permanently (see page 277).

Kaposi's sarcoma can also occur in the bronchus and other airways and have symptoms and signs like lung cancer.

Industrial lung disease

Lung disease can be caused by inhaling (breathing in) dust produced in some work places. These can include mines (especially where hard rock is mined), factories, stone working places (where stone is cut or carved), places where asbestos is used, etc.

Most of these dusts cause the lungs to become scarred or 'fibrotic'. The patient often coughs (and sputum may be coloured by the dust breathed in). The patient becomes more and more short of breath. Crackles may be heard in the chest. Clubbing may be severe. Cyanosis develops. The patient becomes more and more short of breath and thin and wasted and dies.

TB or lung cancer can complicate these illnesses.

Unfortunately, no cure is possible. The patient should stop smoking if he smokes tobacco. Relief of symptoms, including helping with breathlessness at the end of life (e.g. with morphine), is usually all that can be done.

If you think a patient may have an industrial lung disease, refer the patient to the Medical Officer. The patient may be able to be helped. Very importantly, action may need to be taken at the place of work so that other workers do not develop the same disease.

Deep venous thrombosis and pulmonary embolism

Venous thromboses occur when blood clots in a vein and becomes solid. Deep venous thrombosis (DVT) occurs when one of the large veins deep in the leg or pelvis has a clot form in it. This is more likely to occur in certain situations.

1. The blood is flowing more slowly than usual, e.g.:
   • The patient is less physically active than normal, e.g. lying down because of illness, operation, accident, childbirth, etc. or sitting in one position for a long time on a long car, boat or plane trip.
   • The whole circulation is slowed, e.g. heart failure.
2. The lining of the vein has been damaged, e.g. leg injury, especially fracture or operation.
3. The blood is more likely to clot than usual, e.g.:
   • The normal body reaction to when more clotting is needed, i.e. after operation, accident or childbirth.
   • Some blood diseases, e.g. sickle cell anaemia.
   • Some hormone changes, e.g. pregnancy or taking oestrogen-containing oral contraceptive.
   • Malignant cancer anywhere in the body.

DVT often causes no symptoms and signs or only painless swelling of the leg.

Pulmonary embolus (PE) occurs when part or all of a clot from a DVT breaks off and is carried through the veins and then through the right heart and into the pulmonary vein in the lungs (see Figure 27.1 page 456). The clot is stopped by the pulmonary vessels which are becoming smaller and smaller to form the alveolar capillaries. The clot, however, then blocks any more blood flow to that part of the lung. (An embolus (emboli if more than one embolus) is any substance carried by the blood stream until it causes obstruction by blocking a blood vessel.)

Small pulmonary emboli may cause no symptoms or signs. Large pulmonary emboli can cause sudden death by stopping all or most of the blood getting to the lungs. Less large emboli can cause the following.

1. Sudden shortness of breath and increase in breathing rate and cyanosis, as not enough blood can get through the smaller amount of working lung left.
2. Constant central chest pain (heart pain) due to not enough oxygen getting to the heart muscle.
3. Fast pulse (to try to get the rest of the blood around the body quickly enough to give it oxygen) and low BP (as not as much blood to pump around). Shock may occur.
4. Raised jugular venous pressure (JVP) (see Chapter 27 page 462), as the venous blood cannot get into the right heart and blocked up lungs.

If the part of the lung not getting the blood dies, this is called a pulmonary infarction. The dead area may bleed and cause pleuritic pain and/or haemoptysis. Infarction is not common, as the lung has a second blood supply from also the bronchial arteries from the aorta.

DVT and PE are fortunately not as common in developing and tropical countries as in industrialised countries, where they are very common in patients in hospital.

This is fortunate as:

1. Diagnosis needs special blood tests, lung scans, echocardiogram, etc. which are not available in health centres and not available in many hospitals.
2. Treatment needs anticoagulant drugs (heparin and warfarin) to make the blood less likely to clot and allow the normal body mechanisms to be able to dissolve the clot. Treatment may need even thrombolytic drugs to quickly dissolve the clot. These drugs need special blood tests done regularly so that they do not stop clotting so much that they cause bleeding and death of the patient. These drugs and tests are not available in health centres or even many hospitals.

Prevention of DVT and PE is the only thing possible in the health centre. Make sure, therefore, that all of the patients who have any of the conditions mentioned above who are in your health centre:

1. Are kept physically active every day.
   - Do not allow them to lie down all day, even if they have a severe illness or if they have had an injury or operation. They must get up and walk at least twice each day (being helped by one or two other people if needed).
   - Move (wriggle) their toes, feet and legs about 20 times each hour.
2. Do not become dehydrated. Order oral or IV fluids if they are not drinking enough.
3. Take acetylsalicylic acid 100–150 mg each day if they are likely to get a DVT, e.g. more than one of the conditions likely to cause a DVT. Do not give acetylsalicylic acid if the patient has a condition likely to bleed or if the patient may need an operation in the next 10 days. This drug is much better at stopping arterial rather than venous clots and is not very effective for DVT prevention; but until other drugs are available, it is the only one we can use in a health centre.

Some problems of diagnosis and management

Deafness

Causes include:

1. any condition blocking the external ear canal, including wax, foreign body or external ear inflammation;
2. any condition damaging the middle ear, including blocked Eustachian tube and acute and chronic middle ear infection;
3. any condition damaging the inner ear, or the nerve from the ear to the brain, including side effects of streptomycin, gentamicin and trauma of the head;
4. others, including conditions of old age.
5. If not one of the above, see ENT book and refer the patient to the Medical Officer.

Always look in the ear with an auriscope. Do ear toilet or syringing until you can see the ear drum. Treat any condition in the usual way (see Index).

Ear pain

Causes include:

1. external ear infection (otitis externa);
2. foreign body in the external ear canal;
3. middle ear inflammation (otitis media), acute or chronic;
4. mastoiditis;
5. acute parotitis – mumps or acute bacterial;
6. infection of teeth;
7. others, including arthritis of the jaw joint.

If the cause is not one of these see a specialist ENT book and refer the patient to the Medical Officer.

Always look in the ear with an auriscope. Do ear toilet and syringing until you can see the ear drum. Examine behind the ear (mastoid) in front of the ear (parotid) and below the ear (in the mouth and tap on each tooth with a tongue depressor to find if tenderness which would suggest infection in this structure).

Treat any condition in the usual way (see Index).

Ear discharge

Causes include:

1. external ear inflammation (otitis externa);
2. foreign body in external ear canal;
3. middle ear infection (otitis media), acute (with perforated ear drum) or chronic;
4. others.

If the cause is not one of these see a specialist ENT book and refer the patient to the Medical Officer.

Always look in the ear with an auriscope.

Do ear toilet or syringing until you can see the ear drum. Treat any condition in the usual way (see Index).

Nasal discharge – both sides

Causes include:

1. virus infections of the upper respiratory tract including measles (watery discharge);

2. bacterial infections of the upper respiratory tract, e.g. sinusitis, acute, which may become chronic (pus);
3. foreign body in the nose (pus or blood);
4. allergy ('hay fever') (watery discharge) and mucus membrane thick or blueish;
5. irritation by dust, smoke, etc. (watery discharge);
6. others, including tumours.

If the cause is not one of these see a specialist ENT book and refer the patient to the Medical Officer.

Treat any condition in the usual way (see Index). You can usually improve chronic infections by washing out the nose twice daily with normal saline solution ($2\frac{1}{2}$ ml or $\frac{1}{2}$ teaspoon of salt in 200 ml or 1 cup of clean water). Tell the patient to sniff up or squirt in with a 20 ml syringe (without a needle) or pour in the saline through the nose with the head forward and down (top of head pointing to the ground) 20–50 ml; then sit or stand up normally and blow it out or let it run into the mouth then spit it out. This thins the pus or other secretions to make it easier for it to run out and washes it away.

Nasal discharge – from one side only

Always look for a foreign body in the nose (see page 283).

See also nasal discharge both sides (above).

Acute loss of voice or hoarse voice (present for less than 4 weeks)

Causes include:

1. shouting, singing or talking too much;
2. smoking more than usual;
3. acute viral throat/larynx/tracheal/bronchial infections (the patient is usually not 'sick');
4. acute bacterial throat/larynx/tracheal/bronchial infections (the patient is usually 'sick');
5. lung cancer (see page 300);

If the cause is not one of these see a specialist ENT book.

Treat any condition found in the usual way. See Index.

Chronic loss of voice or hoarse voice (present for more than 4 weeks)

Causes include:

1. TB of lung and larynx;
2. cancer of larynx or neck or lung;
3. others.

You must transfer all patients with this so that the Medical Officer can examine the patient's larynx, except patients with sputum-positive TB (who you can treat for TB at the health centre).

Sore throat

Causes include:

1. common cold, and other viral upper respiratory tract infections;
2. acute tonsillitis, and other bacterial upper respiratory tract infections;
3. the same as the causes of a painful ear (see page 302).

Always look in the mouth and throat with a tongue depressor and light, and in the ear with an auriscope.

If these conditions are not present see a specialist ENT book. Treat any condition found in the usual way (see Index).

Cough

The cause is usually obvious from the history and examination.

Do a full history and examination (see Chapter 6). Look at sputum (? mucus ? pus ? blood).

Always ask for how long the cough has been present (see below). If it has been present for more than 2–3 weeks send sputum for examination for AFB.

Cough present for less than 3 weeks

Upper respiratory tract infection

- No other chest symptoms.
- Breathing (respiratory) rate normal and no respiratory distress (see page 270).
- No chest signs.
- Examine carefully all of the URT, including for diphtheria.

Asthma

- Shortness of breath. Episodes of coughing often without sputum, often in late afternoon or night or after exertion. Previous similar attacks.
- Sputum, if any, jelly-like and not made of pus, i.e. not yellow or rusty.
- Wheezes or rhonchi in chest.
- No fever.

Acute bronchitis or pneumonia

- Fever and other general signs of infection.
- Sputum is pus or of rusty colour.
- Breathing (respiratory) rate fast.
- Breathing (respiratory) distress may be present.
- Other chest signs.
- Think of possible underlying HIV infection.

Inhaled foreign body

• Often history of inhalation or choking.

Early cases of prolonged cough. (See below.)

Cough present for more than 3 weeks

Where tuberculosis OR HIV infection is common

Make three sputum smears for examination for AFB – one specimen collected immediately; another specimen collected by the patient the next morning as soon as he wakes; and a further specimen collected when the patient returns with the second one.

Where tuberculosis AND HIV infection are not common

• Treat for 1 week with procaine benzylpenicillin 1 g or 1,000,000 units daily IMI or SMX 800 mg/TMP 160 mg twice a day or alternative.
• If the cough is not cured treat for 1 week with tetracycline *or* doxycycline, but not if pregnant, when use amoxicillin or ampicillin or erythromycin.
• If the cough is still present continue the tetracycline or alternative and send three sputum specimens for examination for AFB.

If sputum is positive for AFB

See Chapter 14 pages 112–126 on Tuberculosis.

If all sputum examinations negative for AFB

1. Repeat sputum for AFB × 3 again if:
   (a) past or family history of TB or other history suggests TB or HIV infection;
   (b) there is wasting or lymphadenopathy or other signs of TB or HIV infection.
2. Otherwise, and if repeat sputum examinations negative for AFB, check for:
   (a) HIV infection with unusual or opportunistic lung infection (see Chapter 19 pages 223–226). Do counselling and HIV blood test. Treat if needed as in Chapter 19 pages 223–226;
   (b) chronic obstructive lung disease, especially if still smoking;
   (c) asthma with cough (especially at night);
   (d) repeated acute upper respiratory tract infections, acute bronchitis or acute pneumonia (especially if underlying HIV infection);
   (e) chronic sinusitis with post-nasal discharge (especially if HIV infection);
   (f) empyema or lung abscess;
   (g) whooping cough (whoop rare in adults);
   (h) bronchiectasis;
   (i) breathing in if stomach acid if reflux or food if swallowing abnormality;
   (j) lung fluke, schistosomiasis, worms migrating through the lungs, etc.;
   (k) certain special infections in certain parts of the world, e.g. fungal infections, melioidosis, etc.;
   (l) lung cancer;
   (m) drugs, especially ACE inhibitors, e.g. enalapril and occasionally beta blockers, e.g. atenolol;
   (n) TB with sputum negative for AFB. If you still suspect TB, transfer non-urgently to the Medical Officer.

Treatment of cough

1. Diagnose then treat the cause (see Index).
2. Explain to patient that he must not smoke or must stop smoking.
3. Physiotherapy often helps; but only if it causes the patient to cough up more than 20 ml of sputum every time. See page 299.
4. 'Cough medicines' do not help.
5. Codeine phosphate 30 mg will decrease cough and help non-productive cough, e.g. whooping cough in adults; but do not give to anyone with sputum.

Sputum

See causes of cough for causes of sputum. Diagnose and treat the cause.

Always find the answers to these three things:

1. Is the sputum from the lower respiratory tract (which is often serious) or from the upper respiratory tract (which is not as serious)?
2. What is the colour of the sputum?
   • Coloured sputum (yellow, green or brown) usually means bacterial infection, e.g. acute bronchitis, bronchopneumonia, lobar pneumonia, bronchiectasis, sinusitis, TB, etc.
   • White or mucoid sputum occurs in viral infections (if there is no bacterial infection as well).
   • White or mucoid sputum is also common from smoking, chronic bronchitis (COLD), asthma and some cases of chronic sinusitis.
   • Bacterial infection needs treatment with antibiotics. Antibiotics will not help other conditions.
3. Is there blood in the sputum (haemoptysis)? If there is blood in the sputum see below.

Blood coughed up – haemoptysis

1. Always check that it is *blood* that is coughed up. Always look at what is coughed up.
2. Always check that the blood was *coughed up*.
   • Check that the blood was not vomited up.
   • Check that the blood was not just from the upper respiratory tract (especially the nose).

3. Always find out *how much* blood was coughed up – if more than one cup, it is an emergency and you must start an IV drip and transfer the patient in case a blood transfusion is needed.

4. Always find out the *cause*. Causes include:
- Tuberculosis. Send sputum for AFB in all cases.
- Lung fluke infection in some areas.
- Any acute lower respiratory tract infection.
- Bronchiectasis or lung abscess.
- Chest injury.
- Lung cancer.
- Bleeding disorder, e.g. snakebite, poisoning with rat poison (warfarin), side effects of some drugs (e.g. quinine), etc. and some blood diseases, e.g. leukaemia.
- Others. If the cause is not one of these, see a specialist book. Causes such as pulmonary embolus are not common in the rural areas of tropical and developing countries but may be common in the towns and cities.

> Tuberculosis is the most common and important cause of haemoptysis.

If you cannot diagnose the cause at the health centre, transfer the patient for investigation.

Treatment of haemoptysis

1. Treat the cause.
2. If there is shock or anaemia, give routine treatment for these (see Chapter 27 page 468 and Chapter 21 page 316).
3. If the patient has difficulty in breathing (because blood is filling the bronchi):
- put the patient on his side, with the diseased part of the chest down or on his underside,
- tip the head of the bed down,
- suck out the pharynx and larynx if necessary,
- give morphine 10 mg (1 ml) by slow IVI or IMI or IVI diazepam 5–10 mg (1–2 ml) 1 mg/minute or (*but* only if does *not* have COLD),
- give intranasal oxygen,
- transfer as soon as possible to Medical Officer care.
4. Wear protective clothing, i.e. gown, mask, goggles, gloves, etc. so that blood does not get into staff members' skin or eyes, mouth, etc.
5. Transfer to Medical Officer urgently if 2 or 3 occur.

Shortness of breath

Do a full history and examination (see Chapter 6).

Look at any sputum (? pus ? blood).

Test the urine for protein and sugar.

Look at the following seven headings to see which paragraphs apply to your patient.

1. With stridor (loud noise breathing in)
Blockage of throat, larynx or trachea by foreign body, acute allergic reaction or acute bacterial or viral infection.
- Emergency. Act immediately.
- If inhaled foreign body or vomit is possible, pull these out of throat. If not successful back slap or do abdominal thrust or if these not successful, lay the patient down and start chest compression. See Chapter 37 pages 606–612.
- If acute allergic reaction is possible, give IM epinephrine/adrenaline 0.5 ml ($\frac{1}{2}$ ml) and IV antihistamine, e.g. promethazine 50 mg immediately. Then see Chapter 10 page 44.
- If infection is possible, give IV (or IM) chloramphenicol 2 g immediately, then 1 g each 6 hours and drain any abscess blocking the airway (see page 285).
- Give intranasal oxygen 4 litres/minute.
- If stops breathing see Chapter 37 pages 606–612.
- Transfer urgently (emergency) unless the patient is cured immediately.

2. With pallor and/or shock (fast PR, low BP, cold hands and feet)
Anaemia ± blood loss.
- If shock or blood loss see Chapter 27 page 468.
- Give routine anaemia treatment to other cases (see Chapter 21 page 316).

3. With fever
Chest infections (cough, sputum made of pus or rusty, crackles or other signs in chest); septicaemia.
- Give penicillin or chloramphenicol (see page 289).
- Send sputum for AFB if cough present for more than 3 weeks. See Chapter 14 page 108.

Malaria if there is no evidence of chest infection.
- Give antimalarials (see Chapter 13, pages 79, 80).

4. With wheezing and rhonchi
Asthma; COLD; acute bronchitis.
- Give inhaled salbutamol or SCI epinephrine/adrenaline *and* ipratropium inhaled and, if needed, oral prednisolone or IV hydrocortisone. (See pages 294–297.)
- Send sputum for AFB if cough present for more than 3 weeks. See Chapter 14 page 108.

5. With oedema, large liver, raised neck veins

Heart failure.

- Give diuretics – IV furosemide/frusemide 40 mg immediately if severe or oral hydrochlorothiazide 50 mg if not severe and see Chapter 27 page 465.
- Treat the cause (see Chapter 27 page 462).

6. And 'sick' but not distressed by shortness of breath

Dehydration usually from gastroenteritis.

- Give IV fluids (see Chapter 23 page 364).

Meningitis or septicaemia.

- Give chloramphenicol by IVI or IMI (see Chapter 12 page 64).

Diabetes mellitus.

- Give IV rehydration and SC or IM insulin. See Chapter 30 page 503.
- Transfer to Medical Officer urgently.

Chronic kidney failure

- See Chapter 26 page 449.

Acidosis

- See Chapter 13 page 83.

Acetylsalicylic acid poisoning

- See Chapter 34 page 562.

7. And very worried by shortness of breath but no abnormalities found on examination

Hyperventilation.

- The patient feels as if he cannot get enough air into the lungs when he obviously is (air hunger) – anxiety/stress.

Obvious 'over-breathing'

- Has a major problem – 'acting out'.

Both often cause dizziness, a strange feeling around the mouth, pins and needles in hands and feet, palpitations, cramps, etc.

See Chapter 35 pages 582–583.

Another classification of shortness of breath

Shortness of breath is of course normal after strong exercise or in high areas (on mountains).

Diseases causing shortness of breath include:

1. Respiratory diseases
    (a) of alveoli
        pneumonia including severe or advanced tuberculous pneumonia – shallow quick breathing

(b) of bronchi
    acute bronchitis
    asthma (deep slow breathing) ⎫ sometimes
    COLD ⎭ wheezing

(c) of throat/larynx/trachea/bronchi
    acute bacterial infections (especially epiglotitis)
    acute viral infections (e.g. 'croup')
    allergy ⎬ often stridor
    foreign body
    cancer

(d) of pleura
    effusion or empyema ⎫ shallow quick
    pneumothorax ⎭ breathing

2. Cardiovascular
    (a) heart failure – shallow quick breathing
    (b) shock – gasping breathing.

3. Anaemia – deep fast breathing.

4. Kidney failure ⎫ deep slow breathing;
   Diabetes mellitus ⎭ but no distress

5. Anxiety – the patient feels as if he can't get enough air into his lungs; but on examination no abnormalities are found.
    'Acting out' – obvious over-breathing.

6. Others.

Stridor

Stridor is noisy breathing *in*. (Noisy breathing *out* is not as important.) Stridor is usually a crowing noise; but sometimes it is more like snoring.

> Noisy breathing is obstructed breathing. Immediately relieve the obstruction.

Stridor is always serious. Stridor is very dangerous if there is rib recession or insuction during breathing in, and/or if the patient uses his neck and abdominal muscles to keep breathing.

Always think of these things and treat any present like this:

1. If the patient is weak or not fully conscious (often like 'snoring'):
    (a) lay the patient on his side, ⎫
    (b) tip his head back, ⎪ See Chapter 25
    (c) pull his jaw forward, ⎬ pages 422–424
    (d) suck out his throat. ⎭

2. Infection of throat and/or epiglottis and/or larynx and/or trachea

(a) IVI (or IMI) chloramphenicol urgently for septicaemia (see Chapter 12 page 64).

(b) if allergy possible, treat (see 4).

(c) Make the patient breathe moist air by boiling water near him if the air is cool and/or dry.

(d) Nurse him carefully (suck out if necessary).

(e) Give intranasal oxygen 4 litres/minute.

(f) Observe him carefully. Transfer urgently (emergency) if he does not quickly improve.

(g) Drain any abscess blocking breathing (see page 285).

3. Foreign body

(a) Tip the patient's head and neck down; hit his back very hard between shoulder blades or try abdominal thrust or do chest compression. See Chapter 37 page 606.

(b) Transfer urgently if he does not cough up the foreign body.

4. Allergy

(a) IMI epinephrine/adrenaline (1:1000 solution) 0.5 ml (1/2 ml) (the essential treatment).

(b) IVI antihistamine, e.g. promethazine 50 mg. Then see Chapter 10 page 44.

(c) IVI hydrocortisone 300 mg if available.

5. Laryngostomy if breathing stops. See Chapter 37 page 613.

Chest pain

Do a full history (see Chapter 6).

Find out all about the pain:

1. Is it 'pleuritic'? i.e.
   • in the chest wall at the side of the chest (or in shoulder or abdomen),
   • worse on coughing or deep breathing,
   • helped by holding that side of the chest or lying on the side of pain.
   See this page.

2. Is it tracheal? i.e.
   • in the neck and front of centre of chest,
   • present only when coughs.
   See page 308.

3. Is it spinal? i.e.
   • also in the back,
   • worse on bending or lifting,
   • tenderness of spine.
   See page 308.

4. Is it cardiac (due to heart or pericardium or blood vessels)?
   • constant in the anterior chest, or
   • crushing type pain like a band around the chest,
   • may also be felt in arm or arms or jaw,
   • constant and not made better or worse by anything (? 'heart attack'); but if comes on exertion and is relieved by stopping the exertion; but comes back again on the same amount of exertion (? angina),
   • middle-aged or elderly person or known high BP, heart trouble or kidney trouble makes it more likely,
   • irregular, slow or fast pulse or shock or heart failure makes it more likely.
   See page 308.

5. Is it constant and in the lower chest, and are abdominal symptoms or signs also present? See Chapter 36 page 593.

6. Is it in the lower chest and comes or goes with eating food? See Chapter 23 page 352.

7. Has it been present for more than 3 weeks, and has cough also been present for 3 weeks? See page 304.

Do a full examination (see Chapter 6).

• Ask the patient to cough.
• Listen to the cough.
• Observe if coughing causes pain (pleuritic or tracheal pain).
• Examine any sputum (? pus ? blood).

Diagnose and manage according to the seven types of pain (see above) that the patient has, like this:

Pain is pleuritic

1. *If* ± cough ± sputum (pus or rusty colour) ± shortness of breath ± fever ± fast pulse ± crackles in chest, *then* pneumonia. See page 287.

2. *If* history of injury to chest, tender place on chest, *then* fracture of rib. Give enough pain relief drug so patient can (and must 5–6 times each hour) take large breaths in and out regularly and cough (to prevent pneumonia).

3. *If* short of breath ± cough ± haemoptysis ± recent other illness or operation or childbirth or even pregnancy ± a recent long trip where the legs were still ± a swollen, tender leg, then ? pulmonary embolus (clot of blood from leg or pelvic veins gone up to the lungs and blocking part of the pulmonary arteries). Exclude pneumonia and pneumothorax (see page 301). Transfer to Medical Officer urgently (emergency).

4. *If* no abnormality found but often one tender area on pressing on chest wall, *then* (not significant) chest wall pain. Give paracetamol and if needed NSAIDs and observe the patient daily for a few days.

Pain is tracheal

1. *If* cough ± sputum ± shortness of breath ± fever ± rhonchi in chest, *then* tracheitis/bronchitis. See page 286.
2. *If* no abnormality found, *then* viral upper respiratory tract infection or too much smoking or shouting, etc.

Pain is spinal

1. *If* pain gets worse over days to weeks then ? staphylococcal abscess. Transfer urgently to Medical Officer.
2. *If* pain gets worse over weeks, *then* ? TB ? cancer. Transfer urgently to Medical Officer.
3. *If* pain is sometimes present and sometimes not present, *then* ? osteoarthrosis. See Chapter 29.
4. *If* spinal tenderness on percussion or stiffness (will not bend properly) especially if lump, *then* ? TB? staphylococcal abscess? cancer? traumatic fracture (if occurred when injury)? crush fracture of vertebra (if suddenly occurred on lifting or bending, especially in middle-aged women or older men and women). Transfer urgently to Medical Officer.
5. *If* weakness of legs, not able to pass urine properly, *then* has pressure on spinal cord.
   Transfer urgently to Medical Officer on stretcher; and held with sand bags so spine cannot move.

Pain is cardiac

1. Give oxygen.
2. Give acetylsalicylic acid 300–500 mg immediately
3. Put a glyceryl trinitrate 0.5 or 0.6 mg or isosorbide dinitrate 5 mg tablet under the tongue and let it dissolve there; repeat in 5 minutes if pain still present and blood pressure above 100.
4. If pain still present, dilute 10 mg of morphine with 9 ml of saline and give 2 ml (2 mg of morphine) IVI each 5 minutes until the pain stops.
5. Give metoclopramide 10 mg IVI if nausea.
6. Treat any heart failure present in the usual way, including oxygen, diuretics and digoxin (see Chapter 27 page 464).
7. If the pulse rate and heart rate (listening at the heart apex with the stethoscope) is 40 beats per minute or less, then (a) lift up the legs (feet above the hips) and tilt the head end of the bed down and (b) give atropine 0.6 mg (1 ml) IVI, then repeat if still needed in 5 minutes and can be repeated in 1 hour and then every few hours to a maximum of 3 mg in 24 hours to try, if possible, to get the heart rate above 60.
8. If the pulse is irregular and fast (over 140) start digoxin (see Chapter 27 page 465) and propranolol 40 mg or atenolol 25 mg.

9. If the patient's heart and breathing stop, give cardiopulmonary resuscitation for 10 minutes. See Chapter 37 pages 607–612.

As soon as possible, you should contact the Medical Officer to ask for advice. Most deaths from myocardial infarctions occur within the first hour and if the patient survives the first hour after the pain starts, the most dangerous period is over.

Pain is constant in lower chest and there is tenderness or mass in upper abdomen

Then abdominal condition with referred pain. See Chapter 36 page 593.

Pain in lower chest that comes or goes with eating

Then peptic ulcer. See Chapter 23 page 352.

Pain and cough present for more than 3 weeks

? TB. See Chapter 14 pages 102–105.
? Lung cancer (see page 300).
? Chronic infection (empyema, etc.). See this chapter.

Appendix 1
Drugs which can be used for asthma and COLD to dilate the bronchi

If using a nebuliser or air pump, the patient should breathe through the mouth at a normal rate and depth.

Metered aerosols are best used through a large volume spacer (see Appendix 2 page 309).

After inhaling a metered aerosol or dry powder, the patient should hold the breath in for 10 seconds.

At one time use only:

- ONE of the short acting beta 2 agonists, and only
- ONE of the long acting beta 2 agonists, and only
- ONE of the anticholinergic drugs, and only
- ONE of the inhaled adrenocorticosteroid drugs.

1. *Short acting beta 2 agonists (about 4 hours)*
   - Epinephrine/adrenaline 1 mg in 1 ml ampoule for injection – 0.25–0.5 ml SCI or IMI.
   - Salbutamol 50 mcg/ml in 5 ml ampoule for injection – 125 mcg or 2.5 ml by SCI.
   - Salbutamol 5 mg in 1 ml solution for nebulisation – 0.5–1 ml 5 mg mixed with 4 ml of 0.9% saline nebulised and inhaled.
   - Terbutaline 5 mg in 2 ml solution for nebuliser – 2.5–5 mg mixed with 4 ml of 0.9% saline nebulised and inhaled.

- Salbutamol 100 mcg/puff metered aerosol for inhalation – 1–4 puffs inhaled.
- Terbutaline 500 mcg/puff metered aerosol for inhalation – 1–3 puffs inhaled.
- Salbutamol 2 and 4 mg tablets – 4 mg (less effective and more side effects than inhaled salbutamol).
- Ephedrine 30 mg tablet (not really a beta 2 agonist and effect tends to wear off and more side effects) – 1 tablet.

2. *Long acting beta 2 agonists (about 12 hours)*
   - Eformoterol/formoterol metered aerosol or powder for inhalation – 6–12(–24) mcg each 12 hours.
   - Salmeterol metered aerosol or powder for inhalation – 25–50(–100) mcg each 12 hours.

3. *Short acting anticholinergic drugs (about 4–6 hours)*
   - Ipratropium bromide 20 mcg/puff metered aerosol – 2–4 puffs inhaled.
   - Ipratropium bromide 250 mcg/ml nebulising solution – 1–2 ml with 4 ml 0.9% saline nebulised and inhaled.

4. *Long acting anticholinergic drugs (24 hours)*
   - Tiotropium bromide (long acting) 18 mcg powder for inhalation – 18 mcg once daily.

5. *Adrenocorticosteroid anti-inflammatory drugs*
   Usually give in one dose in the morning but could be night and morning.
   Use after the above drugs.
   After inhaling have a mouthful of water, gargle and spit this out (as 80% of drug may be in the throat and not the lungs where it is needed and may cause hoarse voice or sore throat or thrush (candida infection) if left in throat).
   Takes days to weeks to be effective.
   Numerous strengths of these available.
   Only the first two are as yet on the WHO list. The others are as effective or more effective:
   - Beclomethasone 100 mcg/puff metered aerosol – 1–5 puffs inhaled daily.
   - Beclomethasone 250 mcg/puff metered aerosol – 1–2 puffs inhaled daily.
   - Budesonide 100–500 mcg inhaled daily.
   - Fluticasone 50–250 mcg inhaled daily.
   - Ciclesamide 80–160 mcg inhaled daily (spacer not recommended).

6. *Non-steroid anti-inflammatory drugs*
   Not very powerful.
   Very safe even for children.
   Takes days to weeks to be effective.
   Used four times a day.
   - Sodium cromoglycate or cromoglycic acid solution 20 mg/2 ml for nebulisation and inhalation.

Give 2 ml with 3 ml 0.9% saline nebulised and inhaled.
- Sodium cromoglycate metered aerosol 1 mg and 5 mg per dose packs. Give 2 puffs of 1 mg four times a day inhaled or 2 puffs of 5 mg twice daily inhaled.
- Sodium cromoglycate 20 mg powder for inhalation. Give 20 mg inhaled four times daily.

7. *Theophylline including aminophylline*
   If full doses of beta 2 agonists and anti-cholinergics and corticosteroids given for asthma, these drugs have usually no further good effect but can have side effects.
   If corticosteroids or anti-cholinergics are not available, these drugs can be used for asthma if beta 2 agonists not effective enough.
   If the patient has COPD they are more likely to be helpful.
   - Aminophylline 250 mg/usually in 10 ml ampoule for injection – see pages 295–296.
   - Theophylline usually 100 mg or 125 mg tablets – dose see pages 295–296 each 4–6 hours.
   - Theophylline slow release tablets usually 200, 250 and 300 mg tablets – dose see pages 295–296 each 12 hours.

8. *Anti-inflammatory drugs for the neutrophil inflammation of COPD*
   PDE4 inhibitors, e.g. cilomilast and rofumilest not yet available.

Appendix 2

A large volume spacer. These are needed by some people to get more of the metered dose aerosol into the lungs (and less into the mouth).

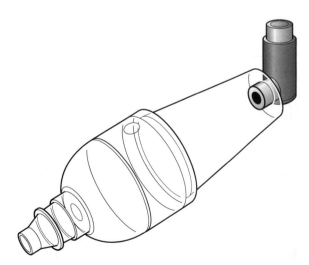

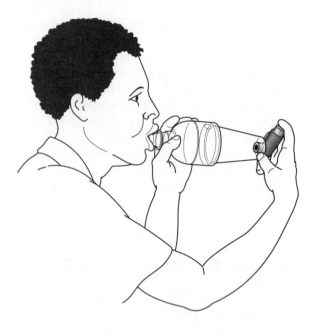

A spacer can be made from a plastic drinks bottle:

- Wash the bottle out with detergent (not soap) and water and allow to dry.
- Cut a hole for the metered aerosol apparatus to just fit into the bottom of the bottle.

Another way of making a spacer is by using a large polystyrene (foam) cup – putting it over the mouth but not the nose.

Use the spacer as follows

1. Breathe out fully.
2. Put the mouth over the bottle opening.
3. Puff the metered aerosol into the bottle.
4. Breathe in deeply and hold the breath for 10 seconds.
5. Breathe out **through the nose**. (Do not blow the air out through the mouth into the bottle.)
6. Breathe in deeply as above from the bottle two more times before having the next puff/dose.

Appendix 3   Peak expiratory flow meter

There are many other models as well as this Mini Wright's Peak Flow Meter.

To get reliable results the meter must be used exactly as directed. See page 311 for diagram and directions.

The patient must take in a full breath, put the mouthpiece inside the mouth (past the lips and the teeth) and on top of the tongue. There must be nothing to block the air going into the mouthpiece. The patient must then blow as hard and fast as he can; but needs to continue for only 2 seconds as the peak flow (fastest flow) is in the first second of blowing. The patient must not cough into the meter or a falsely high reading will be made.

The 'normal' peak flow varies with age and gender and race.

Keep the leaflet (supplied with the meter) with these results in a plastic folder on the wall or other safe place where it can be quickly and easily seen and read.

Appendix 4   H1N1 2009 influenza A ('swine flu')

Since this book was written a pandemic, which may or may not continue, was caused by the above new virus – made of a mixture of human and pig (swine) and bird influenza viruses. It is at present transmitted (spread) only between humans; pigs are not infecting humans; and eating cooked pig meat cannot cause this influenza infection. Only some older people have any immunity to this virus (probably due to infection by a similar virus which was present before 1957). Only new vaccines produced after late 2009 and also proven to be effective in producing immunity to the above virus could give any immunity to this infection.

The infection is similar to usual influenza (see page 278) and at present is not as virulent (likely to cause severe disease) as H5N1 avian influenza A ('bird flu') (see page 279); but the virus could change and become more virulent. At present the disease is 'mild in most, severe in some and moderate overall'. The infection, however, is unusual in the following ways.

1. It is very contagious – it can spread quickly; probably as so few people have any immunity (see above).
2. It tends to infect younger rather than older people (but see above).
3. It may be more dangerous to pregnant than other women (but this is not really unusual).

It, as usual, is most dangerous to the following groups.

1. Those with chronic obstructive lung disease and other chronic lung disease (including asthma).
2. Those with other chronic diseases, e.g. diabetes mellitus, heart disease, kidney disease, obesity, etc.
3. Those with decreased immunity, e.g. HIV infection.

Management is as described on page 279. Only specific new vaccines will help in increasing immunity (see above). Antiviral drugs (see avian influenza), given only if infection occurs, may help pregnant patients and those at risk of dying (see above) but are very expensive and are not usually available.

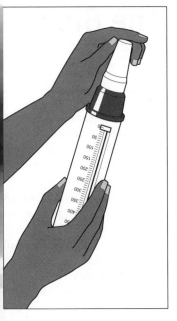

1 *Fit the mouthpiece to the Peak Flow Meter.*

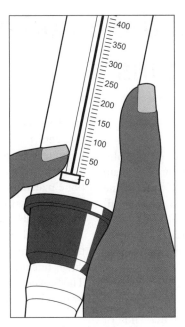

2 *Ensure the pointer is set at zero.*

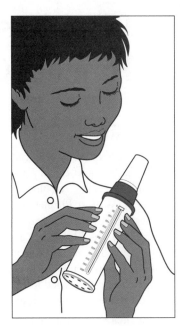

3 *Hold the Peak Flow Meter so that your fingers are clear of the scale and slot. Do not obstruct the holes at the end of the Peak Flow Meter.*

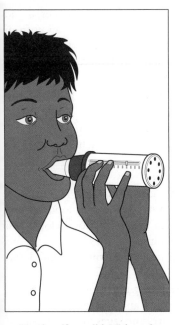

4 *Stand up if possible. Take a deep breath, place the Peak Flow Meter in the mouth and hold horizontally, closing the lips around the mouthpiece, then blow as hard and as fast as you can.*

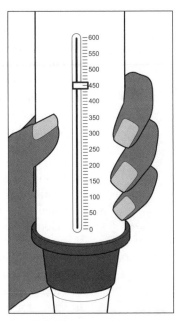

5 *Note the number on the scale indicated by the pointer.*

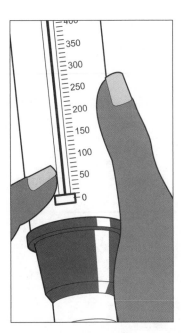

6 *Return the pointer to zero and repeat the procedure twice more to obtain three readings. Mark the highest of three readings on the chart.*

21 Disorders of the Blood and the Blood Forming Organs

Anatomy

Blood is made of many cells, called blood cells and also platelets; and a liquid, called plasma. There are two main kinds of blood cells – red blood cells (RBCs) and white blood cells (WBCs). Platelets are detached (broken off) parts of special cells which stay in the bone marrow. (See Figure 21.1.) The blood cells are suspended (or 'float') in the plasma. The plasma is made of water which carries many things (some dissolved) in it. Proteins, sugars, fats and salts are all carried in the plasma.

Blood is made in the following parts of the body.

1. Bone marrow – the red marrow in the ends of the long bones and in the flat bones (e.g. sternum and pelvis) is most important for making blood. RBCs and most WBCs and platelets are made in the marrow.
2. Spleen.
3. Liver.
4. Lymph nodes.

The bone marrow needs iron, folic acid, vitamin B_{12}, protein and other things to make blood. These things are all in a good diet which includes protein foods (meat, fish, eggs, milk, peanuts, etc.) and protective foods (dark green leafy vegetables, fruit, etc.). Without enough iron and folic acid and protein in the diet, even a normal bone marrow cannot make enough blood.

The spleen is the main organ that gets rid of old or damaged blood cells. When red blood cells get to about 120 days old or before this if they are damaged in any way, the spleen traps them from the blood and breaks them down (including changing haemoglobin into bilirubin). The broken down parts of old cells are then carried away by the blood and most are used to make new blood cells.

Physiology

The heart circulates blood through (i.e. pumps it to and then back from) all of the body's organs. The blood keeps the cells of these organs alive and working properly. Blood takes food and oxygen and hormones to the cells. Blood takes used and waste material and carbon dioxide and sometimes hormones away from the cells. Blood contains many parts of the body's defence system against infection. Different parts of the blood have different functions:

1. Red blood cells (RBCs) containing haemoglobin (Hb) – carry oxygen.
2. White blood cells (WBCs) – fight infection.
3. Platelets – make the blood clot when needed to stop bleeding.
4. Serum proteins include
   - antibodies – to fight infection,
   - albumin – to keep water inside the blood vessels,
   - clotting proteins – to make the blood clot when needed to stop bleeding,
   - body building and repair proteins – to build and repair the body.
5. Sugar (glucose) – for body nutrition and energy.
6. Fats – for body nutrition and energy.
7. Hormones – these carry messages from one part of the body to another part.
8. Salts.
9. Water – suspends or has dissolved in it the other parts of the blood and also makes up the main volume of the blood.

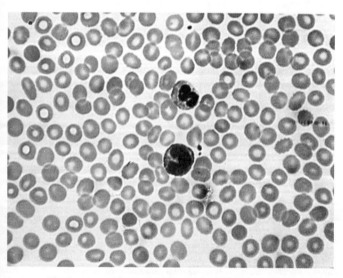

Figure 21.1 *A blood slide as seen through a microscope. The blood was smeared on the slide, dried, fixed and stained. The plasma cannot be seen. You can see many RBCs, two WBCs and some platelets.*

Pathology

Disease may make the blood have too many or too few of one of its parts. Too many or too few of parts of the blood may cause these conditions:

- too few RBCs or low Hb – anaemia
- too few WBCs – infection
- too many WBCs which are cancer cells and do not work as WBCs – leukaemia
- too few platelets – bleeding
- too little antibody protein – infection
- too little albumin protein – oedema
- too little clotting protein – bleeding
- too little body building and repair protein – wasting (body becomes thin)
- too much sugar – diabetes mellitus (see pages 499–504)
- too little sugar – hypoglycaemia – weakness and unconsciousness
- too little fat – wasting
- too much water and salt – oedema, heart failure
- too little water and salt – dehydration, shock

Most of the conditions affecting the blood are caused by:

1. not enough food to eat or not enough of the food eaten absorbed (taken into the body) so that materials for making blood are not available;
2. pathology in the organs which make and destroy the blood (i.e. marrow, spleen and liver);
3. damage to parts of the blood; or loss of parts of or the whole blood from the circulation or body.

Conditions which affect the organs which make and destroy the blood

1. *The marrow*

   The marrow may not make enough blood cells or may make abnormal blood cells because:

   (a) The marrow was abnormal from birth (i.e. the patient inherited an abnormal marrow, e.g. sickle cell anaemia, thalassaemia).

   (b) The marrow does not get enough 'food' to function, e.g. iron deficiency anaemia, folate deficiency.

   (c) The marrow has been affected by disease or drugs, e.g. infection (especially HIV infection), kidney failure, and rarely chloramphenicol.

2. *The spleen*

   If the spleen gets larger than normal for any reason, it may destroy normal as well as old or damaged blood cells.

3. *The liver*

   If disease (e.g. cirrhosis) affects the liver, the liver may not be able to use and store the food absorbed from the intestine properly. This can affect the protein, sugar, fat, salt and water in the blood. If the liver disease partly blocks the blood vessels coming from the gastrointestinal tract to the liver (portal hypertension), the vessels can then burst and bleed into the gastrointestinal tract.

History and examination

The most important disease abnormality of the blood is anaemia (see page 314). Look for anaemia in *all* patients you see.

Symptoms of anaemia include:

1. shortness of breath,
2. weakness and tiredness,
3. dizziness.

The sign of anaemia is 'pallor' (i.e. paleness or whiteness). This may be obvious in the skin even in darkly pigmented skins – especially if there is also low protein in the blood (as occurs with hookworm infestations). But, also look for pallor in those parts of the body which are normally pink or red because you can see the red colour of the blood there. Even in these places there are problems (as follows). However, always look in all of these five places for pallor (Figure 21.2):

1. the conjunctiva under the lower eyelid (but there may be inflammation from conjunctivitis);
2. the mucous membrane behind the lower lip and over the tongue (but the patient may have normal pigment under the lip or have red staining from chewing betel nut);
3. the blood vessels under the fingernails (but the patient may have normal pigment here or might have white nails from liver disease);
4. the palms of the hands including the skin creases (but some patients can get very dark pigmentation of the palms in certain diseases and the skin may be very thick from hard work);
5. the colour of the whole skin.

Test the level of the haemoglobin using a Haemoglobin Colour Scale (Appendix 1 pages 324–326). Tests are needed to find the exact cause of the anaemia if the routine treatment does not work and are listed in Appendix 5 on pages 328–329.

Another important abnormality of the blood is not enough white cells to fight infection. Infection then can start anywhere in the body and be of all types – depending on which white cells are low in number and which infections are common in the area. If someone has an unusual infection or repeated infections or an infection not getting better on powerful antibiotic treatment, and especially a severe throat infection not getting better on treatment, send a blood smear for a full blood count; and the white cell count (total and differential) will show how many of what kind of white cells are present and which ones (if any) are fewer than they should be.

An abnormality of one type of the white blood cells – the CD4 lymphocyte caused by HIV infection can lead to all sorts of infections including pneumonia, TB and also unusual infections. See Chapter 19.

Another important abnormality of the blood is not enough platelets or not enough clotting proteins to stop bleeding. Bleeding is usually from the nose (epistaxis), mouth, lungs (haemoptysis), upper gastrointestinal tract (haematemesis and melaena), lower gastrointestinal tract (melaena), urinary tract (haematuria), skin (pinpoint spots – purpura, larger areas – ecchymoses), conjunctiva, muscles and soft tissues (haematoma), joints (haemarthrosis), etc. The platelets can be looked at on the thin blood smear, but special blood tests are needed to tell if other things are wrong with the platelets or the clotting proteins. If you think the patient is having more bleeding than normal or bleeds for a longer time than normal, then ask the laboratory what blood needs to be sent for screening tests for platelet and clotting abnormalities.

If you suspect anaemia or any other disease of the blood examine very carefully the parts of the body where the blood is made:

1. The bones (which, of course, are around the bone marrow). Look for lumps. Feel gently for tenderness. Examine the sternum carefully.
2. The spleen. See Figure 22.10 (page 343).
3. The liver. See Figure 24.4 (page 393).
4. The lymph nodes. See Chapter 22 pages 330–333.

Tests

1. *Examination of haemoglobin using a Haemoglobin Colour Scale.*
   You can easily do this test yourself. For the method, see Appendix 1 pages 324–326.

2. *Examination of a thin blood film* – full blood count (FBC).
   This test must be done in a laboratory by a trained laboratory worker. If you do not have a laboratory worker to do it, you must make the blood film yourself and then send the blood film to a laboratory with a letter. The letter must state patient's problem and your diagnosis, and ask for both a report and an explanation of the results.
   See Chapter 6 pages 26–29 for the method of making a thin blood film.

Disorders

Anaemia

Anaemia is said to be present when there is not enough red blood cell haemoglobin (RBC Hb) in the blood. Normally, there is more than 11 g Hb in each decilitre (or 100 ml) of blood (written as 11 g/dl or 11 g/100 ml or 11 g% or 110 g/l). In countries that have good public health services, anaemia is diagnosed if the Hb is less than the following:

• men 13 g/dl,
• non-pregnant women 12 g/dl,
• pregnant women 11 g/dl.

Unfortunately, there are no agreed levels of Hb for grading anaemia (there are good reasons why).

The following is a guide.

Hb 3 g/dl or less – anaemia critical or very severe. The heart muscle cannot get enough oxygen to properly pump the blood. Heart failure develops. Death is likely.

Hb 4–5 g/dl – anaemia severe. Respiratory distress can be present. The pulse is fast. If a patient then develops an acute illness, especially malaria which destroys red blood cells, the patient may well quickly get much worse and die.

Hb 6–7 g/dl – anaemia moderate. Shortness of breath at rest can be present. The pulse rate is increased.

Hb 8–11 g/dl – anaemia (moderate to) mild. Shortness of breath on exertion is present. However, if the anaemia has developed slowly the patient may not notice the symptoms.

Anaemia is very common especially in hot wet tropical places where malaria and hookworm are common; in places where malnutrition is common; where HIV infection is common; in women of childbearing age, and in children.

Pathology

The common causes of anaemia include:

1. Not enough haemoglobin to fill the red blood cells has been made by the bone marrow because:
   (a) Not enough iron is in or is absorbed from the food.
   (b) Not enough folic acid or other vitamins are in or are absorbed from the food.
   (c) Not enough protein is in or is absorbed from the food.
   (d) Infection has stopped the bone marrow working properly. HIV infection is a common cause of this. (HIV infection causes anaemia in other ways too – the effect of repeated or chronic infection and the effect of drugs used to treat them on the marrow.) TB also can be a cause.
   (e) Diseases or drugs or chemicals have stopped the bone marrow functioning properly. The most common cause of this is chronic kidney failure (see Chapter 26 pages 449–450); but there are others.
   (f) The patient was born with abnormal bone marrow which cannot make *enough* normal haemoglobin, i.e. thalassaemia (see page 324).
2. Red blood cells are destroyed before they are worn out. This is called 'haemolysis'. When red blood cells are destroyed more quickly than new ones are made, this causes anaemia.
   Reasons for this include:
   (a) Malaria – acute attack.
   (b) Malaria – chronic.
   (c) Malaria – hyperreactive malarious splenomegaly.
   (d) Any cause of a very big spleen as well as malaria, e.g. schistosomiasis, kala azar, cirrhosis.
   (e) Certain drugs or chemicals, especially in patients who were born without enough G6PD (a special part of the red blood cells).
   (f) Sickle cell anaemia – the patient was born with an abnormal bone marrow, which makes an abnormal haemoglobin which causes the red blood cells to become an abnormal sickle shape (called 'sickling') and the abnormal red cells are destroyed quickly by the spleen. See page 321.
3. Red blood cells are lost from the body during bleeding. Reasons for this include:
   (a) Gastrointestinal tract bleeding. This is usually caused by hookworm in the small bowel sucking the patient's blood (see Chapter 23 pages 355–357). This is sometimes due to bleeding from a peptic ulcer (see Chapter 23 pages 352–354). This can be from bleeding veins in the oesophagus from chronic liver disease or schistosomiasis (see Chapter 24 page 395 and Chapter 23 page 374). This can be due to a cancer in the stomach or colon or elsewhere in the gastrointestinal tract.
   (b) Genital tract bleeding in the female. This is usually caused by an ante-partum or post-partum haemorrhage. But it can be caused by having pregnancies close together. It can be caused by having frequent or heavy bleeding with monthly periods. Of course, iron is given to the baby by the mother during pregnancy and many pregnancies can make a woman anaemic.

The common causes of anaemia are:

1. not enough iron, folic acid and protein in the diet,
2. hookworm,
3. malaria,
4. repeated pregnancy,
5. HIV infection,
6. sickle cell anaemia (in Africa and people of African descent only) and thalassaemia.

You must find out the epidemiology of anaemia in your area. If other causes are common in your area, then change this list. The treatment needed will change with the causes in your area.

When you take the history of a patient with anaemia, find out if this patient has any of these common causes of anaemia. Ask about a family history of blood diseases. Ask about a past history of the common causes.

When anaemia is present there is not enough haemoglobin in the blood to carry enough oxygen to any part of the body (hypoxia). No part of the body, therefore, functions properly. The heart pumps the blood through the lungs and through the body more quickly than normal to use the small amount of haemoglobin in the blood to carry oxygen more often – palpitations (feeling the heart beat more quickly or strongly than normal) occur. The patient breathes more deeply or quickly than normal – shortness of breath occurs. Muscles do not get enough oxygen – tiredness and weakness occur. The brain does not get enough oxygen – dizziness or headaches occur. The heart, which is also doing more work than normal, does not get enough oxygen – heart failure can happen.

Symptoms and signs

Symptoms of anaemia include:

1. weakness or tiredness,
2. dizziness,
3. shortness of breath.

Signs of anaemia include pallor (or paleness or whiteness) of:

1. the mucous membrane of the mouth inside the lips,
2. conjunctivae under the lower eye lids,
3. fingernail beds,
4. palms of hands,
5. all the skin.

See Figure 21.2 page 317 and details and exceptions about this on page 313.

Symptoms and signs of

1. the cause of the anaemia (see page 315) (remember HIV infection is present in half of most severe cases of adult anaemia in many areas – look carefully for signs of HIV infection (see Chapter 19 pages 222–233));
2. heart failure (see Chapter 27 page 461) if present.

Haemoglobin estimation (see pages 324–326) should always be made. This:

1. confirms the diagnosis of anaemia,
2. confirms how severe the anaemia is, and
3. gives a starting point to measure the success or failure of treatment.

Management and treatment

Treatment of anaemia will usually cure the anaemia. However, treatment cannot increase the haemoglobin by more than 1 g/dl each week. Often the Hb rises by only 0.5 g/dl each week. As the haemoglobin estimation is often as much as 1(–2) g/dl above or below the real level of the haemoglobin, you cannot tell for at least 4 weeks if the treatment is working (i.e. 0.5 g/dl × 4 weeks = rise of 2 g/dl). After 4 weeks the haemoglobin should have risen by at least 2 g/dl.

However, if the cause of the anaemia is not stopped the anaemia will usually return when the treatment is stopped. Therefore, you must always try to *find out the cause of the anaemia and stop this cause.*

Blood transfusion is not the treatment of anaemia. Blood transfusion does not help the body to make more blood, or stop blood being destroyed, or stop bleeding. Blood transfusion does not stop the cause of anaemia. Blood transfusion is used only if it is needed to keep the patient alive while the cause of the anae-

mia is found and stopped and the treatment of the anaemia is given time to work.

Blood transfusion is given usually only if

- the Hb is 2.5–3 g/dl and there are symptoms and signs of heart failure;
- the Hb is less than 5 and the patient has an acute infection (especially malaria which may make the anaemia worse) or severe illness or needs operation.

Blood transfusion can cause allergic type reactions, heart failure if given too quickly, syphilis, infection with bacteria, etc.; but the most serious thing is viral infection with HIV or Hepatitis B as these are not curable and may lead to the death of the patient. Do not give blood by transfusion unless absolutely essential to keep the patient alive.

Management of anaemia in the health centre is by:

1. Treating the common causes of anaemia correctly.
2. If the anaemia does not get better or if it quickly returns, the diagnosis and/or treatment must be incorrect and the patient needs referring to the Medical Officer for investigation for correct diagnosis and treatment.
3. Do not continue with treatment and in particular do not continue with iron treatment if the patient's anaemia is not cured by the treatment.

Admission for treatment is not needed for many patients. Admit for inpatient treatment *if*:

1. very pale or Hb less than 5 g/dl (until Hb rises to 5 g/dl); *or*
2. a lot of dizziness, shortness of breath, weakness, etc.; *or*
3. heart failure (oedema, etc.); *or*
4. patient may get quickly worse (e.g. acute malaria, recent gastrointestinal bleeding, late pregnancy, etc.); *or*
5. time of stress for patient (e.g. infection, post–partum state, etc.).

---

1. Give routine treatment for the common causes of anaemia in your area to all anaemic patients. This usually includes the following six:
   - antimalarials,
   - iron,
   - folic acid (+/– vitamin A),
   - nutrition education,
   - anti-hookworm drug,
   - advice about family planning and antenatal care if needed.

2. Look for other causes especially HIV infection and TB. Treat any other cause you find.

3. Blood transfusion; but only if essential for special reasons.

4. See the patient and repeat the Hb each 4 weeks until Hb is 10 g/dl.

5. If the Hb does not rise by 2 g in 1 month and eventually reach 10 g/dl (except hyperreactive malarious splenomegaly (HMS)):
   - send blood for special tests[1] with an explanation to your Medical Officer or
   - send non-urgently or refer the patient to the Medical Officer for special tests.[1]

DO NOT CONTINUE IRON TREATMENT IF THE PATIENT'S Hb IS NOT RISING.

---

1 See Appendix 5 for preliminary tests for anaemia not responding to treatment for iron deficiency and malaria.

Give routine treatments for the common causes of anaemia in your area. Your Health Department will have told you what the causes are and how you should treat them. They usually are as follows.

1. *Antimalarial drug*
   (a) Give a curative course (See Chapter 13 pages 79, 80), usually an artemisinin drug for 3 or 7 days depending on which companion antimalarial drug you use with it.

(b) Following this, in the past, routine malaria prophylactic treatment was given until the Hb was 10 g/dl (usually 6–12 weeks). However, because in some places patients did not take the drugs regularly, and also because of the malaria parasites developing resistance to chloroquine and later to sulfadoxine and pyrimethamine, different regimes now apply in different places. In some areas, you may be told to give prophylactic treatment. In some areas, use of insecticide-treated nets and intermittent preventive therapy (IPT see Chapter 13 pages 88, 89) may be used. At the least, arrange for the patient to get early effective curative treatment for any further attack of malaria.

2. *Iron*
Do not start iron treatment until after any infection or illness is first treated.
Give ferrous iron tablet. This treatment is usually ferrous sulfate, usually with 60 mg of elemental iron in it. The ferrous sulfate tablet may be 200 mg or more, as the sulfate is with the elemental iron. Other salts of iron, e.g. gluconate can be used as long as enough mg of elemental iron (about 60 mg) is given. The tablet may also contain 400 mcg of folic acid.
Give ferrous sulfate (60 mg elemental iron) tablets one twice daily for 3 months, although if pregnant for the whole of the pregnancy and for 3 months after delivery.

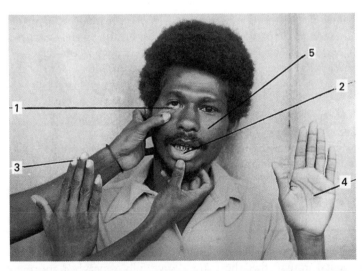

Figure 21.2 *Photograph showing the five places of the body where pallor* must *be looked for in* all *patients. (1) The conjunctivae under the lower eye lid. (2) The mucous membrane inside the lower lip. (3) The fingernail beds. (4) The palms of the hands. Also (5) the colour of the skin. If the skin is very pale, think of hookworm disease as the hookworm makes the patient short of protein as well as haemoglobin and this makes the skin even more pale.*

Give IMI iron dextran in some countries if:

(a) Hb < 5 g/dl or < 7.5 g/dl in pregnant patients; and it is thought the patient will not take the tablets or it is near to delivery of the pregnant woman's baby

(b) The Hb does not rise by 2 g/dl after 1 month of treatment with oral iron and no other cause obvious.

But see Appendix 2 (page 326) at the end of this chapter, *before* giving IMI iron dextran, for contraindications to giving IMI iron dextran and for method of giving IMI iron dextran. *Give* 5 ml daily for:

• 6 days if weight < 40 kg,

• 10 days if weight > 40 kg, and

• 2 days extra if pregnant.

Give IV iron dextran (only preparations not containing phenol) infusion if:

(a) treatment needs to be completed quickly (e.g. outpatient treatment), *or*

(b) patient has little muscle for IM injections,

(c) you have been told by your Medical Officer the preparation of iron you have is safe to give by IV infusion; and you have been trained in this; and you have drugs near the patient in case an anaphylactic allergic reaction occurs.

The total dose required is in the one infusion (TDI). *But* see Appendix 3 (page 326) at the end of this chapter for contraindications to giving IV iron dextran infusion and method of giving IV iron dextran infusion *before* giving it.

Give only half ($\frac{1}{2}$) of these doses of iron if the Hb is 7.5 g/dl or above.

Do NOT give oral iron for more than 3 months unless pregnant or told to do so by the Medical Officer.

Do NOT give a course of iron by injections more than once in any 12-month period.

Do NOT give iron injection (IM or IV) while a patient is very sick or has a fever (above 37.5°C).

Wait until malaria, infections and fever have been successfully treated and then give iron injections or tablets.

---

3. *Folic acid (+/– vitamin A +/– other vitamins)*

Folic acid 5 mg daily for 1 week, *then* 5 mg weekly for 12 weeks.

Some iron tablets also have 400 mcg of folic acid with the 60 mg elemental iron so that the extra treatment of folic acid is not needed.

In some places, vitamin A deficiency is so common that 10,000 IU daily or 25,000 IU weekly needs to be given to help the body use the iron to make blood. In some places, other vitamin B deficiencies and vitamin C deficiency also need treatment before the anaemia improves.

4. *Diet*

Educate to eat enough protein foods (e.g. meat, fish, eggs, peanuts) and protective foods (e.g. dark green leafy vegetables, fruit) daily.

5. *Hookworm treatment*

Give pyrantel 10 mg/kg (maximum dose 1 g) or albendazole 400 mg in one dose orally once, but not if patient could be pregnant, or whatever is your recommended drug for hookworm (see Chapter 23 page 356).

6. *Offer family planning and/or antenatal care advice if required.*

Look for and treat also any other underlying cause found.

Arrange transfer for blood transfusion, but only for the following patients.

1. *If* the haemoglobin is 7.5 g/dl or less *and* *if* the patient is more than 36 weeks pregnant (postpartum haemorrhage possible) *or if* the anaemia is due to haemorrhage which may occur again (e.g. recent haematemesis, melaena, or haemoptysis).

2. *If* the haemoglobin is less than 5 g/dl *and* *if* there is also

• acute malaria (fever), *or*

• heart failure (oedema, etc.), *or*

• severe symptoms of anaemia (dizziness, shortness of breath, severe weakness, etc.), *or*

• pregnancy at any stage, *or*

• a severe infection or other illness, *or*

• other time of stress such as the post-partum state.

3. If the haemoglobin is 3 g/dl or less.

Repeat Hb estimation each 4 weeks until Hb is 10 g/dl.

Send special blood tests (see Appendix 5 page 328) or refer to the Medical Officer if the Hb does not rise.

The haemoglobin should rise by 2(–4) g/dl in 4 weeks. However, this is not true for hyperreactive malarious splenomegaly (HMS) (see page 319) in which it may take 2 years to rise to 10 g/dl.

If the haemoglobin does not rise by at least 2 g/dl, give fully supervised treatment for another 4 weeks including, if available, iron by injection and you yourself watching the antimalarial tablets and hookworm tablets being swallowed.

If the haemoglobin does not rise by at least 2 g/dl, continue treatment and arrange special blood tests or referral or non-urgent transfer to the Medical Officer to find out what the real cause of the anaemia is and what the management should be.

Do not just continue treatment if it is not curing the anaemia. This would allow the cause of the anaemia to get worse and the anaemia to get worse. Incorrect treatment may also make the patient develop a new condition, e.g. iron may cause heart failure if the patient has thalassaemia.

Transfer to Medical Officer care

1. If the haemoglobin does not rise by 2 g/dl after 4 weeks of correct, fully supervised treatment of the common causes (except hyperreactive malarious splenomegaly), as the diagnoses and treatment are wrong. Correct diagnosis and treatment are needed (non-urgent).
2. If blood transfusion is needed (see page 318) (urgent – sometimes emergency).
3. If anaemia has returned after full treatment (see pages 317–318) and if necessary adequate treatment of malaria, before 1 year has gone (non-urgent).
4. If the haemoglobin does not rise by 2 g/dl and the spleen does not decrease in size by 2 cm in 6 months when the patient has hyperreactive malarious splenomegaly and has had correct prophylactic antimalarial drugs regularly (see this page) (non-urgent).
5. If the patient has hyperreactive malarious splenomegaly and becomes pregnant (discuss with Medical Officer first) (non-urgent).

Prevention

Prevention of anaemia is the prevention and treatment of the common causes of anaemia. This includes:

1. Control and treatment of malaria (see Chapter 13 pages 77–89).
2. Control and treatment of hookworm (see Chapter 23 pages 355–357).
3. Good diet with enough iron, folic acid and other vitamins and protein, etc. in it. The diet should be a mixed one which has protein foods (meat, fish, eggs, peanuts, etc.) and protective foods (dark green leafy vegetables, fruit, etc.) (see Chapter 23 pages 376–382).
4. Good obstetrical advice and care. Advice and help with family planning. Antenatal care (see below). Prevention of post-partum haemorrhage.
5. Good health education about the avoidance of HIV and other infections.

Prevention of anaemia in women of childbearing age

1. *Malaria* should be managed by early effective curative treatment with two drugs (at any stage of life). During pregnancy also insecticide-treated nets (ITN) and intermittent prophylactic treatment (for malaria) (IPT) are recommended. (See Chapter 13 pages 87–89.)
2. *Iron and folic acid deficiency.* In areas where anaemia is common, WHO recommends all pregnant women, whether anaemic or not (as many have low iron stores), take ferrous sulfate 60 mg elemental iron and 400 mcg folic acid for 6 months or for all the pregnancy and 3 months after giving birth.

Hyperreactive malarious splenomegaly

Hyperreactive malarious splenomegaly (HMS), previously called tropical splenomegaly syndrome (TSS), is an abnormal reaction of the body to chronic malaria infection. It is present when a person who has had chronic malaria for years has a very big spleen, anaemia, wasting and repeated attacks of haemolysis (see below), and these things are not improving but are worsening.

Pathology

When a non-immune person starts to live in an area where there is malaria, first he gets acute malaria and then he gets chronic malaria. (See Chapter 13.) A person with chronic malaria has a big spleen, anaemia, wasting (or poor growth if a child) and repeated attacks of acute malaria and other infections. If the person does not die from acute or chronic malaria, he develops cellular immunity and antibodies against malaria. After about 4–10 years he develops semi-immunity to malaria. Then his spleen becomes smaller, his haemoglobin rises, his wasting gets less (and he grows better if he is a child) and there are fewer attacks of acute malaria and other infections. However, a few people with chronic malaria do not develop normal antibodies and normal immunity to malaria. These people develop abnormal antibodies (of IgM type) and abnormal immunity to malaria. This causes hyperreactive malarious splenomegaly.

In these people who develop an abnormal immune reaction to malaria, the big spleen stays big and may get bigger. The big spleen (for no other reason than that it is big) destroys normal as well as worn out red and white blood cells more quickly than the bone marrow can make enough new ones.

This causes severe chronic anaemia, low resistance to infections, wasting and chronic ill health. At times, the big spleen may suddenly destroy many more red blood cells than it usually does. This causes acute very severe anaemia (acute haemolysis) and fever and splenic pain.

Clinical features

The patient is usually a young adult, most often female, from a malarious area. The condition happens more commonly in certain places and certain families.

Symptoms include those of:

- anaemia (malaise, inability to work, weakness, dizziness, shortness of breath);
- enlarged spleen (swelling of abdomen, abdominal discomfort); and
- episodes of acute haemolysis (severe weakness, etc. often with fever and sometimes with pain in the abdomen over the spleen).

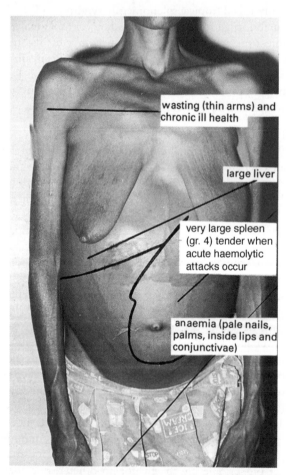

wasting (thin arms) and chronic ill health

large liver

very large spleen (gr. 4) tender when acute haemolytic attacks occur

anaemia (pale nails, palms, inside lips and conjunctivae)

Figure 21.3 *Hyperreactive malarious splenomegaly (previously called tropical splenomegaly syndrome). Note the features in an adult who has lived all her life in an area where malaria is always present.*

Signs include (see Figure 21.3):

- anaemia,
- wasting (thin muscles, little fat),
- spleen very enlarged, firm and usually non-tender,
- liver usually enlarged,
- episodes of fever, jaundice and tender spleen during which the patient is more anaemic than before (acute haemolytic episodes).

The patient has chronic ill health. The patient becomes worse from time to time because of haemolytic episodes. The condition does not improve by itself while the patient stays in a malarious area. Death usually occurs from acute malaria or acute severe bacterial infection or an haemolytic episode.

Management

You are not able to change the patient's abnormal reaction to malaria parasites to normal. You can, however, stop this abnormal reaction, by curing the patient of malaria and then giving malaria prophylaxis so that no more malarial parasites are in the body. The patient must take the malarial prophylaxis until all the symptoms and signs of HMS are gone – this usually takes at least 2 years. After this, the patient will have to take malarial prophylaxis for life if the condition starts to return when the prophylaxis is stopped. Details of the management of a patient with HMS are set out below.

Do an Hb estimation (see page 324). Write down the result. Do this each time you see the patient.

Send a thin blood smear (and if possible 4 ml of blood in an EDTA bottle and enough blood on blotting or filter paper to cover a thumb nail) to the hospital laboratory and ask them to look for sickle cell anaemia, chronic leukaemia, thalassaemia and other rare blood diseases. (Result is not urgent.)

Measure the size of the spleen before starting treatment. Write down the size. Do this again each time you see the patient.

Admit for inpatient treatment if

- the haemoglobin is less than 5 g/dl, or
- the patient has had recent acute haemolytic episode, or
- the patient is sick, or
- the patient is pregnant.

Give routine treatment for anaemia with antimalarials, iron, folic acid, pyrantel or other anti-hookworm drug, education about diet, and family planning (see anaemia pages 317–319). However, do not give total dose infusion of iron during pregnancy if the patient has HMS.

Give explanations and health education about the need for regular treatment for many years. Give whatever drugs your Health Department recommends in your area you use for long-term prophylaxis for malaria.

Before resistance developed, chloroquine was used. The drug to use now will depend on which malaria parasites and to what drugs they are resistant, in your area. A combination of two antimalaria drugs which act in different ways should be used (see Chapter 13 pages 77–79).

You must find out in your area what drugs are recommended and supplied by your health department and give these to the patient. Treatment will be needed for at least 2 years and probably for life.

Give quick, effective treatment for any acute attacks of bacterial infections or malaria as they occur.

Transfer to Medical Officer care the following patients:

1. If the patient has a severe haemolytic episode at any time, but especially during pregnancy (i.e. sudden increase in anaemia often with fever, increased weakness, and possibly jaundice and spleen pain). Transfer for blood transfusion and prednisolone (urgent – at times emergency).
2. If a patient with HMS becomes pregnant. (First discuss with Medical Officer the need for transfer – non-urgent.)
3. If after 6–8 months of treatment the Hb has not risen by 2 g/dl and the spleen has not decreased in size by 1 grade or 5 cm. (Transfer for investigation for other diseases – non-urgent.)

Sickle cell anaemia

Sickle cell anaemia is a severe inherited disease which causes chronic anaemia, episodes of severe pain and tenderness of bones and other parts of the body, and often death.

Sickle cell anaemia is common only in people from parts of Africa and people of African descent. It occurs also in a few parts of the Middle East and India.

Pathology

Sickle cell anaemia is due to a large amount of an abnormal haemoglobin called Hb S, in the red blood cells (instead of normal adult haemoglobin). This abnormality must be partly present in both parents for a child to get the severe abnormality. A small amount of Hb S helps protect a person against malaria. A large amount of Hb S does not protect against malaria but does cause sickle cell anaemia. As the abnormality that makes Hb S (instead of normal haemoglobin) is inherited, there is no cure for the disease.

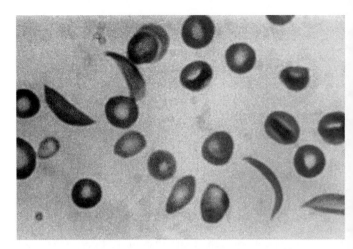

Figure 21.4 *Photograph of normal red blood cells and sickle cells.*

When a red blood cell that has a lot of Hb S in it gives up its oxygen, it changes to an abnormal long thin 'sickle' shape (see Figure 21.4). If the sickled cell is quickly given oxygen again, it goes back to the normal shape. If the sickled cell is not given oxygen for more than a couple of minutes, it cannot ever go back to the normal shape.

Sickling of red blood cells causes two groups of problems.

1. The abnormal red blood cells are destroyed in the body (mostly in the spleen) more quickly than normal red blood cells (called chronic haemolysis). This causes chronic anaemia and a big spleen.
   From time to time, sometimes because of an infection, but often for no obvious reason, the spleen may destroy many more red cells than normal. The anaemia becomes much worse with jaundice and the spleen becomes even larger. This is called a 'haemolytic crisis'. The bone marrow makes as many red cells as it can to replace the ones being destroyed by the spleen. The marrow in the bones gets bigger. This may make the bones get bigger and give an unusual appearance to the bones of the skull and face. The bone marrow often needs more folic acid than it can get to make all the extra blood. All the body then becomes short of folic acid. This shortage of folic acid may stop the patient growing and stop puberty (a child developing into a man or woman). Sometimes a particular virus infection can for a while stop the bone marrow making RBCs – an 'aplastic crisis' – and the patient gets very anaemic.
2. The red blood cells become sickled as they give up their oxygen in the capillaries of the body tissues.

The sickled cells can then get stuck in the capillaries and cannot then return to the lungs to get more oxygen. The blocked blood vessels stop other red cells passing through them and these other red cells give up their oxygen and then sickle. The blood then often clots in the blocked blood vessels. If small veins are blocked, the blood cannot get out of the organ which becomes swollen and filled with sickled RBCs and even death of cells can occur (called also 'sequestration crisis'). If capillaries are blocked, the part of the body which the blocked blood vessels usually supply gets no oxygen and so becomes inflamed and dies. This is often called 'vaso-occlusive crisis'. Death of part of the body like this is called an 'infarction'. The process just described is often called an 'infarction crisis'.

The things which make an infarction crisis more likely are:

(a) infections (bacterial and malarial);
(b) dehydration;
(c) if less oxygen is breathed in than usual, e.g.
  • during an operation,
  • going high in an aeroplane which is not fully pressurised;
(d) if part or all of the body becomes cold and the blood circulation slows down;
(e) if the blood flow to part of the body is stopped, e.g. putting on a tourniquet or tight bandage.

However, many infarction crises happen and no reason can be found.

Some patients have many attacks of infarction – one or two each week. Some patients have few attacks – one or two each year.

The parts of the body most often affected by infarction crises are the bones. In infants, the fingers and toes are the most often affected. In older people, any bone or any other part of the body can be affected. If the spleen has many infarctions, it may become small.

The parts of the body which have been affected by infarction may be infected by bacteria which cause osteomyelitis, etc.

In pregnancy, the above and other severe complications can result in death.

Symptoms and signs

Anaemia and related conditions

The usual symptoms and signs of anaemia are present (see page 316).

The Hb is usually about 8 g/dl. (If a patient's Hb is normal (and the patient is not dehydrated) the patient probably does not have sickle cell anaemia.)

The patient may be mildly jaundiced.

The spleen and liver are usually large; though the spleen may become small.

Sometimes the anaemia may become much worse (haemolytic crisis or aplastic crisis).

The skull and face bones may have an unusual shape because of the large amount of bone marrow.

Growth and puberty may be slow.

Sometimes there are leg ulcers.

Infarction crises

Sudden severe pain and tenderness start in a bone or the spleen or another part of the body; and often fever. With proper treatment, the pain usually greatly improves within 2 days and goes within 7–9 days.

The bones are affected more often than other parts of the body. Any bone can be affected, but often the fingers and toes are most affected. The infected bone becomes painful and tender.

Fat from the marrow of infarcted bones can get into the blood stream and block up capillaries in the lung and cause shortness of breath, injury and death – the sickle chest syndrome.

Old bone infarctions may have made the fingers short and thick with narrow ends. Also, the patient may not be very tall, because the trunk of the body is short.

If a joint is affected, acute arthritis occurs.

If the kidney is affected, there is often blood in the urine.

If the spleen is affected, there is a tender swelling in the left upper abdomen.

If the intestine is affected, there may be acute abdominal pain and tenderness and vomiting.

If the brain is affected, there may be paralysis, etc.

Infections

If pain and tenderness in an area of infarction and fever do not become much better after 2 days of proper treatment, and are not nearly gone after 7–9 days of treatment, then that part of the body probably has developed a secondary bacterial infection. Salmonella infections of bone (osteomyelitis) are common.

Tests

Haemoglobin

The Hb is usually about 8 g/dl.

Sickling test

If you have a laboratory with a microscope, then you can do a simple test for sickling of the blood with sodium metabisulfate.

On one slide a drop of patient's blood is mixed with a drop of freshly prepared 2% sodium metabisulfate solution and placed under a cover slip. The same test is done with normal blood on another slide. Both are examined 20 minutes later. If the patient's blood but not the normal blood shows sickle-shaped or long curved red blood cells, then the patient *has* Hb S in his blood (see Figure 21.4 page 321).

People who have only a *little* Hb S in their blood and do not have sickle cell anaemia *can* still have a positive sickling test.

If the sickling test is *negative*, it is almost certain that the patient does *not* have sickle cell anaemia.

The only *certain* way to diagnose that *the disease* is present is to send the blood to a laboratory where they do a special test for Hb S.

Thin blood smear (send a smear to the laboratory)
You can diagnose sickle cell anaemia fairly certainly in most cases if there is (1) anaemia and (2) a typical thin blood smear for sickle cell anaemia.

White cell count (send blood to the laboratory)
The white cell count is often high (often twice the normal levels) even when there is no infection.

Treatment

There is no cure.

Drugs such as hydroxyurea to increase the other type of haemoglobin in the red cell may help a little but are expensive. More effective drugs on trial may become available.

Treat the anaemia
1. Give regular prophylactic antimalarial drugs for life (if in a malarial area) (see Chapter 13 pages 88, 89).
2. Give folic acid 5 mg (1 tab) daily for life.
3. Do not give blood transfusion unless the Hb suddenly falls to very low levels or before operations, etc.
4. Do not give iron after the first course as it is not usually needed. However, ask the laboratory or Medical Officer to do tests to see if iron is needed if you suspect iron deficiency.

Tell the patient how to avoid infarction crises
1. Take prophylactic antimalarials for life (see page 88) Get proper treatment of malaria infections quickly (see Chapter 13 pages 79, 80).
2. Avoid infections if possible.
   Avoid people with infections.
   Take prophylactic penicillin, e.g. phenoxymethylpenicillin 250 mg bd.
   Get all possible immunisations including pneumococcal and *Haemophilus* vaccines (see Chapter 10).

3. Avoid dehydration – always drink enough to pass a lot of urine (especially if he or she has vomiting or diarrhoea or it is very hot). Never take (and health workers never order) diuretics (e.g. hydrochlorothiazide, furosemide/frusemide, etc.) even for heart failure or high blood pressure, etc.
4. Avoid becoming cold.
5. Avoid tight clothes on the limbs.
6. Do not go on unpressurised aircraft and check if the pressurisation is enough in pressurised aircraft.

Treat infarction crises
1. Give aspirin or paracetamol or codeine as needed (see Chapter 7 pages 32–34). Do not give pethidine or morphine (unless told to do so by the Medical Officer) as the patient may become addicted.
2. The patient must be fully hydrated. Use an IV drip in severe cases (see Chapter 23 pages 364–366).
3. Make the patient rest.

Treat any infection quickly

If pain from an infarction crisis has not improved in 2 days and has not nearly gone in 7–9 days, there is an infection, which you must treat with antibiotics (see Chapter 11 pages 56–61). Osteomyelitis, which could be due to *Salmonella* and may occur again and again, may need repeated long courses of antibiotics (not safe for chloramphenicol). You should urgently discuss what antibiotic to give with the Medical Officer.

Transfer
Transfer patients who need an operation.

The condition the patient has may be because of infarction crisis.

The operation may cause an infarction crisis.

The anaesthetic needs high concentrations of oxygen and may need a pre-operative blood transfusion.

No tourniquets can be used.

Do not operate on patients who have sickle cell anaemia yourself. Transfer all patients with sickle cell anaemia who seem to need an operation.

Transfer pregnant patients

Transfer all patients with sickle cell anaemia who become pregnant to the Medical Officer.

Prognosis

Without treatment, most patients would die before they were adults. If proper treatment is given patients may have a reasonable life, although they may have many attacks of the problems described.

Thalassaemia

Thalassaemia is an inherited disease in which the bone marrow cannot make enough haemoglobin and the patient becomes anaemic. There is no cure.

Thalassaemia occurs in a band from Africa across the Mediterranean to SE Asia. It is most common around the Mediterranean. It can, however, occur in people all over the world.

Thalassaemia must be present, even if only mildly so, in both parents for a child to get severe thalassaemia.

Mild thalassaemia (called 'thalassaemia minor') causes only a few symptoms and signs. There is a mild anaemia with an Hb of 9–11 g/dl, which is like iron deficiency anaemia but which does not improve on routine anaemia treatment (see page 316). If blood tests are sent to the hospital laboratory (a thin blood smear, 4 ml blood in EDTA bottle and blood about 1 cm across on filter or blotting paper) or if the patient is referred or transferred non-urgently to the Medical Officer, the condition can be diagnosed by tests. Although these patients should have an increased resistance to malaria, if they are in a malarious area, it may be recommended to give them regular prophylactic antimalarials (see page 88) for life. Also give folic acid 5 g daily for life. DO NOT GIVE IRON after the first course unless the Medical Officer tells you that the patient also has iron deficiency, as may occur in girls on vegetarian diets, women with many pregnancies, etc. Iron treatment will otherwise damage the heart and other organs and may lead to death.

Severe thalassaemia (called 'thalassaemia major') affects children. They have very severe anaemia which does not improve on any treatment. The spleen becomes larger and eventually very large, also the skull and face bones are large and unusual to look at. You can only keep the patient alive by repeated blood transfusions and treatment as for mild thalassaemia. The iron from the blood transfusions and the food damages the heart and other organs and can cause death, if death is not caused by a complication of the anaemia (usually before adult life is reached).

Moderate thalassaemia (called 'thalassaemia intermedia') is between these two other types. Anaemia is about 7 g/dl and the patient does not usually need transfusion. The spleen is enlarged. Frequent bacterial infections occur. Gall stones are common. Deformities of the bones are seen. Treatment includes malaria prophylactic treatment for life if in a malaria area, full immunisation, attempts to avoid infections, early treatment of any bacterial infection, folic acid daily and in some, removal of the spleen.

Glucose-6-phosphate dehydrogenase deficiency (G6PD)

This enzyme (or chemical) is a part of the outside membrane of red blood cells. It protects RBCs from being damaged and then removed from the circulation by the spleen; or, if the RBC damage is severe, just breaking open in the circulation and releasing haemoglobin into the plasma.

In about 10% of the world's population this enzyme does not work properly – in some people not at all and in others it varies up to working almost normally. The abnormality is most common where malaria occurs as it gives some protection to female carriers of the condition against *P. falciparum* malaria. Males are more affected than females.

In affected people, haemolysis can be caused by

1. drugs, e.g.
   high dose acetylsalicylic acid (aspirin)
   primaquine, quinine, pyrimethamine and some other antimalarial drugs
   sulfonamides
   dapsone
   quinolone antibiotics.
2. certain foods, e.g. the broad bean (*Vicia faba*).
3. bacterial and viral infections.

Patients who have haemolysis get
- anaemia
- jaundice
- dark urine and possibly kidney failure if the RBCs break open in the blood.

> The importance of the condition is that if the severe type is common in the area in which you work, your Health Department will tell you not to use certain drugs which can cause haemolysis, e.g. primaquine.

Appendix 1 Haemoglobin estimation using the WHO Haemoglobin Colour Scale

The Haemoglobin Colour Scale is a small card with six different shades of red on it, which are the same colour as blood with the six different haemoglobin levels of 4, 6, 8, 10, 12 and 14 g/dl. This card is in a booklet which also contains instructions about how to do the test.

Haemoglobin Colour Scale

...a practical answer to a vital need

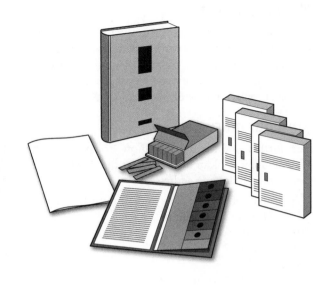

**The Haemoglobin Colour Scale
is a simple, reliable and inexpensive tool
developed by the World Health Organization
to screen for anaemia in the absence of
laboratory-based haemoglobinometry.
(Reproduced from NHO Haemoglobin Colour Scale
information leaflet by permission of the WHO.)**

There is also a dispenser or box in which there are 200 special test strips of paper which will absorb blood well.

Wear gloves so that the patient's blood cannot get onto you.

Use a sterile stilette to prick the patient's finger to get one large drop of blood to form on the patient's finger without squeezing it.

Put the whole drop of the patient's blood directly from the patient's finger on to the test strip of paper.

Wait 30 seconds. Do not try to match the colour before this.

Then hold the test strip of paper next to the six different colours on the Haemoglobin Colour Scale card. Decide which colour the patient's blood matches best. Make sure you do this in good light and not in a shadow.

The colour you have chosen will be opposite the number on the card, which will be the patient's haemoglobin level.

Haemoglobin Colour Scale Starter Kit

• booklet of six shades of red
• instructions for use
• dispenser of 200 specially absorbent test strips in handy box
• 4 spare dispensers (800 tests)

Available in English, French and other languages as required.

Important:
• **instructions for use must be followed**
• **use only approved test strips provided**
  (refill dispensers available).

Quality control

A WHO Collaborating Centre continues to assure quality control for the validation of the printing and accuracy of the six colour shades and the test strips.

How much is it?

The Starter Kit with approved test strips for 1000 tests costs about US$20. This works out at less than 2 cents per test – cheaper than copper sulfate and considerably less than a laboratory test – with the cost per test falling at each purchase of refills.

Find out more ...

For further information on how to procure the Haemoglobin Colour Scale, contact the WHO Secretariat at the following address:

Department of Blood Safety and Clinical Technology
World Health Organization
20 avenue Appia
1211 Geneva 27
Switzerland
Fax: +41 22 791 4836
Email: hbcolourscale@who.int
Web page: www.who.int/bct/

This test gives results very close to those from a laboratory as long as you do the test as above and have had about half an hour's practice training in how to do the test with someone who knows how to do it properly.
(Source: WHO Haemoglobin Colour Scale information leaflet, by permission of the WHO.)

Appendix 2   Method of giving iron dextran by IMI

- Inject only into upper, outer buttock (see Figure 21.5A page 327).
- Use a 19 or 20 gauge needle.
- First, with the fingers of one hand, slide the skin and underlying tissue over the upper, outer buttock away from this area (see Figure 21.5B).
- Insert the needle through the stretched skin (from another area) into the upper, outer buttock (see Figure 21.5C).
- If blood comes back along or through the needle withdraw it and try again.
- Inject slowly.
- Wait 10 seconds after the injection is finished and then withdraw the needle.
- Allow the skin to slide back to its proper place (see Figure 21.5D).
- Make the patient walk around or move the leg.
- Do not rub the site of the injection.

> Do not give iron by injection until malaria, infections and fever have been successfully treated.
> Do not give more than one course of iron by injection in any one 12-month period.

Appendix 3   Method of total dose iron dextran by IV drip

Use only preparations that *do not* contain phenol. Preparations that contain phenol can be used only for intramuscular injections. Check with your Health Department which preparations are safe for you to give by IV as well as IM methods and use only these. New preparations such as sodium ferric gluconate and iron sucrose do not produce the anaphylactic and other reactions which iron dextran can, but are much more expensive and not usually available.

Give only if the patient (1) is past childhood, (2) has no history of allergy or asthma, (3) has no fever or infection and is not sick and also (4) your Health Department and supervising Medical Officer agree with the drug and the technique you use.

Record pulse rate and blood pressure.

Give promethazine 50 mg IMI first.

Insert the drip – 1 litre of dextrose 4.3% in sodium chloride 0.18% (or $\frac{1}{2}$ –1 litre of 0.9% sodium chloride; but only if no heart failure).

Add only one ampoule of the iron dextran to the 1 litre of IV fluid.

Start the drip at 5 drops per minute. Check pulse and blood pressure after 5 minutes and again after 10 minutes.

If
- blood pressure falls more than 15 mm systolic,
or
- pulse rises more than 15 beats per minute, *or*
- patient becomes restless or breathless or coughs, or has chest pains, sweating, nausea or vomiting;

then immediately stop the drip, change both flask and drip set and treat for shock (Chapter 27 page 468).

Give adrenaline (epinephrine) 1:1000 solution 0.5 ml ($\frac{1}{2}$ ml) IMI.

Give promethazine 50 mg (2 ml) IVI if needed.

Also change to IM iron dextran (after patient has fully recovered).

If none of the above signs come, then add the rest of the total dose of iron dextran to the flask. Then

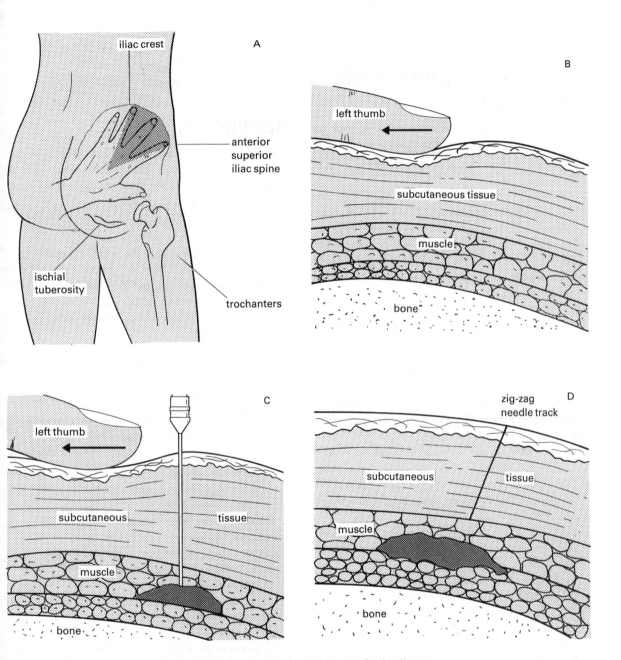

Figure 21.5 *Diagrams to show method of giving iron dextran by IMI. See text for details.*

observe the patient for another 10 minutes as above. Treat as above if signs of shock or allergy occur.

If none of the signs of shock or allergy (above) come, increase the drip rate to 40–60 drops/minute. Check PR and BP each 15 minutes.

The drip should finish in 4–6 hours.

Appendix 4 Notes on blood transfusion

Refer to these notes and any other instructions you have on blood transfusion before giving blood.

1. One unit of blood usually raises the Hb in an adult by 1–1.5 g/dl.
2. Transfuse patients with anaemia until Hb over 5 g/dl – all patients described on page 318. Transfuse until Hb over 7.5 g/dl – (a) patients who may bleed and bleeding could be difficult to control (after 36 weeks of pregnancy, recent gastrointestinal bleeding, etc.) and (b) patients who have severe infections.
3. Use blood only if both the HIV test (see Chapter 19) and the HBV test (see Chapter 24) have been done and are negative and if the donor was not in the period after infection before the test becomes positive. If from an area where *Trypanosoma cruzi* or other serious infections that can be transmitted by blood occur, then tests for these also must have been done and be negative before blood is given. Syphilis tests must be negative.
4. Only use blood which has been properly grouped and cross-matched.
5. Make certain the *correct* bag of blood is given to the patient. The labels, etc. must be checked by two senior health workers.
6. Remove a bag of blood from the Blood Bank refrigerator only when you can start transfusing it immediately.
7. Never transfuse blood that has been out of the refrigerator for more than 4 hours.
8. Take the temperature, pulse rate, blood pressure and breathing rate:
   • before the transfusion is started,
   • 15 minutes after the transfusion is started, and
   • each hour after the transfusion is started.
   A responsible health worker must stay with the patient all the time for the first 15 minutes.
   Observe the patient carefully for any kind of reaction (including low BP, fast PR, back pain,

breathlessness, fever, restlessness, skin rash, etc.).
9. If the patient develops any kind of reaction (as above):
   • stop blood transfusion,
   • give an antihistamine, e.g. promethazine 25 mg (1 ml) IV and 25 mg (1 ml) IM,
   • consult Medical Officer immediately,
   • see Chapter 27 page 468 if shock.
10. Give antimalarial drugs if indicated.

Appendix 5

Laboratory tests needed by Medical Officer to further investigate anaemia (other tests including bone marrow and further blood tests may be needed later).

1. Haemoglobin (Hb), packed cell volume (PCV), mean corpuscular haemoglobin concentration (MCHC) and if available mean cell volume (MCV).
2. Full blood count (FBC) including examination of red blood cells (RBCs) for hypochromia, target cells, anisocytosis and poikilocytosis and of neutrophils for hypersegmentation.
3. Reticulocyte count and reticulocyte index.
4. Malaria smears.
5. Urea/creatinine.
6. Urine microscopy, culture and if needed AFB examination.
7. Tests for any other illnesses, acute and chronic, suggested by examination.

The tests will answer the following questions:

1. Is the anaemia:
   (a) hypochromic (MCHC less than 30–32% and later hypochromic appearance of the RBCs on film)? – see 2, *or*
   (b) normochromic? – see 3.
2. If hypochromic:
   (a) are there numerous target cells and a lot of anisocytosis and poikilocytosis? If so – thalassaemia,
   (b) if not – iron deficiency anaemia or if no response to treatment of this – anaemia of chronic disease.
3. If normochromic (RBCs on blood film normal and MCHC 32–36%):
   (a) is it normocytic (RBCs normal on blood film and MCV 80–100 fl)? – see 4, *or*
   (b) macrocytic (RBCs on films and MCV above 100 fl) – see 5.
4. If normocytic, what is the reticulocyte index?
   (a) if reticulocyte index low (less than 2%) and

normocytic normochromic then –
- bone marrow depression especially drug induced,
- chronic disease,

(b) if reticulocyte index high (greater than 2%) and normochromic normocytic then –
- acute blood loss, *or*
- haemolysis (including malaria, sickle cell, thalassaemia, G6PD deficiency, immune type haemolysis, mechanical, drugs, etc.).

5. If macrocytic, is the marrow:
(a) megaloblastic (more than 30% of the polymorphs with 5 or more lobes)? or

(b) not megaloblastic?
- if megaloblastic macrocytic normochromic, then folate or vitamin B_{12} deficiency and needs trial of a test dose of only 50 micrograms of vitamin B_{12} (this one small dose will not cause acute spinal cord lesion) or only 200 micrograms folinic acid (no more) and then reticulocyte counts to determine which,
- if not megaloblastic but macrocytic normochromic, then consider – alcohol abuse, liver disease, haemolysis, myxoedema, marrow suppression, etc.

(Extract from *Lecture Notes on Tropical Medicine*, Blackwell, 2009.)

22 Disorders of the Lymphatic System and Spleen

The lymphatic system

Anatomy, physiology and pathology

The lymphatic system goes through most of the body. The important parts of it are:

- the lymph vessels,
- the lymph nodes (sometimes called 'lymph glands' or just 'glands'),
- the spleen,
- the tonsils,
- the appendix, and
- collections of 'patches' of lymphoid tissue scattered throughout the gastrointestinal tract and the appendix.

A body fluid called lymph flows through the lymph vessels and lymph glands. The lymph system is connected to the blood circulation system (see Figure 22.1).

Lymph vessels are tubes like the blood capillaries and veins. There is a network of very small lymph capillaries over almost all of the body (see Figure 22.2). These capillaries join to make larger lymph vessels as the vessels go towards the centre of the body.

Lymph nodes are collections of lymphatic tissue along the course of the lymph vessels.

Lymph vessels collect fluid which has come out from the capillaries and is in tissues in the same way as veins. But lymph vessels also collect larger things (such as large proteins and organisms) which

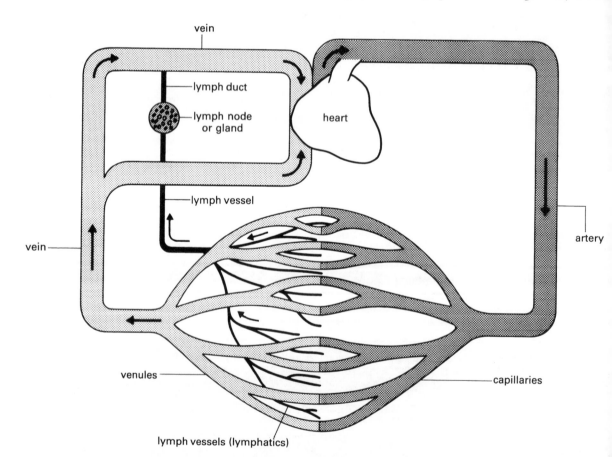

Figure 22.1 *Diagram to show the relationship of the lymphatic system to the circulation of the blood.*

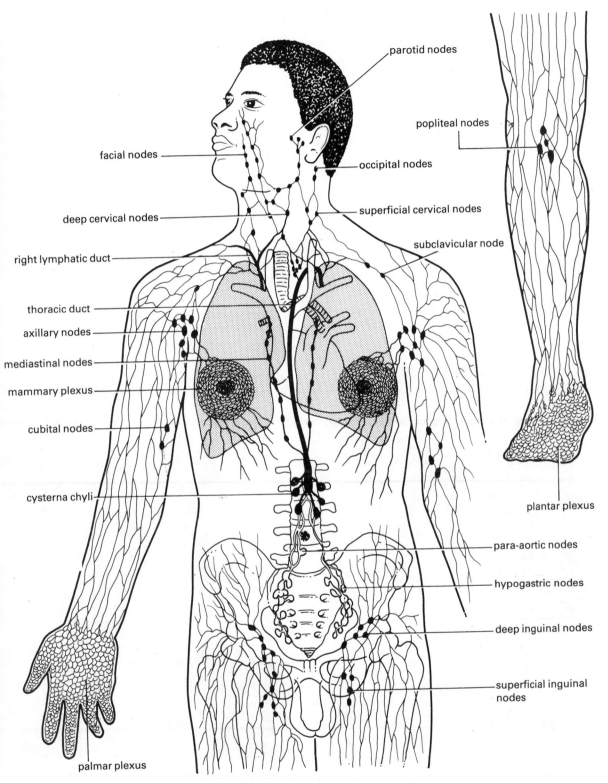

Figure 22.2 *This diagram shows the position of the main groups of lymph glands. It also shows the lymph vessels which carry lymph into the glands. It also shows the lymph glands draining into lymphatic ducts. The largest lymphatic ducts then drain into the large veins.*

331

veins cannot collect. These proteins and organisms are taken to the lymph nodes, where, if necessary, the lymphatic system cells start to make antibodies, etc. against the protein or organism. (See Chapter 10 page 41.)

The protein or organisms travelling in the lymphatic system can sometimes cause inflammation of parts of the lymphatic system. Inflammation of the lymph vessels is called *lymphangitis*. Inflammation of the lymph nodes is called *lymphadenitis*. If the infection is severe, pus may form in the lymph nodes (then sometimes called 'bubos').

If the lymph vessels and nodes are inflamed or destroyed and cannot take fluid and protein from the tissues in the normal way, then the extra fluid and protein in the tissues causes swelling. This is called *lymphoedema*. Lymphoedema is like ordinary oedema except that the fluid has much protein in it, so the oedema does not get a hollow in it, or 'pit', when you press on the area, as easily as ordinary oedema.

History and examination

If you suspect disease of the lymphatic system you must:

1. Examine the lymph nodes in the neck (see Figure 22.3), and axilla (see Figure 22.4), and groin.
   Examine the lymph nodes in the neck and axilla when you examine the head and neck, ENT and thyroid. Examine the lymph nodes in the groin when you examine the abdomen for herniae and lymph nodes. You cannot examine the lymph nodes in the chest or abdomen in a routine physical examination.
2. Examine the related organs:
   • liver (see Chapter 24 page 393),
   • spleen (see this chapter page 343),
   • bone (see Chapter 28 page 476), and
   • blood for anaemia, bleeding or infection (see Chapter 21 pages 313–314).
3. Examine the areas drained by any abnormal lymph nodes for lymphoedema (never forgetting to check the scrotum), infections and cancer.

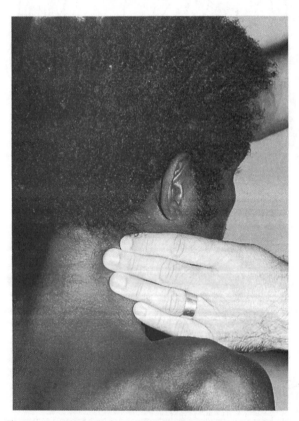 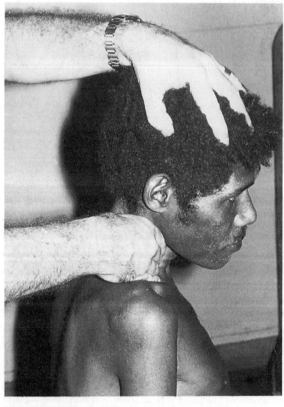

Figure 22.3 *Method of examination of the lymph glands in the neck. The left photograph shows examination of the lymph glands at the back of the neck – from in front of the patient. The right photograph shows examination of the lymph glands at the front of the neck – from behind the patient with the patient's head tipped to the side you are examining to make the muscles relax.*

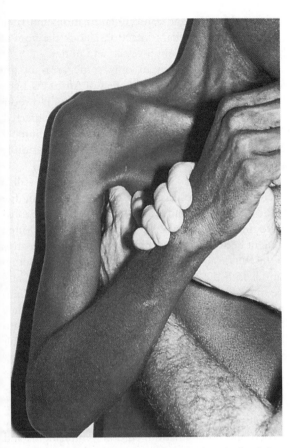

Figure 22.4 *Method of examination of the lymph glands in the axilla. Note that the patient must not hold his arms out so that you can feel under them. That makes the muscles tight and you cannot feel the lymph glands under the muscles. The patient's arm must be at his side as in this photograph.*

Common or important clinical conditions of the lymphatic system

Acute infective lymphangitis and lymphadenitis

Acute infection anywhere in the body may enlarge lymph nodes which drain the area. This may be because the nodes are making antibodies etc. (see Chapter 10 page 41).

But in some infections, the organisms defeat the body defences, and then these organisms may grow and multiply in the lymph vessels and/or lymph nodes, and cause inflammation.

In inflammation of the lymph vessels there is a red, hot, tender, swelling in a thin line between the place where the infection started and the lymph nodes. This is called *acute lymphangitis*.

In inflammation of the lymph nodes the nodes are enlarged and tender (and if they are close to the skin, they may be hot and red). This is called *acute lymphadenitis*.

In severe acute lymphadenitis, pus may form, the nodes be felt to contain fluid (fluctuant) (called 'bubos') and pus may even come out through the skin.

In acute infections of the lymph vessels or lymph nodes, the patient will develop malaise, fever, fast pulse, and the other signs of toxaemia.

Most cases of acute lymphangitis and acute lymphadenitis are caused by bacterial infections. Sometimes they are caused by filarial infection (see page 334) and other causes. Tuberculosis normally causes chronic lymphadenitis, but in an HIV infected person tuberculous lymphadenitis can be acute.

Treatment includes:

1. Antibiotics – usually penicillin (see Chapter 11 pages 57–58).
2. If there is a lot of fluid, use local anaesthetic and aspirate (suck out) the pus through a needle before it bursts through the skin. Do not incise (cut) the skin to let the pus out.

Glandular fever syndrome

See Chapter 16 page 154.

Bubonic plague

See Chapter 17 page 162.

Inguinal bubo (lymphogranuloma venereum)

See Chapter 19 pages 199, 204, 212.

Chronic infective lymphadenitis

Chronic lymphadenitis can be caused by repeated attacks of acute bacterial infection or by chronic infection.

These can cause (1) enlargement of the lymph nodes and/or (2) block of the lymph vessels and the lymph passages in the lymph nodes.

This block of the flow of the lymph can cause lymphoedema. Lymphoedema is swelling of the area drained by the affected vessels and nodes caused by oedema (see Figure 22.7 page 337).

Elephantiasis – chronic severe swelling of the affected body parts with thickening and folding of the skin (see Figure 22.7) – can develop if lymphoedema is present for many years. Lymphoedema and elephantiasis are particularly common in the leg and the scrotum.

Tuberculous lymphadenitis

Tuberculous lymphadenitis is a chronic infection of lymph nodes caused by *Mycobacterium tuberculosis*. Always think of tuberculous lymphadenitis if patient is like this:

1. He is a child or young adult (but can be any age).
2. His neck glands are affected (but can be glands in any other area).
3. He has only one symptom – a lump which does not go away but gets bigger.
4. His only signs are enlarged lymph nodes joined or matted together which are not tender or red or hot. Sometimes there is also a sinus (hole) discharging pus over the top of the nodes.
5. There is no obvious cause of the enlarged nodes (unless other signs of TB are present) (see Chapter 14 page 105).
6. He could possibly have HIV infection.
7. He has a positive tuberculin test (unless he also has HIV infection) (see Chapter 14 pages 109–110).
8. Antibiotic treatment does not cure the infection even if continued for 3 weeks.

If aspiration is negative for AFB and biopsy is not possible and transfer not possible, and after 6 weeks the condition is getting worse, anti-TB treatment could be started. The full length anti-TB treatment must be completed even if the patient quickly improves. Always try at least an aspiration and send for AFB (see Chapter 14 page 110) before giving anti-TB treatment.

Tuberculous lymphadenitis can sometimes be acute (at times with pus formation) in patients who have HIV infection and therefore little cellular immunity.

See Chapter 14 pages 114–120 for management.

Filariasis

Filariasis is a disease caused by infestation with small filarial worms (*Wuchereria bancrofti* or *Brugia malayi* or *timori*). These worms live in the lymphatic vessels and lymph nodes and cause inflammation, and later together with secondary infections, block the flow of lymph through the lymph vessels and nodes.

Filariasis is common in only some areas in the tropical and coastal and island areas of Africa, Asia, the Pacific and the Americas (see Figure 22.6). However, about 120 million people in the world are infected. Also, WHO classifies filariasis as the world's number 2 cause of disability as 40 million people are seriously affected.

The adult filaria worms produce embryos called microfilaria. Microfilaria are carried around in the blood near the skin only at the time when certain mosquitoes in that area usually bite people. This is often at night between 10 p.m. and 2 a.m.; but in some areas of the Pacific about midday. Many kinds of mosquitoes can take up the microfilaria in their blood meal, and the microfilaria then develop in these mosquitoes into infective filaria larvae. These mosquitoes, when they later bite other people, inject the infective larvae into these people, in whom the larvae develop into adult worms (see Figure 22.5).

The adult filarial worms live in and irritate the lymph vessels and lymph nodes. This can cause repeated attacks of acute inflammation, acute lymphangitis and acute lymphadenitis; and eventually also chronic inflammation, chronic lymphangitis and chronic lymphadenitis. As these lymph vessels and glands become so damaged that lymph from the body parts cannot flow through them well, these body parts have more fluid and protein left in them, become swollen, less healthy and are less able to protect themselves from infection. Repeated bacterial and fungal infections start in the skin and can cause cellulitis and then acute lymphangitis and lymphadenitis and a lot more scarring of these tissues. It is these secondary infections – even more than allergic reactions to the worms – which cause the scarring and block of the lymphatics which leads to elephantiasis.

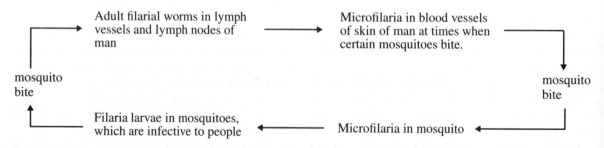

Figure 22.5 *Diagram to illustrate the life cycle of filarial worms.*

Countries and territories with lymphatic filariasis

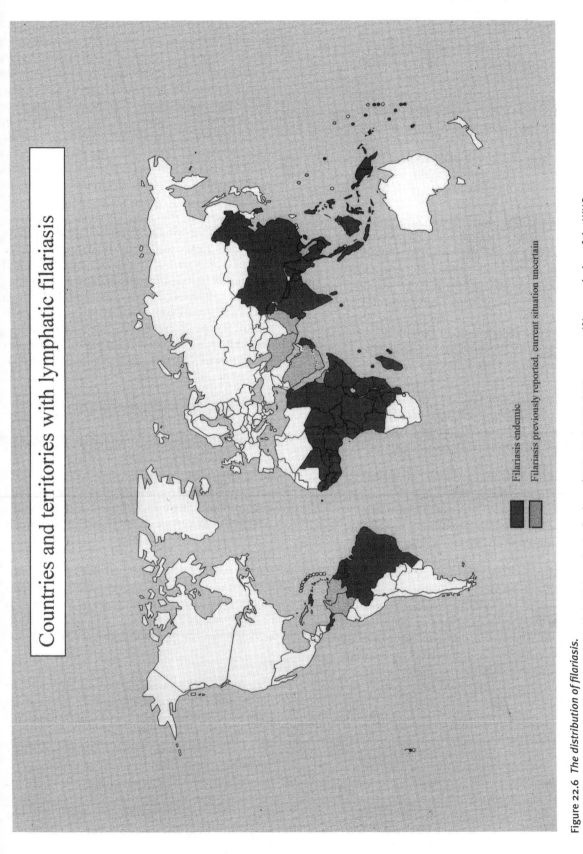

Filariasis endemic

Filariasis previously reported, current situation uncertain

Figure 22.6 *The distribution of filariasis.*
Reproduced from Lymphatic Filariasis http://whqlibdoc.who.int/hq/2001/WHO_CDS_CPE_SMT_2001.7.pdf by permission of the WHO.

Symptoms and signs

1. Allergic type reactions to worms starting to develop in the lymphatic tissues do occur. These cause lymphangitis, lymphadenitis, genital pain (as the scrotal lymphatics are where the *W. bancrofti* prefer to live) and allergic reactions such as urticaria, etc. Surprisingly, however, this is not often seen in the population born in an endemic area and may occur mostly in children. It is most often seen in people who have come recently to the area and have been infected for the first time. It is therefore often called 'expatriate syndrome'.

2. About half of people born and living in endemic areas who are infected have no symptoms. Some of these have no microfilaria in their blood. However, many do have microfilaria. Even in these people without symptoms, their lymph vessels and lymph glands are slowly being damaged and usually also their kidneys. This can be diagnosed by finding blood and protein in their urine.

3. A hydrocoele (collection of fluid in the sac which surrounds the testis) can affect 40–60% of adult males in endemic areas. It usually develops after puberty. The swelling can become huge. This can happen without any lymphoedema or elephantiasis of the penis or scrotum and without there ever having been any recognised acute inflammatory episodes.

4. Lymphoedema can occur in limbs, more often the legs than anywhere else. There may not ever have been any acute episodes of inflammation.

5. Some people, however, do get episodes of acute inflammation in the skin, lymph vessels, lymph nodes, etc. due to bacteria or fungi. These occur probably because the tissues are not healthy and are not able to defend themselves as well as they should, because of the extra fluid and extra protein there from lymphoedema. These episodes of infection scar the already damaged lymph vessels and lymph nodes even more and then block them more.

6. Elephantiasis develops in people who have their lymph vessels initially damaged by the filarial worms and microfilaria and then have them damaged further by these acute bacterial and fungal infections which start in the skin. The oedema does not go away at night time. The tissues become hard. The skin becomes dark. Thick scaly areas of skin develop. Wart-like lumps (which are actually dilated lymph vessels) appear on the surface. In the folds of skin, etc. many bacteria and fungi start to live. At times these get through the surface of the skin and start further episodes of infection, cellulitis, lymphangitis, lymphadenitis and even at times more serious infections. Sometimes the enlarged lymph vessels break open and ooze lymph and so make another place for organisms to get into the body. When these things occur the patient is said to have 'elephantiasis'. In endemic areas 10–50% of men can develop a hydrocoele or elephantiasis of the scrotum and penis, and 10% of the women develop elephantiasis of the vulva or breast and at least 10% of the population have elephantiasis of the leg or arm (see Figure 22.7 page 337).

7. Chyluria occurs when the fat collected from the intestine by the lymphatics drains into the urinary tract when swollen lymphatics burst on the surface of the urinary tract. This causes milky coloured (sometimes blood-stained) urine and malnutrition.

8. An unusual reaction to the parasites can cause asthma (and also a lot of eosinophils in the blood and an abnormal chest X-ray and abnormal blood tests).

9. Tropical arthritis (usually only one joint) and perhaps other unusual conditions may be due to filarial infection.

Other causes of lymphoedema and elephantiasis

1. Chronic infective (bacterial) lymphadenitis including some STDs, especially lymphogranuloma venereum.

2. Tuberculous lymphadenitis.

3. Chronic chemical lymphadenitis from silica absorbed from some soils in some countries through repeated cuts on the feet (podoconiosis) (usually in farmers who work without shoes in the red rocky soil). (See page 341.)

4. Cancer of the lymph nodes themselves (lymphoma); or more likely cancer spread from nearby skin or other organs to the lymph nodes; as well as Kaposi's sarcoma.

5. Lymph nodes removed (surgery or radiotherapy).

Tests

1. A card test (ICT) (immunochromatographic test) can be done on blood in a couple of minutes and gives an immediate answer as to whether an individual patient is infected or not.

2. ELISA tests done in the laboratory can be used for testing blood from large numbers of patients.

3. Microfilaria may be found in thick blood smears collected between 10 p.m. and 2 a.m. or between 10 a.m. and 2 p.m. in the Pacific. This is done on 3 days or nights. The slides have to be sent to the

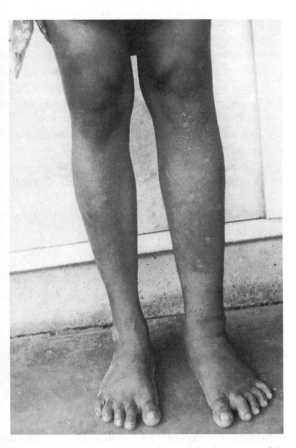

Figure 22.7A *Lymphoedema left leg early in the course of the condition.*

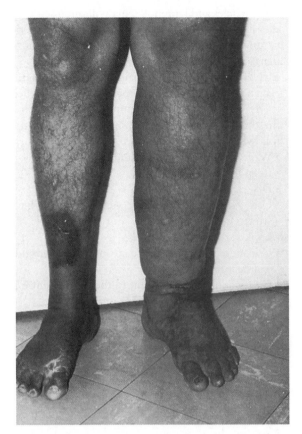

Figure 22.7B *Lymphoedema both legs, 'elephantiasis' left leg.*

laboratory. Microfilaria are no longer seen by the time the patient has developed elephantiasis or if the patient has asthma.

4. Ultrasound tests are done to see the worms themselves, but this requires an ultrasound machine in a hospital.

Showing that a patient is infected with filaria does not of course mean that the patient's symptoms and signs are necessarily due to this infection with filaria.

Do not biopsy the lymph glands as this may make lymphoedema or elephantiasis worse. If the diagnosis is not certain, refer the patient to the next visiting Medical Officer for advice.

Treatment

1. The adult worms are damaged and some killed by doses of diethylcarbamazine (see below) or albendazole 400 mg single dose or ivermectin 100–400 mcg/kg single dose. Doxycycline 200 mg/day for 6–8 weeks stops the adult worms producing microfilaria by killing a bacterium which lives with them

and is needed by the worms. Diethylcarbamazine is cheap. It can, however, cause severe reactions if the patient also has onchocerciasis or *Loa loa* and cannot be used in areas where these occur (which includes significant areas of Africa). In some areas, if the patient has many microfilaria, killing them with drugs can cause significant allergic type side effects such as headache, fever, muscle pains, swollen lymph nodes, rash, etc. which need to be treated with paracetamol, antihistamines and if severe, corticosteroids. An alternative to control these side effects is to start with a quarter of the usual dose and double the dose daily until the normal dose is given; also give these drugs with antihistamines.

The normal dose for diethylcarbamazine is 6 mg/kg/day for 12 days for *W. bancrofti* and 6 days for *B. malayi*, repeated after 6 weeks and again after 6 or 12 months. An alternative is to give diethylcarbamazine 6–8 mg/kg/day for 2 days each month.

Find out from your Health Department and Medical Officer what you should do in your area.

2. Hydrocoeles and lymphoedema will often settle on the above treatment or even on the prophylactic treatment given to the whole population to control filaria infections.

3. Elephantiasis, however, is mainly due to the bacterial and fungal infections. If these can be controlled there is often significant improvement. To stop these infections, the patient should carry out the following management daily.
   • Wash the limbs with soap and water.
   • Keep the nails clean.
   • Dry carefully.
   • Use a moisturiser but not vegetable oil, which attracts cockroaches.
   • Look for any wounds.
   • Use antiseptic or antibiotic cream on any wounds or infections.
   • Go for antibiotic treatment to the health centre if symptoms of infection in leg or fever.
   • Do exercises to encourage the lymph flow.
   • Walk regularly to encourage lymph flow.
   • Keep the legs elevated (as high as possible) by putting them on a stool or chair when sitting and not having them hanging down, and also having the foot of the bed raised at night.
   • Always wear shoes to protect the feet from injury.

   Also (but the above are also essential for a chance of success):
   • Treat with an antihelminthic to damage the adult worm.
   • Give doxycycline for 6 weeks.

4. Hydrocoeles, and much less easily, elephantiasis can be helped by surgery if the above are not effective.

Prevention

1. Kill the organism in the body of the original host.
   • Present drugs do not kill all the adult worms very easily. Long courses or repeated mini-courses are needed.
   • Microfilaria, however, are not produced by the adult worms if they are treated with albendazole and ivermectin or diethylcarbamazine for about 1 year. Adult worms normally live for 4–8 years, although less if treated with drugs.
   • If, therefore, all infected people in the population take drugs once each year for 4–6 years the adult worms produce no microfilaria until they die. In several months, once the already infected mosquitoes have all died, no further mosquitoes will be infected. No further people can be infected. The disease should therefore die out if all infected people are treated each year for about 4–6 years (although it will be many years before all the people with disabilities from filariasis will die). Many infected people, however, have no symptoms. The whole population therefore has to be treated.
   • To be effective, at least 80% of the population needs to actually carry out the programme.
   • This at the moment is the best method of control:
     Albendazole 400 mg AND ivermectin 150–200 mcg/kg where also onchocerciasis and *Loa loa* occur,
     or:
     diethylcarbamazine 6 mg/kg, but only in areas where no onchocerciasis or *Loa loa* occurs
     each year for 5–6 years,
     or:
     diethylcarbamazine put into salt and used each day in cooking and eating by all the population for 1 year. All salt should have 0.2–0.4 mg of diethylcarbamazine per gram of salt. Of course, all salt for all the population would have to have the drug in it and therefore it needs both the salt producers to do this and government legislation to ensure no other salt is used in the community for the year.

2. Stop the means of spread.
   Attempts to kill all the mosquitoes, or greatly reduce their numbers for the 4–8 years before all adult filaria have died, have not been successful.
   Some protection, however, can be obtained by visitors to the area by repellents, protective clothing and the use of insecticide-treated mosquito nets.

3. Raise the resistance of possible new hosts.
   Immunisation or other ways at present do not exist.

4. Give prophylactic treatment.
   This is not normally done; but short-term visitors to the area may be protected by taking diethylcarbamazine 6 mg/kg for 2 days each month.

There are beneficial side effects to the above treatment in populations who are treated each year. There is better nutrition, less anaemia, fewer haemorrhages at childbirth, fewer low birthweight babies and neonatal deaths, better general health of adults, etc. This is due to the effect of the albendazole or ivermectin getting rid of most of the intestinal parasites, and ivermectin also gets rid of scabies.

Burkitt's lymphoma

Burkitt's lymphoma is a common cancer of children, but sometimes young adults, in areas where malaria transmission occurs all the time. It is caused by both infection of the lymphatic cells by Epstein–Barr virus (EBV) and also by other changes in the immune system such as those caused by malaria. Almost everyone gets EBV infection. In early childhood it causes few symptoms, but later glandular fever or infectious mononucleosis (see Chapter 16 page 154). After this, the cells stay infected for life, although in most people in most places where the immune system is not affected by malaria Burkitt's lymphoma does not develop. Some cases are due to EBV and immunosuppression by HIV infection. Some have no known cause.

Burkitt's lymphoma usually causes tumours of the jaw, especially the upper jaw. At first, teeth near the tumour become loose. The tumour grows in the bone and becomes very large very quickly (e.g. in one month). The tumour often pushes the eye forward. It is soft and painless. The skin over the tumour is not ulcerated. The lymph nodes are not enlarged. There is no fever. Apart from the swelling, the patient seems well at first (see Figure 22.8). Dental abscesses can look similar; but an abscess has signs of inflammation and tenderness.

Abdominal swelling due to tumours in any abdominal organ are almost as common as jaw tumours.

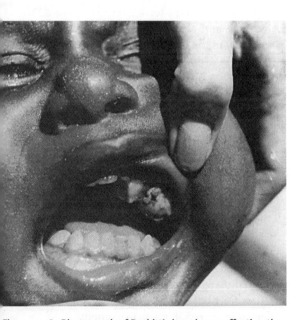

Figure 22.8 *Photograph of Burkitt's lymphoma affecting the upper jaw. The teeth are loose in the swollen gum. If teeth look healthy (no holes in them) but you can very easily push the teeth back and forward in the gum with your finger, without hurting the patient, then it is likely the patient has a Burkitt's tumour.*

Paralysis or other nervous system changes also can occur from the tumour pressing on the brain or spinal cord.

Transfer suspected cases to the Medical Officer as soon as possible for diagnosis by biopsy and treatment with anti-cancer drugs, as patients can get very much worse and die in a few days; however, good early treatment can quickly remove all signs of the tumour in many patients (although it may come back later).

Vaccines to prevent Epstein–Barr virus infection and this tumour are being tried.

Cancer of the lymph nodes

There are two kinds of cancer that affect the lymph nodes.

The first kind is a *primary cancer of the lymph nodes called a lymphoma.* You will most often diagnose lymphoma when you get the result of a biopsy of one of a group of large, firm, non-tender lymph nodes (often biopsied because of suspected TB). Some names of lymphomas are Hodgkin's disease or non-Hodgkin's lymphoma. These and other lymphomas are primary cancers of the lymphatic system and lymph vessels. Some are caused by viruses, e.g. EBV or HIV infections. Sometimes lymphomas can be much improved (even cured) by special treatment.

The other sort of cancer of lymph nodes you may diagnose is when cancer from the skin or an internal organ spreads to the lymph nodes, i.e. *secondary cancer of the lymph glands.* These nodes are often hard, irregular or lumpy and fixed or stuck to each other or the skin or muscles or other structures near them. One particular site for a primary cancer which spreads to the lymph glands of the neck is the back of the nose or throat (nasopharyngeal carcinoma). This tumour is also related to EBV infection and perhaps diet in people who have come from southern China. Often this cancer cannot be seen without special instruments or X-rays. It is anaplastic, meaning very malignant, and is often called 'anaplastic nasopharyngeal carcinoma'.

Always try the effect of two different types of antibiotics on enlarged lymph nodes before considering aspiration, or if this does not give the diagnosis, then biopsy as very often they are enlarged because of bacterial infection.

Refer or non-urgently transfer such patients to the Medical Officer. Do not yourself biopsy lymph nodes unless they are very near the surface and you have been taught how to do it and you have actually done it under supervision (it is often much harder to do than it looks). You can, however, do an aspiration (see Chapter 14 page 110).

Enlargement of the lymph nodes

Do a full history and examination (see Chapter 6). See which of the following your patient has:

1. Enlargement of a lymph node or some lymph nodes *and* tenderness of enlarged nodes *or* fever (see below).
2. Enlargement of a lymph node or some lymph nodes *but* no tenderness of enlarged nodes *and* no fever (see below).
3. Enlargement of *most* of the lymph nodes of the body *but* no tenderness of enlarged nodes *and* no fever (see below).

Enlargement of a lymph node or some lymph nodes and tenderness of enlarged nodes or fever

1. *Acute bacterial lymphadenitis*
   An infected lesion of some sort in the part of the body drained by the affected lymph nodes is usually present (the lesion may be very small).
   Treat with antibiotics (see page 333 and Chapter 11 pages 56–61).
2. *Acute filarial lymphadenitis*
   • The patient is from or in an area where filariasis occurs.
   • He has sometimes had previous attacks.
   • There may be positive tests for filariasis (see page 336).
   Treat as for acute bacterial lymphadenitis (as most are due to bacterial infection) and see page 337 for treatment of the filaria.
3. *Acute viral infections* such as rubella (German measles).
   • Usually the patient is young.
   • Sometimes there is an epidemic.
   • Often the nodes affected are in the neck and not acutely inflamed.
   • Sometimes there are other symptoms and signs (especially a rash).
   • Usually the patient is not very sick.
   Give symptomatic treatment only and observe.
4. *Glandular fever syndrome*
   • Often young.
   • Often sore throat with swollen tonsils with white material on them.
   • Often enlarged liver and spleen.
   • Sometimes rash.
   • Give symptomatic treatment only and observe.
   Do not give ampicillin or amoxicillin, which may cause a rash in these patients.
   See Chapter 16 page 154.

5. *Bubonic plague*
   • The patient is in or has been in an area where plague occurs.
   • Sometimes there is an epidemic; but could be first case.
   • Usually there have been recent rat deaths.
   • The nodes usually severely inflamed and soon become large (bubo), fluctuant and discharge pus.
   • The patient is very sick, with fever, rigors, etc.
   • Septicaemia often develops.
   • Pneumonia may develop.
   • The patient often dies within a week.
   If plague is a possible diagnosis, see Chapter 17 page 162 urgently for diagnosis and management.
6. *Some sexually transmitted diseases* especially:
   • Lymphogranuloma venereum.
   • Chancroid.
   • Donovanosis.
   • Herpes simplex,
     – lymph nodes in groin affected,
     – may be genital lesion.
   See Chapter 19 pages 199, 204.

Enlargement of a lymph node or some lymph nodes but no tenderness of enlarged nodes and no fever

1. *HIV infection* (PGL) see Chapter 19 page 223.
2. *Repeated acute or chronic bacterial infection*
   • Usually in the legs of a person who does not wear shoes.
   • Often there is a history of repeated injury or infection of feet, with swelling of lymph nodes in groin.
   • Chronic infection may still be present.
   • The nodes are hard and smooth.
   • Often there is lymphoedema.
   Management. Give antibiotics and see page 338.
3. *Filariasis (usually with bacterial infection)*
   • The patient is in or from an area where filariasis occurs and usually other people near where he lives are affected.
   • There is often a history of repeated attacks of acute lymphangitis and lymphadenitis.
   • The nodes are hard and smooth.
   • Often there is lymphoedema.
   • Tests for filariasis may be positive.
   See pages 337–338 for management.
4. *Tuberculosis*
   • The affected patient is often young (but not always) and could have HIV infection.
   • The affected nodes are often in neck (but can be anywhere).

- A node may be joined to other nodes under the skin.
- Sometimes there is a sinus (hole) discharging pus over the node.
- There is no infection or other cause for the node enlargement in the area of the body drained by the node.
- Sometimes chronic cough or other symptoms or signs of TB are present.
- Sometimes there is a family history of TB.
- The tuberculin test is usually positive (unless for HIV infection).
- Treatment for 3 weeks with antibiotics does not cure the disease.

Aspirate or biopsy all such glands.

See page 334 and Chapter 14 pages 105, 110, 114.

5. *Some sexually transmitted diseases*

See 'Enlargement of a lymph node and tenderness', No. 6 (page 340) as nodes are normally but not always tender.

6. *Chronic chemical lymphadenitis* of the groin nodes *(podoconiosis)* (see pages 336, 338)
   - Only in some countries where some soils have a lot of silica (e.g. red clay soil from basalt volcanic rocks).
   - Patients are usually members of farming families who have not worn shoes and have had numerous cuts on feet over years.
   - Often lymphoedema or elephantiasis of leg.
   - No filariasis or bacterial infection or other cause.

7. *Cancer of the nodes*
   - Often as for TB (see 4 pages 340–341) except no history suggesting TB and the tuberculin test may be negative, *or*
   - The nodes are often hard and lumpy and stuck to each other or the skin or the nearby muscles, *or*
   - There are other lesions which could be cancer in the area drained by the nodes.
   See page 339 for management.

8. *Trypanosomiasis*
   Often mostly affected are the neck nodes.
   See Chapter 18 pages 181–186.

9. *Visceral leishmaniasis*
   Usually all nodes are affected but sometimes it is mostly in one part.
   See below and Chapter 18 pages 175–181.

Enlargement of most of the lymph nodes of the body but no tenderness of nodes and no fever

1. *HIV infection (PGL)*
   - The patient is usually aged 15–50 years.

- Unsafe sexual practices, blood transfusion, IV drug abuse, etc. in last few years.
- Nodes 1–3 cm in diameter not getting larger after 3 months.
- No other cause obvious.
- May have other symptoms and signs of HIV infection, although often none.
- Blood test for HIV, if available, is usually positive.

See Chapter 19 page 223.

2. *Syphilis*
   - The patient has had sexual intercourse with a possibly affected person some weeks or months before.
   - There was a chancre (sore on genitalia) for 2–6 weeks about 6 weeks before.
   - Skin rashes are sometimes present.
   - Condylomata lata are sometimes present.
   - Mucous patches are sometimes present.
   - Malaise is sometimes present.
   - The serological test for syphilis is positive.
   See Chapter 19 pages 208–210.

3. *Lymphoma (cancer of lymph glands)*
   - The spleen is often enlarged.
   - The liver may be enlarged.
   - Anaemia is often present.
   - Wasting is often present.
   See page 339 for management.
   Make certain that the patient does not have severe TB.

4. *Visceral leishmaniasis (kala azar)*
   - The patient is in or from an area where kala azar occurs.
   - There may be a fever.
   - The spleen is enlarged, often very enlarged.
   - The liver is enlarged, but not very enlarged.
   - Anaemia is present.
   - Repeated attacks of diarrhoea often occur.
   - Wasting is often present.
   - Lumps on skin are sometimes present.
   - There are leishmania organisms in an aspirate or a biopsy.
   - The formaldehyde gel test is positive after a few months but the immunochromatographic test is much more accurate.
   See Chapter 18 pages 175–181 for management.

5. *Trypanosomiasis*
   - The patient is in or from an area where trypanosomiasis occurs.
   - There was a sore (in Africa) or a swelling (in America) at the place of the bite.
   - A fever may develop later.

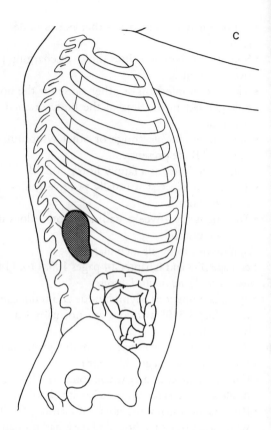

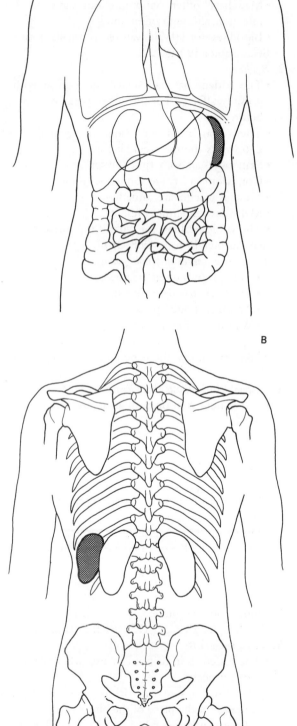

Figure 22.9 A, B and C. *These diagrams show the normal position of the spleen (slightly enlarged). (A) Anterior or front view. (B) Posterior or back view. (C) Left lateral or side view. Note that the spleen is a posterior organ. Note that a normal spleen cannot be felt on examination of the abdomen. When a spleen enlarges it enlarges forwards, downwards and to the right. At first you can feel it right under the ribs on the left side, in the front. See Figure 22.10. Note also that the spleen is just under the ribs which protect it. If the left lower ribs are damaged (especially if they are fractured) the spleen is likely to be damaged too.*

- Neck lymph nodes most often affected (in Africa).
- The spleen is enlarged.
- The liver is enlarged.
- Anaemia is present.
- The pulse is fast.
- There may be meningitis or encephalitis or psychosis or unconsciousness (in Africa).
- There are trypanosomiasis organisms in blood or aspirate from lymph gland.
- CIATT test positive.

See Chapter 18 pages 181 and 186.

Swelling of one limb

Causes include:

1. injury,
2. infection,
3. chronic lymph vessel and lymph node disease with blocked lymph node channels (see this chapter),
4. clots in the main deep vein ('deep venous thrombosis' or DVT) (see Chapter 20 page 301),
5. varicose veins, and
6. snakebite or allergic reaction to sting or toxin, etc.

Swelling of both legs

See 'Generalised oedema', Chapter 36 pages 588–590.

The spleen

Anatomy, physiology, pathology

The spleen (Figure 22.9) makes some of the white blood cells and also some antibodies. The spleen also takes 'worn out' red blood cells from the blood, breaks them down and saves most of the parts for the bone marrow to make new red blood cells.

If the spleen collects and breaks down many more red blood cells than normal (e.g. in a patient with malaria which damages red blood cells), then the spleen enlarges. If the vein from the spleen (which goes through the liver) becomes blocked by disease of the liver (e.g. cirrhosis or schistosomiasis), then the spleen becomes too full of blood and enlarges.

Anytime the spleen enlarges, it can start taking normal red blood cells, normal white blood cells, and normal platelets out of the blood (as well as the 'worn out' red blood cells). The body may then not have enough of some or all of these blood cells.

An enlarged spleen is more likely to rupture (break open) and bleed than a normal spleen.

Symptoms and signs

Disease of the spleen may cause these *symptoms*.

1. Pain in the left upper abdomen. This is usually caused by trauma or inflammation or sudden haemolysis

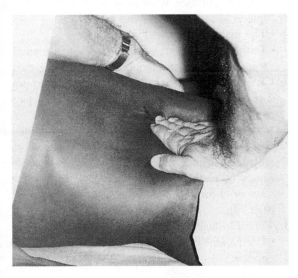

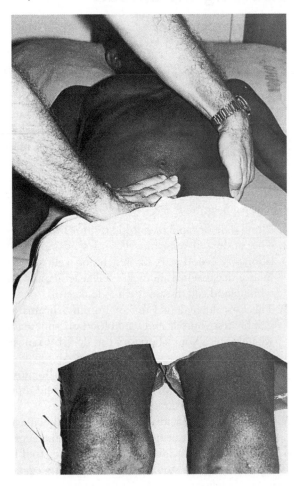

Figure 22.10 A and B *These photographs show how to feel for a spleen. Place the left hand behind the left side of the patient's abdomen. Lift it upwards (forwards). Place the right hand with the palm flat on the patient's abdomen and the fingers pointing to the left upper abdomen. Start in the right lower abdomen (or you may not feel a very large spleen). Tell the patient to take slow deep breaths in and out. If the spleen is enlarged to where your fingers are you will feel it hit the tips of your fingers as the patient breathes in. If you do not feel the spleen, move the fingers towards the ribs and tell the patient to breathe deeply again. Keep moving the right hand up until the spleen is felt or you have felt along the edge of the ribs, and found no enlargement of the spleen.*

(suddenly processing a lot of the contents of many broken open red blood cells).

2. Swelling of the left upper abdomen; or if the spleen is very enlarged, swelling of the whole abdomen.

3. Anaemia (and other blood disorders), if the spleen is enlarged and takes normal blood cells as well as 'worn out' red cells from the blood.

4. Shock and anaemia, if the spleen is ruptured and bleeds.

Disease of the spleen may cause these *signs*.

1. Tenderness in the left upper abdomen (see symptoms, 1).

2. Enlargement of the left upper abdomen or the whole abdomen (see symptoms, 2).

3. Anaemia (and other blood disorders) (see symptoms, 3).

4. Shock and anaemia (see symptoms, 4).

Common conditions affecting the spleen

Very large spleen

A very enlarged spleen may be caused by many conditions. In some areas, some of these causes do not occur. Do not worry about causes that do not occur in your area or areas where your patients may have been.

Your patient may have more than one cause for a very enlarged spleen. It is not always possible to know what causes a patient's enlarged spleen. But you must always try to find out.

If possible, do these tests on your patient (do not do the test if the disease does not occur where your patient has been):

1. Blood slide or rapid diagnostic test for malaria.

2. The sickle cell test yourself; and send blood for laboratory blood tests for red blood cell diseases such as thalassaemia and sickle cell anaemia, and for white blood cell diseases such as leukaemia.

3. The formaldehyde gel test or immunochromatographic test yourself; and send blood or aspirate for whatever tests your laboratory can do for diagnosis of leishmaniasis.

4. The card CIATT test; or send to the laboratory tests for trypanosomiasis on blood and fluid aspirated from lymph node.

5. Urine test for miracidia yourself; and send urine to the laboratory for urine test for schistosome eggs.

6. Stool test for miracidia yourself; and send stool to the laboratory for stool test for schistosome eggs.

Some of the causes for a very big spleen are:

1. *Chronic malaria*
   - The patient is in a malarial area; but he has not been there for long enough to have developed (semi-) immunity to malaria (which needs 4–10 years of continuous exposure).
   - He has repeated attacks of acute malaria.
   - Anaemia is present.
   - An enlarged liver is present.
   - Wasting is present.
   Treat acute attacks of malaria as soon as they start (see Chapter 13 pages 79, 80).

2. *Hyperreactive malarious splenomegaly* or *tropical splenomegaly syndrome*
   - The patient has lived in an area of stable malaria for some years.
   - The spleen keeps on enlarging.
   - The liver is enlarged.
   - Anaemia is present.
   - Wasting is present.
   - There are episodes of haemolysis, when there is fever, jaundice, worsening of anaemia and the spleen becomes painful and tender.
   - The malaria smear is often negative.
   - Tests for schistosomiasis and visceral leishmaniasis, trypanosomiasis and blood diseases are negative.
   Give prophylactic antimalarial drugs for at least 2 years, and probably for life (see Chapter 21 pages 319–321).
   In an area where malaria occurs *always think of this condition* in any patient who has a chronically enlarged spleen as HMS is one of the few treatable causes of very enlarged spleen. But do not treat cases of chronic malaria as HMS (see Chapter 13 page 74).

3. *Visceral leishmaniasis (kala azar)*
   - The patient is in or from an area where kala azar occurs.
   - There may be fever.
   - The lymph nodes are enlarged.
   - Anaemia is present.
   - Diarrhoea is present.
   - Wasting is present.
   - Sometimes skin rash is present.
   - Formaldehyde gel test is positive and the immunochromatographic test or laboratory test for leishmania in blood test is positive.
   Management. See Chapter 18 pages 175–181.

4. *Trypanosomiasis*
   - The patient is in or from an area where trypanosomiasis occurs.

- Sore or swelling at the site of the infecting bite.
- Fever, fast pulse, swelling of lymph nodes and liver as well as spleen.
- A card (CIATT) or blood tests or lymph node aspirate are positive for trypanosomiasis.

Management. See Chapter 18 pages 181–186.

5. *Schistosomiasis*
- The patient is in or from an area where schistosomiasis occurs.
- He has a past history of blood in the urine or dysentery.
- There may still be urinary or intestinal symptoms and signs.
- Late in the disease he may vomit blood or pass melaena (black tarry stools).
- Late in the disease the abdomen may be full of fluid (ascites) and there may be some swelling of legs and back (oedema).

Diagnose and treat as soon as possible. Once late stages are reached treatment is not likely to help as much. See Chapter 18 pages 187–191.

6. *Chronic liver disease usually of undiagnosed cause (cirrhosis)*
- No evidence of schistosomiasis is present.
- A lot of ascites and some oedema are present with wasting of the muscles most noticeable around the shoulders.
- Sometimes the patient may vomit blood or pass melaena (black tarry stools).
- There may sometimes be a change in behaviour or level of consciousness; sometimes jaundice; sometimes bleeding, from anywhere.

Diuretics help the ascites and oedema; but no treatment is much help. See Chapter 24 pages 395–398.

7. *Blood diseases*
- *Leukaemia* – The report of the laboratory blood film suggests this.

Refer or non-urgently transfer to Medical Officer for diagnosis and possible treatment.
- *Thalassaemia* – The report of the blood film and examination for abnormal haemoglobin from the laboratory confirms diagnosis.

See Chapter 21 page 324.
- *Sickle cell anaemia*:
  - The patient is usually an African.
  - Anaemia is present.
  - The patient has repeated infarction crises.
  - The spleen may become smaller.
  - The sickling test you do or the report of the blood film and examination for abnormal haemoglobin confirms diagnosis.

See Chapter 21 pages 321–323.
- *Lymphomas*
  - Cancers of the lymphatic system.
  - Can be caused by HIV or EBV infection.

See page 339.

8. *Many infections*
- Spleen usually not very large.
- Diagnosis made by other symptoms and signs and tests.

Painful or tender spleen

There are many causes of an enlarged, painful or tender spleen in tropical and developing countries. You can usually use other symptoms and signs to make the diagnosis. But never forget to check for the following conditions.

Traumatic rupture of the spleen

Small injuries can cause the spleen to rupture (or burst open).

Be very suspicious of ruptured spleen if there has been a left-sided chest or abdominal injury.

Sometimes there is a haematoma (bruise) under the capsule (or covering) of the spleen for some hours or days after the injury before the capsule bursts and the spleen then bleeds a lot.

The patient will become paler, the pulse rate faster and the blood pressure lower if the spleen is bleeding.

Generalised abdominal tenderness and later shifting dullness (see Chapter 36 pages 593–598 and 603) will develop.

Transfer urgently all suspicious cases to Medical Officer care after you have started an IV drip and any other necessary treatment (see Chapter 27 page 468).

Acute malaria

Always give antimalarial treatment (see Chapter 13 pages 79, 80) to any patient in a malarial area with a tender spleen, especially if also a fever, unless you are certain he does not have malaria.

Septicaemia and especially typhoid fever

Always think of septicaemia in any patient who is very sick. Unless another cause for the illness can be found, treat for septicaemia (see Chapter 12 page 64).

Sickle cell anaemia

See Chapter 21 page 321.

Acute haemolytic episode

See Chapter 21 page 315.

23 Disorders of the Gastrointestinal System and Nutrition

Anatomy, physiology and pathology

Food consists of proteins, carbohydrates, fats, salts, vitamins and water. Food is used as fuel for the muscles and other working parts of the body, and for growth and repair of the body.

Before body cells can use food, it must be crushed, digested (or broken down into simpler substances) and then absorbed (taken) into the body.

The parts of the gastrointestinal canal in which foods are crushed, digested and absorbed are the mouth, the oesophagus, the stomach, the small intestine and the large intestine.

First the food is crushed by the teeth, and mixed with saliva, which is a lubricant that also starts di-

gestion of the food. The saliva is made by three sets of paired salivary glands. The parotid glands are on both sides of the jaw in front of the ears. The submandibular glands are on both sides under the jaw. The sublingual glands are under the tongue. (See Figure 23.1.)

Then the food is swallowed. The oesophagus has muscles in its wall which move the food into the stomach.

The stomach is a storage bag. It lets small amounts of food into the intestine every few minutes until it is empty, which takes a few hours after filling it by eating. In the stomach the food is mixed with two very powerful digestive juices – hydrochloric acid and pepsin. These are made in glands in the mucous membrane of the stomach.

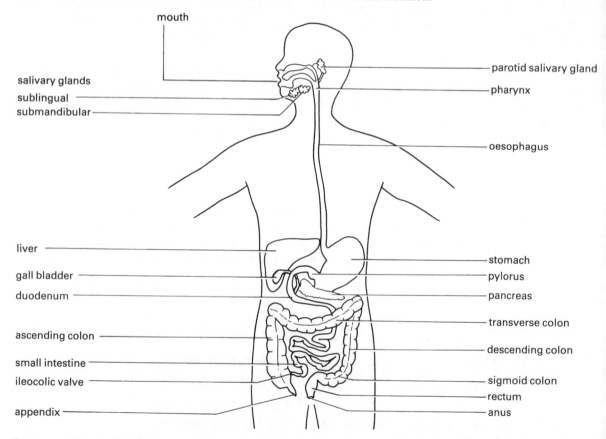

Figure 23.1 *Diagram of the main parts of the gastrointestinal system.*

When the food has been partly digested by the acid and pepsin, the ring of muscle at the outlet of the stomach (which is called the pylorus) opens a little. This allows the muscular contractions of the stomach (called peristalsis) to push a little food into the first part of the small intestine (called the duodenum).

In the duodenum the food is mixed with other digestive juices. Bile, made in the liver and stored in the gall bladder, is added and helps fats to be absorbed. Pancreatic juice from the pancreas is added and this contains an enzyme (trypsin), which breaks down proteins, and other enzymes, which break down carbohydrates and fats (see Figure 23.2).

The food is moved through the duodenum and the small intestine by contractions of the small intestine (also called peristalsis). The small intestine is about 6–7 metres long.

As the food travels along the small intestine, more digestive juices are added from glands in the mucous membrane of the intestinal wall. All these digestive juices break down (or digest) the food into simpler compounds.

These simpler compounds are then absorbed by the special mucous membrane of the intestinal wall. The digested and absorbed food is put into the blood, which goes to the liver through the portal vein (see Figure 24.3 page 391).

When the remains of the food reach the large intestine, also called colon, it is only the fibres and hard parts, which cannot be digested and absorbed by the small intestine, that are left. The remains of the food have been mixed with bilirubin (which is the remains of haemoglobin from worn out red cells which is excreted in the bile). This bilirubin gives the faeces their brown colour. The food remains are also mixed with many bacteria (both dead and alive) which normally live in the intestine. There is also a lot of water from food, drink and the digestive juices mixed with the food remains.

As all this material goes through the large intestine, most of the water is absorbed through the mucous membrane of the large intestine.

The lower part of the large intestine is called the rectum. The rectum is a storage bag for the remains of the food until it can be passed through the anus into the toilet.

The unabsorbed remains of the food and the other materials are called faeces or stool. If the faeces stay a long time in the rectum, they become hard and difficult to pass. This is called constipation. If food is not absorbed in the small intestine and/or the remains of the unabsorbed food go through the large intestine very quickly, there is not enough time for the water to be absorbed. The stools are then soft, watery, large in volume and frequent. This is called diarrhoea.

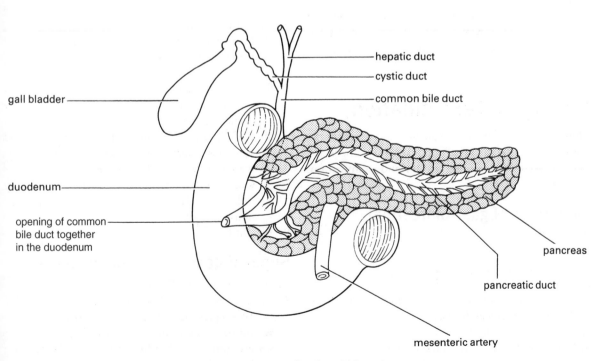

Figure 23.2 *The duodenum and how bile and pancreatic juice flow into the intestine.*

The peritoneum

The peritoneum is like a very large thin balloon or bladder of a football inside the abdominal cavity. The diaphragm, liver, spleen, pancreas, kidneys, blood vessels, etc. below the diaphragm and on the posterior (back) abdominal wall are above and behind it. The bladder, uterus, fallopian tubes, etc. in the pelvis are below it. There are no organs on the back of the anterior (front) abdominal wall in front of it.

The small intestine and some other organs push in so far that the peritoneum comes together behind them and the outside walls of the peritoneum stick together behind the intestine; but the intestine is still outside of the peritoneum. Like a balloon or football bladder from which all the air is let out and it is squashed and then tied off or sealed, the peritoneal cavity has nothing inside it.

The inside surface of the peritoneum makes a covering of slippery fluid so that it and the organs outside it can easily slip or slide over each other if they move.

If organisms get into the peritoneum, pus is made and can collect inside the peritoneal cavity (called peritonitis). If an organ outside the peritoneum is broken, tearing the peritoneum, and bleeds, blood can collect inside the peritoneal cavity (called haemoperitoneum). If the peritoneum becomes oedematous, fluid could seep into the peritoneal cavity and collect (called ascites).

There is no way for pus, blood or fluid to get out of the closed peritoneal cavity unless the blood can absorb it into itself; or it is removed by a needle or surgery.

History and examination

These symptoms and signs can be caused by conditions of the gastrointestinal system. Always check for those marked* in a routine history and examination. See Figure 23.3.

Symptoms of gastrointestinal disease

1. Fever* – if there is infection.
2. Painful mouth or salivary glands.
3. Difficulty in swallowing (dysphagia).
4. Chest pain usually worse on swallowing or lying down (oesophageal disease).
5. Change in appetite.*
6. Vomiting*/haematemesis (blood vomited).*
7. Diarrhoea*/dysentery (blood in loose stool).*

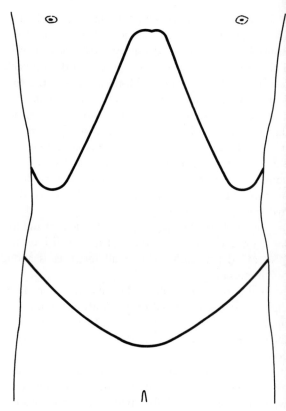

Figure 23.3 *Use a simple diagram like this and mark the findings of your examination on it.*

8. Abdominal pain.*
   (a) Epigastric (upper central abdomen) and if related to food (made worse or eased by food) – usually caused by stomach or duodenal disease.
   (b) Colic in epigastrium and around umbilicus – usually inflammation of or obstruction of the small intestine.
   (c) Colic in the side or lower part of the abdomen and around the umbilicus – usually caused by inflammation of or obstruction of the large intestine.
   (d) Constant in any area – usually caused by inflammation of or stretching of the peritoneum in that area.
9. Weight loss.*

Signs of gastrointestinal disease

1. Temperature raised* – if there is infection.
2. Dehydration and/or shock* – inelastic skin, fast pulse, low blood pressure, little or no urine passed, etc.
3. Wasting/malnutrition* – if not eating; or chronic vomiting; or not absorbing food (malabsorption); or chronic diarrhoea.

4. Pallor* – if gastrointestinal bleeding, acute or chronic; or poor absorption of iron, vitamin B group, etc.

5. Inflammation of the mouth or salivary glands.

6. Enlarged lymph glands above the clavicles – some cancers in the abdomen spread to here.

7. Abdomen (details in Chapter 36 pages 593–605):

- (a) Inspection
  - size*
  - shape*
  - surface for scars*
  - movement when breathing*
- (b) Palpation
  - tenderness*
    - – rebound tenderness
    - – guarding
    - – rigidity
  - enlarged organs*
  - lumps or masses*
- (c) Percussion (if necessary)
  - organs
  - masses
  - fluid (shifting dullness)
- (d) Auscultation (if necessary)
  - bowel sounds
    - – increased
    - – absent
  - splash
- (e) Pelvic examination through the rectum ('PR') (if necessary) (see Figures 26.6–26.9 pages 442–444)
  - tenderness
  - enlarged organs
  - masses
  - faeces, blood or pus in rectum
- (f) Pelvic examination through the vagina ('PV') (if necessary) (see Chapter 26 page 443)
  - tenderness
  - enlarged organs
  - masses
  - blood or pus in vagina or from uterus

Disorders of the gastrointestinal system

Parotitis

Parotitis is usually caused by mumps (see Chapter 16 page 155) in people who were healthy before.

Parotitis can be caused by acute bacterial infection (see below) in people who were already sick before. See Figure 23.4 for the position of the parotid glands.

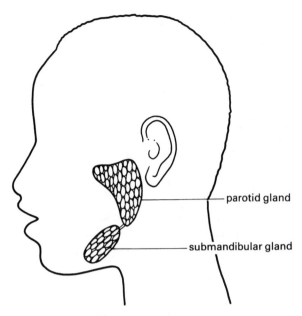

Figure 23.4 *The anatomical position of the parotid and submandibular glands.*

Acute bacterial parotitis

Acute bacterial parotitis usually occurs in sick people who are not eating, drinking or caring for their mouths properly. (See also 'Melioidosis' Chapter 17 page 161.)

Symptoms include pain in the side of the face (which is made worse by movement) and swelling of the parotid area.

Signs include:

- The parotid gland at the side of the face is swollen, hard, tender, often hot and sometimes red. It is difficult for the patient to open his mouth. The swelling is sometimes very large.
- The pulse is fast and the temperature is raised.

Differential diagnosis includes: parotid tumour (which is not acute); and mumps (see Chapter 16 page 155).

Treatment includes:

- antibiotics (start with penicillin),
- pain relief,
- mouth toilet, and
- proper hydration (intravenously, if necessary).

Prevention is by doing a mouth toilet for and making sure that sick patients have enough fluids.

Peritonitis

Peritonitis is an inflammation of the peritoneum (or lining of the peritoneal cavity) in all parts of the abdomen. The inflammation is usually acute and is usually caused by bacterial infection, most commonly from the bowel when acute appendicitis or peptic ulcer or typhoid fever or diverticulitis ruptures (breaks open) the bowel wall. Blood in the peritoneal cavity can cause similar symptoms and signs (see below). The inflammation is occasionally chronic, and is then usually caused by TB (see Chapter 14 page 107).

There may be a history or symptoms or signs of the condition which caused the peritonitis, e.g.

- inflammation of the bowel wall, e.g. acute appendicitis, typhoid fever, enteritis necroticans (pigbel) or diverticulitis;
- a bowel obstruction, especially if strangulated;
- an abdominal wound, e.g. spear or knife;
- a peptic ulcer that has ruptured (eaten through stomach or duodenal wall);
- a genital tract infection in the female, e.g. gonorrhoea or post-partum infection;
- liver abscess which ruptured (burst).

Symptoms and signs (see also Chapter 36 pages 593–598)

Symptoms may include:

- constant abdominal pain made worse by movement,
- vomiting, and
- constipation, usually.

Signs may include:

- temperature usually above normal,
- pulse usually fast,
- blood pressure low, especially late in the disease,
- the breathing rate may be fast, especially late in the disease,
- dehydration may be present,
- the patient looks 'sick',
- the abdomen:
  – distension after some hours,
  – no movement on breathing,
  – tender all over with rebound tenderness, guarding and rigidity,
  – bowel sounds absent.

Tests

No tests are usually possible in a health centre.

If you do a white cell count, it is usually increased, with an increased percentage of neutrophils.

Treatment

Urgent (emergency) transfer to hospital is necessary if the patient agrees to surgery (to treat the cause; and to remove the pus, faeces or blood from the peritoneal cavity; and to give powerful antibiotics).

While waiting for transfer, treat like this:

1. IV fluids as necessary for dehydration or shock (see pages 364–365 and Chapter 27 pages 468–470) and then give maintenance fluids.
2. Nil orally. Insert a nasogastric tube, and aspirate all the fluid every hour.
3. Antibiotics: chloramphenicol 1–2 g immediately and every 6 hours by IVI (or IMI).
4. Morphine 7.5–10 mg if necessary for pain while waiting for, and during, transfer.

Haemoperitoneum

Haemoperitoneum is the collection of blood in the peritoneal cavity.

Blood can get into the peritoneal cavity only if one of the organs which the peritoneum covers ruptures (bursts) and bleeds. The most common causes in tropical countries are:

1. ruptured ectopic pregnancy (pregnancy in the fallopian tube);
2. ruptured spleen;
3. ruptured liver;
4. other traumatic injuries and only very rarely blood vessels (e.g. aneurysm) bursting.

Blood causes severe irritation of the peritoneum. Blood loss affects the circulation.

Symptoms and signs include the following.

- Generalised severe constant abdominal pain; often sudden in onset (when the blood first gets into the peritoneum); worse on movement; sometimes shoulder tip pain (from peritoneal irritation under the diaphragm).
- No movement of the abdomen on breathing.
- Abdominal generalised tenderness, guarding and rigidity.
- Bowel sounds absent.
- Abdominal distension later.
- Pulse fast. Blood pressure low when sitting at first and later when lying. Pallor. Low haemoglobin later. Shock (see Chapter 27 pages 466–470).
- Temperature normal and no signs of infection.
- Symptoms and signs of chest or abdominal trauma or of an enlarged spleen or of a late or missed menstrual period, etc. may be present.

Treatment includes:

1. Insert an IV drip and treat blood loss (see Chapter 27 pages 468–470). Blood transfusion will be needed if surgery is not carried out soon.
2. Immediately contact the Medical Officer to arrange emergency transfer for surgery.

3. Give pain relief.
4. Give nothing to eat or drink (before surgery).

Intestinal obstruction

Intestinal obstruction is present when the food and fluids in the intestine cannot go through a part of the intestine. The intestine above the part that is blocked contracts more than usual and secretes more fluids than usual, and then dilates (get bigger).

There may be a history or symptoms or signs of the disease which caused the obstruction, e.g.

• hernia (especially if recently won't go back),
• previous abdominal operation (a loop of bowel may get stuck in or around a peritoneal scar),
• enteritis necroticans ('pigbel') (leaving narrowed bowel),
• cancer of the intestine (blocking the bowel passages),
• previous vomiting or passing of roundworms (*Ascaris*), especially if this followed a dose of tetrachloroethylene (TCE) (a mass of worms blocking the passage),
• the swallowing of a large foreign body.

Symptoms and signs (see also Chapter 36 pages 593–598)

Symptoms include:

• abdominal pain, usually central, which lasts for about half a minute and which then goes away, only to come back every few minutes, often with loud intestinal sounds,
• repeated vomiting and
• constipation (no faeces or flatus (i.e. wind or gas) passed).

Signs include:

1. Dehydration occurs if the condition has been present for more than a couple of hours (fast pulse, low blood pressure, inelastic skin, little or no urine passed, etc.).
2. Abdomen
   Inspection:
   • distension of the whole abdomen,
   • the abdominal wall does not move well with respiration,
   • intestinal movements can sometimes be seen through the abdominal wall,
   • you must *always* look for hernias and scars (in case these are the cause).
   Palpation:
   • Tenderness is not present. (Tenderness is present only if the obstruction is strangulated. Strangulation occurs when part of the bowel is twisted or pressed

on in such a way that no blood can get through to that part of the bowel and that part of the bowel starts to die. It is then attacked by bacteria from inside the bowel which spread through the bowel wall into the peritoneal cavity, causing inflammation first of the strangulated bowel and then of the peritoneum. At first, tenderness is only over the strangulated area. Later, when general peritonitis develops, the tenderness spreads to the whole abdomen.)
   • You may feel a mass. It may be the affected length of intestine or a cancer or other mass which is causing the obstruction.
   Auscultation:
   • Intestinal sounds are increased (and pain occurs during the sounds).
   • You can hear a loud splash if the abdomen is shaken while you listen with the stethoscope.
3. General signs of peritonitis (see page 350) are not present. These occur only if the obstruction is strangulated.

Treatment

If the patient will agree to surgery, transfer to hospital urgently (emergency) is necessary for operation to remove the cause of the obstruction.

While waiting for transfer, treat like this:

1. Nil by mouth. Insert a nasogastric tube into the stomach, and leave the end open and lower than the patient so that fluid can drain from it; but also aspirate all the fluid every hour.
2. IV fluids (see: IV fluids therapy – dehydration and shock, page 364 and Chapter 27 page 468).
3. Treat for peritonitis if this is present (see page 350).

Gastro-oesophageal reflux

Gastro-oesophageal reflux (GOR) is said to happen when acid, pepsin and food from the stomach come back into the oesophagus. This happens if the 'one-way' valve into the stomach does not work properly (e.g. when there is a hiatus hernia and the stomach can partly slide through the bigger than normal hole in the diaphragm into the chest).

Acid and pepsin cause inflammation and even ulceration of the oesophagus; and of the lungs if they get up as far as the mouth and are then aspirated (breathed in) during sleep.

Symptoms and signs can include:

1. Pain in the front of the chest behind the sternum, often called 'heartburn'. This is felt especially after

meals or on bending or lying down, at times acid reflux gets into the mouth. It may be relieved by drinking any fluids or swallowing antacids.

2. Haematemesis and melaena if the acid makes a peptic ulcer in the oesophagus and eats into an artery which bleeds.

3. Difficulty in swallowing if an ulcer causes scarring and then obstruction of the oesophagus.

4. Cough, sputum, haemoptysis, shortness of breath, wheezing, etc. if acid etc. is aspirated into the lungs and causes asthma, bronchitis, pneumonia, etc.

Diagnosis can be proven only by special tests (barium swallow, endoscopy, etc.) by a Medical Officer.
Treatment includes:

1. Keep upright as much as possible (it is harder for the acid to flow upwards):
   • do not lie down soon after meals,
   • sleep with the head end of the bed higher than the foot end.

2. Have small meals and small volumes of fluid often rather than large meals and drinks less often.

3. Lose weight if overweight and do not use tight clothes around the abdomen (these, and pregnancy, push acid, etc. up into oesophagus).

4. Drugs as for peptic ulcer (especially, if available, H_2 blockers or PPIs). See page 353.

Peptic ulcer

A peptic ulcer is an acute or recurring acute or chronic ulcer of the wall of the stomach or duodenum caused by acid and pepsin and other factors.

Acid and pepsin are normally made by the stomach to digest food. But they do not normally digest the wall of the stomach or duodenum and do not cause a peptic ulcer as these walls can protect themselves against acid and pepsin. The most common cause of the stomach and duodenal walls not being able to protect themselves is infection with a special bacterium (*Helicobacter pylori*), which damages the mucous membrane. Other causes may be taking acetylsalicylic acid or other NSAIDs. Drinking alcohol, smoking tobacco, high-dose adrenocorticosteroids, possibly worrying and unknown causes may help cause ulcers.

Peptic ulcer occurs everywhere; but it is common only in some areas.

Symptoms and signs

The main *symptoms* include.

1. Epigastric pain (i.e. in the upper central abdomen) related to food (i.e. pain made worse *or* better by

food). The pain may wake the patient at night after the food has gone from the stomach and duodenum. At first the pain may occur for only a few days or weeks, and then get better. *Epigastric pain related to food is the main symptom.*

2. Later the pain may be there most of the time and may radiate (spread) to the back.

3. Sometimes there is vomiting after food (if food causes pain, the vomiting usually relieves the pain).

4. Weight loss (especially if food causes pain and there is vomiting).

The *signs* include:

1. 'The pointing sign'. When the patient is lying on a bed and you ask him to point with one finger to where the pain is, the patient points to one place, usually between the umbilicus and the lower end of the sternum. If the patient does this, there is usually a peptic ulcer. If the patient does not point to one place but instead rubs his hand in different parts of the abdomen, or if the pain is not between the umbilicus and the lower end of the sternum then there is usually not a peptic ulcer.

2. Epigastric tenderness. This is the main sign.

3. Weight loss (if there is pain and vomiting after food).

4. Anaemia (if the ulcer has bled).

Complications which the ulcer can cause include:

1. Penetration of (i.e. the acid and pepsin 'eating' through) the posterior (back) wall of the stomach or duodenum into the liver or back – this causes back pain which is there all the time.

2. Perforation of (i.e. the ulcer eating through) the front wall of the stomach or duodenum – the food and acid inside the stomach or duodenum then go out into the peritoneal cavity. This causes *sudden severe abdominal pain* and peritonitis.

3. Ulceration of a blood vessel – this causes bleeding into the stomach or duodenum with vomiting of blood (haematemesis); or digested black, tarry blood in the stool (melaena); also anaemia; and sometimes shock.

4. Obstruction of the stomach outlet so that food and later fluid cannot go from the stomach into the duodenum – this causes vomiting and wasting (called 'pyloric stenosis').

The *differential diagnosis* includes all other causes of upper abdominal pain (see Chapter 36 pages 593–598). Sometimes an infection with many hookworms or the protozoal organism called *Giardia* in the duodenum or a cancer in the stomach may cause symptoms similar to a peptic ulcer.

Treatment

The treatment depends on how severe the attack is.

Mild attack:

- The epigastric pain is usually made better or worse by food.
- The epigastric tenderness is mild.
- There are no complications.

Treat as an outpatient.

1. Antacids.
   - Aluminium hydroxide (compound) tablet or oral suspension (i.e. liquid); or magnesium hydroxide suspension; or calcium or other antacid tablet or liquid. (Magnesium may cause diarrhoea; calcium may cause constipation.)
   - Give 2 tablets or 10–20 ml liquid 1 hour after every meal, and at night before sleeping, and at any other time if necessary for pain. Give this treatment regularly for 3 weeks.
   - If the patient gets better then give 2 tablets only if necessary for pain.
   - If no antacid tablets or liquid are available, give 1 cup of full cream milk (instead of 1–2 antacid tablets).
2. Tell the patient:
   - not to take acetylsalicylic acid or NSAID containing tablets or any other tablets for pain or arthritis except paracetamol, and
   - not to smoke,
   - not to drink alcohol,
   - not to drink strong coffee or tea or cola drinks,
   - not to eat foods that he knows cause pain.
3. Tell the patient to eat at the same time every day (and, if possible, to eat 3–6 small meals every day rather than fewer larger meals).
4. Give no acetylsalicylic acid and as few other drugs as possible (many drugs can cause the symptoms of peptic ulcer). Give paracetamol if needed for other pain.
5. Give anti-hookworm drug (see page 356).
6. Treat anaemia if present (see Chapter 21 pages 316–319) but do not give oral iron while the pain is still present.

Severe attack:

- The epigastric pain may be present a lot of the time or keep coming back after treatment.
- The epigastric tenderness is marked.
- There are no complications.

The cause of the ulcer needs treatment.

1. Treat as for mild attack and especially make sure the patient is not taking acetylsalicylic acid or NSAIDs. The proper treatment of a peptic ulcer is to treat the cause.
2. Treat the *Helicobacter pylori* infection.
   This is done by a combination of two (or three) antibiotics. The first is amoxicillin 1 g twice daily for 1 week. The second is clarithromycin 500 mg bd but this is not usually available, and instead metronidazole 400 mg three times a day for 1 week can be given; but some *H. pylori* are now resistant to metronidazole. Another combination is tetracycline 500 mg four times a day and metronidazole 400 mg three times a day for 2 weeks.
3. Give also during this time a drug to decrease the acid secretion (as well as treating the infection) as this will allow the ulcer to heal more quickly. Ranitidine 300 mg twice daily is such a drug. Alternative drugs are:
   - Histamine$_2$ (or H$_2$) blockers, which include famotidine 40 mg twice daily, nizotidine 300 mg twice daily, cimetidine 800 mg twice daily (as well as ranitidine).
   - Proton (acid) pump inhibitors (PPIs), which are more effective but more expensive and not usually available, include omeprazole 40 mg twice daily, lansoprazide 30 mg twice daily, pantoprazole 40 mg twice daily, esomeprazole 20 mg twice daily and robepazole 20 mg twice daily.
4. Following the 1–2 weeks of antibiotics and high-dose drug to decrease acid, it is best if the H$_2$ blocker can be continued once daily at night for 4–6 weeks or the PPI once daily in the morning for 2–4 weeks (i.e. in half of the previous dose).

If the essential drugs are not available and the patient cannot be transferred to Medical Officer care, try the effect of the following:

1. Admit the patient to the health centre. Make sure he gets rest in bed for 3 weeks. Give diazepam 5 mg three times a day if the patient will not rest.
2. Give whichever of the above treatments you have; the patient must not take acetylsalicylic acid or other NSAID and must swallow a lot of antacid or milk.
3. Make as sure as possible that the patient does not have another disease causing upper abdominal pain and tenderness (see Chapter 36 page 593), but especially peritonitis, acute cholecystitis, liver abscess, pancreatitis, injury or disease or spleen, etc.

and make sure treatment of hookworm and *Giardia* (see page 356 and page 373) has been given.

4. Treat any other condition the patient has.

Note that actual rest in bed is needed for this treatment to work. It was used before effective drugs were available. It is not known why this helps. It does, however, often stop the patient's symptoms and signs at least for a while.

Transfer
Transfer to Medical Officer care if:

1. Severe pain is not relieved by treatment for severe attack (non-urgent).
2. The pain comes back many times (non-urgent).
3. Perforation causing peritonitis occurs (urgent – emergency).
4. Haematemesis (vomiting blood) or melaena (black stool which looks and smells like tar) occurs, even if there is no shock or anaemia (urgent – emergency).
5. There is vomiting and weight loss caused by obstruction of stomach outlet (non-urgent).
6. There is constant pain in the back caused by penetration of the pancreas or back (non-urgent).

Prevention
Prevention is by not taking drugs (such as acetylsalicylic acid) when they are not needed and by not smoking. Not drinking too much alcohol is wise.

Carcinoma (cancer) of the stomach
Usually, old people or people of a particular race or people eating a particular diet are affected. Early symptoms and signs include:

• epigastric pain and/or
• a feeling of fullness after only a little food and/or
• anaemia.

Later symptoms and signs include:
• all of the above, and/or
• epigastric mass, and/or
• obstruction of the stomach outlet, and/or
• weight loss, and/or
• enlarged lymph glands above the clavicle.

If cancer of the stomach is suspected, treat as a peptic ulcer for 3 weeks. If the patient is not cured after 3 weeks, transfer him to hospital for investigation. Surgery does not often cure the patient.

Roundworm (*Ascaris lumbricoides*)
Infestation (infection) with roundworms is very common everywhere.

The adult worms are about 15–25 cm long. They live inside the tube of the small intestine.

The female adult roundworm puts about 200,000 eggs into the patient's intestine every day. These eggs are then passed in the patient's faeces. Inside fertilised eggs, infective larvae develop after about 2 weeks. The larvae will grow best when the patient passes faeces in those places where it is cool, shady and moist; but eggs can survive in other places for years. If an infective egg from dirt or in food is swallowed, the larva hatches and travels through the small intestinal wall, portal vein, liver, right heart, lungs, bronchi, trachea and then oesophagus and stomach into the small intestine, where it develops into an adult roundworm. (See Figure 23.5.)

Symptoms, signs and complications
Symptoms, signs and complications are all uncommon.

1. Usually there are no symptoms or signs. You can only make the diagnosis if an adult worm is seen in the stool or is vomited up or if eggs are seen when the stool is examined under the microscope.

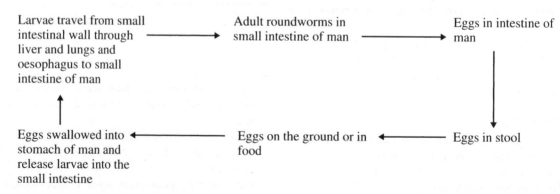

Figure 23.5 *The life cycle of the roundworm.*

2. If there are many worms, abdominal discomfort or mild colic and distension (swelling) sometimes occur.
3. If there are many worms, especially in children who eat a poor diet, malnutrition or anaemia can occur.
4. If there are many worms, especially in children and especially if tetrachloroethylene is given (which irritates but does not kill the worms), a tangled mass of worms can cause intestinal obstruction (this is rare). (Obstruction of other organs such as bile ducts, pancreatic duct or appendix, etc. by a worm which wanders there, does occur; but is rare.)
5. Pneumonia and asthma can be caused as the larvae travel through the lungs. (This may not be rare but the diagnosis is not often made.)

Treatment

Treat only if:

1. roundworms are vomited or passed in stool; or
2. you are giving tetrachloroethylene (TCE) to children (give roundworm treatment before giving the TCE); or
3. there is malnutrition; or
4. there is abdominal discomfort and you can find no other cause; or
5. the whole community is being treated (as is sometimes done if 50% or more of the population has infection).

Treat as an outpatient.

Use whichever of the following drugs (see Table 23.1) is cheapest and is available.

- Albendazole (200 mg and 400 mg tablets).
  For children 2–5 years 200 (possibly 400) mg once.
  For patients over 5 years 400 mg once.
  Side effects are usually mild and include gastrointestinal symptoms and occasionally mild hepatitis or blood cell changes.
  Do not give during pregnancy (especially in the first 3 months) or 7 days after last normal menstrual period or in the first 6 months of life.

- Mebendazole (100 mg tablets).
  A single dose of 500 mg once only is best. A dose of 100 mg twice daily is usually adequate, especially if given for 3 days. Side effects are mild, like albendazole. Do not give if pregnant (especially in the first 3 months) or more than 7 days after the last normal menstrual period or in the first 6 months of life.
- Pyrantel (pamoate or ambonate) (250 mg base tablets or 250 mg/5 ml of syrup).
  Give 10(–20) mg/kg (maximum dose 1 g) once.
  Side effects are very rare.
  This drug can be used during pregnancy after the first 3 months.
- Levamisole (40 mg, 50 mg and 150 mg tablets and 40 mg/5 ml syrup).
  A dose of 2.5–5 mg/kg (maximum dose 150 mg) once only. Do not give during the first 3 months of pregnancy. Side effects include gastrointestinal symptoms, headache and dizziness.
- Piperazine (numerous strengths of tablets and mixtures).
  A dose of 75 mg/kg of the hydrate (maximum 4 g of the hydrate or maximum 5 g of the citrate or other salts) once between meals or half of this dose for 2 days. Note that piperazine is not effective against the other parasites and is now more expensive than the above drugs and often needs more than one dose and has more side effects.

Prevention

Tell the patient, family and village about the life cycle of the worm and that prevention is by the use of proper toilets by everyone (including children) always.

Hookworm (*Necator americanus* or *Ancylostoma duodenale*)

Infestation with hookworm is very common. The adult worms are about 1 cm in length. They live in the upper small intestine attached by their mouths to the intestine wall. They suck blood and protein from the intestine wall.

Table 23.1 Effect of drugs on internal parasites.

	Levamisole	Pyrantel	Mebendazole	Albendazole
Ascaris lumbricoides	+++	+++	+++	+++
Necator americanus	++	++	++	+++
Ancylostoma duodenale	+++	+++	+++	+++
Trichuris trichiura	++	++	+	++
Strongyloides stercoralis	+	+	+	++

+++ very effective   ++ moderately effective   + not very effective

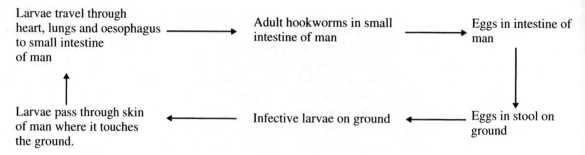

Figure 23.6 *The life cycle of the hookworm.*

The female adult puts eggs into the patient's bowel. These eggs are then passed in the patient's faeces. In shady moist soil, fertilised eggs develop into larvae. After about 1 week the larvae can pass through the skin of a person who touches them. The larvae travel through the blood vessels, right heart, bronchi and trachea, and then the oesophagus and stomach into the small intestine where they develop into the adult worms (Figure 23.6).

Symptoms, signs and complications

1. Anaemia. This causes weakness, tiredness, dizziness, shortness of breath, pallor, etc. (see Chapter 21 page 316). It is caused by the loss of the blood that the hookworms suck from the intestine wall. (Some hookworms can suck 0.5–1 ml blood daily. Some patients have up to 1000 worms.) The body stores of iron are soon used up by the bone marrow making new blood. When this happens the bone marrow cannot make as much blood as before.
   Anaemia is the only common and important result of hookworm.
   Anaemia occurs usually only if there are a large number of hookworms in the patient and the patient also has a poor diet.
2. Heart failure (if the anaemia is severe).
3. Oedema (if the anaemia or protein loss is severe or heart failure).
4. Sometimes there is epigastric pain like the pain of a peptic ulcer. Sometimes there is just a little abdominal discomfort.
5. Sometimes a rash occurs (an itchy red rash which may be hard to see and lasts for only a few days) where larvae went through the skin (usually between the toes) at the time of infection.
6. Sometimes a cough or wheeze (like bronchitis or asthma) can be caused by the worms travelling through the lungs soon after infection.

You cannot be certain of the diagnosis of hookworm in the intestine at a health centre as you cannot normally examine the stool by microscope. But if you examine the stool under a microscope, you can see the eggs if the patient has hookworm.

Assume hookworm infestation is present in all patients who have anaemia.

Treatment

1. Give drugs to kill hookworms (Table 23.1). See page 355.
   Use whichever of the following drugs is the cheapest and available.
   • Albendazole (see page 355).
     A single dose of 400 mg will remove 80% of the worms and 200 mg daily for 3 days will remove almost all of the worms. Do not give if pregnant (especially in the first 3 months of pregnancy) or more than 7 days after the last normal menstrual period or if less than 6 months old.
   • Mebendazole (see page 355).
     A single dose of 500 mg is effective. A dose of 100 mg twice daily for 3 days is very effective against both types of hookworm. Do not give if pregnant (especially in the first 3 months of pregnancy) or more than 7 days after the last normal menstrual period or if less than 6 months old.
   • Levamisole (see page 355).
     Give 2.5–5 mg/kg, maximum dose 150 mg. This drug is less effective against *N. americanus*. A second dose after 7 days may be needed. Do not give in the first 3 months of pregnancy.
   • Pyrantel (pamoate or ambonate) (see page 355).
     Give 10(–20) mg/kg, maximum dose 1 g. Do not give in the first 3 months of pregnancy.
     In heavy hookworm infestations, a further dose on each of the next 3 days may be needed.
   • Tetrachloroethylene (TCE) (not recommended as above drugs better and safer).

Treat for roundworm first (see page 354) as otherwise these roundworms are not killed but are irritated and may cause intestinal or other obstruction. The patient should not eat on the night before and on the morning of the treatment, although he can have water. Give TCE 0.1 ml/kg (one tenth of a ml/kg of body weight) to a maximum dose of 6 ml. Do not give TCE to a patient whose haemoglobin is less than 5 g/dl or who is jaundiced or sick or who is in the first 3 months of pregnancy.

2. Give routine anaemia treatment.

Give antimalarials if needed, iron, folic acid, good diet (containing iron, protein and vitamins) and advice on family planning if needed. (See Chapter 21 pages 316–319.)

Prevention

Tell the patient, family and village about the life cycle of the worm and that prevention is by the use of proper toilets by everyone (including children) always. Wearing proper shoes to stop larvae going through the skin is important; but for some populations, not practicable.

Threadworm (*Enterobius vermicularis*)

Threadworm infestation is very common, especially in children.

Adult worms are up to 1 cm in length. They live in the large intestine and cause no pathology.

The fertilised female comes out through the anus at night, and lays eggs on the skin around the anus. This causes itching and scratching.

The eggs are taken by fingers or clothes from the skin around the anus to the mouth and are swallowed. Then they pass into the intestine where they hatch and grow into adults.

Management of the patient includes:

1. Treat the *whole family* with an anti-threadworm drug (as all are soon infected).
2. Cut the fingernails short and keep them short.
3. Wash the whole body every morning.
4. Wash clothes and bedclothes often.
5. Apply ammoniated mercury or any thick ointment to the anus every night (while taking the anti-threadworm drug) to stop the worm getting out through the anus.
6. Wash hands well when get up in the morning and after using the toilet and before preparing or eating food.
7. Drugs for treatment: see page 355.
   - albendazole 10–40 mg/kg to a maximum dose of 400 mg once only,

- mebendazole 100 mg once only, and
- pyrantel (pamoate) 10 mg/kg to a maximum dose of 1 g once only.

Note that albendazole and mebendazole should not be given to a pregnant woman or 7 days after the last normal menstrual period or to children less than 6 months of age, and pyrantel should not be given in the first 3 months of pregnancy. These drugs may have to be repeated in 6 weeks, as well as all the other treatment carried out, to get rid of the infection in the family.

Whipworm (*Trichuris trichiura*)

The whipworm is 2.5 cm long with a thin front half and lives in the mucosa of the large intestine of humans and pigs.

Whipworm may cause gastrointestinal symptoms and signs, but only if they are present in large numbers, and even then, usually only in children. These include diarrhoea with blood, prolapse of the rectum and anaemia.

Treatment is needed only if there are symptoms and signs. Treatment is with mebendazole 100 mg twice daily for 3 days, although for adults 500 mg once is just as effective, or albendazole in a single dose of 400 mg. Do not give if the patient is pregnant or more than 7 days after the last normal menstrual period or the child is less than 6 months old. See page 355.

Strongyloides

Strongyloides is a very small worm which lives in the upper small intestine but can spread through the whole gastrointestinal tract, and also sometimes through it to other parts of the body.

Strongyloides has a life cycle similar to roundworm and hookworm; but as well can also reproduce inside the body (usually bowel and lung) and also in the soil (without having to pass through man).

Symptoms are not usually caused, but there may be abdominal discomfort, diarrhoea, failure to absorb food, allergic type skin rashes and another unusual rash with an inflamed line in the skin which disappears after a few hours.

However, if a patient has a decrease in their immune system caused by (1) drugs given for cancer or adrenocorticosteroid drugs (such as cortisone and prednisolone) or (2) severe malnutrition or (3) HIV infection, then worms may get through the bowel wall and then spread through the whole body, causing severe generalised symptoms, pneumonia, empyema, meningitis, septicaemia, etc. as well as severe diarrhoea or bowel obstruction (paralytic ileus). These are caused by the spread and growth of both the worm and the bacteria (usually from the patient's bowel) that are in the worm.

Treatment is not usually given unless there are some symptoms; but **it is given if worms are in the bowel, before adrenocorticosteroid-like drugs or anti-cancer drugs are given** or if the patient has HIV infection. Albendazole 400 mg once daily (or thiabendazole if not pregnant 25 mg/kg up to 1.5 g twice daily) for 3 days – is the usual treatment. Ivermectin in a single daily dose of 200 micrograms/kg for 3 days is very effective.

Prevention is by all people, including children, always using proper toilets and by washing hands after going to the toilet and before preparing and eating food.

Tapeworm and cysticercosis

Two large tapeworms, the beef tapeworm (*Taenia saginata*) and the pork tapeworm (*Taenia solium*), and a number of very small tapeworms affect man.

The adult *Taenia* live in the gastrointestinal tract of man.

They can become metres long, but the adult worms do little harm. The patient usually diagnoses the condition when a part of the worm forces itself out of the anus or he sees part of the worm wriggling in his faeces. You can see eggs if the stool is examined under the microscope.

If the eggs in the stool are not passed into a proper toilet, the eggs may be swallowed by beef cattle or pigs. The larvae travel through all of the animal but most go into the muscles. When the animal is killed you can see the larvae as little white marks in the meat. If the

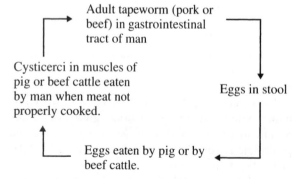

Figure 23.7 *The normal life cycle of the pork and beef tapeworm.*

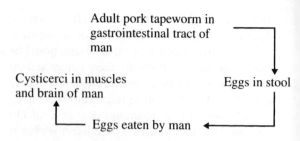

Figure 23.8 *How the pork tapeworm causes cysticerci in man. The beef tapeworm cannot cause cysticerci in man.*

meat is not properly cooked (and the larvae not killed) before it is eaten, then the larvae develop into an adult worm in the intestine. (See Figure 23.7.)

The big danger to man from tapeworms is from the pork tapeworm, if the pork tapeworm eggs get into the upper gastrointestinal tract. This occurs (1) if a person gets some of his own faeces onto his food or into his mouth, or (2) if a person gets someone else's faeces containing the eggs on uncooked vegetables, etc. into his mouth or (3) possibly during vomiting when the contents of the small intestine return to the stomach (Figure 23.8). If the eggs of a pork tapeworm get into the upper gastrointestinal tract of man, then the larvae develop and travel all through the body (just as they do in pigs). The larvae cause painful muscles, fever and later muscle lumps. More importantly, the larvae also go to the brain. If very many go to the brain, then a meningoencephalitis (see Chapter 25 page 415) develops, often with epilepsy. If only a few go to the brain, there is often little trouble for some years. But, when the worm dies, the cyst it formed starts to swell. This causes symptoms and signs like a brain abscess or a brain tumour, with epilepsy or headaches or psychosis, etc. (see Chapter 25 page 421). This condition, where pork tapeworms cause cysts in the muscle and brain, is called 'cysticercosis'.

You can diagnose the type of tapeworm infection a person has by examining the worm. But if the worm is a pig tapeworm, the worm and stools are dangerous to the patient and others. In the health centre *treat all cases immediately* as if the worm is a pork tapeworm.

Give niclosamide 2 g for a large adult or 1.5 g for a small (less than 34 kg) adult in a single dose. Previously, an anti-emetic 1 hour before and a laxative 1 hour after the niclosamide was given, but this is no longer thought needed.

Praziquantel 10 mg/kg in one dose once (or albendazole) can be used instead of niclosamide for treatment of the worm. These drugs in repeated doses can also be used in the treatment of human cysticercosis as they also kill the cysticerci. However, they must not be given in a health centre if cerebral cysticercosis is possible as the dying cysticerci may swell and may make the patient worse at first, and special drugs and even surgery on the brain may be needed.

Make sure no stools from the patient get on anyone at any time and all go into a safe toilet.

Send the stool to the laboratory for a test for ova 3 months later to see that the worm is not present.

Prevention of tapeworm infection includes:

1. Kill the parasite in the original host. Treat all patients.
2. Stop the spread:
   (a) All people must use a proper toilet at all times.
   (b) All meat must be properly inspected for cysticerci, and not sold if cysticerci are seen.
   (c) All meat should be properly cooked. All the red colour all the way through the meat must go before the meat is eaten.
   (d) Hand washing after using the toilet and before preparing or eating food.

Hydatid disease

Echinococcus granulosus is a very small tapeworm of dogs. When the dog passes faeces onto grass, the faeces break down and get into the soil, but the eggs are left on the grass and may be eaten by sheep or cattle. The eggs hatch in the animal's bowel and an infective organism gets carried in the portal vein to the liver, but sometimes through the liver to the lung and occasionally to the brain, bone or other places. It grows in these places to a large fluid-filled cyst, sometimes many centimetres in diameter, with organisms infective to dogs on the inside of the cyst. When the animal is killed for meat or dies, if a dog eats these infective organisms in the cyst when it eats the rest of the organ, these organisms form into the small tapeworms in the dog's bowel.

Man can be infected instead of sheep or cattle if he gets eggs from dog faeces in his mouth. Cysts in the person's liver, and also lung, brain, bone or elsewhere, can then develop. Children who spend a lot of time with dogs and sheep and on grass are infected most.

The cysts can cause the following:

• painful enlargement of the liver, if in the liver;
• cough and shortness of breath, if in the lung;
• symptoms like a brain tumour, if in the brain;
• pain and fracture of bone, if in a bone;

• allergic reactions if fluid from the cyst gets into the circulation – these reactions can range from just urticaria to allergic type shock;
• sudden death if the cyst ruptures and a severe allergic reaction develops;
• typical X-ray changes, eosinophils in the blood and positive serology tests for circulating hydatid antigen if these tests are available.

If you suspect the patient has a hydatid cyst because it occurs in your area and the patient has suspicious symptoms and signs, do not try to aspirate the cyst (as this may cause death from an allergic reaction or spread the infected material to other parts of the body where new cysts will form) but transfer the patient to the Medical Officer for investigations and, if necessary, treatment with albendazole and cutting out the cyst without letting it burst.

Prevention is by not allowing dogs to eat animal offal (i.e. internal organs such as liver, lung, etc.) from animals killed for meat or which die. If possible, dogs should be de-wormed regularly with drugs and all people should wash their hands after touching dogs as well as before preparing or eating food.

Larva migrans

Cutaneous larva migrans occurs when the larvae of the dog hookworm (*Ancylostoma braziliansis* or *A. canium*) get through the skin of people but are not able to develop any further as they are not in a dog. The larvae wander (or migrate) under the skin (cuta) at a rate of a few mm daily for weeks to months. They cause a rash which follows a line shaped like a moving snake and which is red and itchy. Treatment is with a single dose of albendazole 400 mg (although daily for up to a week if one dose not effective) (see page 355) or ivermectin 12 mg.

Visceral larva migrans cannot be diagnosed in the health centre, but you may hear of patients with it. This occurs when the eggs or ova of roundworms of dogs or cats (*Toxocara canis* or *T. cati*) are swallowed by people. The worms (larvae) are not able to develop into adults in the bowel as they are not in dogs or cats. The larvae wander (migrate) around in the organs (viscera) of the person. This causes fever; enlarged and tender organs such as the liver, spleen, lymph glands, muscles, etc.; nerve and brain damage; serious changes in the retina of the eye which not only can cause blindness but can be mistaken for a malignant melanoma; more eosinophils and gamma globulin in the blood than normal, etc. Treatment is with albendazole 10 mg/kg for 5 days.

Gastroenteritis (or acute diarrhoeal disease)

Definition

Gastroenteritis is a very common and sometimes serious or fatal syndrome. (It is not a specific disease with only one cause; there are many causes.) About 8 million people die of gastroenteritis each year (mostly children, but also adults).

Gastroenteritis is diagnosed when there is:

1. diarrhoea (more than three loose bowel motions in a day), and
2. abdominal pain of bowel (i.e. intestinal) colic type (usually), and
3. vomiting (usually), and
4. other symptoms and signs such as fever (in some but not all).

Causes

(see Table 23.2 page 363)

Causes of gastroenteritis include:

1. *'Food poisoning'*
   - Poisonous foods, especially certain fish and certain plants.
   - Poisons or chemicals in food (including large volumes of alcohol).
   - Drugs (including antibiotics given for infections).
   - Toxins in food made by organisms which have grown in the food but may be dead or cannot cause infections in the intestine (e.g. streptococci and staphylococci).
   - Organisms in food which can cause infections in the bowel (see below).
2. *Infections in the intestine (do not try to remember all the names)*
   - Viruses (especially rotavirus and calicivirus/norovirus mainly in children; but in HIV patients, cytomegalovirus and Epstein–Barr virus).
   - Unusual types of normal intestinal bacteria (e.g. *Escherichia coli*, i.e. *E. coli*).
   - Special bacteria, such as:
     - *Shigella* (bacillary dysentery organisms).
     - Salmonellae (other than *S. typhi*) (non-typhoid salmonella or NTS) which cause gastroenteritis (especially common in HIV patients).
     - *Salmonellae typhi* which cause typhoid fever.
     - Clostridia which cause enteritis necroticans ('pigbel').
     - *Campylobacter* which causes dysentery.
     - *Vibrio cholerae* which causes cholera.
   - Protozoae
     - *Entamoebae histolytica* (amoebic dysentery organisms).
     - *Giardia*.
     - Cryptosporidium.
     - Cyclospora.
   - Worms.
     Schistosoma mansoni and *Schistosoma japonicum*. Sometimes other worms.
3. *'Medical causes'*
   - Any cause of fever, but especially malaria.
   - Any acute infection, but especially middle ear infection, pneumonia, and urinary tract infection.
   - Many chronic infections, especially visceral leishmaniasis.
   - Malnutrition.
   - Malabsorption, especially lactose intolerance and tropical sprue.
   - Change of diet.
   - Anxiety.
4. HIV infection.
5. *'Surgical' causes*
   - Enteritis necroticans ('pigbel').
   - Intestine obstruction – early or incomplete.

HIV is really a 'medical' cause; but not only does the HIV itself damage the bowel wall and can cause diarrhoea; it also allows all the above infectious organisms as well as other organisms which do not normally cause infection to easily cause infection and gastroenteritis (especially diarrhoea, especially chronic diarrhoea).

Usually, you cannot find the cause of gastroenteritis at a health centre, unless there is a medical or surgical cause. But you must always look for evidence of the cause. (Details of some of the causes are found above.)

You must also ask if other people are affected, because this is the only way to diagnose 'food poisoning' in a health centre. You may need to control an epidemic.

Epidemiology

The *spread* of gastrointestinal infections is usually:

- *From* the faeces (occasionally vomit) of an infected case or carrier.
- *To* the mouth of a susceptible person.
- *By* direct contact (personal contact) *or* vehicles (food or milk or water) into which organisms from faeces were introduced (put) by fingers or flies, or improper or dirty toilets. See Figure 23.9.

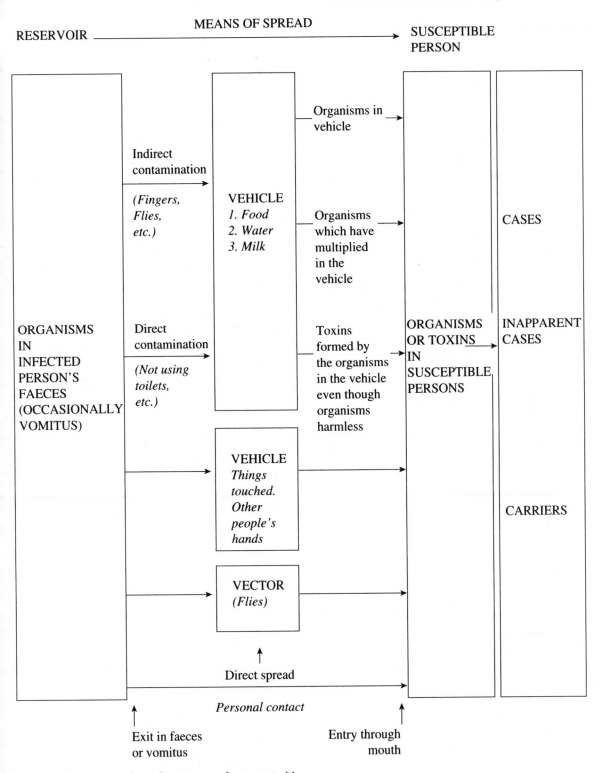

Figure 23.9 *The epidemiology of most cases of gastroenteritis.*

Symptoms

Symptoms include:

1. Diarrhoea (frequent watery stool),
   Dysentery (diarrhoea with blood and pus as well) if the intestine wall is ulcerated.
2. Abdominal pain
   Pain due to gastroenteritis is bowel colic, i.e. it comes for some seconds and then goes away for some minutes. The pain is usually in the centre of the abdomen, but large intestinal colic can be at the side low down.
   Constant abdominal pain is NOT usually caused by gastroenteritis.
   Cramps in the abdominal and limb muscles if the patient has severe diarrhoea suggest cholera.
3. Vomiting
   This is not always present; but it can be frequent. You must find out how often vomiting is occurring and how much fluid is being lost in the vomit each time.
   This helps you to know if dehydration will occur. Vomiting is dangerous, because it stops fluid from entering the body, and means dehydration will occur much more quickly and be more serious than if the patient can drink and absorb fluids.
4. Symptoms of infection in the gastrointestinal tract or elsewhere or of an underlying disease, may or may not be present.
5. Symptoms of the cause – always remember HIV infection.

The following will give you an idea of what part of the gastrointestinal tract is most affected and this often gives an idea of the cause.

- If the small bowel affected – large size or volume stool but bowels move not very often.
- If the large bowel affected – small size or volume stool but bowels move often.
- If the large bowel infected/inflamed – dysentery (blood/pus in stool) and pain when or after passing stool.
- If bowel wall infected/inflamed – fever often present.
- If the whole gastrointestinal tract affected – vomiting and diarrhoea.

History

Ask if the patient has eaten possibly poisonous food, 'bad' foods, pig meat or other high protein food when this is not usually in the diet, food that was cooked a long time before it was eaten; or if he has taken drugs, etc.

Family and contact history

Ask about contacts with similar disease.

> You can usually only diagnose 'food poisoning' at a health centre if a group of people develop gastroenteritis together. Always ask if other people are affected. You may need to control an epidemic.
> Think of cholera if there is an epidemic in which there are some cases of very rapid dehydration and death.

Signs

1. *Signs of dehydration* (these develop if a large volume of fluid is lost and not replaced quickly enough):
   - the number of times the patient has had vomiting and diarrhoea and the volume of the vomitus and stool – each time you check a patient ask about these during the last 6 and the last 24 hours,
   - urine volume small and urine of dark colour (concentrated urine),
   - rapid loss of weight (more than 5% of body weight),
   - loss of full consciousness,
   - decreased elasticity of skin (the pinch test), especially the skin of the neck (but do not mistake the inelastic skin of old age or of malnutrition or wasting for the inelastic skin of dehydration),
   - sunken fontanelle (babies only),
   - sunken eyes,
   - dry mouth,
   - fast pulse,
   - low blood pressure,
   - cyanosis,
   - fever.

> PR, BP, skin elasticity and urine volume and colour are the best signs of dehydration in adults.

2. *Signs of gastroenteritis:*
   The abdomen
   - is normal in shape and moves normally on breathing;
   - has no marked tenderness and definitely no guarding or rigidity;
   - has increased intestinal sounds (which can be heard at the same time as the patient gets pain).
3. *Signs of cause of gastroenteritis:*
   You must look for all medical causes, especially malaria, other infections and malnutrition.
   You must look for all surgical causes, especially the signs of intestinal obstruction and peritonitis.
   You must think of possible HIV infection.

Complications

Look for these especially in the old, children, those with malnutrition, and if certain virulent infections.

Complications include:

- dehydration which can cause shock and death – *dehydration is the usual cause of death*;
- dysentery, with the loss of large amounts of blood, causing anaemia or shock;
- septicaemia which can cause infections in other organs or shock or death;
- paralytic ileus – loss of potassium causes intestinal muscle paralysis; this causes vomiting, abdominal distension, constipation but not colic (see page 385);
- continuing diarrhoea, because of lactose intolerance (i.e. damage to the bowel wall caused by the gastroenteritis means lactose cannot be absorbed; but milk with lactose in it is still in the diet);
- malnutrition;
- anaemia.

Diagnostic features

Diagnostic features are:

- diarrhoea or dysentery,
- colicky (not constant) pain, usually in the centre of the abdomen,
- vomiting (not always),
- no significant signs in the abdomen except increased intestinal sounds,
- sometimes an underlying cause not in the gastro-intestinal tract,
- dehydration (if vomiting; or if diarrhoea is often or is of large volumes or goes on for a long time).

See Table 23.2 about differential diagnosis; but these things do not need to be known to treat the patient correctly.

Treatment

Treatment includes five things:

1. Treat dehydration by oral fluids *or* by IV then oral fluids (page 364).

2. Treat any underlying surgical or medical disease (page 360).
   Treat for malaria if it is a possible cause.

3. If necessary, treat any infection in the intestine (page 360).
   Most cases do NOT need chloramphenicol or other antibiotics or metronidazole.

4. Treat symptoms; but only if necessary and only after you have done the other three things (page 362).

5. Maintain nutrition. Do not stop the patient eating.

Table 23.2 The likely causes of gastroenteritis/diarrhoea/dysentery according to the length of time these symptoms present and whether blood is in the stools (dysentery) or not. However, the cause of gastroenteritis cannot be known and does not need to be known for proper treatment to be carried out in the health centre (see text).

Diarrhoea/Dysentery/Gastroenteritis – acute (less than 2 weeks)				Diarrhoea/dysentery – chronic (greater than 2 weeks)
Fever & dysentery (often vomiting)	Fever and no dysentery (often vomiting)	No fever Dysentery	No fever No dysentery (often vomiting)	
Shigella	Malaria	Amoebic (Entamoeba histolytica)	Poisonous foods	Giardia lamblia
Campylobacter	Any infection – especially upper respiratory tract infection, lower respiratory tract infection and urinary tract infection	Balantidium coli	Preformed toxins, e.g. Staphylococci;	Amoebic (Entamoeba histolytica)
Salmonella		Schistosomiasis	Clostridium perfringens	GI roundworms
Escherichia coli		Trichuris and other GI worms	Escherichia coli	Schistosomiasis
Visceral leishmaniasis		Antibiotic caused (Clostridium difficile)	Viral, e.g. rotavirus (endemic; mostly children), norovirus (epidemic; mostly adults)	Many systemic infections
	Salmonella		Cholera	HIV infection
	Shigella		Incomplete bowel obstruction	Visceral leishmaniasis
	Campylobacter			Lactose intolerance
				Post-infective malabsorption
				'Tropical sprue'
				Bowel cancer

1. Treat dehydration

In *all cases*, look carefully for signs of dehydration:

• fast pulse (if severe),
• blood pressure low (if severe),
• inelastic skin,
• sunken eyes,
• dry mouth, and
• urine volume small and colour dark.

Mild case, with no or mild dehydration:

• treat as an outpatient;
• tell the patient to return if he does not improve and especially if vomiting is repeated.

Severe case, with definite signs of dehydration:

• treat as an inpatient.

Oral rehydration (See page 366 for fluids.) If

• there is no clinical dehydration, or
• only mild clinical dehydration, or
• moderate clinical dehydration but the vomiting is not repeated, and
• the abdomen is not distended (swollen),
then give oral rehydration fluid (see below).

Give the patient 2–4 large cups (400–800 ml) of fluid to drink. Tell the patient to drink it immediately if he has no nausea or vomiting. Tell the patient to sip it slowly over the next hour if he has nausea or vomiting.

If the patient has moderate dehydration, he must continue to drink till the signs of dehydration are gone (100 ml/kg or 3–6 litres). The patient can do this as quickly as he can if he has no nausea or vomiting. He should do it slowly over 6 hours (i.e. sip 2–4 cups during each hour for 6 hours) if he has nausea or some vomiting.

When the patient has no (or only mild) clinical signs of dehydration and does not vomit (or only vomits a little), the patient can then go home. Tell the patient to drink at least 2–4 cups of fluid in every 3-hour period (i.e. 3–6 litres/day) until the diarrhoea and/or vomiting stops.

If most of the oral fluids are refused or vomited or they are not effective, or abdominal distension (swelling) develops or there is severe dehydration, *then* admit for IV fluids.

Intravenous rehydration. If

• there is shock, *or*
• severe dehydration, *or*
• repeated vomiting, *or*

• abdominal distension (swelling), *or*
• the patient does not improve after oral fluids, *or*
• oral fluids are vomited or refused,

The method for IV rehydration is as follows:

(a) *Give Ringer's lactate (Hartmann's) or Darrow's solution or if not available 0.9% sodium chloride solution*[1] '*fast*'.
Give 40 ml/kg (2 litres) as fast as possible (e.g. in 1 hour).

(b) *Review the hydration of the patient after (a).*
• If he has improved, start (c).
• If he is still shocked or very dehydrated, give another 40 ml/kg (2 litres) of Ringer's lactate or Darrow's solution or 0.9% sodium chloride solution[1] as fast as possible. Then review the hydration of the patient again.
• If he still has shock, see Chapter 27 page 468.
• If he has improved, start (c).

(c) *Give Ringer's lactate or 0.9% sodium chloride solution*[1] more slowly to complete rehydration in 6 hours.
• Give 60 ml/kg (3 litres) over the next 4–5 hours.
• When the signs of dehydration have gone, start (d).

(d) *Give 0.18% sodium chloride in 4.3% dextrose solution.*
Give 1 litre every 6 hours.

(e) *Start oral rehydration solution.*
When you have done (a) to (c) or earlier if possible (i.e. the patient has stopped vomiting) start oral rehydration fluids 400–800 ml every 3 hours. This is especially important if you have used 0.9% saline as it has no potassium in it, but oral rehydration fluid does, and the patient needs potassium.

(f) *Stop IV fluids.* When the patient can take enough oral fluids (400–800 ml every 3 hours) to maintain hydration, stop IV fluids.

If the patient possibly has cholera, always use IV Ringer's lactate (Hartmann's) solution. Only if you have no Hartmann's, use 0.9% sodium chloride and start oral rehydration solution as soon as possible.

---

1 Hartmann's solution (lactated Ringer's solution) is better than 0.9% sodium chloride solution; but it is not usually available. But 0.9% sodium chloride solution is not good for cholera. If the patient has cholera you must try to get Hartmann's solution or another special IV fluid for cholera.

2. Treat any underlying medical or surgical disease

- Antimalarial drugs must *always* be given, unless you are certain that the patient does not have malaria.
- Give at least the first dose by injection.
- See malaria (Chapter 13 page 80).

3. If necessary treat any infection of the intestine

If the patient has

- severe dehydration with shock, *or*
- severe toxaemia which continues after correction of dehydration and injection of antimalarials (i.e. after 6 hours), *or*
- fever of unknown cause for more than 2 days, *or*
- new red spots appearing on the skin of the trunk, *or*
- spleen getting larger, *or*
- more than mild abdominal tenderness, *or*
- severe dysentery (blood and/or pus in the stools which does not improve after a few days or returns),

then give chloramphenicol 25 mg/kg every 6 hours for 10–14 days (14 if could be typhoid), *either*

- 1 g every 6 hours until the patient can take it orally, by
  - IVI if there is shock, *or* by
  - IVI or IMI if there is vomiting, or severe diarrhoea, or the patient is very sick, *or*
- 1 g orally every 6 hours if there is no shock, no vomiting and diarrhoea not severe, the patient is not very sick or the patient has improved after IV chloramphenicol,

or

instead of chloramphenicol if the organisms in your area are resistant to chloramphenicol, you may be told (*but only if told*) to use a quinolone, e.g. ciprofloxacin 500 mg orally or a cephalosporin, e.g. ceftriaxone 1 g IV or IMI twice daily.

> Note that **most** cases do **not** need antibiotics.

If:

- dysentery does not get better during the course of chloramphenicol, *or*
- dysentery returns after the course of chloramphenicol, *or*
- dysentery has occurred a number of times before the present attack, *or*
- dysentery has been present for 5–7 days already,

or

- diarrhoea does not stop after 2 weeks,

then give metronidazole 800 mg t.i.d. for 5 days (possible amoebic or *Giardia* infection).

If there is another infection or infestation, especially schistosomiasis (see Chapter 18 pages 187–191), shown by tests *then* give the necessary treatment for this.

4. Treat symptoms if necessary

Treat symptoms only after you have done rehydration, given antimalarial injection and treated any other medical condition and excluded surgical conditions, especially peritonitis and intestinal obstruction.

(a) If there is severe colic, cease oral food and fluids, and give IV fluids only.

(b) If there is severe abdominal colic or severe diarrhoea (and also vomiting), you can give morphine 10 mg and atropine 0.6 mg IMI once.

(c) If there is abdominal colic or diarrhoea (but no vomiting), give codeine phosphate 30 mg every 4–6 hours if necessary.

(d) If there is repeated vomiting, give metoclopramide 10 mg or chlorpromazine 0.5 mg/kg but not more than 12.5 mg IMI every 6 hours if needed. Do not give more than two doses. Look instead for the cause of the repeated vomiting.

5. Maintain nutrition

Once vomiting has ceased encourage the patient to eat good food and as soon as possible in a normal amount. Do not 'rest the bowel' by stopping the patient eating – this is not needed and harms the patient's nutrition.

Zinc sulfate, up to 20 mg daily, has been shown to reduce diarrhoeal disease in children. This has not yet been proven in adults. Watch to see if this later will be a treatment worthwhile for adults, especially those with prolonged diarrhoea.

Transfer these cases to Medical Officer care

1. If a surgical condition is possible – peritonitis, enteritis necroticans ('pigbel'), intestinal obstruction, etc. (urgent).
2. If vomiting continues for more than 2 days after you give IV fluids and IV or IM drug treatment (and stop oral food, drugs and fluids) (urgent).
3. If abdominal distension develops, especially if there is also constipation and repeated vomiting (paralytic ileus) (urgent).

4. Diarrhoea which does not improve after the proper treatment (non-urgent).

5. Dysentery which does not stop after treatment with chloramphenicol and then metronidazole (non-urgent).

Oral rehydration solution (in order of preference)

1. Oral Rehydration Salts (for a glucose/electrolyte solution): 1 packet dissolved in water (boiled, if possible) in the volume as directed on the packet. Use a special bottle from the Medical Store, if available.
Throw away any you have not used after 24 hours. Wash the bottle carefully, and if possible sterilise it, before using it again.
or

2. Especially if cholera a possibility

Sodium chloride (common salt)	2.6 g
Trisodium citrate	2.9 g
Potassium chloride	1.5 g
Glucose	13.5 g

Rice powder 50 g boiled in
1 litre water,
then allowed to cool
or   1 litre
$\frac{1}{2}$ cup rice boiled in 1 litre of
water and water tipped off
and allowed to cool
or

3.

Sodium chloride (common salt)	3.5 g
Sodium bicarbonate	2.5 g
Potassium chloride (each tablet of potassium chloride is 0.5 g)	1.5 g
Glucose	20 g
Clean water (boiled, if possible)	1 litre

or

4. 1 pinch of salt (only what you can hold between *one* finger and the thumb) and
1 teaspoon sugar and
1 cup clean water (boiled, if possible) or tea and
a little lemon juice (if possible)
or

5. Coconut water

Control and prevention

Control and prevention includes giving health education about hygiene, especially food cooking and handling, plentiful supply of safe water, toilets which are safe and used by all the community including children, and hand washing on getting up in the morning after going to the toilet before preparing or eating food, etc. This needs to be given to the patient, his family and his village.

It is important to recognise any epidemic of gastro-enteritis. An epidemic is usually caused by a common source of the disease. This is usually food or water. You must discover the cause of any epidemic so that you can stop it.

You must think of cholera if there is an epidemic of very rapid dehydration and early deaths. Special treatment and control methods are necessary (see page 367).

Methods of control and prevention of gastroenteritis caused by infections include:

1. Kill the organism in the body of the original host or reservoir (e.g. treat infected persons with antibiotics).
You cannot usually do this. If you treat all cases and carriers with antibiotics, then soon many of the organisms become resistant to the antibiotics.

2. Stop the spread of the organism.
Cases and carriers
• do not allow them to handle food,
• they must wash their hands after using the toilet.
Proper disposal of faeces
• proper toilets so that faeces do not contaminate water,
• proper toilets so flies, etc. cannot walk on faeces and later walk on food.
Provide a large supply of safe water.
Cook food properly. Keep food covered and cool after cooking; but it is best to eat it immediately.

3. Raise the resistance of susceptible persons.
Improve nutrition and health.
• People with good nutrition usually have mild attacks.
• People with malnutrition often have severe attacks.
Immunisation against cholera and typhoid are available; but these immunisations are expensive and would need to be given repeatedly and are not usually used.
Immunisation against some viral diseases are likely to be used routinely later. At present, effective immunisation against rotavirus infections is possible; but it is as yet too expensive to be used routinely anywhere in the developing world. Hopefully, this will soon change.

4. Prophylactic treatment.
Do not give prophylaxis, except to special groups of people in a cholera epidemic.

For details of descriptions of special kinds of gastro-enteritis, see pages 367–375 and a reference book.

Cholera

Definition and cause

Cholera is an acute illness caused by the cholera bacterium *Vibrio cholerae*. There are a number of different types of this bacterium, including the 01 or El Tor type and now also the 0139 type which cause epidemics. If the organism grows in the small intestine, it can cause severe diarrhoea and vomiting, with rapid dehydration and often shock and death.

Frequency

Cholera is endemic in India and Pakistan in the Ganges basin, but it has now spread to many other parts of the world where sanitation, water supplies and personal hygiene are poor, especially at the time of war or disaster.

Epidemiology

Man was originally thought to be the only host. The reservoir includes cases, inapparent cases and carriers. The cholera organism is passed from the gastrointestinal tract in the faeces or in the vomit. The organism then spreads to the mouths of other people. The usual way this happens is when the faeces or vomit contaminate drinking water. Contamination of food by contaminated water, hands and flies can also occur. Direct spread from person to person can occur; but is not common.

Cholera organisms have now been found to also have another life cycle in brackish water in association with small water organisms. This accounts for cholera being endemic in some areas.

All people are susceptible if there is an epidemic in a new area. But many infected people do not develop the clinical disease. And many people who do develop clinical disease have only mild disease. In endemic areas, most of the clinical cases are children. (Only one in every 100 infected persons gets severe disease.)

A person can be a carrier for months.

Immunity after an attack lasts only for a short time.

The disease occurs mostly in countries where there is poor sanitation and the water supplies are not safe.

Pathology

Cholera causes no pathological changes in the structure of the gastrointestinal tract. The organism does not get into the blood or other parts of the body. The toxin from the cholera organism makes the small bowel wall secrete very large volumes of salt and water. These are then lost by continuous vomiting and diarrhoea. This causes rapid dehydration (within hours), shock and death. If the lost salt and water is replaced quickly enough in the right quantity, this is all that is needed for the patient to get better.

Symptoms

If cholera comes to an area where it is not endemic, the first thing you will notice is a *group* of people with gastroenteritis. Some of the people will develop significant symptoms and some quickly die.

At first, all of the normal faeces in the bowel are quickly passed. Then large amounts of watery stool are passed repeatedly, or almost continuously. Several litres may be passed in the first few hours. The stools often look like the water in which rice has been boiled and may smell like fish; but sometimes they are different.

There is usually no abdominal pain or colic.

Vomiting usually occurs after the diarrhoea, but sometimes occurs first. There is little nausea. Large volumes of fluid are vomited. The vomit is usually clear and watery.

Cramps in the muscles of the abdomen (and other areas) can cause severe pain.

Signs

When you see a patient with these symptoms, he is usually severely dehydrated, shocked and cyanosed and often unable to speak.

Signs may include:

1. The patient at first is conscious, but restless and thirsty and very weak. Soon he may become unconscious.
2. The temperature is not raised; it may be lower than normal.
3. The pulse is very fast and weak; or you cannot feel it.
4. The blood pressure is very low; or you cannot record it.
5. The breathing rate is fast.
6. The weight is decreased.
7. Severe signs of dehydration are present with wrinkled skin with no elasticity, sunken eyes and cheeks, etc.
8. There is cyanosis.
9. The abdomen
   • is sunken,

- is not tender, guarded or rigid,
- has bowel sounds which are loud,
- is usually soft; but sometimes there is spasm of all of the muscles of the body which may seem like guarding of the abdomen.

10. Spasm (tightening) of muscles, with cramps in the hands and feet and the calves of legs is quite common.

11. No urine is passed.

Course and complications

The disease has a course of 2–7 days.

Without treatment, over 50% of severely affected cases will die. Death can occur within a few hours.

With proper treatment, less than 1% of these cases will die.

After proper rehydration, vomiting usually stops.

Diarrhoea (of up to 60 litres a day) may continue for some days before it stops.

Miscarriage or premature labour is common if the patient is pregnant.

Affected children may not be fully conscious, may fit and the temperature may be raised.

Without antibiotic treatment, many patients become carriers for some days or weeks or months.

Many mild cases and many unnoticed cases occur for every severe case.

Tests

There is no test for the disease that you can do at the health centre.

If you suspect cholera, you must take specimens to send to the laboratory urgently (stools, rectal swabs and vomitus) to confirm the diagnosis. If antibiotics are given before the laboratory tests are collected, the chance of a positive culture is less; so you must collect at least one specimen before you start the antibiotic treatment.

Collect faeces in a sterile pan which is free from disinfectant or antiseptic. Avoid contamination with urine if possible. Use a sterile wooden spatula or a spoon to put 10–15 ml of faeces (two or three tea-spoonfuls), containing blood and mucus, if present, into a sterile screw-topped glass or plastic container and send this to the laboratory. Put the spoon into antiseptic. When the patient is incontinent, put a sterile, stiff-walled, 1.5 cm wide, 15 cm long, rubber or plastic tube, which is cut at an angle at the end and well lubricated, into the rectum (with the lubricated angled end in the rectum) and drain the faeces into a

sterile container. If you take swabs, take them from the rectum, not only the anus.

Send the specimen to the laboratory *immediately* If the laboratory is not close to the place of collection send for a suitable transport medium such as alkaline peptone water. Put 1–3 grams of faeces ($\frac{1}{2}$ teaspoonful) into 10 ml of the medium in a screw-topped bottle and mix it thoroughly.

Send a letter with the specimen which gives all the details of the specimen, full clinical notes, and a request for examination for cholera organisms. If you could not collect a specimen before you gave antibiotics, then the request form must give the name of the antibiotic, the dosage and how long the patient has been having it.

You must also make a request for a microscopic examination and culture of the specimen for all other organisms which could cause a similar disease.

Differential diagnosis

This is the same as for gastroenteritis (see page 360 and Table 23.2 page 363).

Diagnostic features

Suspect cholera if:

1. A single patient who has returned from a cholera area within the last week develops gastroenteritis of *any* type; but especially if they have the typical signs and symptoms, *or*

2. There is an epidemic of gastroenteritis with some cases with the typical signs and symptoms, especially if some quickly die.

Treatment

Treatment includes three things:

1. Treat and prevent dehydration and shock.
   - Correct the dehydration and loss of salts.
   - Replace continuing loss of water and salts.
   - Give maintenance fluids.
2. Treat the infection in the intestine.
3. Treat symptoms if necessary, and give good nursing care.

Treat and prevent dehydration and shock
First you should correct the dehydration (loss of water and salts).

For severe dehydration use IV Hartmann's solution (also called lactated Ringer's solution).

For moderate or mild dehydration, use Oral Rehydration Solution (see page 366).

Table 23.3 Treatment of dehydration. For severe dehydration use IV Hartmann's solution. For moderate or mild dehydration use Oral Rehydration Solution.

Dehydration	Route	Adult	Child
Severe	IV	40 ml/kg *very fast* Then 60 ml/kg *over 2 hours*	40 ml/kg *very fast* Then 60 ml/kg *over 4 hours*
Moderate	Oral	25 ml/kg/hour *for 4 hours*	25 ml/kg/hour *for 4 hours*
Mild	Oral	15 ml/kg/hour *for 4 hours*	15 ml/kg/hour *for 4 hours*

Note about children. Hartmann's solution does not contain enough potassium or sugar or water for children. As soon as they can drink at all, give children as much Oral Rehydration Solution (see page 366, but not just salt and glucose and water) as they can drink *and* the IV Hartmann's solution.

Note: If you have no Hartmann's solution – use WHO IV diarrhoea treatment solution or dextrose 2.5% in half strength Darrow's solution; or if you do not have these, use 0.9% sodium chloride. If you do not have Hartmann's solution start Oral Rehydration Solution (see page 366, but not just salt, glucose and water) as soon as possible, as the other IV fluids do not contain everything (especially potassium) the patient needs. This is especially important if you give 0.9% sodium chloride.

The best signs to use to judge hydration are:

- pulse volume and rate,
- blood pressure,
- skin elasticity,
- normal fullness of neck veins,
- loss of cramps, nausea and vomiting,
- weight increased,
- urine passed, and
- loss of thirst.

After 2–4 hours of intravenous hydration the patient will become alert and look well. Vomiting will stop and he will start to pass urine. But diarrhoea will continue for 1–3 days; but it should become less, and the stool less watery.

After correcting the dehydration you should *replace continuing loss of salt and water, and give maintenance fluids.*

Maintain the rehydrated state during the continuing diarrhoea by oral fluid.

Check the patient's hydration every 2 hours (see above). Keep a record of all the fluid you give (intravenous and oral). Also record the stool volume, appearance (clear, whitish, watery, yellow-watery, faecal) and frequency and how much urine is passed.

Order oral fluids every 4 hours. Give a volume of $1\frac{1}{2}$ times the stool volume passed over the previous 4 hours. Continue this until the diarrhoea stops. Give Oral Rehydration Solution (see page 366, but not just salt, glucose and water), which is either drunk or else put down an intragastric tube. If the stool loss is not more than 500 ml per hour, further intravenous fluids are not necessary.

Only rarely will further IV fluid be necessary; but you may continue it at 10–20 ml/kg each hour for the 4 hours after rehydration if it is really necessary, while you start oral fluids.

If you do not have much intravenous fluid, you can use oral fluids immediately for most moderately or mildly dehydrated patients, and even in severely dehydrated patients immediately after they have been rehydrated intravenously. In most cases, you can replace the continuing stool loss with an oral rehydration solution.

Treat the infection in the intestine with antibiotics

Give doxycycline or tetracycline. Start the drug only when the patient has been rehydrated and is taking oral fluids, so that the antibiotic will not be vomited.

The dose of doxycycline for adults is 300 mg once or tetracycline 500 mg every 6 hours for 2 days.

If the organisms are resistant to tetracycline you will be told to give erythromycin, co-trimoxazole, ciprofloxacin, chloramphenicol or other antibiotics.

Antibiotics help to reduce the time and volume of diarrhoea, and the time the patient continues to pass the bacteria in the stool (and be infectious).

Treat symptoms if necessary

This is not usually necessary. The above treatment will usually cure the symptoms.

- *Do not* give diuretics – rapid rehydration will make the patient pass urine.
- *Do not* give chlorpromazine for vomiting – rapid rehydration will stop the vomiting.
- *Do not* give morphine or analgesics for muscle cramps – rehydrate (and then if necessary give calcium gluconate 10% solution, 10 ml IV slowly).
- *Do not* use stimulants like adrenaline.
- *Do not* use adrenocorticosteroids.
- *Do not* use plasma volume expanders.
- *Do not* use oxygen to try to correct cyanosis.

These complications all improve with rapid IV rehydration. For the above symptoms give more IV fluid.

Nurse patients on a bed with the mattress made of a waterproof sheet or mat with a 22 cm (or nine inch) hole in it. Place his buttocks over the hole, with a bucket under the hole. Measurement of stool volume is then easy.

The patient can start to eat when the vomiting stops.

1. In an epidemic, check that every patient has cholera and not another disease.
2. Repeated vomiting is usually caused by not enough of the right IV fluid.
3. Watch for overhydration and heart failure in children.

Control of epidemic

You must immediately find out how the disease started and how it has spread so that you can use the correct methods of control. The usual means of spread is water.

Kill the organism in the body of the original hosts and the reservoir.
Admit patients. Isolate patients. Start treatment with doxycycline or tetracycline when vomiting stops. This will make the patient non–infectious and stop him becoming a carrier.

Close contacts of patients (i.e. family and others who may have been infected by the same reservoir of infection (usually water)), may develop the disease or be mild cases or carriers. Treat them also with doxycycline or tetracycline (or erythromycin if pregnant).

The usual reservoir is contaminated water. Chlorinate all water supplies and boil all water used for drinking, cooking, preparing food, washing dishes, etc.

Stop the means of spread.
Use all usual methods of stopping faecal-oral spread.

Disinfect the faeces and vomit and articles used by patients.

Staff must practise good hygiene, especially removing gowns before leaving the ward and washing hands after nursing patients and before eating or drinking. (No eating or drinking by staff is allowed in the ward.)

Check that everyone uses proper toilets.

Tell everyone to wash their hands after using the toilet and before preparing or eating food.

Protect and chlorinate all water supplies.

Tell people to boil all water used for drinking or cooking or putting on food or washing dishes, etc.

Tell people to cook all seafood or food which comes from water very well.

Tell everyone about hygiene and safe cooking, handling, storing, serving and eating of food.

Try to reduce the number of flies, and keep flies away from all toilets and food.

Raise the resistance of susceptible persons.
The previously available injectable vaccine was of little help. New oral vaccines are of killed organisms or of an avirulent cholera organism and are effective. However, they are expensive and boosters are needed and they are not completely protective. Their place in epidemics is not yet clear. They are used by travellers. However, staff at health centres in affected areas may well be given some protection if given these vaccines.

Prophylactic treatment.
During an epidemic, staff at the health centre should be told to take doxycycline or tetracycline or, if pregnant, erythromycin to kill any cholera organisms that enter their gastrointestinal tracts.

Prevention
Quarantine procedures may be carried out at border posts, ports and airports to try to stop cholera entering a country.

Good sanitation and a plentiful supply of safe water and good general hygiene would stop any case which did enter a country causing an epidemic.

Immunisation gives some personal protection.

Notification
You should report all suspected cases of cholera *immediately* to the Health Officer, by telephone or radio or fast transport.

Cholera is an 'Event of Public Health Concern'. The Government will immediately report to the WHO and neighbouring countries if any case occurs.

Enteritis necroticans (pigbel)
Pigbel occurs in the Highlands of Papua New Guinea, especially in children if the diet is poor in protein and high in sweet potato. Similar cases have also been reported from Uganda and Ghana, Thailand and India and no doubt occur in other places.

The cause is a special type of special bacteria (*Clostridium*).

These organisms live in the intestines of animals or man or in the soil.

If these organisms

1. contaminate food, and
2. are not all killed by proper cooking, and
3. are eaten,

then they may

1. grow in any protein food in the intestine, and
2. produce a toxin in the intestine.

If the toxin (which is a protein) is not destroyed because there is

1. little of the digestive juice (trypsin) which digests protein (because of little protein normally in diet) and
2. sweet potato or other food present in the intestine which stops what little protein digestive juice there is from working,

then the toxin damages the bowel wall causing inflammation or even necrosis (death) of the bowel wall.

History

The history is usually of a person who:

• is usually a child from a known place for the disease, e.g. the Highlands of Papua New Guinea;
• usually does not have much protein in the diet;
• has eaten pig meat or other high protein food ½–4 days before;
• then develops one of the four syndromes listed below.

Symptoms, signs, course and complications

1. As for gastroenteritis (see page 362) (diagnosis of enteritis necroticans is not made)
   or
2. • Severe upper abdominal pain which is constant, but there is also colic.
   • Vomiting; and vomitus soon becomes dark fluid (from blood) with flecks or spots in it (dead mucous membrane).
   • Blood in the stool, sometimes with diarrhoea (this has often stopped by the time the patient has come to the health centre).
   • Raised temperature, fast pulse and dehydration.
   • Upper abdominal distension, with loops of the intestine visible under the abdominal wall.
   • Upper abdominal tenderness, often with guarding and rigidity.
   • Intestinal masses may be felt.
   • Bowel sounds are decreased, though occasionally increased.
   • Death occurs in a few days if the patient does not get proper treatment.
   or
3. Soon after the start there is rapid development of severe general symptoms and signs of infection (septicaemia) and death.

also

4. Patients who get better may have an incomplete intestinal obstruction or have malnutrition. These are caused by a narrowing of the affected intestine.

Treatment

Treat as for acute gastroenteritis (see pages 363–365) if there is no definite abdominal tenderness or distension. Give also albendazole 400 mg once.

Treat as for peritonitis if there are definite signs of enteritis necroticans 'pigbel' (i.e. 2 above) (nothing by mouth, IV fluids, IV penicillin or if severe, chloramphenicol, IM morphine) (see pages 349–350).

Transfer

You should arrange transfer to *Medical Officer care* when:

1. The patient has a severe case: i.e. his abdomen is very swollen, and he has black flecked vomit and marked general symptoms and signs (urgent – emergency).
2. The patient has only a mild case (only some abdominal swelling, not toxic, no black flecked vomit), but does not improve after 2 days of treatment.

Control and prevention

1. Kill the organism in the reservoir.
   This is not possible.
2. Stop the means of transmission.
   Proper cooking of *all* foods to kill all organisms would stop most cases. It is difficult to get people always to do this.
3. Raise the resistance of susceptible persons.
   More protein in the diet and not eating sweet potato can increase the activity of the digestive juices from the pancreas. But it is also difficult for people to afford the first and often impossible to do the second thing.

People can be immunised against the disease. You should give immunisation if you work in a place where the disease is common and are told to do so. Give a dose of 0.5 ml of vaccine by IMI at the same time as each dose of DPT or triple antigen (i.e. at 2 months of age, 2 months after the first dose and again 2 months after the second dose).

Amoebiasis

Amoebiasis is an infection with special amoebae (*Entamoeba histolytica*). These amoebae are protozoal organisms that usually live in the large intestine.

The amoebae in the large intestine make cysts, which are passed in the stool. These cysts are infective if swallowed. Direct faecal-oral spread can occur, but much more commonly, faeces with cysts contaminate water or sometimes food. When the water or food is swallowed, the cysts develop into amoebae in the intestine.

Most infected people have no symptoms or signs. The amoebae eat only bacteria and surface cells of the mucous membrane. But these persons are infective to others.

Sometimes the amoebae eat into the intestinal wall and form ulcers. This is more common if the immunity is decreased, e.g. pregnancy or the patient is given adrenocorticosteroid drugs (e.g. prednisolone or cortisone, for e.g. treatment of a leprosy reaction or asthma) or has HIV infection. Sometimes the ulceration is started by other infections, e.g. bacteria or worms (e.g. *Schistosoma* or *Trichuris*).

The invading amoebae can cause any or all of the following types of diarrhoea and dysentery.

1. Short periods of diarrhoea over many years; but examination shows nothing abnormal *or*
2. More severe attacks with malaise, fever, severe bowel colic and dysentery (frequent bloody stools). Examination shows general abdominal tenderness and often an enlarged liver. There may be fever, dehydration or anaemia. Chloramphenicol does not cure the dysentery.
3. Sometimes very severe attacks with complications.
   • Peritonitis from perforation of (the amoebae eating through) the bowel wall (see page 349).
   • Bleeding when amoebae eat through a blood vessel wall causing anaemia or shock.

Sometimes large masses of chronic inflammatory tissue (granulation tissue) form in the intestinal wall. Symptoms and signs similar to cancer or obstruction of the intestine can occur. You can often feel the mass made by the amoebae on examination of the abdomen, or on pelvic examination PR.

The amoebae can travel up the portal vein to the liver and cause liver abscess (see Chapter 24 page 398).

The amoebae can live on the skin and produce ulcers around the anus, or on the genitalia (see Chapter 19 page 215).

Diagnosis can be proven by seeing the amoebae under the microscope in stool samples; but a harmless protozoa (*E. dispar*) looks the same and an ELISA test for the proteins (antigens) of *E. histolytica* would also be needed. These tests are not usually available. Treat the condition on the clinical diagnosis.

Treatment to kill amoebae in all parts of the body is metronidazole 750–800 mg three times a day for 5 days (400 mg three times a day for 10 days if nausea

from the larger dose). Tell the patient not to drink alcohol (see Chapter 11 page 60).

Albendazole in a large dose for 5 days, although not when possibly pregnant, is said to be as effective. You can also use chloroquine, tetracycline and emetine but only in certain circumstances (see Chapter 24 page 398 or a reference book for special doses of these).

If reinfection is not likely, then, and especially if previous attacks have occurred, it is best to ensure no amoebae are left alive in the bowel by following this treatment with diloxanide 0.5 g tablets one three times a day for 10 days (but if unavailable tetracycline may be effective).

Give treatment for gastroenteritis (see pages 363–365) or other conditions if present.

Control and prevention is the same as for all gastrointestinal infections. See page 366.

Shigella infection (bacillary dysentery)

Shigella infection causes acute inflammation of the large bowel wall and then diarrhoea or dysentery (frequent stools with blood and mucus), abdominal pain and fever. Sometimes mild cases with just diarrhoea occur and many infected persons have no symptoms. But, severe cases with complications can also occur.

The usual reservoir is man. Spread is from infected faeces to the mouth of another person. This spread is direct or in contaminated food or by flies.

In a health centre, there is no way that bacillary dysentery can be distinguished with certainty from other causes of acute diarrhoeal disease or gastroenteritis which have caused dysentery. However, if the dysentery does not need metronidazole to cure it (if metronidazole is needed it was probably due to amoebae) it may be assumed that the cause was the bacillary dysentery organism.

For symptoms and signs, course and complications, treatment, control and prevention, see pages 362–366 or a reference book. Antibiotics should not be given unless the bacteria (1) invade deeply into the intestinal wall and cause severe disease with dysentery or abdominal tenderness or (2) spread into the bloodstream and cause symptoms and signs of septicaemia. *Shigella* are often resistant to many antibiotics; but fortunately most cases do not need antibiotics.

Salmonella causing typhoid

Typhoid is caused by only the very special *Salmonella typhi* organisms.

Infection with these organisms causes malaise, fever, abdominal pain and constipation with a slow pulse during the first week of the disease. During the second week the patient gets worse and diarrhoea, enlargement of the spleen and rash occur. In the third week intestinal haemorrhage or perforation and severe general symptoms and signs of infection may occur and the patient may die. (See Chapter 18 pages 173–174 for details.)

You are not likely to mistake typhoid for one of the usual or undiagnosable forms of gastroenteritis.

Non-typhoid salmonella (NTS) infections

Salmonellae are bacteria that very often cause gastroenteritis. They can cause a mild or moderate or severe attack of acute diarrhoea and sometimes dysentery. The patient usually has a fever. There are no specific symptoms and signs which you can use to make the diagnosis in the health centre.

In some patients, especially those with decreased immunity, especially those with HIV infection, septicaemia occurs.

The reservoir of the salmonellae is the gastrointestinal tract of many animals and man. Spread can be direct, but it is usually by food or drink which is contaminated with the faeces of an infected man or animal. The organisms multiply in the food (especially milk, meat, chicken, eggs, fish, etc.), especially if it is stored warm for a time before eating. Very commonly most, but not all, the salmonellae are killed by cooking which is not hot enough or not long enough to kill them all. If this cooked food is not stored in a cold refrigerator (which slows their growth), these remaining salmonellae rapidly multiply. Many salmonellae are then in the food or drink later swallowed. If enough organisms are swallowed (a large number are needed), acute diarrhoeal disease with fever occurs, after an incubation period of 4–48 hours.

If a group of people eat the infected food, there will be an epidemic of acute diarrhoeal disease with fever 4–48 hours later.

Treatment is as described for gastroenteritis (see pages 363–365). Do not give antibiotics unless (1) the conditions described on page 365 develop, especially spots on the skin of the trunk, increasing splenomegaly or fever for more than a few days or (2) the patient becomes very ill or septicaemic.

However, antibiotics are important if (1) the patient has HIV infection and does not quickly improve (as salmonella infections are very common in HIV patients and can cause severe illness, septicaemia and death, and often come back again and again after

treatment (in which case antibiotic prophylaxis may be worthwhile)), or (2) if the patient has sickle cell anaemia (to stop salmonella causing osteomyelitis in the sickle cell patient).

Toxin type of food poisoning

If staphylococci or streptococci get into food or drink (especially milk), they grow in it and produce a toxin. The toxin is not destroyed by later cooking the food or boiling the drink.

If the food or drink is swallowed, the bacteria do not cause disease; but the toxin causes acute gastroenteritis. There is usually the sudden onset of severe vomiting only. There is no fever. The other usual symptoms and signs of gastroenteritis can be present. The gastroenteritis usually gets better after a few hours, even without treatment.

The reservoir is the infected respiratory tract or skin of patients or carriers. These people contaminate food or drink with the organisms when they cough into or handle food. Enough toxin can form to cause disease, especially if the food is milk, and especially if it is kept warm before drinking or eating. The incubation period is 1–6 hours. There is no infection of the patient by the organisms.

If a group of people eat the infected food there will be an epidemic of acute gastroenteritis without fever (probably just vomiting) 1–6 hours later.

Treatment is the same as for gastroenteritis (see pages 363–365). Do not give antibiotics.

Giardiasis

Giardiasis is an infection of the duodenum and small bowel with the protozoal organism, *Giardia lamblia*. It is a parasite of humans only. When the organism is carried into the lower bowel, it forms cysts which are able to survive outside the body for several weeks and are infective to other people as soon as they are swallowed. Infection is therefore common where sanitation is poor, water supplies are not protected from faeces and personal cleanliness is not good.

The organism in the small bowel causes diarrhoea with pale, large, smelly stools often with a lot of flatus (gas). There may be abdominal distension. There may be bowel sounds able to be heard by the patient and others; as well as burping bad tasting and smelling gas; as well as passing a lot of flatus. There may be loss of appetite and weight loss. Diarrhoea may continue for weeks or months. It is thought that eventually most adults start to lose their symptoms. However, if the patient has any abnormality of immunity, especially HIV infection, the giardia infection and its symptoms may become very severe.

The diagnosis may be made by finding the cysts on a microscopic examination of the stool. This is not usually possible in the health centre and the patient will be treated for gastroenteritis with metronidazole 800 mg three times a day for 5–10 days because he had diarrhoea which did not stop after 2 weeks of treatment. Metronidazole usually cures this condition.

See 'Gastroenteritis' pages 360–366 and 'Post-infective malabsorption' below.

Prevention is by good sanitation, a plentiful supply of safe water and good personal hygiene, especially handwashing.

Schistosomiasis

See Chapter 18 pages 187–191 for details if *Schistosoma mansoni* or *S. japonicum* affect people in your area.

Intestinal symptoms and signs start between 2 months and 2 years after infection.

There is often diarrhoea with blood and mucus in the stools and intestinal colic. All of these can be severe. These conditions can improve after some days or weeks; but they return some weeks later. On examination of the abdomen, you can often feel the thickened large intestine and it may be tender.

After some time, masses of infected tissue can form inside the intestine. You can often feel these masses on abdominal or pelvic (PR) examination and they can prolapse (come out) through the anus.

It is difficult to tell the difference between amoebic infection and cancer of the large intestine and schistosomiasis, without tests.

Later, the eggs travel to the liver and damage the liver blood vessels, causing portal hypertension with ascites and a large spleen (see Chapter 24 page 395).

If patients have only a few worms or if they do not have repeated infections, they may not have these or any symptoms and signs.

See Chapter 18 pages 190–191 for diagnosis and treatment and control.

Hypolactasia (lactose intolerance), post-infective malabsorption syndrome and tropical sprue

After some viral, bacterial, protozoal or worm infections of the gastrointestinal tract, patients may not be able to absorb the sugar called lactose which is in milk. Lactose is then broken down in the bowel by organisms and these chemicals cause chronic diarrhoea with a large amount of watery stool. If the patient drinks milk or eats a milk product, he may get abdominal colic and swelling and pass a lot of flatus and watery stool. This can be diagnosed by testing the stool for sugar with a Benedict's test or tablet test for sugar. However, many of the stick tests for glucose do not work, as they do not show lactose (only glucose). Fortunately, most of these people get better without treatment if milk is kept out of their diet for a month or so and then only slowly put back into it. Fortunately, many adults in developing countries do not drink milk and this condition is not a problem to them. The condition is called 'hypolactasia' or 'lactose intolerance'.

In the same sort of way, after many acute viral, bacterial, protozoal or parasitic infections of the bowel, other patients do not absorb fat, vitamins, electrolytes, protein, etc. properly. They develop chronic diarrhoea with large fatty stools which smell bad and pass a lot of flatus. They also lose weight as they do not absorb fat, and develop a sore mouth and anaemia as they do not absorb vitamins. This condition is called 'post-infective malabsorption'.

In some areas, a similar condition can occur suddenly and even in epidemics, and it is thought that this may be due to a bacterial infection. This condition is often called 'tropical sprue'. It is especially common in the Indian subcontinent and in the north part of South America as well as around the Mediterranean Sea.

It may well be that the 'post-infective malabsorption syndrome' and 'tropical sprue' are due to certain organisms being in the wrong parts of the bowel. A similar clinical state, however, may be caused by continuing infection with organisms such as *Giardia*, *Strongyloides*, HIV, TB, etc. The problem can also be due to lack of the enzymes in bile, pancreatic secretion and intestinal secretions (which help break down food so it can be absorbed) and can therefore occur in pancreatitis, liver disease, or if parts of the bowel have been surgically removed, etc.

Because of the difficulty of such cases, you need to refer them to the next visiting Medical Officer or transfer them non-urgently to the Medical Officer for investigation. Before doing this, however, you should test the stool for sugar and send stool tests for examination for AFB, ova, cysts and parasites and send blood for tests for HIV antibodies, full blood count, electrolytes, liver function tests and glucose. Ask the Medical Officer the meaning of the test results; and if you should try treating the patient with metronidazole for 10 days and then with tetracycline 250 mg four times a day for a month before sending the patient.

Appendicitis

Appendicitis is an acute inflammation of the appendix. The inflamed appendix may burst and cause a localised abscess or general peritonitis if it is not treated. (See a specialist surgery book for details.)

The patient usually complains of a central abdominal pain at first. After some hours the pain moves to the right iliac fossa and is constant. The patient loses his appetite from the start of the disease.

On examination there is usually:

1. mild fever,
2. pulse faster than normal,
3. abdomen:
   • not distended,
   • may not move well on breathing,
   • tenderness and rebound tenderness and guarding in the right iliac fossa, and tenderness on the right side on pelvic examination through the rectum.

Later, if it is not treated, an abscess with a tender mass in the right iliac fossa, or general peritonitis, develops.

Treatment is urgent; transfer to Medical Officer care, if patient agrees to surgery, to remove the appendix.

Meanwhile give:

• nil by mouth;
• IVI fluids, 1 litre of 4% dextrose in 0.18% sodium chloride each 8 hours;
• IVI or IMI chloramphenicol 1 g each 6 hours;
• morphine 10 mg IMI before transfer.

Cancer (carcinoma) of the intestine

See a specialist surgery book for details.

Cancer of the intestine occurs more often in old people or in people with schistosomiasis.

Cancer of the intestine may cause any of these:

• anaemia from bleeding into the bowel;
• blood in the stool;
• attacks of constipation and diarrhoea (one after the other):
• intestinal colic and later obstruction of the intestine;
• an abdominal mass you can feel; and
• weight loss and malaise.

It may be difficult to distinguish cancer of the intestine from amoebic dysentery and amoeboma and schistosomiasis, which can have similar chronic histories and similar signs.

If cancer of the intestine is suspected, give the patient a full course of anti-amoebic treatment (metronidazole 400 mg three times a day for 10 days preferably with tetracycline (500 mg 6 hourly) and if the patient is in or from an area where schistosomiasis occurs, give praziquantel 30 mg/kg twice with 6 hours between doses.

If the disease does not improve rapidly and get completely better after some weeks, transfer the patient non-urgently to hospital.

Nutritional disorders

Major problems are:
(1) undernutrition, especially because of drought or famine or the effects of war or government policies which result in starvation; and on the other hand, (2) overnutrition which results in obesity.

Likewise, (1) deficiency of simple vitamins leads to vitamin deficiency diseases which are easily preventable but can cause things such as blindness or heart failure; and on the other hand, (2) inappropriate excesses of certain foods or alcohol lead to conditions such as heart disease, cancer and alcoholism.

These can be a major problem for a whole community. However, at times, only certain parts of the community or only a certain family or only one member of the family are involved.

There are formulas for working out the exact amount of energy from food that people need. These vary according to gender, body weight, amount of exercise to be done, etc. In general, however, the following is a rough guide.

Table 23.4 Daily energy requirements of men and women.

Circumstances	Healthy adult females	Healthy adult males
At rest	6.7 MJ (1600 kcal)	8.4 MJ (2000 kcal)
Light work	8.4 MJ (2000 kcal)	11.3 MJ (2700 kcal)
Heavy work	9.4 MJ (2250 kcal)	14.6 MJ (3500 kcal)

Food to provide at least 2100–2400 kcal per day in an average population is a minimum. Protein requirement in the diet is about 6 g/kg ideal body weight or 10–14% of calories from protein. Fat intake, on the other hand, when food is plentiful, should be less than 30% of calories. At least 55% of the calories should be from carbohydrates. Water is needed at least 1–1.5 ml/kcal; but in a hot climate or on exertion or if illness especially vomiting or diarrhoea is present, many times this amount may be needed. Vitamins and minerals of at least the known daily requirements are also needed. Many factors including growth, body size, physical activity, pregnancy, lactation, disease, drugs, etc. alter these requirements. If a therapeutic feeding programme is needed in your area, experts should work this out for you and work out what food will provide these requirements.

The relationships between nutrition and infection are of vital importance. Infection increases the nutritional needs because of fever, need for repair of the body, etc. Infection decreases nutrition, however, by a decrease in appetite, less intake of food, loss of food or fluids by vomiting or by being not absorbed or by having diarrhoea or dysentery. Malnutrition decreases the body's defences against infection and increases the likelihood of infection. There is therefore a vicious cycle of malnutrition leading to infection and infection to more malnutrition and more malnutrition to more infection … The relationship of malnutrition and infection may affect the whole population or just certain communities or certain families or just one member of the family.

The health worker usually should be involved with other members of the health department as well as social and agricultural and other workers in diagnosing, treating and preventing nutritional problems.

The health worker usually has to start with the individual patient who comes to him and then work back to the family and then to the community diagnosing and treating nutritional disorders.

Investigation of a person's nutritional status is done in four ways.

1. Dietary history. Both quantity (amount) and quality (type) of food needs to be known. As the patient's memory is often not accurate, it may be better to get the patient to write down for a few days exactly what he has eaten and bring this for you to see.
2. Clinical examination. Although it is important not to wait until the signs of nutritional abnormality develop before doing something about the diet, of particular importance are:
   • muscle wasting, especially of the muscles above the jaw and around the shoulders,
   • oedema,
   • pallor,
   • weakness.
   (Figure 23.10 shows other things which may be found and their causes.)
3. Anthropenometry (measuring the body).
   Body mass (weight) is determined by:
   (a) the amount of water in the body and
   (b) the energy balance.
   If there is no loss of water, loss of 1 kg is equivalent to 25–29 MJ (6000–7000 kcal) of food.

The body mass should always be measured. It does however, depend not only on the above but varies with height, gender, race, etc. and other factors such as childhood nutrition.

Weight for height compared with the usual weight for that height in healthy members of the population is usually used for assessment of adolescents. An adolescent whose weight is less than 70% of that predicted for his height has severe malnutrition and needs admission to a therapeutic feeding programme.

Body Mass Index is more reliable than just weight as a predictor, as it takes into account the patient's height. It can be used only for adults (i.e. not for children and adolescents). It is calculated by measuring the person's body weight in kg and dividing that by the patient's height in metres^2, i.e. BMI = kg/m × m. The usual interpretation is:

Body mass index (weight/height^2)

Underweight	< 18.5
Normal	18.5–24.9
Overweight	25.0–29.9
Obese	30.0–39.9
Extremely obese	> 40

Mid-arm *muscle* circumference in cm, as well as the mm measurement of triceps skin fold, would be helpful except that it requires a special caliper to measure the skin fold thickness and then a calculation to work out the mid-arm muscle circumference. A simple measurement of just mid upper arm circumference is less accurate, but it can help tell who has severe malnutrition (see page 379).

4. Laboratory investigations. Many are helpful. Unfortunately, no simple ones, apart from Hb, are available in the health centre.

Protein calorie malnutrition in adults

Causes include:

• insufficient food
• loss of appetite including psychiatric disorder
• vomiting
• malabsorption (the bowel not properly digesting and absorbing (taking into the body) the food eaten)
• increased energy requirements such as in thyrotoxicosis
• fever
• trauma
• cancer

Weight Chart

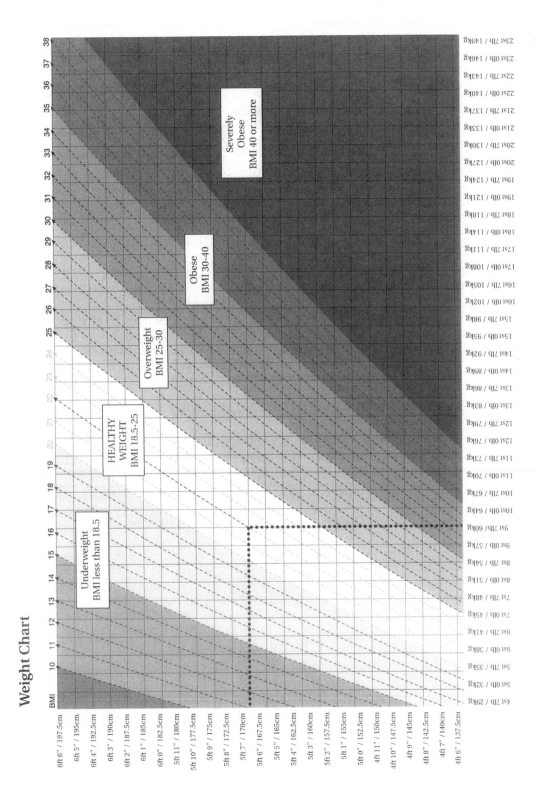

Table 23.5 Body weights corresponding to specified BMI (body mass index) for given height (BMI for adults = W/H²) (Reproduced by permission of vertex42.com)

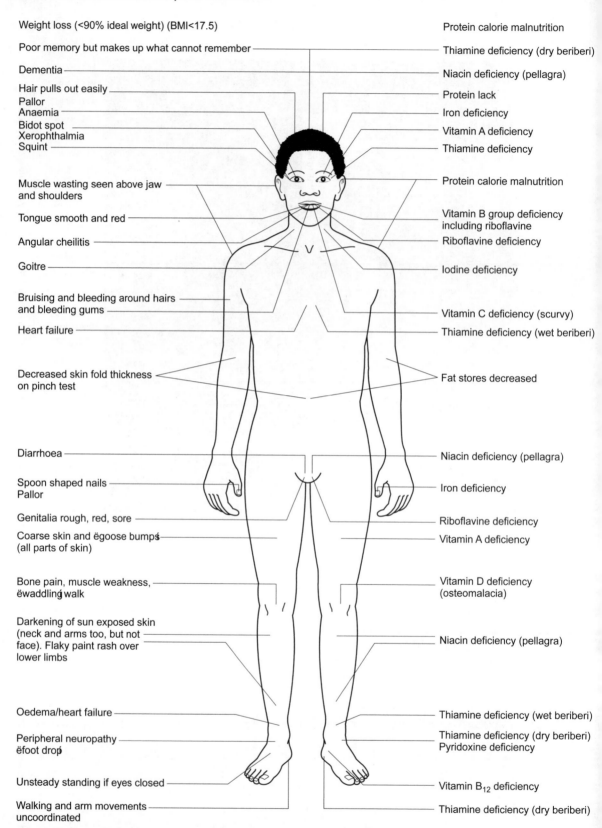

Figure 23.10 *Some signs (patient's right) seen in malnutrition and their causes (patient's left).*

- infections especially TB, HIV, trypanosomiasis, visceral leishmaniasis, etc.
- increased energy loss such as diabetes with sugar in the urine and
- the need to do a large amount of physical exertion.

Findings include:

- craving for food
- thirst
- nocturia
- weakness
- impotence (a man not able to have sexual intercourse) or no menstrual periods
- loss of weight with BMI < 18.5, especially if < 16
- uncorrected middle upper arm circumference of < 16 cm or 15 cm in the elderly; or < 18.5 cm or 17.5 cm in the elderly together with oedema of the lower limbs or inability to stay standing or obvious dehydration
- temperature decreased
- pulse slow
- blood pressure low
- dry, pale inelastic skin
- thinned hair (except adolescents)
- feeling cold and cold hands and feet
- muscle wasting most easily seen in the temporal muscles above the jaw and in the shoulder
- loss of fat best seen or felt by pinching the upper arm and around the abdomen
- oedema
- distended abdomen
- apathy and depression
- possibly an infection present.

Patients with mild starvation are in no danger, but patients with moderate starvation need extra feeding and patients with severe starvation need admission and supervised feeding.

Because the intestinal mucosa and pancreas and liver have not been working properly for some time in severely malnourished people, when feeding commences, they cannot immediately start to digest and absorb food properly. The initial re-feeding is to get these metabolic functions back to normal. Once this has been done, the next aim is to improve weight. Too much food too quickly can cause diarrhoea, vomiting, low blood sugar, heart failure, low body temperature during the night and dehydration, etc. Food should taste good and preferably have a cereal similar to the one the patient normally eats and also have in it milk powder, oil, sugar, vitamins (especially B group

vitamins but do not give large doses of vitamin A to pregnant women) and minerals. This should be given in six small meals rather than three large meals daily and another meal given during the night. If needed, therapeutic milk may have to be given and if the patient is not able to drink this, it may have to be given by nasogastric tube. The requirement initially is 40(–55 for adolescents) kcal per day. Once recovery has started, the requirement is increased to 80 (100 for adolescents) kcal a day. A weight gain would not be expected to be more than 5% per month.

Other treatment of severely malnourished people includes the following:

- Treat malaria if this could possibly be present.
- Give antibiotics only if an infection is found.
- Treat intestinal parasites with albendazole 400 mg or mebendazole 500 mg after 1 week (but not if pregnant).
- Give ferrous sulfate 200 mg (60 mg elemental iron) twice daily; but not until after 2 weeks.

Hypo-vitaminosis

Vitamins are organic substances (proteins) in the food, which cannot be made by the body. Although they are present in very small amounts they are essential for the proper functioning of the body. Vitamins A, D, E and K dissolve in fat but not water and are called 'fat soluble vitamins'. The B group and C dissolve in water but not fat and are called 'water soluble vitamins'. A decrease in any of these vitamins can cause a specific disease; but if one is decreased often others are too and mixed diseases occur. If vitamins are taken in tablet form in larger doses than would be in a good diet, side effects or specific diseases can be caused – especially for vitamins A, B and D.

Vitamin A

Vitamin A is in animal foods, especially liver, but is also made in the body from carotene in green vegetables and yellow or orange fruit. Vitamin A is needed for the part of the retina used to see at night to work, for mucous secretory cells to work and for normal growth.

Vitamin A deficiency causes:

- night blindness, conjunctival dryness and Bitot's spots – white plaques on the conjunctivae just outside the lateral edge of the cornea (see Chapter 31 page 514)
- dull or hazy and dry cornea
- corneal ulcer

- keretomalacia with perforation of the cornea and blindness
- skin being dry and having little lumps ('goose bumps').

Treatment is by vitamin A (retinol). Pregnant women are given only 5000(–10,000) units daily for 3 weeks (or 25,000 units weekly for 3 weeks). Others are treated with 200,000 units immediately and again the next day and again in 2 weeks.

High doses of vitamin A can be used to treat skin conditions (e.g. acne). High doses of vitamin A given to pregnant women can cause abnormalities in her baby (pregnant women need only normal amounts of vitamin A). Very high doses of vitamin A, e.g. eating large amounts of shark or turtle liver can cause hepatitis and death.

Vitamin D

Vitamin D is normally made in the skin when sunlight falls on the skin.

Vitamin D deficiency causes ricketts in children and osteomalacia in adults (see Chapter 28 page 477).

Vitamin K

Vitamin K is present in green leafy vegetables and liver in the diet, but is also made by bacteria in the bowel. It is used by the liver when making blood clotting proteins. If it is low, bleeding can occur. Warfarin stops vitamin K working and is a drug that is used in small amounts to stop abnormal clotting in the body, but it is also used in large amounts as a rat poison. The treatment of vitamin K deficiency and the antidote to bleeding from warfarin is oral or IM vitamin K.

Thiamine (vitamin B$_1$)

Thiamine is in many foods but most comes from cereals. However, if the cereals are treated in certain ways, e.g. making polished rice, the thiamine is lost. Thiamine deficiency occurs if only certain cereals such as polished rice are still eaten; it also occurs in alcoholics on a poor diet.

Thiamine is needed for the body to be able to use sugar to provide energy. Because the heart and the nervous system use a lot of sugar, they are particularly affected by a thiamine deficiency.

Thiamine deficiency causes:

1. Dry beriberi when the nervous system is affected. There may be a peripheral neuropathy (page 420) with the motor nerves affected (with wrist drop and foot drop) and the sensory nerves affected (with uncomfortable feelings and later on loss of sensa-

tion of the hands and feet and later arms and legs). Encephalopathy may also occur with paralysis of the eye muscles.

2. Wet beriberi when the heart and blood vessels are affected. There is high output heart failure with fast pulse, large pulse volume, oedema, etc. (see Chapter 27 page 461).

Treatment is by thiamine 50–100 mg IVI or IMI; or if unavailable, orally three times a day for a week; then give lower doses orally for some weeks. Dry beriberi however, usually needs the other vitamin B group as well and general improvement in the diet before it improves.

Riboflavin (vitamin B$_2$)

Riboflavin is in milk but not much in cereals until the seeds sprout (start to grow).

Deficiency causes:

- glossitis with a red/purple sore tongue,
- sore red lips,
- angular stomatitis (or cheilitis) with cracking at the corners of the mouth,
- at times genital and facial roughness and soreness and redness.

Treatment is by riboflavin 10 mg daily.

Niacin (nicotinic acid and nicotinamide)

These vitamins are usually made in the body from tryptophane, which is in foods such as eggs and cheese. It is used by the body cells to metabolise. Niacin deficiency occurs in those on a diet of maize or sorghum with little other food, as well as in alcoholics on a poor diet.

Niacin deficiency causes pellagra, a disease of the 3 Ds (or the 4 Ds):

- D – dermatitis – on the exposed areas like the neck, hands and feet a sunburned appearance with the skin becoming swollen, itchy, blistering and becoming scaly and later pigmented or dark (see Figure 32.30 page 548).
- D – diarrhoea; and also non-infectious inflammation and discomfort of the whole gastrointestinal tract.
- D – dementia but in acute cases, even delirium.
- D – death.

Treatment is with nicotinamide 100 mg each 8 hours. Improvement should occur rapidly (see Chapter 32 page 547).

Vitamin B₆ (pyridoxine)

Vitamin B_6 is in many foods but especially meat, fish, potatoes and bananas.

Dietary deficiency is rare but isoniazid (and some other drugs) stop it working.

Peripheral neuritis and occasionally encephalopathy can occur if isoniazid is given without extra pyridoxine.

Treatment is with 50–100 mg of pyridoxine daily; but if very large doses are given for a very long time, pyridoxine also can cause a peripheral neuritis.

Vitamin B₁₂ and folic acid

Vitamin B_{12} is found only in animal products, and people who eat no animal products are at risk of deficiency. The most common cause of deficiency, however, is an autoimmune disease of the stomach (pernicious anaemia), when vitamin B_{12} is not absorbed even though it is in the diet. Fish tapeworm infection can also cause this deficiency.

Folic acid is found in green leaves, etc.

Vitamin B_{12} and folic acid are used to make blood. If either are missing, at first the red blood cells become large (macrocytes) and later anaemia develops. They are also used in the nervous system. If vitamin B_{12} is absent then peripheral neuropathy or severe spinal cord damage can occur and later dementia and loss of vision.

Folic acid is needed to help the unborn baby's nervous system develop properly especially in early pregnancy. Folic acid is therefore given together with iron in pregnancy.

Vitamin B_{12} can be given only by injection if the patient has pernicious anaemia, as it cannot be otherwise absorbed. Special tests may be needed by the Medical Officer to diagnose pernicious anaemia. Discuss cases of anaemia and peripheral neuritis and spinal cord lesions with your Medical Officer, about the possible need for vitamin B_{12} treatment. If you suspect a patient does have peripheral neuropathy and spinal cord damage due to vitamin B_{12}, do not give folic acid but transfer the patient immediately; as the folate without vitamin B_{12} may make the nervous system condition get worse.

Vitamin C or ascorbic acid

Vitamin C is found in fresh fruit and vegetables. It is used to make collagen, the supporting tissue of the body.

If fresh fruit and vegetables are not eaten for a couple of months, scurvy occurs and causes:

- weight loss, weakness, aching of limbs especially at night
- swollen and spongy gums which bleed and the teeth become loose
- bleeding around hairs, but also other bleeding into the skin including larger areas (ecchymoses)
- bleeding into the gastrointestinal tract
- anaemia
- wounds do not heal.

Treatment is by Vitamin C 100 mg three times a day until 4 g has been given.

Obesity

Fat is stored by the body if the amount of energy used (especially exercise done) is less than the amount of energy taken in (food eaten). A person is overweight if his BMI (see page 377) is above 25 and obese if above 30 kg/m².

Causes include:

1. decrease in the amount of exercise done now in comparison to the past.
2. increase in the food eaten caused by
   - food eaten being high in fat (which does not make the patient feel satisfied as other foods do)
   - snacks – food is more available
   - energy dense foods and drinks – high in fat and sugar but low in bulk
   - alcohol intake
   - giving up smoking (which causes a fall in energy used up and increase in appetite).
3. genetic factors; but it is mainly eating habits that are passed on by parents.
4. endocrine factors – hypothyroidism. Other diseases can cause obesity; but they have other endocrine symptoms and signs and are very rare causes of obesity.
5. drugs
   - antidepressants
   - sulfonylureas for diabetes
   - oral contraceptives
   - corticosteroids and
   - sodium valproate for epilepsy

can all cause weight increase.

Weight gain around the abdomen is more dangerous than weight gain around the hips and is more likely to cause heart disease, diabetes, etc. The waist circumference for a male should be < 90 cm and for a female < 84 cm.

Complications of weight gain include the following:
- For young adults the gain of each 0.5 kg increases the risk of death by 1%

- For older adults the gain of each 0.5 kg increases the risk of death by 2%
- Diabetes mellitus Type 2
- Hypertension
- Stroke
- High fats in the blood
- Coronary heart disease
- Gall stones
- Cancers, especially of the colon in men; and gastrointestinal tract, breast and uterus in women
- Dyspnoea or shortness of breath
- Menstrual disorders and hairiness in women
- Pregnancy complications
- Arthritis
- Stress incontinence
- Obstructive sleep apnoea.

If a person loses weight, there is a significant improvement even if the weight loss is not down to the ideal for his height, e.g. a 10% weight loss will produce a 20% fall in mortality.

Fall in weight can be done if the patient carries out the following.

1. Reduce energy intake. (The theoretical first aim to reduce by 2.5 MJ (600 kcal) per day.)
   Fatty and oily foods especially should be avoided.
   Return to a more traditional diet as long as cereals and in particular vegetables form a major part, although if possible some fruit and some animal protein should be included.
2. Increase exercise. Walking for half an hour quickly each day can result in the loss of 1 kg in one month.
3. Join a group of people trying to lose weight.
4. Drugs are too expensive to have any real part to play in the loss of weight and are not needed if the above can be done.

Alcohol and alcoholism

Ethyl alcohol or ethanol is the alcohol contained in intoxicating drinks (see Figure 24.6 page 397). (Methyl alcohol or methanol is a severe poison which may be put with ethyl alcohol so that it will not be drunk; and is then called 'methylated spirits'. Drinking methanol is very dangerous and likely to lead to blindness and probably death.)

Ethanol in small doses of less than two standard drinks a day may have some beneficial effects on vascular and other diseases. In larger doses, however, it damages many body systems. Heavy drinking takes about 10 years off the life of all men and women who do so.

Ethanol itself has no nutritional value apart from one standard drink or 10 g providing 300 kJ or 70–100 kcal. It is absorbed quickly from the bowel unless food, especially fat, is also present. About 2–10% is excreted in the air breathed out and in the urine; the rest is destroyed by the liver.

Blood alcohol levels of 20–30 mg/dl (i.e. 1–2 drinks) cause changes in behaviour, muscle control and thinking; 80–100 mg/dl intoxication and drunkenness; 160–200 mg/dl deep but disturbed sleep; and 300–400 mg/dl, death. The effects of alcohol depend on the rate the blood alcohol level rises; whether it is actually rising or falling at the time; whether other drugs are affecting the body and in particular the brain at the same time; and the fact that tolerance to the brain effects of alcohol develop, so that after regular drinking less noticeable changes occur, although of course the dangerous side effects continue.

Ethanol affects all body systems.

In the gastrointestinal tract there is irritation, often with vomiting and with bleeding, and oesophageal tears can occur. Acute pancreatitis is three times more common than in non-drinkers. Hepatitis and later cirrhosis develops in one fifth of alcoholics.

Cancer increases as the amount of alcohol increases. Breast cancer is one and a half times more common in women who drink 1 ½ standard drinks a day. Other mainly gastrointestinal cancers increase up to five times the rate of non-drinkers when a person has 7–8 standard drinks a day.

Blood changes of the red blood cells (become larger or macrocytes) and white blood cells occur, as does decreased immunity.

Cardiovascular changes include an increase in blood pressure. Heavy drinking causes heart failure by damaging the heart muscle and causing an irregular heart beat and at times clots within the heart itself.

Sexual drive may be increased by ethanol, but ability to have sexual intercourse is decreased. Heavy drinking causes permanent damage to the testes, impotence and large breasts in men; and irregular periods, decreased fertility and if pregnant at times damage to the baby (fetal alcohol syndrome) in women.

Muscle weakness and arthritis (gout) are common.

Brain damage is of many kinds. Acute intoxication is well known. Chronic heavy drinking is accompanied by 'blackouts' with complete forgetfulness of what happened during drinking, poor sleep, obstructive sleep apnoea, peripheral neuropathy, a number of different kinds of encephalitis (Wernicke's syndrome has paralysis of some eye muscles and unsteadiness in walking also), dementia, poor memory, and all sorts of psychiatric abnormalities

Alcohol intoxication is well known as are its effects, especially motor vehicle accidents.

Alcohol abuse is said to occur when there is repetitive drinking that has bad effects on social, family, work or health.

Alcohol dependence is said to occur when the person continues to look for and get alcohol despite its bad effects. Criteria for alcohol dependence include drinking being more important than other activities, tolerance to the effects of alcohol, repeated alcohol withdrawal syndrome when alcohol is not drunk, relief of withdrawal symptoms by further drinking, a feeling that the patient has to drink and going back to drinking even if the patient stops for a while.

Alcohol withdrawal syndrome is a serious sometimes fatal illness. If a person has had his whole body, and in particular his whole nervous system depressed by alcohol for months or years, then the activity of the nervous system has had to be increased so that it can still function (work). The withdrawal syndrome occurs if the alcohol is then suddenly stopped (e.g. admission to the health centre for treatment of an injury or illness), the depressant effect of the alcohol goes within hours but the increased activity of the nervous system takes about a week or more to settle. This increased activity of the nervous system causes tremor or shaking; agitation and anxiety; nervous system cause of increased pulse rate, breathing rate and temperature; insomnia or not being able to sleep, usually with frightening dreams; and being unable to eat properly. These symptoms start by 6–12 hours, are at their worst at 2 or 3 days and improve by the fourth or fifth days. In its most severe form this alcohol withdrawal syndrome causes delirium tremens (called DTs) with delirium (see Chapter 35 pages 568, 575) and severe tremor and other symptoms as above, including terrifying hallucinations and delusions. At times, even epileptic fits can occur. Death is not uncommon.

Social problems caused by alcohol include not going to work, unemployment, marriage problems, child abuse, money problems and getting into trouble with the law, including violence and traffic offences.

The so-called 'CAGE' questions are helpful insofar as one 'yes' response from a patient should raise the suspicion of alcohol being a problem, and more than one 'yes' to these questions is a strong indication of abuse or dependence.

C Have you ever felt you ought to **C**ut down on your drinking?

A Have people **A**nnoyed you by criticising your drinking?

G Have you ever felt **G**uilty or bad about your drinking?

E Have you ever had a drink first thing in the morning to steady your nerves or get rid of a hangover (**E**ye-opener)?

Education about alcohol, i.e. no more than 1(–2) standard drinks at a time or 7(–14) in a week for a woman, or 2(–3) at a time or 14(–21) in a week for a man, is important. This needs to be explained to all people, especially young people, and especially to people who may have a problem with alcohol.

Acute intoxication should be managed by making sure that there is no other injury or illness present, and checking that the cardiovascular, respiratory and nervous systems are stable. It is best that the patient be just kept quiet until the effects wear off. If a drug has to be used, a benzodiazepine (although the only one you are likely to have available is diazepam) would be safer than using other drugs. It is important the patient be checked regularly in case there is a head or other injury or meningitis, malaria, pneumonia or other condition which may cause his death.

Withdrawal syndrome needs urgent treatment. Make sure no other condition is present such as liver failure, gastrointestinal bleeding, heart irregularity, etc. Give all patients thiamine 50–100 mg daily and if possible other vitamin B vitamins. The patient is likely to have tremor, hallucinations and at times even fitting. These are treated by giving a safe nervous system depressant drug such as diazepam, in doses 5 up to 20 mg each 4–6 hours to control these symptoms and then when they are controlled, slowly reducing the diazepam over 5–7 days. Besides all the usual physical conditions to check for, if there is deterioration, do not forget to check the blood sugar (glucose) for low levels which need treatment.

Rehabilitation of alcoholics is difficult in the health centre. It is important to gain the trust of the patient and try to work out with them how they are going to cope with the problem of not drinking again. It is important to get the family involved so that they can support the patient. It is very worthwhile going to a group such as 'Alcoholics Anonymous', if such a group exists in your area, as reformed alcoholics in these groups can probably give the patient the best support and advice.

Some common symptoms and signs and their management

Pain or difficulty swallowing (dysphagia)

Do a full history and examination (see Chapter 6).

Weigh the patient, test the urine and do the haemoglobin estimation.

Look for evidence of these conditions:

1. *Foreign body in throat or oesophagus*
   - often history of having swallowed bone or other object
   - sudden pain when swallowing
   - feeling of something stuck in the neck or chest
   - vomiting at first; and if complete block cannot swallow saliva
   - no fever or other abnormal signs at first
   Urgently transfer to Medical Officer if you cannot see and remove the foreign body; as severe, usually fatal, neck or chest infections can develop.
2. *Snakebite*
   - cannot swallow
   - cannot open eyes, talk or cough properly
   - history of snakebite
   - sometimes pain near the bite or abnormal bleeding from many places
   See Chapter 33 page 554 urgently and give antivenom.
3. *Infection in the mouth or throat*
   - pain on swallowing
   - acute start
   - inflamed mucous membrane with patches of *Monilia* (thrush); or ulcers in the mouth; or pus on the tonsils which are enlarged; or tender swelling of abscess in throat or neck
   - sometimes fever
   - lymph nodes in neck often enlarged
   See Chapter 20 pages 284–285.
4. *Diphtheria*
   - things swallowed come back through the nose
   - difficulty seeing
   - other parts of the body paralysed at times
   - often no diphtheria immunisation
   - grey material stuck on to red inflamed throat (or sores on skin)
   See Chapter 20 page 284.
5. *HIV infection with oesophageal thrush or CMV infection or Kaposi's sarcoma, etc.*
   - age 20–50
   - other history or examination suggests possible HIV infection
   See Chapter 19 pages 226–227.
6. *Rabies*
   - a history of dog (or bat) bite
   - symptoms and signs of encephalitis (Chapter 25 page 415) with episodes of over-activity or some paralysis
   - even the sight of water may cause spasms of throat muscles
   See Chapter 25 pages 416–417.
7. *Tetanus*
   - starts over a few days
   - if asked to do so, cannot open mouth widely
   - spasms of rest of body may come and go
   - often recent wound
   - no tetanus immunisation
   See Chapter 25 pages 419–420.
8. *Diseases of the oesophagus* including cancer, Chagas' disease, achalasia, acid reflux, stenosis, etc.
   - slow start of difficulty in swallowing – at first only solid food; but later also soft food, then fluids
   - may vomit food and fluid eaten, but no bile in vomitus
   - weight loss
   Transfer all such cases to a Medical Officer at a hospital.
9. *Acting out*
   - the patient has a big problem
   - the patient has no abnormal signs on examination
   - the condition gets better if you discover his problem and solve it
   Discover and help solve the patient's problem.

Transfer

Transfer patients to Medical Officer care when there is:

1. a foreign body (urgent),
2. tetanus or diphtheria (urgent),
3. no improvement after treatment of the suspected cause (non-urgent), or
4. you cannot find the cause after observing the patient for a week (non-urgent).

Nausea or vomiting

Causes include:

1. Irritation of the gastrointestinal tract.
   (a) All causes of gastroenteritis (see page 360).
   (b) Alcohol. Some foods. Some drugs.
   (c) Peptic ulcer (see page 352).
2. Block or paralysis of the gastrointestinal tract.

(a) Intestinal or 'pyloric' obstruction and gastro-oesophageal reflux (see pages 351 and 352).

(b) Paralytic ileus (like obstruction but no colic)
- 1–3 days after abdominal operation or prolonged gastroenteritis or peritonitis or haemoperitoneum
- transfer to Medical Officer.

(c) Peritonitis (see page 349).

(d) Haemorrhage into peritoneum (e.g. ectopic pregnancy or ruptured spleen) (see page 350).

3. Irritation of vomiting centre in brain.

(a) From disease of brain:
- cerebral tumour or tuberculoma or abscess, etc. (see Chapter 25 page 421),
- meningitis (see Chapter 25 page 409),
- encephalitis (see Chapter 25 page 415).

(b) From changes in blood going to the brain:
- any fever (including malaria),
- any infection (especially middle ear inflammation),
- pregnancy (or other hormone changes),
- chemicals – drugs, poisons, toxins,
- kidney (renal) failure,
- hepatitis,
- diabetes.

(c) From 'higher' centre in the brain:
- fear,
- worry,
- severe pain of any cause.

Diagnosis

Do a full history and examination (see Chapter 6). Test the urine for protein, sugar, bile and pus. Diagnose the cause by the other symptoms and signs the patient has. Then treat the cause.

Which of these seven groups of symptoms and signs does your patient have?

1. Vomiting and
- constipation *and*
- abdominal pain, which is colic, *and*
- abdominal swelling (distension).

Then: intestinal obstruction. See page 351.

If he *also* has constant abdominal pain or a tender area in the abdomen especially over a hernia.

Then: strangulated obstruction. See page 351.

2. Vomiting and
- constipation *and*
- abdominal pain, which is constant, *and*
- abdominal swelling (distension) *and*
- abdominal tenderness all over.

Then: paralysis of the intestine because of pus or blood in the peritoneal cavity (peritonitis or haemoperitoneum).

See pages 349–350.

3. Vomiting and
- diarrhoea *and*
- abdominal pain, which is colic, *but*
- no abdominal tenderness.

Then: gastroenteritis. See pages 360–366.

4. Vomiting after food and
- abdominal pain (in epigastrium, worse after food, relieved by vomiting)
- abdominal tenderness only in epigastrium.

Then: peptic ulcer. See page 352.

5. Vomiting and
- headache *or*
- stiff neck *or*
- confusion *or*
- fitting *or*
- paralysis *or*
- unconsciousness.

Then:
- meningitis, *or*
- cerebral malaria, *or*
- encephalitis, *or*
- head injury, *or*
- brain tumour, etc.

If the condition is acute and the patient is very 'sick' (but not if he has a head injury), do a malaria smear, give IV or IMI artesunate or quinine, do a lumbar puncture and see Chapter 25 pages 409–414 and 421–425.

If the condition is chronic and the patient is not acutely 'sick' or if he has a head injury and is not improving, transfer to the Medical Officer.

6. Vomiting and
- conditions found that would affect blood going to brain.

Then:
- fever of any cause (especially malaria) (see Chapter 36 pages 585–587), *or*
- infection of any type (especially middle ear infection) (see Chapter 20 pages 280–281), *or*
- if menstrual period/s have been missed: pregnancy (see an obstetrics book), *or*
- if jaundice: hepatitis (see Chapter 24 page 393), *or*
- if wasted, anaemic, BP high, protein in urine: kidney failure (see Chapter 26 page 449 and a medical reference book), *or*

- if glucose in urine and blood glucose high: diabetes. (See Chapter 30 pages 499–504.)

7. Vomiting and
- pain *or*
- fear *or*
- worry *but*
- no other abnormalities found on physical examination.

Then:
- pain (see Chapter 7 pages 32–34), *or*
- fear or worry (see Chapter 35 pages 569, 577 and 582).

Vomiting blood (haematemesis)

If a patient has recently vomited blood, then:

- Immediately start an IV drip (before doing the history and examination).
- Do a full history and examination and test the urine (see Chapter 6).
- Find out the answers to these four questions.

1. *Did the patient really VOMIT the blood?*
   Check that the patient vomited blood and did not:
   (a) cough up the blood, or
   (b) vomit up blood swallowed after coughing up blood (haemoptysis) or bleeding from the upper respiratory tract (e.g. bleeding nose).
   Look at the blood.
   (a) If it is brown it is from the stomach (the acid turns it brown).
   (b) If it is bright red it is more likely to be from haemoptysis or the upper respiratory tract; but if there is a lot of gastrointestinal bleeding the blood can be bright red.
   If the patient has blood in the gastrointestinal tract he will later pass melaena (black, smelly stools like tar).

2. *How much blood has been vomited up?*
   If more than 300 ml (1 cup), it is an emergency. Put in an IV drip *immediately*, in case the patient bleeds again and needs resuscitation.

3. *Is the patient shocked?*
   If he is shocked, start intravenous resuscitation immediately (see Chapter 27 page 468) and make arrangements for emergency transfer or blood transfusion.

4. *What is the cause of the bleeding?*
   (a) Stomach and duodenal diseases.
      - Peptic ulcer.
         - History of epigastric pain related to food.
         - Tenderness in the epigastrium.
      - Peptic ulcer caused by acetylsalicylic acid (or anti-arthritis tablet (NSAID)) or alcohol.
         - The recent taking of acetylsalicylic acid or other NSAID (even only a few) or alcohol (usually a lot).
      - Cancer of the stomach.
         - Older person.
         - Feeling of fullness soon after eating.
         - Weight loss.
         - Not cured by proper treatment for severe peptic ulcer.
   (b) Oesophageal diseases.
      - Cirrhosis of the liver with varicose veins in the oesophagus.
         - Ascites, often marked.
         - Some oedema.
         - Wasting and other signs of liver failure.
      - Schistosomiasis with liver disease and varicose veins in the oesophagus.
         - From area where schistosomiasis occurs, bowel symptoms, usually blood in the stool in the past.
         - Anaemia and ascites may not be present.
      - Tear in the oesophagus after vomiting from any cause.
         - Bleeding started AFTER vomiting.
   (c) Bleeding disease.
      - Snakebite.
         - History of being bitten by a snake.
      - Rare blood diseases.

If the patient:
- has vomited more than 1 cup of blood and/or
- has vomited blood more than once and/or
- has melaena too and/or
- is anaemic and/or
- is shocked;

then manage as follows:

1. Set up an IV drip. Give IV fluids/plasma volume expanders/blood as necessary (see Chapter 27 pages 468–470).
2. Give sedation – diazepam 5–10 mg (1–2 ml) IMI; or if you are certain the patient does not have cirrhosis, morphine 10 mg (1 ml) IMI.
3. Insert an intragastric tube and aspirate till the stomach is empty; then aspirate hourly. When no blood comes back, give antacids every hour.
4. Transfer the patient to Medical Officer care in case he bleeds again and needs blood transfusion.
5. See Index for other treatment of the diagnosed condition.

Diarrhoea or dysentery

Diarrhoea (frequent (>3 in a day) soft or watery stools) is a symptom – not a disease. You must try to find out the cause. Diarrhoea can cause dehydration and death.

Dysentery (diarrhoea with blood and often mucus) is a symptom – not a disease. You must try to find out the cause. Dysentery can cause: dehydration and death; but also anaemia and shock from blood loss; and also allow infection into blood (septicaemia).

Diarrhoea and dysentery usually occur with intestinal colic (often), vomiting (sometimes) and other symptoms and signs (sometimes), i.e. gastroenteritis.

Often you cannot find the cause in a health centre.

But it is always important to do the following three things:

1. Look for dehydration of the patient (see page 362). Prevent or treat dehydration (see page 364).
2. Try to find the cause (see below).
   Treat any cause you find.
3. Find out if others are also affected (i.e. an epidemic). Control and prevention may be necessary.

Do these things by doing a full history and examination (see Chapter 6) and see pages 360–366.

Causes to look for include:

1. 'Food poisoning'
   Often there is a history of others who ate the same food also being affected (i.e. an epidemic).
   Sometimes there is a history of eating food which may be poisonous (certain fish or plants); or food which did not look, smell and taste as it should; or food which was not eaten soon after it was cooked.
   Sometimes there is a history of taking drugs.
2. Infections in the intestine.
   These include viruses, bacteria (*Escherichia coli*, *Shigella*, *Campylobacter*, *Salmonella typhi*, other *Salmonella*, *Clostridium*, *Vibrio cholerae*), amoebae, e.g. *Giardia* and helminths, e.g. *Schistosoma*.
   Dysentery is caused by some of these infections.
   Fever is often caused by infections.
3. 'Medical' causes include:
   • any cause of fever, especially malaria,
   • any acute infection, especially middle ear infection,
   • any chronic infection, especially visceral leishmaniasis and HIV infection,
   • malnutrition,
   • lactose intolerance (if the patient has also drunk milk), or malabsorption including tropical sprue,
   • change in diet, and
   • anxiety.

4. 'Surgical' causes:
   • intestinal obstruction, early or incomplete,
   • enteritis necroticans.
5. HIV infection (especially if chronic diarrhoea and weight loss) must always be remembered.

See also Table 23.2 page 363.

Management includes:

1. Prevent or treat dehydration (see page 364).
2. Treat any underlying cause you find (see above). Always give antimalarial drugs (see Chapter 13 pages 79, 80 unless you are certain that the patient does not have malaria).
3. Give chloramphenicol or other antibiotic and metronidazole only if necessary (see page 365).
4. Transfer to Medical Officer care if necessary (see page 365).
5. Do any control and prevention that is necessary (see page 366).

Persistent or recurrent diarrhoea or dysentery

Diarrhoea or dysentery may last for more than 2–4 weeks. It may start as acute gastroenteritis and persist or continue; it may start as acute gastroenteritis and seem to go away but then come back again and again; and it may just start without an acute attack but not go away.

These conditions may occur in otherwise normal people but are much more common in patients with HIV infection.

Causes include:

1. Continuing infection
   • Viruses especially
     HIV which itself can damage the bowel wall.
     Cytomegalovirus in HIV patients.
   • Bacteria, including
     non-typhoid *Salmonella*, especially in HIV patients.
     Shigella
     E. coli special types
     Campylobacter
     Clostridium difficile
   • Protozoa, especially
     Entamoeba histolytica in anyone.
     Giardia in anyone.
     Cyclospora, especially in children.
     Cryptosporidium, *Isospora belli* and *Microsporidia*, especially in HIV patients.
     Leishmania (kala azar) in anyone, but especially HIV patients.
   • Worms, especially

Schistosoma mansoni and *japonicum*.
Strongyloides, but also others.

2. Delayed recovery from an acute infection
   Malnutrition
   Zinc deficiency.
3. The effect of previous infection in the bowel
   Hypolactasia
   Post-infective malabsorption
   Tropical sprue.
   See page 374.
4. Repeated new infections
   This can occur if sanitation (disposal of faeces) is not good, flies are many, personal hygiene (washing hands after toilet, etc) is not good or if water drunk is not safe (contaminated with faeces).
   See page 366.
5. Others
   • Pancreatic disease if not enough pancreatic juice made to help digestion and absorption.
   Chronic calcific pancreatitis (see Chapter 24 page 401) is common in some areas.
   • Liver disease if not enough bile made to help digestion and absorption.
   • Short bowel when not enough bowel left for digestion and absorption, e.g. after enteritis necroticans or surgery when a large part of the gastrointestinal tract had to be removed.
   • Infection damaging the bowel, especially HIV and TB.
   • Tumours damaging the bowel, especially lymphomas and carcinoma (cancer of bowel).
   • Inflammatory bowel diseases which are special kinds of (possibly autoimmune) inflammation of the bowel which need Medical Officer diagnosis by special tests, e.g. endoscopy or colonoscopy and biopsy.

Management

1. Treat any dehydration as for acute gastroenteritis.
2. Treat any infection.
   If possible, after discussing how to do this with the Medical Officer, send three lots of stool specimens for microscopy (including for TB, worms and amoebae, etc. and also culture and sensitivity tests) and blood for HIV test, full blood count, urea, electrolytes, liver function tests. Ask the Medical Officer to tell you what the results mean and what you should do, or if the patient needs to be sent for other tests (e.g. endoscopy or colonoscopy to look at the gastrointestinal tract; faecal fat tests to see if fat malabsorption; INR and other tests to see if vita-

min malabsorption; glucose and xylose tests to see if carbohydrate malabsorption; Schilling test to see if vitamin B_{12} malabsorption due to ileal disease, etc.).
If transfer not possible, the following could be tried:

(a) TMP 160 mg and SMX 800 mg twice daily for 7 days for *Salmonella*, *Shigella* and some of the protozoa; and if not effective:

(b) Chloramphenicol 500–1000 mg orally four times daily for 7–10 days for *Salmonella, Shigella* and some other bacteria (in some areas you may be told because of sensitivity tests to use a different antibiotic such as ciprofloxacin).

(c) Metronidazole 400 mg three times a day for 10–14 days for *Clostridium difficile*, some protozoa, but especially *Giardia* and *Entamoeba histolytica*.

(d) Tetracycline 500 mg four times a day together with the metronidazole for some infections such as *Campylobacter* and tropical sprue and to help treat *Entamoeba histolytica*.

(e) Albendazole 400 mg daily for 3 days. Give before the above if worms known to be present. This dose will treat strongyloides and most other worms but you may be told to give a larger dose of 800 mg twice daily for 4 weeks for microsporidia or other protozal infections. Do not give albendazole in a large dose unless told to do so, and do not give albendazole if pregnant or could be pregnant and especially in the first 3 months of pregnancy.

(f) If schistosomiasis give (before the other drugs) praziquantel 40 mg/kg as a single dose (see Chapter 18 page 190).

(g) Anti-retroviral drugs if HIV infection and stage 3 or 4 may need consideration.

3. Treat any underlying medical or surgical case.
4. Treat symptoms.
   If after all investigation and treatment possible has been done and diarrhoea continues, codeine phosphate 30–60 mg each 4 hours may be needed.

Blood in stools

Always look at stools:

• to check there is blood in the stools, and
• to see what kind of blood there is, and
• to see where the blood is.

1. If fresh blood is on the outside of the stool, then it is probably due to:

- haemorrhoids (see a surgery book), or
- anal fissure (see a surgery book).

2. If blood is mixed with diarrhoeal stool, then it is:
   - dysentery (see gastroenteritis pages 387–388) for cause (note especially – bacterial dysentery, amoebic dysentery, and schistosomiasis); or
   - cancer of the intestine (see page 375).
3. If blood is mixed with solid stool, then it is most likely to be:
   - cancer of lower large intestine (see page 375).
4. If black smelly stools like tar (melaena), then it is:
   - upper gastrointestinal tract bleeding (see haematemesis, page 386).

Constipation

Constipation is present when the patient does not pass faeces for longer than is normal for that person.

Complete constipation:

- no faeces or flatus (gas) passed,
- usually serious and needs immediate management,
- causes – bowel obstruction (see page 351) or paralytic ileus (see pages 363, 385).

Incomplete constipation:

- less frequent bowel movements than normal,
- usually not immediately serious; but may be indication of serious underlying disease,
- causes – not eating much, dehydration (see page 362), incomplete bowel obstruction (especially bowel cancer, page 351), drugs, e.g. codeine or morphine.

If, however, no cause can be found and the constipation continues for more than 2 weeks, or is getting worse, then transfer the patient for Medical Officer investigation and treatment (as could be incomplete bowel obstruction from cancer or amoeboma or schistosomiasis or other bowel condition).

Abdominal pain – tenderness – guarding – rigidity

See Chapter 36 pages 593–598.

Abdominal swellings

See Chapter 36 pages 598–604.

Loss of weight

See Chapter 36 pages 590–591.

24 Disorders of the Liver, Bile Ducts and Pancreas

Anatomy

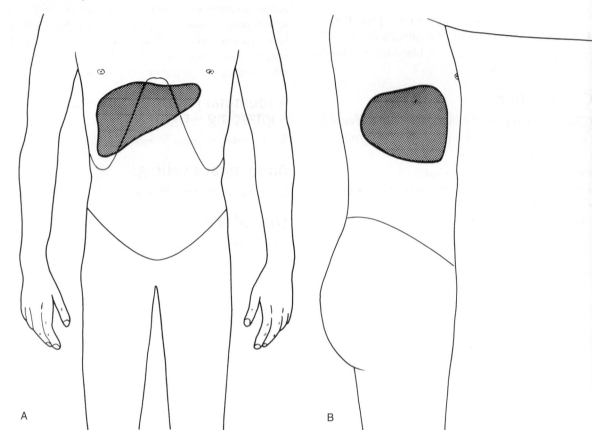

Figure 24.1 A and B (above) *The normal position of the normal liver (A) on the front of the body and (B) on the right side of the body. Note that most of the normal liver is under the right ribs. In the mid-clavicular line at the right side the liver is almost as high as the nipple and is only about 1 cm below the edge of the ribs.*

Physiology and pathology

The liver has many functions including:

1. manufacturing and storing bile;
2. storing sugar and controlling the amount of sugar in the blood;
3. manufacturing proteins and other substances; and
4. removing toxins, poisons, drugs and hormones, etc. from the blood.

Manufacturing and storing bile

The liver cells make bile. Small tubes or ducts take the bile from the liver cells. These join to form larger tubes, until they all join into one large tube called the common hepatic duct. The cystic duct goes from this to the gall bladder (see Figure 24.2) where the bile is concentrated and stored. When a person eats, the gall bladder squeezes the bile back through the cystic duct to the common bile duct which takes the bile into

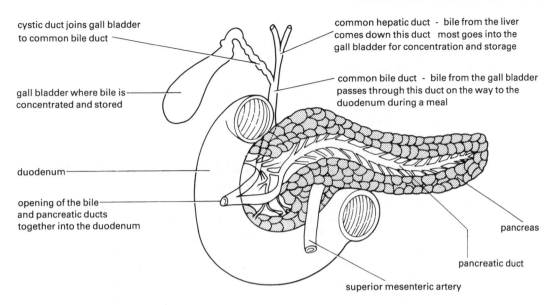

cystic duct joins gall bladder
to common bile duct

common hepatic duct - bile from the liver
comes down this duct   most goes into the
gall bladder for concentration and storage

common bile duct - bile from the gall bladder
passes through this duct on the way to the
duodenum during a meal

gall bladder where bile is
concentrated and stored

duodenum

opening of the bile
and pancreatic ducts
together into the duodenum

pancreas

pancreatic duct

superior mesenteric artery

Figure 24.2 *The anatomy of the bile ducts, pancreas and duodenum.*

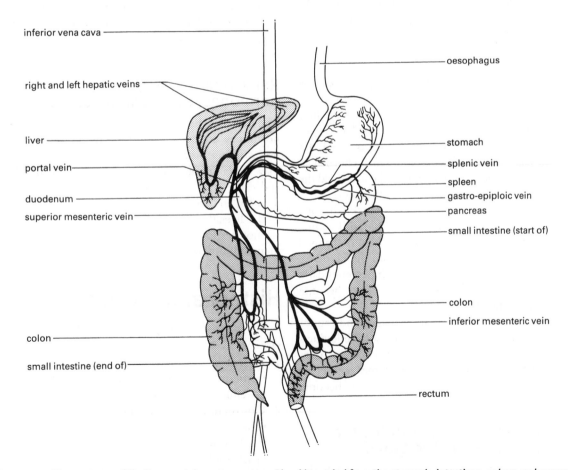

inferior vena cava

oesophagus

right and left hepatic veins

liver

stomach

portal vein

splenic vein

spleen

gastro-epiploic vein

duodenum

pancreas

superior mesenteric vein

small intestine (start of)

colon

inferior mesenteric vein

colon

small intestine (end of)

rectum

Figure 24.3 *The anatomy of the liver portal venous system. Blood is carried from the stomach, intestines, spleen and pancreas into the liver by the portal vein. Hepatic veins then carry the blood from the liver to the inferior vena cava. The liver also has its own supply of arterial blood from the hepatic artery.*

the duodenum. In the duodenum the bile mixes with the food.

Bile contains bile salts which help the fat in the food to be digested and absorbed. Bile salts are reabsorbed further down the intestine so that they can be used again.

Bile also contains bilirubin. Bilirubin is a yellow waste product from worn out or damaged red blood cells. These red blood cells are usually destroyed in the spleen. The spleen then puts the bilirubin into the blood. This bilirubin is insoluble (not able to dissolve) and cannot get into the urine from the blood. The liver cells therefore take it out of the blood, change it to make it soluble, and then put it into the bile. When the bilirubin in the bile reaches the intestine it becomes brown, and makes the faeces brown. If any of this changed bilirubin in the bile gets back into the blood, it is soluble and is taken out of the blood by the kidney and passed in the urine. The urine then looks brown or black (like tea or coffee without milk or like 'cola' drinks), though many patients say it looks 'red'. (Also the colour of the froth on the urine shaken in a test tube is yellow – normally urine froth is white, even if the urine is yellow.)

In haemolytic conditions, when many red cells are destroyed, much bilirubin goes into the blood. If the amount of bilirubin in the blood is more than the liver can take out, the amount of bilirubin in the blood rises. The patient therefore looks yellow; he is jaundiced. But the urine colour and the faeces colour remain normal (as the insoluble bilirubin cannot get into the urine and the faeces cannot be any more brown than they are).

In conditions which obstruct (or block) the bile ducts, the bile is reabsorbed into the blood. The bile salts cause itch. The bilirubin, which is the sort changed by the liver to be soluble, is taken from the blood by the kidney and put in the urine, which becomes dark. No bile reaches the intestine so the faeces become light or even white.

In hepatitis, the liver cells are damaged and cannot take all the bile out of the blood. The small bile ducts are also damaged, and bile with changed bilirubin goes back into the blood. The patient becomes jaundiced. The urine becomes dark. The faeces may become lighter; but they do not become white.

Storing sugar and controlling the amount of sugar in the blood

The blood which comes to the liver through the portal vein (see Figure 24.3) after eating is often full of sugar absorbed from the intestine. The concentration of sugar is often far more than the body needs. The liver cells receive messages from the pancreas (through a hormone called insulin) to remove much of the sugar and store it. When the concentration of sugar in the blood falls, the pancreas makes less insulin and the liver puts some of the sugar back into the blood. In that way the body does not have too much sugar after eating and not enough between meals.

Manufacturing proteins and other substances

The liver is the main place for building up the proteins the body needs. These proteins are built up from the substances which the intestine absorbs from the food, and which come to the liver in the portal vein (see Figure 24.3). Some of these proteins (albumin) stay in the blood to hold water inside the blood vessels, and stop it going out of the blood vessels and causing oedema and ascites. Other proteins made in the liver have other functions, including helping blood to clot.

If the liver does not work properly, the person may develop oedema and ascites, wasting of muscles and bleeding.

Removing toxins, poisons, drugs and hormones, etc. from the blood

The liver also destroys many poisons, toxins, drugs and hormones, etc. which enter the blood. If the liver is not working properly, ordinary doses of some drugs may be dangerous; hormones may stay in the blood and cause such things as enlargement of the breasts in men; and toxins from the intestines which come to the liver through the portal vein (see Figure 24.3) are not destroyed and may damage the brain, causing mental disturbance or unconsciousness.

History and examination

If you suspect liver disease or jaundice, try to find out if there is:

1. Liver structure abnormality
   - pain or tenderness of the liver
   - swelling of or lumps in the liver.
2. Obstruction of the bile ducts
   - jaundice
   - dark urine
   - pale stools.
3. Liver cell failure (failure of the liver cells to do their work)
   - jaundice

• fluid in the body tissues – oedema and ascites
• wasting of muscles
• bleeding
• loss of full consciousness or abnormal mental state.

4. Haemolysis, if jaundice is present
   • anaemia
   • enlarged spleen, etc.

5. Infection in the liver or other parts of the body
   • fever, malaise, etc.
   • temperature raised
   • fast pulse   } general symptoms
   • symptoms and   and signs of infection
     signs of hepatitis,
     pneumonia, malaria
     or septicaemia.

6. Signs of high pressure in the portal vein
   • ascites (high pressure pushes water out of the portal vein and the 'oedema fluid' collects in the peritoneal cavity).
   • gastrointestinal bleeding usually with vomiting of blood if one of these veins under high pressure bursts.

In the routine clinical examination of a patient, you may find these things in liver disease or jaundice:

• Loss of full consciousness } if there is liver
• Mental abnormality   } (cell) failure.
• Temperature raised, if there is infection.
• Pulse fast, if there is infection; but sometimes the pulse is slow in deep jaundice.
• Wasting usually, if there is chronic liver failure.
• Oedema usually, if there is chronic liver failure.
• Pallor, if there is haemolysis or bleeding.
• Jaundice if there is haemolysis or liver cell disease or obstruction of the bile ducts.
• Bleeding if there is liver failure (and especially gastrointestinal bleeding if there is high portal venous pressure).
• Ascites if there is liver failure (especially if there is high portal venous pressure).
• Liver enlargement (see page 401 for causes).
• Liver tenderness (see page 401 for causes).
• Splenomegaly if there is haemolysis or high portal venous pressure (but the spleen may be enlarged because of other causes, e.g. malaria or kala azar).
• Enlarged veins on the abdomen suggest high pressure in or obstruction of the portal vein.
• Urine – dark (like tea) and bile present on testing, which suggests liver cell disease or obstruction of the bile ducts (urine is normal in haemolysis).
• Faeces – light or white if there is obstruction of the bile ducts.

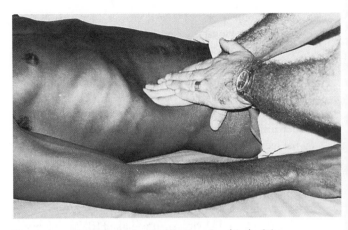

Figure 24.4 *Method of palpating for the edge (size) of the liver. See text for description of the method.*

Method of examination of the liver

Gently put the right hand with the fingers pointing to the patient's head flat on the right lateral abdomen. Place the hand outside the rectus muscle (the long strong muscle which runs down the middle third of the abdomen). Put the other hand either on top of the right hand or at the back of the patient to hold the liver forward. Ask the patient to take a deep breath. As the patient breathes in, gently press the hand inwards and upwards. (See Figure 24.4.)

Start low down in the abdomen (in the right iliac fossa). Move the hand up a little each time the patient breathes out until the fingers reach the edge of the liver, on the edge of the ribs. The edge of the liver hits the ends of the fingers as the patient breathes in.

The gall bladder can be felt at the lower edge of the liver in the mid–clavicular line if it is enlarged due to a block in the common bile duct in a jaundiced patient. It may not be felt, but there may be tenderness in this area if the gall bladder is inflamed (acute cholecystitis due to infection and a gall stone blocking the cystic duct).

Feel the surface of the liver for tenderness and lumps.

If you are not sure about the size of the liver, percuss in the mid–clavicular line from high up in the chest down to the dullness of the liver. (Just below the right nipple.) Check how far down the dullness of the liver goes.

Disorders of the liver and bile ducts

Acute viral hepatitis

Viral hepatitis is a viral infection of the whole body, but it causes mainly inflammation of the liver.

The *cause* is one of several viruses. Hepatitis A virus (HAV) (previously called infectious hepatitis virus) spreads by faecal–oral means. In many developing countries, most adults have had HAV infection during childhood and are immune. As health standards improve, fewer adults will be immune and epidemics will occur. Hepatitis B virus (HBV) (previously called serum hepatitis virus) spreads mainly from blood, semen, vaginal secretions or saliva. This happens at the time of birth or during childhood (when there is close skin contact, sores, scratches, etc.) or during sexual intercourse or when blood is transfused or from unsterilised needles and syringes at health centres or among IV drug addicts. Hepatitis C and D viruses, spread like HBV; and hepatitis E virus like HAV; but these are much less common. In many developing countries, most adults have had HBV or HCV as an infant or in childhood and most are immune to HBV infection. However, up to 15–30% may still in fact carry the virus in their blood, as up to 90% of infected infants and up to 10% of infected older children and adults become carriers.

Other viruses (cytomegalovirus, Epstein–Barr virus, arboviruses, e.g. yellow fever virus and other viral causes of haemorrhagic fevers) cause hepatitis; but yellow fever and haemorrhagic fever are severe acute diseases (see Chapter 17 pages 170–172).

The incubation period for HAV is long (2–6 weeks) and for HBV very long (6 weeks to 6 months).

Symptoms and signs

For the first week the patient complains of:
• mild fever (a high fever is not common),
• malaise,
• loss of appetite, nausea, vomiting, etc.,
• mild right upper abdominal pain (over the liver).

After the first week
• dark urine (like tea – test for bilirubin positive),
• jaundice (yellow skin and sclera),
• liver smooth enlarged and tender (but not very enlarged or very tender).

The patient feels much better soon after the jaundice appears; but he may not feel completely well for months.

The jaundice usually gets worse for about 2 weeks and then slowly (sometimes very slowly) gets better.

Hepatitis B or C is a more serious disease. The patient may die from severe acute hepatitis with liver failure. Some patients do not fully recover and have a continuing mild chronic hepatitis. After some years some patients develop chronic liver disease (see page 395). After some years, some patients develop hepatoma, i.e. primary cancer of the liver (see page 399).

Some patients with hepatitis B or C infection cannot destroy all the virus in their body even when they become well. The virus stays in their blood. They are then 'carriers' of hepatitis B or C.

Differential diagnosis

See jaundice page 401; tenderness of liver page 401; or fever with jaundice Chapter 17 pages 170–172 if the patient is very sick or has bleeding.

The condition you are most likely to confuse with viral hepatitis is hepatitis caused by drugs, especially drugs for leprosy, tuberculosis, schistosomiasis, HIV infection or chlorpromazine given for psychosis or vomiting. If a patient on such drugs becomes jaundiced or develops hepatitis, stop all drugs, discuss the problem with a Medical Officer but transfer tuberculosis, HIV and leprosy cases for new treatment – do not just stop their drugs.

Treatment

There is no cure.

Admission is not normally necessary.

If he is 'sick', the patient must rest in bed.

If he has repeated vomiting, give IV fluids for dehydration and maintenance fluids (see gastroenteritis Chapter 23 page 364).

Encourage the patient to drink as much sugary fluid and eat as much good food as possible. Tell him not to drink beer or other alcohol.

Give antimalarial drugs if malaria is a possibility. (See Chapter 13 pages 79, 80.)

Do not give drugs which could affect the liver, especially chlorpromazine or TCE (tetrachloroethylene). Stop all drugs the patient is taking, including oral contraceptives. If the patient is taking tuberculosis, HIV or leprosy drugs, stop ALL of these drugs and transfer the patient to the Medical Officer urgently. (Do *not* just stop TB, HIV or leprosy drugs and take no other action.)

Control and prevention

1. Kill the organism in the body of the original host and reservoir. This is not possible (even with the people who are carriers of HBV or HCV).
2. Stop the means of spread.
   (a) Stop faecal–oral spread
       See Chapter 23 page 366.
       Check then advise about toilets, water supply, hand washing and personal hygiene if an epidemic occurs.

(b) Stop spread by sexual intercourse. Advise about 'safe sex'.
See Chapter 19 pages 256–257.
See also about immunisation.

(c) Stop spread by blood in the health centres (see Chapter 19 page 257). If an epidemic occurs, check that your staff are doing proper sterilisation.

(d) Stop spread by transfusion of infected blood. Do not transfuse blood unless the test for HBV has been done and is negative. See Chapter 19 page 257.

(e) Stop the spread by IV drug addicts.
See Chapter 19 page 258.

(f) Stop the spread in the home.
See Chapter 19 page 258.

(g) Isolation of the patient does not help. The patient with HAV is infectious before the jaundice appears, but for less than 1 week after it appears. Carriers of HBV and HCV are infectious for life.

3. Raise the resistance of susceptible people.

(a) Normal human immunoglobulin (gamma globulin) contains antibodies against HAV.
A killed HAV vaccine exists and live HAV vaccines are being tested.
Immunisation is helpful in areas where contacts of patients are not likely to be immune. HAV vaccine is likely to be helpful if a non-immune person is going to an area where there is much HAV infection. These situations are uncommon in many developing countries at present.

(b) Hepatitis B immunoglobulin (HBIG) is made from the serum of people previously infected with HBV and now immune and not carriers of HBV.
Killed HBV vaccines are effective.
HBIG should be given to HBV non-immune people who are exposed to HBV infection (e.g. health worker with needle stick injury and newborn children if the mother is HBV patient or carrier).
HBV vaccine should be thought about for:
- all newborns but see Chapter 10 pages 44 and 46 (as well as HBIG if the mother is a carrier of HBV),
- all health workers (together with HBIG if exposed to infection),
- all persons in institutions or where HBV infection commonly occurs,
- all sexual and household contacts of HBV positive patients,
- all patients with decreased immunity,
- persons in high risk groups (e.g. IV drug addicts, sex workers, STD patients, male homosexuals, prisoners, etc.).

However, apart from the newborn, many of the above reasons for giving HBV vaccine do not apply in many developing countries as many people have already been infected.

What should be done in your area will depend on the prevalence of infection, the availability of blood testing for infection or to detect carriers, and the availability of immunoglobulin and vaccines. The WHO recommends that all infants receive vaccination for HBV at birth and later or as in Chapter 10 pages 44 and 46. **Find out what the policy of your health department is, and write it in the book here.**

Cirrhosis of the liver (chronic liver disease)

Cirrhosis of the liver is a disease which slowly destroys liver cells in all parts of the liver. Fibrous scar tissue forms and some, but not enough, new liver cells grow. All this slowly destroys the structure and function of the liver.

Cirrhosis is a common disease. It usually affects middle-aged adults; but it can also affect the young and the old.

Pathology and clinical features:

When a patient has cirrhosis, liver cells die. After a long time there are not enough liver cells for the liver to function properly (see pages 390–392).

The following very important *effects of liver failure* occur:

1. If the liver does not make enough of the serum proteins (albumin) which hold fluid inside the blood vessels; fluid goes out of the blood vessels causing oedema and ascites.

2. If the liver does not metabolise hormones, hormone levels get too high and this causes changes in the sexual characteristics of the patient.

3. The liver does not metabolise drugs; the effects of some drugs are increased or last a very long time.

4. The liver does not metabolise toxins from the intestines; and these toxins may stop the brain working properly.

The new fibrous scar tissue presses on the portal veins (see Figure 24.3). The *pressure in the portal vein is more than normal* and the vein becomes overfilled and stretched.

1. Fluid from the vein goes into the peritoneum causing ascites.
2. Sometimes the vein bursts and the blood goes into the gastrointestinal tract, causing vomiting of blood (haematemesis) or passing of faeces which are made of digested blood and so are black, tarry and smelly (melaena).

You cannot find out the *cause of cirrhosis* in a health centre. Previous infection with hepatitis B virus is the most common and important cause in a health centre. Drinking a lot of alcohol most days for a long time can cause cirrhosis. Toxins which form in badly stored grains or groundnuts can cause cirrhosis. In parts of the world where schistosomiasis occurs, schistosomiasis is the common cause of liver damage; but the damage is mostly to the portal vein, not the liver cells.

Symptoms usually include:

1. swelling of the abdomen (usually the first symptom),
2. swelling of the legs,
3. malaise, weakness, etc.
4. haematemesis (vomiting blood) or melaena (black tarry smelly bowel motions made of digested blood).

Signs (Figure 24.5) usually include:

1. Wasting. This is not marked at first; but later it is very severe. You can see it most in the arms and shoulders (as the legs are swollen with oedema). (This is caused by liver cell failure.)
2. Oedema of the legs and back. (This is caused by low protein in the blood from liver cell failure.)
3. Very swollen abdomen caused by ascites. (This is caused by both low protein in the blood from liver cell failure and high portal vein pressure.)
4. The spleen is enlarged. (This is caused by high portal vein pressure; but there are often other causes for an enlarged spleen as well.)

Note two things.

1. The liver is often not enlarged.
2. Jaundice is not common until late in the disease.

Check the patient does not have one of the other common causes of these symptoms or signs.

• Oedema see Chapter 36 page 588.
• Wasting see Chapter 36 page 590.
• Splenomegaly see Chapter 22 pages 344–345.
• Ascites see Chapter 36 pages 602–605.

Check the patient does not have abdominal tuberculosis, which causes ascites *but*:

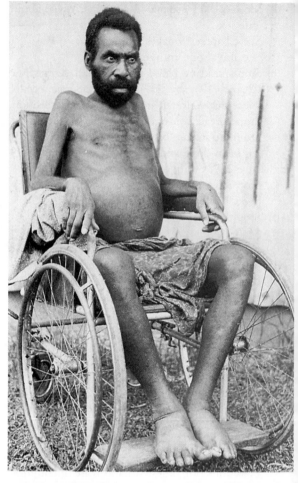

Figure 24.5 *A typical patient with cirrhosis: an adult, very swollen abdomen (ascites), some swelling of the legs (muscle wasting but hidden by oedema), very thin arms and shoulders (muscle wasting).*

• little or no oedema,
• abdominal pain or tenderness (sometimes),
• abdominal masses (sometimes), and
• no help from diuretic treatment.

Test the stools and the urine for schistosomiasis to see if this is the cause (see Chapter 18 pages 189–190).

Complications may develop:

1. Gastrointestinal bleeding
   This comes from burst varicose veins in the oesophagus or stomach caused by high portal pressure. Haematemesis, melaena, anaemia or shock may develop. In most places there is nothing the Medical Officer can do to help, so do not transfer the patient. Find out what you should do in your area in case injection of the oesophageal veins through

an endoscope (sclerotherapy) or even an operation is available, as these can help especially if the cause is schistosomiasis. Treatment at the health centre is with IV fluids. See Chapter 27 pages 468–469 but do not give morphine. Treat also for peptic ulcer in case the patient has bled from an ulcer. See Chapter 23 page 352. Be ready to treat for brain disturbance (see 2 below).

2. Brain function disturbance

   If there is high protein food or blood in the gastro-intestinal tract, toxins made during its digestion and absorption may go past the liver (as there are not enough liver cells left to take the toxins out of the blood) and these toxins can stop the brain working properly. The patient may become psychotic or unconscious. If this happens, give proper nursing care; and give neomycin or streptomycin powder for injection (not by injection) 1 g or amoxicillin 1.5 g *orally* or down an intragastric tube every 6 hours until the patient improves. Give enough magnesium sulphate (e.g. 10–15 mg or ml in water) as often as needed to make the patient pass faeces 2–3 times every day to get rid of the high protein food or blood from the bowel.

Treatment

Cure is not possible.

If the cause is schistosomiasis, give praziquantel. Do not give the previous drugs used for treatment for schistosomiasis as these are dangerous if the patient has liver disease. See Chapter 18 page 190.

Manage complications as described above.

Routine treatment is for the ascites and oedema to make the patient feel better for the rest of his life.

1. Diuretics – hydrochlorothiazide 25–100 mg should be given every morning.
   - You can also give furosemide/frusemide 40–160 mg every morning if hydrochlorothiazide alone is not effective.
   - You can give furosemide/frusemide 20–60 mg by IVI every morning for some days if the tablets are not effective.
   - Sometimes other diuretics which act in another way and can be more effective (e.g. spironolactone or amiloride or triamterene) could be given instead of, or as well as, the hydrochlorothiazide and frusemide.
   - Always give a small dose of each drug first. If the drug is not effective after 3–4 days, increase the dose. If large doses do not help, stop these drugs.

2. If the patient is not eating a tuber diet (i.e. sweet potato, yam, taro, etc.) or if you have given him frusemide, then add potassium chloride 1200 mg three times a day. Do not give potassium if giving the spironolactone, amiloride or triamterene group of diuretics (as these increase potassium).

3. The patient must eat food with high protein but no added salt. He should not eat tinned meat or fish as these contain a lot of salt. He should eat fresh foods if possible.

4. Usually you should *not* drain the ascitic fluid through a needle. See a medical reference book.

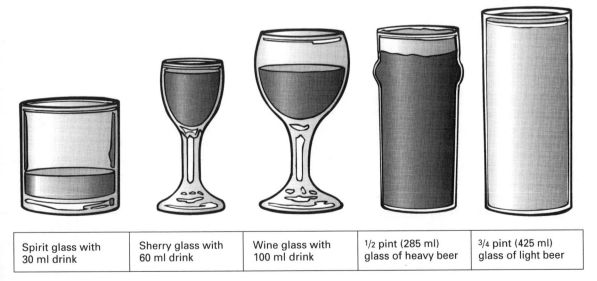

| Spirit glass with 30 ml drink | Sherry glass with 60 ml drink | Wine glass with 100 ml drink | 1/2 pint (285 ml) glass of heavy beer | 3/4 pint (425 ml) glass of light beer |

Figure 24.6 *Standard drinks. From left: one standard drink, 30 ml of spirits or liquers, 60 ml of fortified wine, 100 ml of wine, 285 ml of heavy beer or 425 ml of light beer.*

Check the effect of the treatment every time you see the patient by measuring his:

1. weight,

2. amount of oedema of legs and back, and also,

3. the abdominal circumference with a tape measure, at the level of the umbilicus.

After some months or years, even increased doses of diuretics will not help the oedema, and the patient will die.

Note that if you give large doses of diuretics quickly this may damage the brain function and cause death.

If the patient has only ascites, or if intravenous diuretics do not cure the ascites, refer or transfer (non-urgently) the patient to a Medical Officer to check if he or she has another disease (e.g. tuberculosis of the abdomen or ovarian cyst).

Prevention (1) Prevention of the main cause of chronic liver disease, i.e. hepatitis B infection, is now possible with immunisation. See Chapter 24 page 395. (2) Prevention of schistosomiasis is also possible (see Chapter 18 page 190). (3) Dry storage of grains and groundnuts (so that toxins do not form in them) may help. (4) Educate people not to drink more than 1(–2) standard alcoholic drinks per day if a woman, or 2(–3) if a man (Figure 24.6).

Liver abscess

Liver abscess is an acute or chronic infective inflammation of the liver. It is often caused by amoebae. Acute abscesses are also caused by bacteria. TB is a rare cause but is more common in HIV infected people. The TB infecting organism causes inflammation, then pus and then an abscess forms in the liver.

A liver abscess is not very common; but it is important. If it is treated, it is cured. If it is not treated, the patient dies.

The organisms usually spread to the liver from the intestine through the portal vein. The patient with an amoebic abscess often does not have symptoms or signs of amoebic infection in the intestine (or a history of these).

Symptoms include:

1. Pain and swelling of the abdomen, especially the right upper part. Right shoulder tip pain can occur.

2. The general symptoms of infection – malaise, weight loss, fever, etc.

Signs include:

1. The liver is tender and enlarged. Sometimes you can feel a soft area. Percussion of the right lower ribs *gently* causes pain (see Figure 24.7).

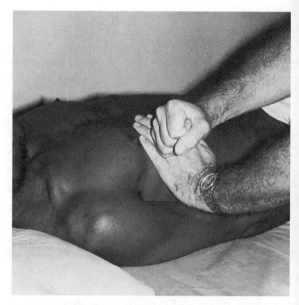

Figure 24.7 *Method of examining for tenderness of the liver (which is under the ribs) by gently percussing over the ribs. It is usual for the liver to be tender if a liver abscess is present. Sometimes you can find the tender area in the liver caused by an abscess by palpating with the fingers between the patient's right ribs, low down at the side or the back.*

2. Fever, fast pulse, anaemia, weight loss, etc. may be present. Jaundice is not common.

3. A right pleural effusion with cough or right sided pneumonia may develop.

The patient gets progressively worse and dies.

Hepatoma causes a similar clinical appearance. TB in the liver occasionally can cause similar symptoms and signs.

Management includes:

1. Check there is not another cause for the enlarged, tender liver (e.g. malaria, acute heart failure, hepatitis).

2. Admit for inpatient treatment.

3. Take 10 ml of venous blood and send the serum to the hospital laboratory with a request for examination for alpha-fetoprotein (AFP). (AFP is positive if it is hepatoma.) In some places an ELISA test on stools or blood diagnostic for amoebic infection is available.

4. Give treatment for abscess while waiting for the result of the AFP. Note the effect of the treatment.

(a) Metronidazole 800 mg three times a day for 10 days. If this dose causes nausea, reduce the dose to 400 mg three times a day for 20 days. Advise the patient not to drink alcohol until the treatment is finished.

(b) Chloroquine 600 mg daily until cured, transferred, diagnosed as hepatoma, or finished 3 weeks' treatment.

(c) Chloramphenicol 1 g four times a day until cured, transferred, diagnosed as hepatoma, or finished 2 weeks' treatment.

5. If AFP is positive, stop this treatment. Inform the patient's relatives of the diagnosis (hepatoma) and prognosis (see below). Allow the patient to go home if he wants to. Give analgesics (see Chapter 7) as necessary at home, or in the hospital, or health centre.

6. If the patient is cured, treat with diloxamide 500 mg three times a day for 10 days to kill all the *E. histolytica* organisms in the bowel.

7. Transfer these cases to Medical Officer care:

(a) High fever, toxicity, etc. (i.e. general symptoms and signs of severe infection) which do not improve after 2 days or are not cured after 5 days of treatment (? pyogenic liver abscess). (Urgent.)

(b) If signs develop suggesting the abscess is about to burst, i.e. fluctuant area in liver, as aspiration of the pus may help (urgent).

(c) Not cured by treatment and AFP is negative. This is especially important in the first 4 months of pregnancy or HIV infection. TB should be a consideration. In other cases a liver biopsy will probably be necessary. (Non-urgent.)

Hepatoma

Hepatoma is a primary cancer of the liver cells themselves. It is common in many tropical countries. It affects young people as well as older adults.

The usual cause is now known to be infection with the hepatitis B virus, usually many years before. Some cases may be caused by toxins in badly stored groundnuts or grains.

Symptoms usually appear and get slowly worse over weeks or months and include:

1. pain in the right upper abdomen,
2. abdominal swelling, and
3. weight loss and weakness and malaise.

Signs include:

1. wasting, and
2. an enlarged hard lumpy liver, which is usually very tender.

Late in the disease liver failure with oedema, ascites and jaundice may occur.

The alpha-fetoprotein (AFP) test is positive. Send the serum from 10 ml of clotted blood to the hospital laboratory for this test immediately if you suspect hepatoma.

The patient usually gets quickly worse and dies in a few months.

Check the patient does not have a liver abscess.

1. Send blood for AFP.
2. Meanwhile treat for liver abscess (see page 398).
3. If AFP comes back positive, stop liver abscess treatment.
4. If AFP comes back negative and the liver abscess drugs have not cured the patient, transfer him to hospital for tests and possibly liver aspiration or biopsy. See liver abscess management (7 this page) for details of the above.

No cure is possible. But paracetamol (or acetylsalicylic acid), with if needed codeine, can be given for pain as necessary. Give morphine regularly (only if the diagnosis is confirmed by AFP). (See Chapter 7 page 32.) Arrange for care and analgesics with the relatives at home; or, if the patient prefers, in the health centre.

Biliary colic, acute cholecystitis and obstructive jaundice

If something suddenly blocks the bile duct (which goes from the liver to the duodenum) or the cystic duct (which goes to and from the gall bladder), the patient feels severe pain called *biliary colic*. If the obstruction remains, infection may occur behind the obstruction. *Obstructive jaundice* may also occur when the patient will become yellow, the stools will become pale and the urine will become dark. These conditions are uncommon. They can be caused by gall stones or sometimes by a liver fluke or a roundworm going from the duodenum into the bile ducts.

The patient feels *biliary colic* as a sudden upper central abdominal pain that gradually increases in waves and usually moves to the right upper abdomen. He may feel it in the back, the right side and the right shoulder. The pain is extremely severe and may cause vomiting. The pain usually lasts several hours and then suddenly stops, leaving a feeling of soreness in the right upper part of the abdomen. During the attack, there is some muscle spasm and guarding in the right upper part of the abdomen, but no fever.

Give an injection of pethidine 100 mg or if not available morphine 10 mg and atropine 0.6 mg for biliary colic. If the pain stops, the patient needs nonurgent transfer to a hospital for investigation. If the pain does not stop after one or two injections, you must refer the patient to the Medical Officer urgently.

If obstruction and infection of the gall bladder occurs it is called *acute cholecystitis*. In acute cholecystitis following an attack of biliary colic, some pain remains. The patient develops both the general symptoms and signs of infection and the localised symptoms and signs of infection over the gall bladder in the right upper part of the abdomen. There is fever and a fast pulse. There is tenderness and guarding over the gall bladder.

Transfer a patient with acute cholecystitis urgently to hospital. Meanwhile manage like a case of peritonitis – nil by mouth, intravenous fluids, pethidine or morphine and chloramphenicol. (See Chapter 23 page 349.)

Slow obstruction of the bile duct which finally becomes complete occurs when a cancer presses on the main bile duct. This does not usually cause pain or infection. It causes *painless obstructive jaundice* with marked jaundice with itching, very dark urine and pale or almost white faeces. The liver may be enlarged. If the obstruction is in the common bile duct past the gall bladder (see Figure 24.3), the gall bladder may be enlarged: you may feel it as a soft lump underneath the front of the liver. Cancer of the pancreas is a more common cause of this than cancer of the bile ducts.

You should transfer the patient non-urgently to hospital to confirm the diagnosis, and for surgery if necessary, as some cases are due to gall stones or other curable causes.

Liver flukes

Liver flukes with the names *Clonorchis* and *Opisthorchis* are small worms about 10–25 mm long which live in the bile ducts of dogs, cats and other animals. Eggs are passed through the bile ducts and bowel. If they reach fresh water, they develop in certain snails and then attack certain fish and crayfish and live in their muscles. Dogs and cats then eat these fish and the larvae hatch in the bowel and eventually become worms in the liver. Humans are also affected when they eat uncooked freshwater fish or crayfish.

Other liver flukes with the name *Fasciola* are larger flat worms of cattle and snails especially in South America. Humans are also infected when they eat raw water vegetables.

Symptoms include a feeling of something moving about in the liver and episodes of fever, enlargement and tenderness of the liver and jaundice. If a worm completely blocks a large duct, obstructive jaundice can occur.

The *diagnosis* is made by finding the ova or eggs in the stool.

Treatment is with praziquantel 40 mg/kg once or 25 mg/kg three times a day after meals for 1–3 days. For *Fasciola*, triclabendazole 10 mg/kg with food once or twice in a day is most effective.

Prevention is not eating uncooked fish or crayfish, even if they are pickled or eating raw water vegetables.

The pancreas

The pancreas (see Figure 24.2 page 391 for anatomy) has two functions.

Firstly, *the pancreas makes insulin*, which keeps the blood glucose at the best level for the body to use glucose. If the pancreas is damaged in certain ways it does not make enough insulin to keep the blood glucose normal and diabetes mellitus develops (see Chapter 30 page 499).

Secondly, *the pancreas makes enzymes* (especially lipase, trypin, amalyse and others), which help the bowel digest and absorb fat and protein. These enzymes flow into the duodenum at the same place as the bile after a person eats. (See Figure 25.2.) If the pancreas is damaged so that it does not make enough enzymes or if the pancreatic duct is blocked so that the enzymes do not get into the duodenum, fat and protein are not digested and absorbed properly and the patient becomes thin and wasted and the fat, etc. in the bowel causes chronic diarrhoea (malabsorption syndrome – see Chapter 23 page 374).

Diseases of the pancreas are very difficult to diagnose in a health centre as thick muscles and the spine are behind it and muscles and the stomach and small and large bowel are in front of it. Special blood tests and X-rays are needed to diagnose the diseases accurately. Fortunately, this does not matter as much as would be expected as pancreatic disease is not very common in developing countries.

Acute pancreatitis is acute inflammation of the pancreas. It is usually caused by overwork by the pancreas (e.g. after large alcohol intake); viral infections (including mumps); block of the pancreatic duct (by gall stones or liver flukes, or wandering roundworm (*Ascaris*)); drugs (including some used for HIV treatment); and other and unknown causes. It causes constant upper abdominal and often back pain, nausea and vomiting. The patient often sits up leaning forward. There is epigastric tenderness but no guarding (as the pancreas is behind the peritoneum). In some cases the patient becomes shocked and cyanosed. Treatment is with nil orally; IV fluids; pethidine 100 mg or morphine 10 mg and atropine 0.6 mg 4 hourly for pain; IM or IV metoclopramide 10 mg and/or IM chlorpromazine 12.5–25 mg if needed for vomiting and IV antibiotics if evidence of infection. If the patient does not improve in a day or is very sick from the beginning, transfer to the Medical Officer in case there is another diagnosis which can be effectively treated.

'Chronic calcific pancreatitis' or 'fibrocalceous pancreatitis of the young and malnourished' causes chronic upper abdominal and back pain; malabsorption with poor growth and nutrition (see Chapter 23 page 374); and diabetes (see Chapter 30 page 499). The cause is somehow related to poor nutrition. Treatment is very difficult. Pain relief is needed or suicide often occurs (non-steroidal anti-inflammatory drugs should be tried to avoid morphine). Pancreatic extracts to help digestion and absorption need to be taken with every meal and are usually not available. Treatment of diabetes with insulin injections is needed. Refer such patients to the Medical Officer for advice.

'Chronic pancreatitis strongly associated with alcohol abuse' (i.e. too much alcohol too often for too long) causes abdominal and back pain, attacks of acute pancreatitis after drinking alcohol and at times malabsorption with diarrhoea. Treatment is by stopping drinking any alcohol at all; and if needed treatment of acute pancreatitis and malabsorption and pain (see above).

Cancer of the pancreas causes pain, weight loss, obstructive jaundice (by pressing on and blocking the common bile duct – see page 392) and many unusual symptoms and signs (including clotting of blood in veins). Refer all such cases to the Medical Officer for diagnosis and advice or management as curative treatment (surgery) is rarely possible.

Diagnosis of symptoms and signs in liver, gall bladder, pancreas

Enlargement of the liver

The normal liver is not more than 1 cm below the ribs of the right side of the chest.

Causes of enlarged liver include:

1. Malaria. Where malaria is common 70% of the normal population has an enlarged smooth non-tender liver. The liver functions normally. No treatment is needed for this liver enlargement.
2. Unknown. Up to 20% of normal people in tropical developing countries have an enlarged smooth non-tender liver even in areas where malaria is not common. The liver functions normally. The cause is not known. No treatment is possible or needed.
3. Other diseases.
   - viral hepatitis
   - amoebic or bacterial liver abscess
   - tuberculosis of liver
   - hepatoma
   - secondary cancer
   - hydatid cyst
   - heart failure
   - kala azar – visceral leishmaniasis
   - trypanosomiasis
   - brucellosis
   - schistosomiasis
   - sickle cell disease
   - rare blood diseases
   - others – see a specialist reference book.

Tenderness of liver

The liver may be tender for any of these reasons:

1. Enlargement which happened quickly, e.g. acute heart failure.
2. Acute inflammation, e.g. liver abscess, viral hepatitis, infarction in sickle cell anaemia.
3. Hepatoma (tenderness is unusual if it is a secondary cancer).
4. Acute injury.
5. Others – see a specialist reference book.

Jaundice

There are three types of jaundice (see page 392). There may be more than one type at the same time in a patient (see below, four groups).

Do a full history and examination (see Chapter 6).
Test the urine for protein and bile (Chapter 26 page 445).
Look at the colour of the stools.
Diagnose and treat the cause.

Find out which of the four groups of symptoms and signs your patient has.

1. *Acute severe infections with red blood cell and liver cell damage* (i.e. acute haemolysis and acute hepatitis in varying degrees)
   The *symptoms* and *signs* are:
   - fever, often high,
   - 'sick',
   - sometimes diagnostic symptoms and signs of the cause,
   - sometimes diagnostic tests, if available, of the cause,

- jaundice,
- dark urine with bile,
- stools not white.

Causes include:
- malaria,
- pneumonia,
- relapsing fever,
- yellow fever,
- septicaemia, etc.

See Chapter 17 page 170.

Treat with antimalarials and antibiotics if diagnosis is not possible (see Chapter 12 page 64 and if haemorrhagic fever Chapter 17 page 171).

2. *Hepatitis caused by a hepatitis virus or a drug*
The *symptoms* and *signs* are:
- feels sick with nausea or vomiting,
- right upper abdominal pain,
- dark urine,
- stools not pale,
- fever (not high),
- tender enlarged liver (not severe),
- bile in urine.

Treat like this:
(a) If he feels 'sick', the patient must rest in bed.
(b) If he has repeated vomiting, give IV fluids for dehydration and maintenance fluids (see Chapter 23 page 362).
(c) Encourage him to drink as much sweet fluid and to eat as much good food as possible.
(d) Give an antimalarial drug if malaria possible (see Chapter 13 pages 79, 80).
(e) Stop all drugs including oral contraceptives.
If the patient is on TB or leprosy or HIV treatment, stop all drugs and urgently transfer the patient to Medical Officer care.
Give no drugs which could affect the liver, especially not chlorpromazine or TCE (tetrachlorethylene).
(f) Check the patient's home and village sanitation and water supply if possible HAV infection.
Check sterilisation procedures of the patient's health workers if the disease could be HBV infection. Give health education about these things if required.
(g) If a case of viral hepatitis occurs in a closed community (e.g. college) consult with the Medical Officer about using immunisation or immunoglobulin to prevent an epidemic.

3. *Obstructive jaundice*
The *symptoms* and *signs* are:
- jaundice,
- urine dark and test for bile positive,
- stool light colour or white,
- often an itch.

Causes include:
- cancer ⎱ pressing on and
- enlarged lymph nodes ⎰ blocking the bile duct,
- gall stone or liver fluke or roundworm in the bile ducts,
- some drugs including chlorpromazine.

Treat like this:
(a) Stop all drugs except antimalarials.
(b) Transfer to Medical Officer care – urgent if the patient has a fever or is sick or was on drugs for TB, HIV or leprosy, non-urgent if he has no fever and is not sick.

4. *Haemolytic jaundice*
The *symptoms* and *signs* are:
- jaundice,
- stools normal colour,
- urine normal colour and test for bile negative.

Causes include chronic haemolytic anaemias including:
- hyperreactive malarious splenomegaly
- sickle cell anaemia and
- thalassaemia.

Causes also include acute haemolysis in hyperreactive malarious splenomegaly or sickle cell anaemia as well as drugs, snakebite, etc.

Find and *treat* the cause if possible.
Transfer to Medical Officer if treatment or a blood transfusion is necessary.

25 Disorders of the Nervous System

Anatomy and physiology

The nervous system consists of three parts:

1. the brain and spinal cord – the central nervous system;
2. the peripheral nervous system; and
3. the special sense organs (organs of sight, hearing, smell, taste).

The nervous system is made of nerve cells and some other cells which support and help the nerve cells. The nerve cells have a body, and some have very long extensions (like tails) called axons (see Figure 25.2). These axons conduct (or carry) messages from one part of the nervous system to other parts of the nervous system, or to other systems (in a way similar to the wires which carry electrical messages in a telephone system).

The nerve cells in the nervous system that have the same function are grouped together in one or more areas.

In the brain the bodies of the nerve cells which deal with speech or movement or sensation, etc. are grouped together in special areas on the surface (or cortex) of the brain, and these areas are called the speech area, motor (movement) area, sensory area, etc. (see Figure 25.3).

In the *spinal cord* the bodies of nerve cells which deal with movement are in the front of the cord, and

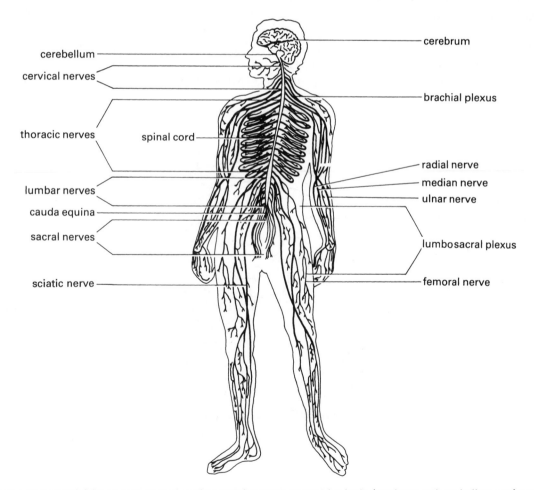

cerebellum
cervical nerves
thoracic nerves
spinal cord
lumbar nerves
cauda equina
sacral nerves
sciatic nerve

cerebrum
brachial plexus
radial nerve
median nerve
ulnar nerve
lumbosacral plexus
femoral nerve

Figure 25.1 *Two parts of the nervous system. 1. The central nervous system, i.e. brain (cerebrum and cerebellum, etc.) and the spinal cord. 2. The peripheral nervous system, i.e. the peripheral and cutaneous nerves.*

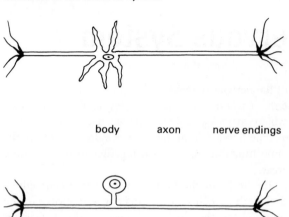

body   axon   nerve endings

Figure 25.2 The microscopic structure of two types of nerve cell.

those which deal with sensation are in special extensions of the spinal cord, called 'dorsal root ganglia', attached to the back of the cord (see Figures 25.4, 25.5 and 25.10).

The *axons* of nerve cells which run from one part of the nervous system to another are also grouped together (like the wires of a telephone system, which run in a cable). These groups of axons are called '*tracts*' if they are in the central nervous system. They are called '*nerves*' if they are in the peripheral nervous system (see Figure 25.4, 25.5 and 25.6).

The central nervous system

The central nervous system consists of the brain and spinal cord.

The central nervous system is like a telephone exchange. Messages about sensation travel from many parts of the body through nerves, called 'sensory nerves', to the central nervous system. These messages are then sent to other parts of the central nervous system and/or to the nerves which go from the central nervous system to other parts of the body. The nerves that go from the central nervous system are called 'motor nerves' because they carry messages to make parts of the body move.

The sensory system

Sensory messages coming into the central nervous system can go to three different places.

1. Sensory messages can go up the spinal cord to the cerebral cortex of the brain. The person then knows what is happening and can decide to do something or not.

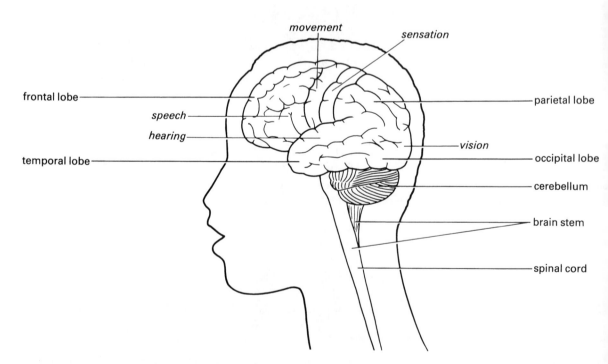

Figure 25.3 The anatomy of the cortex or the outer layer of the brain. Note the positions of the groups of bodies of nerve cells that have the same special function (e.g. hearing).

2. Sensory messages from joints and muscles, about the position of limbs, can go to the cerebellum. The cerebellum then sends messages back to the muscles to help the person stand or move properly (the way he has decided in the cerebral cortex).

3. Sensory messages coming into the spinal cord do not all go up the spinal cord (to the cerebral cortex or cerebellum). Some go to other nerves in the spinal cord and may cause reflex action. For example, if a sensory message comes into the cord that says the hand is being burned by fire, the message immediately goes to the correct nerve in the spinal cord to pull the hand away from the fire. This reflex action pulls the hand away before the person feels the pain and thinks about pulling the hand away.

Usually, when a sensory message comes into the central nervous system, it causes all these things as necessary:

- reflex action,
- control of movement by the cerebellum, and
- decision about action by the cerebral cortex.

The motor system

The cerebral cortex controls movement through motor nerve cells whose fibres go from the cortex through the brain to the spinal cord. In the spinal cord, they pass the message to other motor nerves which go to muscles. Motor messages travel in tracts and nerves to the muscles in the same way that sensory nerve cells take sensation to the brain from the body.

Note that *movement and sensation of one side of the body are controlled by the opposite side of the brain.* This is because the nerve axons cross over to the other side of the body where the cerebellum and spinal cord meet (at the brain stem) or in the spinal cord. See Figures 25.4 and 25.6.

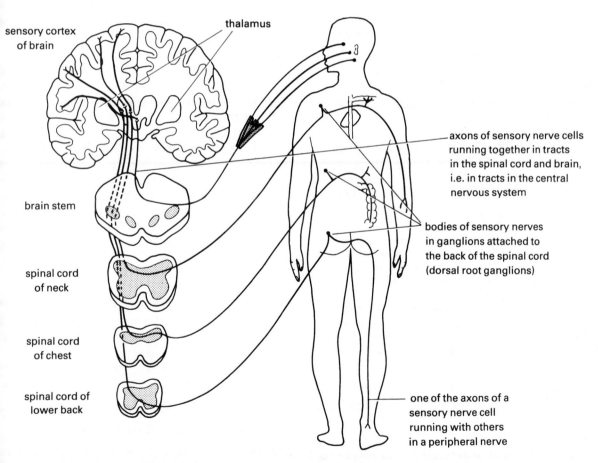

Figure 25.4 *This diagram shows how one of the sensations of the body (pain) is taken from the skin to the cerebral cortex of the brain where the person can feel it. Pain nerve cell axons are all grouped together in one tract after they enter the central nervous system. Other sensations have other tracts. Note that tracts also go to the cerebellum (not shown).*

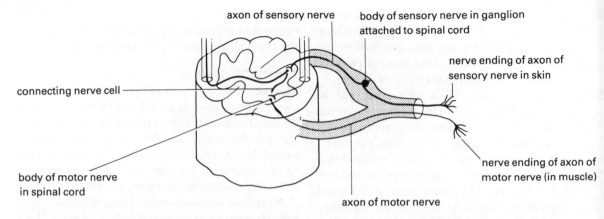

Figure 25.5 *Diagram showing the spinal cord and a reflex arc. Pain sensation from sensory nerve endings in the skin goes along the axon of the sensory nerve and into a connecting nerve cell. The message then goes into the motor nerve cell. The motor nerve cell then sends a message to the muscle to move that part of the body away from what is causing the pain. The sensation of pain is also sent up to the cerebral cortex of the brain (see Figure 25.4) and the cerebellum.*

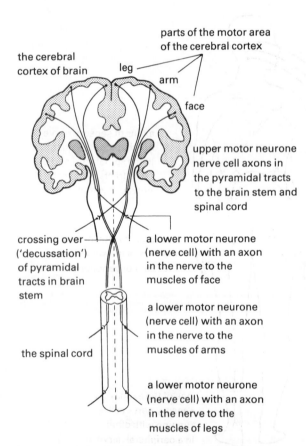

Figure 25.6 *Diagram to show the axons of the nerves in the motor area of the cerebral cortex which go in tracts to the brain stem and spinal cord. Note that the motor tracts cross to the other side of the body in the brain stem.*

Note also that the *control of the body in the brain is upside down*, i.e. the sensation and movement of feet are at the top of the brain, and the face at the lower part. See Figures 25.7 and 25.8.

Note also that there are large areas of the brain connected to the parts of the body that have many sensations and many complicated movements (e.g. face and hands). See Figures 25.7 and 25.8.

Damage to the special motor or sensory parts of the cerebral cortex will cause loss of sensation or movement on *the opposite* side of the body. Damage to the spinal cord will cause loss of movement and loss of joint and touch sensation on *the same* side of the body but pain sensation on *the opposite* side of the body below the lesion. Damage to the brain stem (where the cross–over of nerve fibres occurs) may cause a mixture of motor and sensory losses on different sides of the body and face.

The meninges

The *meninges* surround the whole of the central nervous system. The meninges are three layers of membranes (see Figures 25.9 and 25.10). In the middle layer, there is a meshwork of fibres in which circulates a fluid called the cerebrospinal fluid (CSF). The meninges and CSF protect and give food to the central nervous system.

The peripheral nervous system

Nerves are the white cords which take messages between parts of the body and the central nervous system. They go to and from the spinal cord and brain through gaps between the vertebrae of the spine or

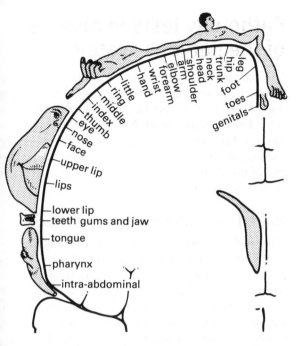

Figure 25.7 *A diagram of a section cut through one half of the brain at the level of the sensory cortex (see Figure 25.3). This diagram shows which parts of the sensory cortex make the person aware of sensation in various parts of the body.*

Figure 25.8 *A diagram of a section cut through one half of the brain at the level of the motor cortex (see Figure 25.3). This diagram shows which parts of the motor cortex move the various parts of the body.*

holes in the skull. They consist of very many axons (thin fibres which are the tails of nerve cells which are in the spinal cord or in ganglia). (Ganglia are special groups of nerve cells attached to the spinal cord.)

Most nerves contain both sensory and motor fibres. Most nerves therefore both take sensation to the central nervous system and take motor messages back to parts of the body. The small nerves in the skin are called *cutaneous nerves* and contain only sensory nerve fibres.

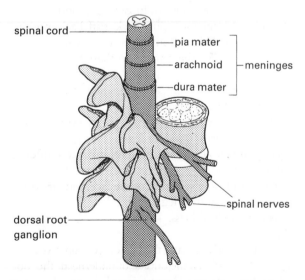

Figure 25.10 *The vertebrae from the neck to the sacrum have a body in front (which carries the weight of the person) and plates of bone at the sides and back which form the spinal canal through which the spinal cord runs. The spinal nerves run to and from the cord between the side plates, which have notches (or hollows) in them to make room for the nerves.*

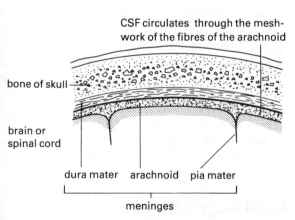

Figure 25.9 *Diagram showing the structure of the meninges around the brain and spinal cord.*

Symptoms and signs of disease of the nervous system

Note that you will find only those symptoms and signs marked with an asterisk (*) in a routine history and examination. If you have a special reason to suspect nervous system disease, then check for the other symptoms and signs too.

Symptoms

- Headache
- Fits or convulsions
- Change or loss of sight, hearing, smell or taste
- Weakness or paralysis of arm/s and/or leg/s
- Weakness of the bladder
  - retention of urine (the patient cannot pass urine)
  - incontinence of urine (the patient cannot stop the passing of urine)
- Change or loss of sensation
- Clumsiness
- Fever and general symptoms* (if there is infection)

Signs

- Change in level of consciousness*.
- Confusion*. Poor memory. Disorientation. Not thinking properly, sometimes with mixed up thoughts, hallucinations or delusions (organic psychosis).
- Meningeal irritation* (stiff neck, stiff back, positive Kernig's sign, bulging fontanelle but only in infants). See page 428 for the ways to do these tests.
- Fitting*.
- Change or loss of sight, hearing, smell or taste.
- Change or loss of speech.
- Stiffness or weakness or paralysis of eye/s and/or face, and/or arm/s, and/or leg/s.
- Paralysis of the bladder, with retention or incontinence of urine.
- Change or loss of sensation of the face, and/or arm/s, and/or trunk and/or leg/s.
- Shaking or clumsiness.
- Reflexes
  - plantar – if abnormal, the big toe goes up if you scratch the outside of underneath the foot
  - tendon – decreased or increased
    - right side not equal to left side
    - arm not equal to leg on same side } if abnormal
- Fever*, fast pulse, etc., if there is infection.

Pathology tests in diseases of the nervous system

You can get CSF for examination with the naked eye and with certain 'dip stick' rapid bedside tests and, if possible, in the laboratory by doing a lumbar puncture (LP). (For the proper method of doing a lumbar puncture, see Appendix 1 page 429, and for the laboratory examination of CSF, see Appendix 2 page 435, at the end of this chapter.) See below for rapid bedside tests of the CSF using dip sticks.

Naked eye examination of the CSF

Normal CSF should look clear like clean water.

If CSF does not look clear, assume that it contains pus, and treat for bacterial meningitis. In viral meningitis and encephalitis the CSF usually looks clear (because there are not enough mononuclear cells for you to see with the naked eye). The same is true for some early cases of tuberculous meningitis. Unfortunately, in up to one in three patients with early bacterial meningitis, the CSF can look clear (but become cloudy by another day if the patient is not treated; but this delay may lead to death).

Sometimes a few red cells can make the CSF look cloudy and you may treat some patients for meningitis who do not have it. But this is better than not treating some patients with meningitis.

Sometimes the CSF is red and obviously has red blood cells in it. Find out if this is caused by a 'traumatic tap' or if there is blood in all the CSF (see page 435).

Sometimes the CSF is clear but yellow. This is called 'xanthochromia'. Xanthochromia is caused by red blood cells that are destroyed and release their haemoglobin and other pigments into the CSF, i.e. there has been a haemorrhage into the CSF. Xanthochromia appears 4 hours after the haemorrhage. There are also other causes of yellow CSF including tuberculous meningitis, cerebral tumours, etc. So, unless the patient has clinical evidence of a haemorrhage, transfer him for tests to find the cause of the 'xanthochromia'.

If you leave the CSF for a day in a cool area, a clot (sometimes like a spider's web) may form. This is not normal. There are various causes for this, including tuberculous meningitis.

Rapid diagnostic tests on the CSF

If you have dip sticks to measure glucose, protein and pus cells, you may be able to use these dip sticks to measure levels of these in CSF. Most dip sticks are reasonably accurate for protein and sugar; but not reliable for pus cells. Check with your Medical Officer to see if the ones you have can be used or not; and if so, for what tests. **Do not use the dip sticks if you are told the ones you have are not suitable.**

If the CSF glucose is low (e.g. less than the 2.2 mmol/ml or 40 mg/dl and especially if you have measured the blood glucose at the same time and the CSF glucose is lower than the blood glucose) or if the protein is above 0.5 g/l or if the leucocyte (pus cell) patch is suitable and the patch is positive; ANY of these make it likely that there is an infection in the CSF even if the CSF looks clear.

Remember that the tests could be positive because of tuberculosis or other chronic types of infections causing meningitis as well as acute bacterial meningitis; and the protein high but other tests normal in viral meningitis, encephalitis, cerebral tumour, haemorrhage and at times even cerebral malaria, etc.

NEVER USE A NEGATIVE RESULT (i.e. normal results) on a dip stick to decide not to treat a patient for meningitis. USE A POSITIVE RESULT (i.e. abnormal test for protein high and glucose low and, if reliable, pus cells present) only to decide to treat for meningitis when otherwise (because of clear CSF) you may not have started meningitis treatment. Hopefully, much more reliable and helpful rapid diagnostic tests for CSF will soon become available.

If it is possible, keep the CSF cool and send it to the hospital laboratory for examination for cells, organisms, protein, sugar and culture with sensitivity testing (see Table 25.1 page 436).

If you strongly suspect acute bacterial meningitis in a very sick patient, give an extra dose of chloramphenicol or penicillin by IMI immediately (while you are doing the lumbar puncture and starting the IV drip).

Common conditions affecting the nervous system

Acute bacterial ('purulent') meningitis

Acute bacterial meningitis is an acute bacterial infection of the meninges (the coverings) of the brain and spinal cord. This infection causes:

1. acute inflammation with pus in the meninges, and
2. damage to the brain, and
3. toxaemia or septicaemia.

It is a common disease and often causes death. The *cause* is one of many bacteria including:

1. *Neisseria meningitidis* (the meningococcus) – the most common cause of epidemics.
2. *Streptococcus pneumoniae* (the pneumococcus) – now the most common cause, especially in populations where there is decreased immunity, especially HIV infection.
3. *Haemophilus influenzae* – mainly in children.

Many healthy people carry these organisms in their throats. Most of these people slowly develop resistance to the organisms and eventually get rid of them. While this is happening these carriers can pass the organisms to non-immune people by direct but mostly droplet means. If people are going to get meningitis from these organisms they usually do so within a couple of weeks of the organisms getting into their upper respiratory tract.

In the meningitis belt of Africa (the semi-arid sub-Saharan part) and now south of it too, epidemics of meningococcal meningitis occur every 2–5 years in the dry season. This could be due to immunity becoming less in people and new babies, but probably also to damage to the lining of the upper respiratory tract by the dry dusty air, as the epidemics stop as soon as it rains. Viral infections of the respiratory tract and smoking, etc. may similarly help the organism to spread to the brain. Pneumococci spread more easily if immunity is decreased, such as in patients with HIV infection, splenectomy, sickle cell anaemia, etc. when meningitis may complicate pneumonia, otitis media, sinusitis, etc. Any organism may get to the meninges if there has been a fracture of the nose or skull and also a break made in the overlying mucosa or skin making a path for bacteria from the inside of the nose or the outside of the skin straight into the meninges. In many cases, however, the reason the organism has spread to the brain is not clear.

Meningitis is usually a disease of children; but anyone can be affected. Young adults recently crowded together (e.g. army recruits or children in boarding schools) are commonly affected. Regular huge epidemics occur in Africa and Asia and small epidemics occur elsewhere.

Symptoms and signs
Symptoms may include:

• Headache
• Fever
• Photophobia (dislike of light as there is pain in the eyes and head if the eyes are open in the light)

- Pains often in the legs at the beginning of the infection but then, as expected, also in the head, neck and back
- Nausea and vomiting.

(In children there may be few symptoms.)

Signs (see Figure 25.11) include any of these:

1. Signs of damage to the brain.
   - Any loss of full consciousness, e.g. sleepiness, drowsiness, unconsciousness, etc.
   - Any irritation of the brain, e.g. restlessness, irritability, confusion, delirium, psychotic behaviour, muscle twitching, fitting, etc.
2. Signs of inflammation of the meninges.
   - Full or bulging fontanelle (infants only)
   - Stiff neck
   - Stiff back
   - Positive Kernig's sign

   (In children these signs may not be present.)
3. • General signs of infection are usually present, e.g. fever, fast pulse, fast breathing, dehydration.
   - Signs of septicaemia may be present, especially haemorrhagic rash, which may be only pin point dots of bleeding (i.e. purpura) that are difficult to see on dark skin (but may be able to be felt), but may be seen in the mucosa of the conjunctiva and inside the mouth; and soon after, shock, etc.
   - Cold hands and feet and abnormal skin colour are said to be early signs which should make you think of meningitis.
4. Signs of an underlying condition, especially
   - HIV infection
   - Sickle cell anaemia
   - Splenectomy
   - Otitis media, sinusitis, pneumonia
   - Broken nose or compound fracture of the skull.

Tests

You must do a lumbar puncture on *every* person who has symptoms or signs which could be caused by meningitis.

Do a lumbar puncture for anyone who:

1. is not fully conscious or is unconscious, or
2. has fitted (and is not known to be epileptic), or
3. is not mentally normal (and is not known to suffer from a mental disease), or
4. has signs of meningeal irritation (neck stiffness, back stiffness, etc.), or
5. is 'sick' and has a rash with bleeding into the skin or mucous membranes,
6. is sick with leg pains, cold hands and feet and abnormal colour of the skin,

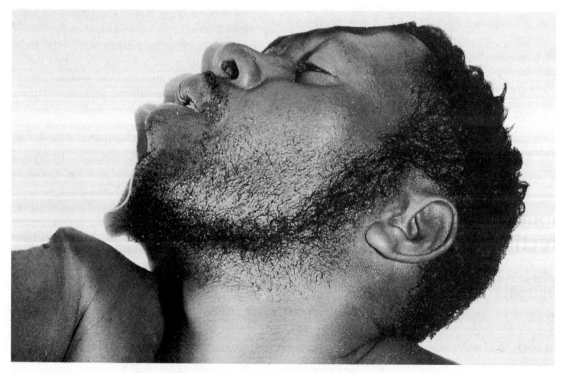

Figure 25.11 *This patient has meningitis. Not only does he have a stiff neck but he also lies with his neck bent backwards (sometimes called 'neck retraction'). This is a sign of severe meningeal irritation.*

7. has a severe illness with a fever which you cannot diagnose.

If the CSF is hazy or turbid or cloudy or like pus, treat as bacterial meningitis.

If the CSF is blood-stained, treat as bacterial meningitis.

If you do not get any CSF (lumbar puncture failed), treat as bacterial meningitis.

If the CSF is clear but the patient has the clinical signs of meningitis, he must have:

- cerebral malaria, or
- viral meningitis, or
- encephalitis, or
- TB meningitis, or
- very early bacterial meningitis (before much pus has formed).

} Sometimes (in up to $\frac{1}{3}$ of cases) the CSF may look clear

If you have suitable rapid diagnostic test dip sticks and the CSF is clear, do the test. Treat for meningitis if the test shows +/− pus cells (only if dip stick suitable for this test), low sugar in comparison to blood sugar +/− high protein (see pages 408–409).

Management

Treat for meningitis if:

- CSF is not clear,
- CSF is bloody,
- CSF clear but gives a positive result on dip stick test for protein and low sugar and pus cells (if dip stick suitable),
- CSF is clear but the patient is very ill and no other cause is found,
- you cannot get CSF (LP failed) but you strongly suspect meningitis.

Treat all cases of meningitis also for cerebral malaria with an artemisinin drug or quinine and a companion drug (see Chapter 13 page 80) unless you are sure that the patient is not in or has never been to an area where he could get malaria.

If the CSF is clear and the CSF glucose not low, treat only for cerebral malaria. But, if there is no improvement after 12–24 hours, repeat the lumbar puncture.

Treatment includes five things:

1. An antibiotic, preferably chloramphenicol, in the correct large dose, for 10 days to 14 days (see right)

2. IV fluids; but only if necessary

3. Anti-convulsants if necessary

4. Antimalarial drugs – an artemisinin drug or quinine and companion drug

5. Care of unconscious patient if necessary.

1. *Antibiotics*

Give chloramphenicol (*or* powerful alternative).

(a) Chloramphenicol – 25 mg/kg each 6 hours
For an adult of average weight give 2 g immediately then 1 g every 6 hours.
Give it by IVI *if*:
- there is shock (essential), or
- an IV drip is needed for another reason and is running.
Give by IMI to *all other cases* until they can take oral doses.
Give orally *only if* the patient:
- is not shocked, and
- is not very sick or after he improves (when oral drugs are reliable enough), and
- can swallow, and
- has no vomiting or severe diarrhoea.

(b) Benzyl (crystalline) penicillin
You can give penicillin *instead of* chloramphenicol if it is likely the organism is sensitive to penicillin, or chloramphenicol is not available or is contra-indicated. Chloramphenicol is better if these are not so, as penicillin resistant organisms cause meningitis; but meningococci are sensitive to penicillin.
Give 1.2 g or 2,000,000 units by IVI immediately. *Give 1.2 g or 2,000,000 units by IVI every 3 hours after the first dose.*
Give by IMI if a drip is not running. However, IVI is essential if the patient is in shock.
If you cannot give injections every 3 hours then give 2.4 g or 4,000,000 units *slowly* (at 1 ml/minute) by IVI or by IMI every 6 hours instead.

(c) Continue the antibiotic for at least 10 days or for 1 week after the fever stops – whichever is longer.
Do *not* reduce the dose of chloramphenicol unless the patient appears to be cured very quickly (see Chapter 12).
You can reduce the dose of penicillin to 1.2 g or 2,000,000 units every 6 hours when the patient appears to be cured.

(d) In epidemics of proven meningococcal meningitis (but not in pneumococcal or other or unknown types) treatment is effective with 3(–5) days of penicillin as above; or one dose of a mixture of short and long acting penicillin; or with one dose of long acting oily preparation of chloramphenicol which is safe for only *IMI*. This oily IMI chloramphenicol contains 250 mg in 1 ml. The dose for an adult, 3 g or 12 ml (i.e. 2 ampoules), is administered as 6 ml IMI into the upper outer quadrant of each buttock. If the patient is not improved in 24 hours a second IMI dose of the penicillin mixture or oily chloramphenicol is needed.

(e) If available, a third generation cephalosporin, e.g. ceftriaxone 2 g IV (or IMI after first dose) each 12 hours for 10–14 days is very effective treatment for most infections including chloramphenicol resistant ones; but is not needed if meningococci are isolated (see above), and is usually much more expensive. It is safer for pregnant women and children under 2 years of age (50 mg/kg twice a day).

2. *IV fluids* if necessary

Do not give more IV fluids than necessary. Too much IV fluid can cause cerebral oedema with convulsions and death.

If shock is present, see Chapter 27 page 468. If dehydration is present, see Chapter 23 page 364. If only maintenance is needed, or if there is a drip to allow repeated IV instead of IM injections, give 0.18% sodium chloride in 4.3% dextrose solution – 1 litre each 8–12 hours.

3. *Anti-convulsant drug* if necessary for fitting or restlessness

Immediately give rectal diazepam for adult 10–20 mg injected using a 5–10 ml syringe without a needle. If available, you could give paraldehyde 0.2 ml/kg (5–10 ml) using a glass syringe IMI. Then see Convulsions page 424.

Do not use phenobarbitone if you are giving the patient chloramphenicol (because it may reduce the concentration of chloramphenicol in the body).

4. *Antimalarial drug* as for cerebral malaria.

Give IVI or IMI artemisinin drug or IMI quinine and companion drug (see Malaria Chapter 13 page 80).

5. *Routine care of unconscious patient* if necessary. See pages 422–424.

Prognosis

Without treatment most patients die within a couple of days. With treatment 10% with meningococcal to 50% with pneumococcal disease can still die or have permanent brain damage. However, the sooner the treatment is started the better the prognosis.

If a patient could have meningitis it is an extreme emergency. Give chloramphenicol and antimalarials immediately. Do a lumbar puncture.

Transfer

Transfer to Medical Officer care if the patient:

1. is still unconscious after 24 hours of full treatment (urgent).
2. is not improving after 2 days of full treatment (urgent).
3. still has a fever after 1 week of full treatment (urgent – but not emergency).
4. is not cured after 2 weeks of full treatment (urgent – but not emergency).
5. any complications develop which you cannot manage in the health centre (urgent).

Prevention

1. *Kill the organism* in the body of the original host or reservoir.

It is not possible to kill the organisms in the reservoir as most carriers are completely healthy and do not know they have the infection; and after passing it to others most probably develop immunity and get rid of the organism themselves.

2. *Stop the means of spread.*

Carry out all the usual means of stopping direct and droplet spread of respiratory infections.

In an epidemic in an institution, avoid overcrowding and separate people's eating and especially sleeping quarters as much as possible and ventilate the rooms as well as possible. (See Chapter 14 page 124.)

3. *Raise the resistance* of possible new hosts.

Immunisation against meningococcal infection is effective but usually is not long lasting and is at present not used routinely. It is used to control epidemics. If 10–15 cases of meningococcal meningitis or septicaemia occur in 2 weeks for each 100,000 of the population or more than the usual number of children older than 5 are affected, then immunisation with the appropriate meningococcal vaccine, and in some cases chemoprophylaxis, will be very effective in controlling the epidemic, as long as it is started early enough. If, therefore, you have such an outbreak of meningitis, always immediately notify your Medical Officer and ask him to see about urgent control measures including immunisation.

Samples of CSF sent to the laboratory for culture and sensitivity tests are essential to guide the choice of vaccine and drugs for the control programme. *Haemophilus influenzae* type b (Hib) vaccine and a conjugate (combined) DPT-Hib vaccine are effective in protecting against *Haemophilus influenzae* infections in children. Doses should be given to all at 6, 10 and 14 weeks of age.

Pneumococcal vaccines have been developed and in some populations are given to prevent pneumococcal pneumonia. They could also be given to patients at risk of any pneumococcal disease and to HIV infected people.

4. *Prophylactic antibiotics* for other members of the family who live in the same house as the patient, or who live in a closed community with them (e.g. boarding school) or staff who have close personal contact with an untreated patient (e.g. who do mouth-to-mouth ventilation) seems sensible. Unfortunately, most antibiotics which cure the disease do not get rid of the carrier state except very expensive antibiotics or ones which should not be used for other reasons. Ampicillin, amoxicillin, tetracycline or doxycycline for 5 days is not very effective. A more effective alternative is to check close contacts daily. Educate all contacts and the public to come for examination and if needed treatment at the first sign of meningitis or septicaemia.

Cerebral malaria

Cerebral malaria is the acute damage of the brain (encephalitis) and meninges caused by falciparum malaria parasites and their toxins in the blood vessels of the brain.

Cerebral malaria is clinically similar to acute bacterial meningitis (see page 409) but there are some differences.

The *history* is similar *but* the history may also suggest malaria, e.g.

• the patient is a non-immune person recently in a malarial area,
• the person in a malarial area may have been semi-immune but may have lost some of their immunity, e.g. pregnancy, HIV infection, etc.
• the patient has had recent attacks of fever.

The signs of brain damage are similar, i.e.

• loss of full consciousness,
  e.g. the patient may be sleepy, drowsy, unconscious, etc.
• irritation of the brain,
  e.g. the patient may be restless, irritable, confused, delirious, psychotic, twitching, fitting, etc.

The *signs of inflammation of the meninges* are similar, although not as definite, e.g. stiff neck, stiff back, etc.

The *general signs of infection* are similar, e.g. fast pulse, fast breathing, dehydration, etc. *but* there are no signs of septicaemia.

There may be other signs of acute or chronic malaria, e.g. anaemia and/or jaundice, enlarged tender spleen, or enlarged liver.

But you cannot tell the difference between acute bacterial meningitis and cerebral malaria without a lumbar puncture.

> Always do a lumbar puncture if you suspect cerebral malaria *or* meningitis.

In cerebral malaria the CSF will be normal and look clear. The CSF will also look clear in:

• viral meningitis,
• encephalitis,
• tuberculous meningitis (sometimes), and
• a very early acute bacterial meningitis (in a worrying number of cases).

In cerebral malaria the CSF glucose should be normal or only slightly low, the protein usually not high and the pus cell test (if suitable) negative on urine dip stick testing (see pages 408–409). If the CSF glucose is low or absent or protein high or pus test positive then treat for meningitis also.

Treatment

Treatment includes five things (see also Chapter 13 pages 77–87):

1. Antimalarial drugs *immediately* by IV or IM injection (see Malaria, Chapter 13 pages 80–81).
   Give artesunate 2.4 mg/kg usually 120–180 mg IV or IM; or artemether 3.2 mg/kg usually 160–240 mg IMI; or quinine not IVI but IV infusion or IMI 20 mg /kg usually 900–1200 mg.
   Then see Malaria Chapter 13 pages 80–83.
2. Anti-convulsants if there is fitting.
   Give diazepam 1 mg/minute (no more quickly) maximum dose 10 mg; but stop if fitting stops or breathing slows. Diazepam IMI is too slow acting to use but can give IMI paraldehyde 0.2 ml/kg (5–10 ml usually) using a glass syringe. Otherwise, give rectal diazepam 0.5 mg/kg, maximum dose 20 mg using a 5–10 ml syringe without a needle pushed in 4–5 cm.
   Then see Convulsions page 424 for details about giving and continuing these drugs.

3. As both malaria and quinine can cause low blood glucose, *immediately* do a test for blood glucose. If it is low (less than 2.2 mmol or 40 mg/dl) or if you cannot do the test, give glucose 50 ml of a 50% solution glucose stat and use 5% or 4.3% dextrose in the drip for the quinine (not 0.9% saline).

4. If the patient is unconscious, give routine care for unconsciousness.

   See pages 422–424 for details. Patients may be unconscious for some days and still make a complete recovery.

5. Reduce temperature if 40°C or above.

   See Chapter 13 pages 81–82 for details.

6. IV fluids if necessary.

   Do not give more fluid than necessary. Too much fluid can cause cerebral oedema and death. See meningitis page 412. Use 5% or 4.3% glucose.

Transfer patients to Medical Officer care:

1. if unconscious for more than 1 day;
2. if they are not greatly improved after 2 days; or
3. if they are not cured in 2 weeks.

Tuberculous meningitis

See also Chapter 14 pages 106–107.

Tuberculous meningitis is a subacute or chronic infection of the meninges with TB organisms.

Tuberculous meningitis is in some ways clinically similar to acute bacterial meningitis; but it develops much more slowly and at first is much less severe (see pages 409–410).

Symptoms and *signs* include:

• at first only headache;
• then slow loss of being fully alert and conscious; and later other symptoms and signs of brain damage;
• eventually coma and/or paralysis and then death;
• signs of meningeal irritation, with stiff neck, stiff back, etc. but may not be marked and at first can be absent;
• general symptoms and signs of infection, especially fever which may be mild and not marked until late in the disease;
• abnormal CSF, but sometimes you cannot see this without a microscope (see below).
• eventually paralysis of eye, face and mouth muscles, difficulty walking, dementia, vomiting, coma and death. (This may happen over days but usually weeks and occasionally months.)

There are differences from acute bacterial meningitis.

• The history is often longer (days or weeks or months; not hours or days).

• The patient is often not 'sick' at first.
• Evidence of tuberculous infection is sometimes present in other parts of the body.
• Evidence of HIV infection may be present.
• The CSF may look almost clear; or may be yellow; or, when left standing for some hours, form a spider's web type clot. The test for glucose will be low, protein will be high and increased cells will be present. Some patients with HIV infection early in the disease will have almost normal CSF tests even when tuberculous meningitis.
• Proper routine antibacterial meningitis treatment causes no improvement in 2 days, no loss of fever in 1 week and no cure in 2 weeks.

The tuberculin test is often negative.

The condition is more common in patients with HIV infection. HIV patients often have only few or no symptoms of meningitis at first.

Suspect tuberculous meningitis if any of these above. *Transfer* all suspected cases urgently to the Medical Officer for diagnosis and treatment with (usually 2(EHRZ)S/1(EHRZ)/5(HR)E) (no S if pregnant) and possibly at first corticosteroids.

Cryptococcal meningitis may have the same symptoms and signs as TB meningitis, except the diagnosis is made by special India ink stains on the CSF, which show the fungal cryptococcal organisms; and positive cryptococcus blood and CSF serology tests. Brain infections such as toxoplasma and nocardia and viruses and other organisms can cause a similar clinical meningitis. Blood tests exist for toxoplasma, some viruses and others.

In areas where African trypanosomiasis (sleeping sickness) occurs, this may cause similar signs and symptoms. This patient needs urgent transfer to the Medical Officer for diagnosis and treatment. A lumbar puncture should not be done until after diagnosis and the start of treatment (see Chapter 18 pages 181–183).

Whenever you see meningitis that does not respond to treatment or is chronic, ask yourself if there is any history or signs that would suggest TB infection.

Cryptococcal meningitis

Cryptococcus is a fungus in soil, especially soil contaminated by droppings from pigeons or eucalyptus trees. If inhaled, it can cause pneumonia which may have so few symptoms that it is not noticed and may get better without treatment. The cryptococcus, however, may still be carried by the blood to the brain where it causes a subacute or chronic meningitis and encephalitis, with progressively more and more symptoms and signs, and leads to death any time from 2 weeks to a couple of years later. Occasionally, skin and other organs are infected.

Many people (but not all) with normal immunity get better from the pneumonia, although a few do develop meningitis. People with decreased immunity, but especially those with HIV infection (but also those on prednisone or other corticosteroid drugs or on cancer chemotherapy), often develop meningitis and encephalitis.

Cryptoccal meningitis and encephalitis have symptoms and signs like tuberculous meningitis (see page 414). At first, there may be only a headache but fever and neck stiffness may be very mild or not present. Other signs of meningitis and encephalitis then slowly develop. Some or even complete loss of sight, severe headache, fever, nausea, clumsiness and falling when walking, paralysis of eye or face muscles, twitching, confusion, coma, etc. and eventually death, develop.

Diagnosis is made by doing a lumbar puncture. Laboratory tests are needed to show the diagnosis by (1) an 'India ink' stain which often shows the cryptococci in the CSF, (2) a test for cryptococcal antigen in the CSF which is usually positive (it is less often positive in the blood and a positive blood test does not always mean infection is still present). The other typical abnormalities of meningitis in the CSF may not be marked or even present – especially in patients with HIV infection.

Treatment with drugs (such as IV amphotericin B) is possible but very expensive, can have severe side effects and takes a long time. Then, even if the patient is cured, if the patient has HIV infection and the CD4 count does not improve enough on ART, he may need drug prophylaxis (e.g. oral fluconazole) to be continued for the rest of his life to stop the condition returning.

The differential diagnosis includes not only TB but also toxoplasma and nocardia and viral and other infections of the meninges.

The Medical Officer will diagnose the condition and tell you what to do after you transfer patients with possible chronic meningitis to him for diagnosis and management.

Viral meningitis

Viral meningitis is an inflammation of the meninges caused by infection with one of many viruses. It is clinically similar to acute bacterial meningitis (see pages 409–410), *but*

1. The CSF looks clear and the glucose is not low, although the protein may be high. The leucocytes are not a lot in number and are lymphocytes.
2. Most cases get better with no treatment. Antibiotics do not help. If the virus is HIV or the virus is an opportunistic infection because of HIV, the patient will get worse and die.

You will diagnose most cases in a health centre (where laboratory tests are not available) incorrectly as cerebral malaria. This does not matter as the management is as for cerebral malaria.

Treat as for cerebral malaria (but do not give antimalarial drugs if malaria is not possible) (see pages 413–414).

Transfer to Medical Officer care if the patient is unconscious for more than 1 day, *or* not improving after 2 days, *or* not cured after 2 weeks.

African trypanosomiasis (sleeping sickness)

See Chapter 18 pages 181–183 for details.

The patient is in (or from) an area where African trypanosomiasis occurs.

Early *signs* may be:

1. fast pulse, and perhaps heart failure,
2. anaemia,
3. enlarged lymph glands (especially in the back of the neck),
4. enlarged spleen, and
5. proteinurea.

Chronic meningoencephalitis follows and causes:

1. headache;
2. tiredness, sleepiness and no interest in anything (the patient may not even eat);
3. sleeping in the day, but sometimes not at night;
4. changes in personality, confusion, and development of organic psychosis (see Chapter 35 pages 572–573) (these may be the first signs);
5. shaking, weakness, pains, difficulty in walking;
6. coma and death.

Transfer all such cases for diagnosis and treatment by the Medical Officer. Do not do a lumbar puncture if you suspect African trypanosomiasis before the patient is put onto effective treatment.

Encephalitis

Encephalitis is inflammation of the brain itself, usually caused by one of many viruses.

Most patients have a fever, headache, decrease of brain function (with loss of alertness and full consciousness or paralysis) or irritation of the brain (with fits or abnormal behaviour). Often the meninges are also inflamed (i.e. it is meningoencephalitis). The CSF looks clear and glucose is normal (although the protein may be high and leucocytes are most likely lymphocytes).

Many cases get better with no treatment. Some cases may have permanent brain damage. A few cases (and any case due to rabies) die. Antibiotics do not help.

You will diagnose many cases incorrectly as cerebral malaria; but this does not matter because management is as for cerebral malaria (see pages 413–414). If you could be certain that the patient did not have malaria, you would not give the antimalarial drugs.

An occasional case is due to hyperpyrexia from people being in the sun or exercising during a hot humid time when they are not used to these things. Take the rectal temperature in all patients with acute encephalitis of unknown cause. See Chapter 13 pages 72 and 81.

Arboviruses (see Chapter 17 pages 166–172) are a common cause, especially if there is an epidemic. Japanese encephalitis is the most severe with one in five cases dying and half of the patients developing some permanent brain damage. Effective immunisation for Japanese encephalitis exists.

However, always think of rabies (see below) if you are in an area where rabies occurs.

HIV infection itself can cause encephalitis. (See Chapter 19.) Opportunistic viruses such as CMV and herpes also cause encephalitis in HIV infected patients.

Cases may be caused by malaria, African trypanosomiasis (see page 415), American trypanosomiasis (see Chapter 18 page 183), cysticercosis (see Chapter 23 page 358) relapsing fever or typhus fever (see pages 158, 164).

Encephalitis due to an immune reaction can occasionally occur several weeks after some viral infections and some vaccinations.

Transfer to Medical Officer care if the patient is: unconscious for more than 1 day, *or* not improving after 2 days, *or* not cured after 2 weeks.

Rabies

Rabies is an acute viral disease of the brain (encephalitis) and of the salivary glands of animals, which sometimes affects man.

It is spread from one animal to another animal by infected secretions (usually saliva). The means of spread is usually a bite by an infected animal. All warm-blooded animals can be infected with rabies.

Rabies occurs in most countries. Find out if it occurs in your area.

Symptoms and *signs* of rabies in man include:

1. There is a history of an animal bite, usually from a dog which was behaving abnormally (but at times other animals or patients with rabies). Bites from, or the inhalation of faeces from infected bats can also cause rabies.
2. The disease has a long incubation period (1 week to more than 1 year), before the first signs appear.
3. The patient becomes 'sick' for a few days with fever, headache, etc.
4. The patient then has a period of encephalitis.
   This produces over-activity or paralysis or a mixture of both. Some patients become very anxious. Sudden noises and lights, etc. cause strange behaviour. There are episodes of wild behaviour and muscle spasms and fear. The patient cannot swallow because of the spasms of the throat muscles. Even the sight of water causes these spasms. The spasms can cause 'foaming at the mouth'. Other patients become very depressed and quiet, and become paralysed. But even they can get spasms of the throat and cannot swallow.
5. The patient dies, usually within 10–15 days (but it can be shorter or longer).
6. Cases that are not typical may be common. Suspect rabies in any unusual disease of the nervous system in an area where rabies occurs.

Signs of rabies in the dog or other animals are similar to those in man.

Confirmation of the *diagnosis* is by special tests.

If you strongly suspect rabies in a patient or an animal, notify the nearest Medical and Veterinary Officer urgently.

No *treatment* can cure rabies once it has developed. Give morphine, chlorpromazine and diazepam in large regular doses each 4–6 hours to relieve the distress and pain.

Prevention of rabies includes:

1. Kill the organism in the body of the original hosts (reservoir).
   In areas where rabies occurs:
   (a) All dogs without owners should be killed.
   (b) All dogs with owners should be immunised against rabies.

(c) If wild animals in the area carry the disease they can be immunised by spreading live virus vaccines on baits.

2. Stop the means of spread.

Control dogs.

Do not get bitten by dogs, cats or bats or go into bat caves.

When nursing patients with rabies, use strict barrier nursing, including use of gloves, masks and goggles as the saliva is infectious if it gets into the eyes or mouth as well as through the skin – and the patients sometimes spit. All staff should also be immunised.

3. Raise the resistance of persons who are bitten.

Give passive immunisation with anti-rabies hyperimmune serum, preferably from humans, but if not available, from animals. However, it is probably needed only if there has been a large dose of virus from a large bite or many bites, or if the bite was in a central part of the body. Give half of the dose by infiltration around the wound.

Give active immunisation with whatever is available. Brain tissue vaccine is effective, but quite a number of patients develop encephalitis from the vaccine. Purified duck embryo vaccine is safer. The best, however, are tissue or cell culture vaccines, e.g. HDVC, PCECV and PVCU but they are very expensive.

Give only according to the direction with it immediately and then e.g. on days 3, 7, 14 and 20. This gives good protection.

Find out what is available in your area and what you should do.

Give active immunisation to any staff or family member caring for the patient.

If a person is bitten by an animal, manage as follows:

1. *Give proper treatment for the bite*
   - Wash the wound with a lot of soap and water.
   - Rinse with a lot of water.
   - Then apply iodine in spirit.
   - Then do the necessary surgical toilet.
   - Do not stitch the wound.
   - Infiltrate around the wound with half the dose of rabies immunoglobulin if available.
   - Give the rest of the immunoglobulin by IMI.
   - Dress the wound and apply a compression bandage to stop bleeding.
   - Start antibiotics, e.g. co-amoxyclav if needed.
   - Give tetanus prophylaxis (see page 420).
2. *Try to find out if the animal has rabies and transfer the patient for immunisation if necessary.*

(a) If the animal looks healthy, lock it up for 10 days. If it is still alive and well after 10 days, the animal did not have rabies and no immunisation of the patient is necessary. If the animal shows any sign of sickness before the 10 days are finished, start immunisation or transfer the patient immediately for immunisation.

(b) If the animal has disappeared, start immunisation or transfer the patient for immunisation.

(c) If the animal has been caught and looks sick, lock up the animal carefully (make sure that it does not bite anyone) and inform the local Veterinary Officer. Transfer the patient for immunisation.

(d) If the animal has been killed leave the body for the Veterinary Officer. If the Veterinary Officer cannot come and you do not have special ways of removing animal brains, or cutting off the head and keeping it in ice without infecting yourself, bury the animal carefully. Start immunisation or immediately transfer the patient for immunisation.

Poliomyelitis

Polio is an IHR 'disease under surveillance' by WHO and it was hoped to eradicate it by the year 2000. Unfortunately, cases still occur in a few countries. All cases must be notified immediately to your Medical Officer so that the government can control the disease and notify the WHO. Most of such rare cases now will turn out to be diseases similar to that caused by the polio virus that are caused by another virus such as Echo or Coxsackie and need the same treatment; but they do not cause major epidemics like the polio virus.

Poliomyelitis is an acute inflammation of parts of the brain and spinal cord caused by one of the polio viruses. Polio viruses are spread by the faecal–oral route or, less often, by respiratory secretions.

Infection can cause one or more of the following:

1. An asymptomatic infection.
2. A non-specific viral gastroenteritis or febrile illness.
3. In only a very few of the above, clinical virus meningitis (see page 415).
4. In only a very few of the above, an infection of the brain and spinal cord (encephalitis and myelitis). This can cause sudden paralysis of groups of muscles in 1 or 2 days. Other groups may then be paralysed in the next week or so. Often a number of limbs are partly paralysed. This is different from a stroke or injury where usually the whole of one limb or the whole of one side of the body is para-

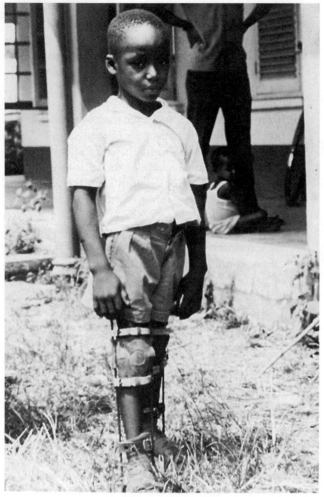

Figure 25.12 *A boy who had polio affecting both legs and could not walk – he could only crawl. Calipers were made for him in a health centre at a cost of about US$1. He can now walk without help.*

lysed. There is often severe pain and aching in the affected muscles. There is no loss of sensation. If the muscles used for breathing are affected, the patient will die because he cannot breathe. If the muscles which are used to swallow are affected the patient may die because saliva, food, etc. will be breathed into the lungs and cause pneumonia.

No treatment to kill the infection or cure the encephalitis and myelitis is possible. However, if the patient can be kept alive, considerable improvement of muscle paralysis may later occur with physiotherapy, exercises, etc.

If you have a patient who could have poliomyelitis contact the Medical Officer urgently about *care* and *transfer* of the patient, as breathing may later become

affected and there will be the need for vaccination of contacts.

Killing the parasite in the body of the original host or reservoir is not possible. Stopping the means of spread by reducing faecal–oral spread and respiratory secretion spread helps. However, the main way of control is by raising the resistance of all people to polio. If everyone is made resistant to polio, the disease will have to die out. Sabin trivalent live attenuated oral polio vaccine (OPV) should be given at birth in polio endemic countries and then to all children everywhere at 6, 10 and 14 weeks of age with the DPT or triple antigen and again twice 1 month apart to all children under 5 years (no matter how many previous doses) in polio eradication campaigns. All non-immunised adults should be given three doses of the vaccine. In an epidemic all contacts should be given a dose of the vaccine. If the contacts were not previously immunised, the vaccination course should be completed. In polio eradication programmes, extra doses will be given even if the person has been immunised before.

Polio can cripple people so that they cannot care for themselves (see Figure 25.12). Many people who have suffered from polio become beggars. You can make cheap surgical aids to help these people care for themselves again (see Huckstep, R.L, 'Orthopaedic appliances for developing countries' *Tropical Doctor* 1971; **1**: 64–7).

Cerebrovascular disease (stroke)

A stroke is a sudden paralysis or loss of one of the other functions of the body controlled by the brain. This is caused by disease of the blood vessels that bring blood to the brain.

When people get old, their blood vessels get narrower; and the blood in them flows slowly and may clot. If a person has high blood pressure, it can damage the blood vessels; one of these damaged blood vessels may burst or the blood in one of them clot. Some people are born with weakness in part of a blood vessel (called an aneurysm); the weak blood vessel can burst. Diseases, especially diabetes but also meningitis and syphilis and especially atheroma (due to age but worse if poor diet, lack of exercise, obesity or smoking), can damage blood vessels; and then the blood in these blood vessels can clot. A clot of blood from a diseased heart can break off and suddenly block a normal blood vessel. All of these blood vessel conditions can stop the flow of the blood to a part of the brain which then does not work and then dies, i.e. they can cause strokes.

Prevent strokes by treating patients with high blood pressure and diabetes and giving health education about diet, exercise, obesity and smoking.

A mass in the skull pressing on the brain can look like stroke. Blood can collect after head injury (from artery in minutes to hours and from veins in days to weeks) and be cured by a simple operation. Masses from TB, cysticercosis, schistosomiasis and nocardia infections can be cured.

Always get the Medical Officer urgently to see a patient who seems to have had a stroke after a head injury, or non-urgently to see a patient who could possibly have an infection causing a mass in the brain. These patients may be able to be cured.

The *symptoms* and *signs* depend on which blood vessel disease is the cause and what part of the brain is affected.

If a haemorrhage occurs the stroke usually starts suddenly. If the blood goes into the subarachnoid space, it will cause symptoms and signs of meningeal irritation like meningitis (see page 410), i.e. a severe headache, stiff neck, etc. A lumbar puncture will show blood in the CSF which does not decrease as each bottle of CSF is collected.

If a blood vessel clots then the stroke will start slowly over a few hours; and there will be no signs of meningeal irritation.

If the part of the brain which controls movement is affected, then the patient will have paralysis.

If other parts of the brain are involved, the patient will have loss of sensation, blindness, loss of speech, etc.

Do a lumbar puncture to check that the patient does not have meningitis. If the patient could have had an STD, do a serology test for syphilis (see Chapter 19 pages 208–210) to check that the patient does not have syphilis.

The patient often dies in the first few days to weeks. If the patient lives for the first few days, he can often greatly improve for the next 6 months or more (sometimes even up to 24 months).

Treatment includes:

1. Nursing care as necessary. If the patient is unconscious, see pages 422–424.
2. Physiotherapy. All limb joints must be moved 10–20 times each, twice daily. If the patient cannot do this, the nurse or orderly must do it for them.
3. Early mobilisation. The patient must get out of bed as soon as possible after the first 2 days. Help the patient to walk as well as he can even if it takes two strong people to hold him up while he tries. The patient must not stay in bed all the time. If he does,

many complications will develop, and he will not get better.

4. If the patient and the relatives force the paralysed or affected parts of the body to try to work *all the time* for the first year, great improvement may occur (even return to normal).
5. If the patient's blood pressure stays high (more than 160/90), then see Chapter 27 page 470.

Tetanus

Tetanus is an acute disease of the nervous system caused by tetanus toxin. Tetanus toxin is made if tetanus bacteria grow in the body. *It usually causes a painful death. It is very difficult and expensive to treat. It is easily and cheaply prevented by immunisation.*

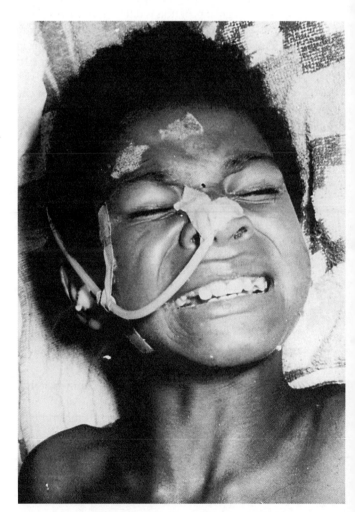

Figure 25.13 *Tetanus. Note the muscles of the body are all in spasm, the head is bent backwards and the lips are pulled back (as in a smile). The patient is in great pain.*

Tetanus bacteria (*Clostridium tetani*) normally live in the intestines of animals and in dirt. They can get into a person's body when dirt gets into the body, e.g. through wounds or burns, the female genital tract at delivery, and the cut end of a baby's umbilical cord at birth. Usually, the tetanus bacteria grow and make the toxin only in special types of wounds: puncture wounds, wounds or burns that get dirt in them and wounds infected by other bacteria.

The first *symptoms* are usually pain and stiffness of the jaw, difficulty in opening the mouth wide and difficulty in swallowing. The pain and stiffness then spread to the whole body. Several days later, spasms of the whole body usually occur (Figure 25.13). The spasms last from a few to many seconds. Movement of the patient's body or a sudden noise can sometimes start the spasms. During the spasms the patient is conscious and in great pain (this is different from 'fits'). The nervous system controlling the heart, blood pressure and temperature may be affected and changes occur in these. The condition may continue to get worse for 10 days and take 4 weeks to go away after treatment.

Very occasionally, the stiffness may be only in the muscles near the infection, e.g. in a limb near a wound or in the face if ear infection; but this can spread to involve the whole body.

There are *no tests* to make the diagnosis. If you have real doubt about meningitis or cerebral malaria, do a lumbar puncture and a blood slide, and start treatment as on page 411. Muscle spasms can sometimes be caused by drugs such as chlorpromazine. If you suspect this, see Chapter 35 page 581. You can only diagnose tetanus from the history of the wound; the symptoms of jaw stiffness; and the signs – the mouth will not open wide, general body stiffness and later spasms; in a patient who was not properly immunised.

Treatment at a health centre is not usually possible. If you make the diagnosis, immediately arrange urgent transfer of the patient to hospital. Management before transfer includes:

1. Give IMI chlorpromazine 100 mg immediately.
2. Give IMI phenobarbital 100–200 mg *or* paraldehyde from a glass syringe 10 ml immediately or diazepam rectally as below.
3. Start an intravenous drip. Give maintenance fluids.
4. Also give, when necessary to control the spasms, rectal diazepam 10 mg (2 ml) in 8 ml of 0.9% saline and if needed IVI diazepam 5–10 mg very slowly.
5. Give IMI human tetanus immunoglobulin 500 units (2 of the 250 international units vials) immediately.

(In hospital a 3000–6000 unit dose will be added. Give this if available.)
6. Give benzylpenicillin 2,000,000 units (1.2 g) immediately by IVI and continue 6 hourly.
7. Nurse the patient on his side with the head lower than the feet. Gently suck out the patient's airway if it is blocked, or he is breathing noisily. Do not disturb the patient if possible.
8. Give nothing to eat or drink by mouth.
9. Clean and dress any wound.
10. A good health worker must go with the patient to the hospital. This person will care for the patient's airway, suck out the airway if necessary and give more of the above drugs (a different one each 2-4 hours) for spasms if necessary.

Prevention includes:

1. Immunise all children with DPT or triple antigen and all adults (especially pregnant women to stop tetanus in her newborn child if the umbilical cord is infected) with DT or tetanus toxoid three times (see Chapter 10 pages 44 and 46–48) and then give tetanus toxoid each 10 years.
2. Treat wounds and burns properly. Clean them all well, and remove all dead tissue from wounds.
3. If the wound is:
   (a) a deep wound, a puncture wound or a compound fracture;
   (b) a wound which has a lot of dead tissue in it;
   (c) a wound which has foreign bodies, especially wood, dirt or manure (animal faeces) in it;
   (d) many hours old before you treat it, or is already clinically, infected:
   then
   • give antibiotics,
   • give tetanus toxoid 0.5 ml IMI and complete the course, if not immunised,
   • give human tetanus immunoglobulin, if not immunised, (250–)500 IU (or animal tetanus immunoglobulin 1500–5000 units) with precautions about allergic reactions – see Chapter 10 page 44) in different limb from toxoid.

Epilepsy

See Convulsions (fits) and epilepsy pages 424, 425.

Peripheral neuritis or peripheral neuropathy

These are the names for the condition when the nerves (page 406) that run to the edges of the body do not work properly.

Usually (but not always) the longest nerves in the body are the most affected and therefore the legs and then the arms are usually the most affected parts.

If the nerves do not work properly, sensation from the part of the body to the brain may not be normal.

1. The patient may complain of numbness or not being able to feel things in the affected area.
2. The patient may get injuries or burns without feeling them and therefore they let the cause continue until large injuries or burns or ulcers form. Even then they do not cause the pain that would be expected.
3. On the other hand, if the nerves are not completely stopped from working, the patient may feel pains or a burning sensation or a 'pins and needles' sensation or a 'crawling' sensation in the areas supplied by the nerves.
4. On examination there will be loss of some touch and pain and other sensations in the area (see Chapter 15 pages 133–135) for ways of testing sensation.

If the nerves do not work properly the muscles that are supplied by the affected nerve may become weak and wasted and eventually paralysed unless the cause is stopped.

See Chapter 15 pages 135–137 for ways of testing for some of the muscles.

Causes of peripheral neuropathy are many but include the following:

• Traumatic injury including just pressure on them as when lying still during drunkenness or general anaesthesia and also if the nerve is trapped by normal structures at the wrist, elbow, neck or knee if the patient gets oedema, obesity or arthritis, etc.
• Infections especially: leprosy, HIV, diphtheria, typhoid.
• Post-infectious (after infections) immunological reactions (Guillain–Barré syndrome) which causes both legs to start to get weak about 3 weeks after a viral type infection and the weakness slowly goes up the legs and into the trunk and can cause death if it reaches the breathing muscles and this is not treated.
• Non-infectious immunological inflammatory conditions, especially leprosy reactions.
• Autoimmune diseases, especially rheumatoid (arthritis) disease.
• Drugs especially isoniazid if given without pyridoxine and some anti-HIV drugs.
• Vascular causes, especially diabetes mellitus.
• Vitamin deficiencies, especially some of the vitamin B group deficiencies (e.g. pellagra, beriberi), folic acid and vitamin B_{12} deficiency (see page 380).
• Poisons especially alcohol excess.

• Effects of cancers elsewhere in the body.
• Many other causes known.
• Many other causes not known (up to 50% of cases have no cause found).

If a patient has a peripheral neuropathy:

1. Treat any cause you can, especially:
   • stop any drug which could be cause;
   • give pyridoxine 100 mg daily if on isoniazid;
   • give vitamin B group vitamins and improve diet if any suggestion of malnutrition or alcoholism;
   • advise patient to stop any excess alcohol intake;
   • treat any leprosy reaction quickly and transfer if you are not successful;
   • control any diabetes better;
   • treat any diphtheria and transfer for anti-toxin.
2. Discuss the case with your Medical Officer to see if there are any special tests you should do or special treatment you should give or if the patient should be transferred for further investigation.

Brain tumour/Intracranial mass

Brain tumours or intracranial masses are lumps of tissue within the skull (cranium) that progressively become larger. As the bony skull cannot enlarge to make room for the mass, the mass has to press on and damage the brain. This diagnosis is suggested by:

1. slowly increasing loss of some part of the brain's function, e.g. slowly increasing paralysis starting in the thumb and then slowly involving more of the hand, arm, etc. and/or
2. onset of epilepsy in someone previously not epileptic and/or
3. generalised abnormality of brain function, e.g.
   • headache especially on coughing, sneezing, straining, etc. or lying down including on waking in the morning; the attacks of headache gradually getting longer and at times being accompanied by vomiting,
   • change of personality,
   • development of dementia or coma.

The diagnosis can be made only by special X-rays or scans in a hospital. If this condition is strongly suspected and there is not a strong suspicion of some type of meningitis, a lumbar puncture should not be done in a health centre as this could make the condition quickly worse. Instead, the patient should be transferred to the hospital.

If the condition is due to a primary cancer of the brain cells or of secondary cancer spread from elsewhere in the body to the brain, no curative treatment is possible.

If, however, the mass is due to:

1. a tuberculoma – a mass of tuberculous inflammation tissue,
2. schistosomiasis – a mass of inflammation around schistosome eggs (see Chapter 18 pages 187–191),
3. cysticercosis – a pig tapeworm cyst (see Chapter 23 page 358),
4. a pyogenic bacterial abscess from infection in the nose or ear or blood stream or head injury,
5. syphilis (see Chapter 19 pages 208–210),
6. toxoplasma causing one or many masses of inflammatory tissue (see Chapter 19 pages 228–230) very common in patients with HIV infection but rare if immunity normal,
7. nocardia causing inflammatory masses (see Chapter 19 pages 228–230),
8. others,

then, for each of the above; treatment with:

1. anti-TB drugs,
2. praziquantel,
3. praziquantel or albendazole; but transfer for corticosteroids, etc., also,
4. chloramphenicol; or penicillin probably with metronidazole,
5. penicillin or chloramphenicol,
6. sulfadoxine 500 mg and pyrimethamine 25 mg tablets, two tablets twice daily for 6 weeks (but not in the first 14 weeks of pregnancy and preferably with also folinic acid); and if not available SMX/TMP as below.
7. co-trimoxazole SMX 1600 mg and TMP 320 mg 3 times a day for small adults and four times a day for large adults for 3 weeks,
8. or other drugs

may help.

An intracranial haemorrhage with a haematoma hours after a head injury if an artery is bleeding, or days or weeks after if a vein is bleeding, can cause a similar condition and be able to be cured by simple surgery. Transfer all such cases as emergencies.

High dose corticosteroids (e.g. dexamethasone 4 mg tid or prednisolone 50 mg daily, slowly reducing to zero over 4 weeks) usually decreases oedema and swelling in the brain and improves the patient. Prophylaxis against TB and malaria, etc. is needed if not supplied by the other treatment.

Similar conditions may affect the spinal cord.

Discuss such patients with your Medical Officer or transfer.

Diagnosis and management of common symptoms and signs

Unconsciousness (coma)

Causes of unconsciousness include (look up these conditions):

1. Disease of the brain and meninges.
   - head injury
   - meningitis – all types
   - cerebral malaria
   - hyperpyrexia (temperature over 40°C)
   - encephalitis – all types
   - intracerebral masses and cerebral tumours – all types
   - haemorrhage with haematoma
   - malnutrition with beriberi.
2. Abnormality of the blood going to brain.
   - alcohol, drugs, poisons
   - toxins from infections, especially septicaemia and pneumonia and typhoid
   - toxins, etc. from the body – chronic kidney failure, chronic liver disease
   - low oxygen from anaemia, shock, heart failure, lung diseases
   - high sugar from diabetes; low sugar from too much insulin
   - eclampsia
   - small volume of blood circulation because of severe dehydration, especially cholera.
3. Non-organic mental illness.
   - acting out.

Management of the unconscious patient

Management of unconsciousness includes:

1. Give routine nursing care to the unconscious patient.
2. Record the level of consciousness hourly.
3. Diagnose and treat the cause.
   Take a full history from the patient's relatives or friends.
   Do a full physical examination.
   Do blood glucose. Give glucose (or insulin) if needed.
   Make a malaria smear and give treatment for cerebral malaria.
   Do a lumbar puncture. Treat for meningitis if necessary.
   Test the urine.

4. Transfer to Medical Officer care if the level of consciousness gets worse, if complications develop or if the patient is still unconscious after 24 hours.

1. *Routine nursing care of the unconscious patient*

Maintain the airway (check that the patient can breathe):
- lay patient on his side (never on his back) (see Figure 25.14),
- bend his head back,
- pull his jaw forward,
- suck out his pharynx every hour and also any time when there is noisy or blocked breathing (noisy breathing or snoring means blocked breathing),
- raise the foot of the bed if needed and if no head injury; to let secretions run out of his mouth,
- insert 'airway' if necessary, and
- give artificial ventilation if the patient stops breathing because of something you can treat (e.g. snakebite, poisoning by drugs, etc.).

Care of pressure areas – turn every 2 hours.

Give intravenous fluids if necessary. If you give intragastric fluids nurse the patient with his head down and the patient on the side, and maintain his airway carefully.

Use an indwelling catheter if the bladder becomes distended and cannot be emptied by gentle pressure every 2–4 hours (bladder distension is one of the common causes of restlessness in an unconscious patient).

2. *Record the level of consciousness*

You should also record the size of the pupils of the eyes.

Repeat these observations every hour to see if the patient is improving or getting worse.

Observations will show if the patient:
- is fully conscious, or
- answers only simple questions, or
- obeys only simple commands, or
- responds (moves) only if hurt,
- does not respond (move) if hurt, or
- is dead.

3. *Diagnose and treat the cause*

(a) Always take a full *medical history* from the patient's relatives or friends (see Chapter 6). Ask about the possibility of drug overdose or poisons (including alcohol) or if he has had recent treatment for an illness (including insulin) or a head injury.

(b) Always do a full, careful *physical examination* of the patient. (See Chapter 6.)

- Smell the breath for alcohol, diabetes and kidney failure.
- Look carefully for a head injury.
- Check the BP (especially if pregnant (eclampsia)).
- Check for shock, especially from bleeding or severe dehydration (cholera), and treat if present (see Chapter 27 page 468).
- Check for severe infection (e.g. septicaemia), and treat if present (see Chapter 12 page 64).
- Check for chronic conditions (e.g. cirrhosis, kidney failure, African trypanosomiasis).

(c) Always do a malaria smear and *give antimalarials* for cerebral malaria (see page 413) unless you are certain that the patient does not have malaria. Give IV or IMI artesunate 2.4 mg/kg (120–180 mg) or IMI artemether 3.2 mg/kg (160–240 mg) or IMI quinine 20 mg/kg (900–1200 mg) and see Chapter 13 pages 80, 82.

(d) Always do a *lumbar puncture*. Treat for meningitis if:
- the CSF is cloudy, or
- the CSF is blood-stained, or
- the CSF looks clear but a rapid diagnostic test suggests meningitis or
- the CSF is not obtained (failed LP).

(e) Always *test urine* for sugar, protein and bile (diabetes, eclampsia and chronic kidney failure).

(f) Always do a *blood glucose test*. If glucose low (less than 2.2 mmol/l or 40 mg/dl) or you cannot do the test, give 50 ml of 50% glucose IV and repeat blood glucose test 2 hourly.

(g) Try to find out if patient has a psychiatric condition ('acting out') (see Chapter 35 page 579). But do not diagnose this until the patient is fully conscious and recovered again.

4. *Transfer*

Transfer to Medical Officer care:

(a) if the level of consciousness gets worse every hour for 4 hours (urgent – emergency) (especially important if the cause can be treated); or

(b) if the size of one pupil does not stay the same as the size of the other pupil (urgent); or

(c) if another complication develops which you cannot treat at the health centre (e.g. the patient is not breathing enough) (urgent); or

(d) if the patient is still unconscious after 24 hours and not obviously improving (urgent).

Do not transfer if the cause is known and it cannot be treated.

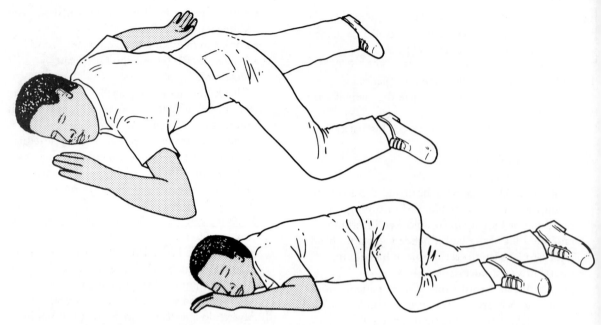

Figure 25.14 *Diagram showing the position in which you should nurse an unconscious patient (the recovery position).*

Simple faint (syncope)

In a faint (or attack of syncope), the patient feels light headed, is not able to see properly, has muscle weakness, cannot stand, and loses full consciousness.

If you lay the patient down, he will recover quickly – in 1–3 minutes.

Check that the patient does not have another condition, especially a fit.

Look for and treat the cause:

1. diseases of the brain,
2. abnormality of the blood going to the brain, or
3. mental disturbances.

See Unconsciousness page 422 for a list of causes. Most cases are caused by:

1. standing still for a long time (blood stays in the legs and not enough goes back to the heart to go to the brain);
2. anaemia (not enough oxygen in blood going to the brain); and
3. fear, worry, disgust or pain.

Dizziness (vertigo)

This is a feeling of movement (e.g. things going around) often with faintness and nausea or vomiting.

Causes include:

1. diseases of brain (see Unconsciousness page 422 for list);

2. abnormalities of blood going to brain (see Unconsciousness page 422 for list);
3. some eye conditions; and
4. some ear conditions.

Treat the cause if it can be found. Symptomatic treatment would be something such as prochlorperazine 5–12.5 mg, chlorpromazine 10–12.5 mg, promethazine 10–25 mg or chlorphenamine 4 mg, as long as the blood pressure was not already low, each 4–6 hours if needed.

Convulsions (fits) and epilepsy

Convulsion (fit)

In a 'generalised' ('grand mal') convulsion or fit, the patient suddenly loses consciousness, and falls. All the muscles of his body suddenly contract and stay contracted. The face and the limbs become stiff. The patient cannot breathe and goes blue. He may pass urine and faeces. Usually after about 30 seconds, muscles relax. Then the muscles start to contract and then relax again and again quickly. This makes the patient's limbs jerk and his mouth and eyes open and close. Often the patient bites his tongue. Breathing starts again but it may be very noisy. This period can last a very short or very long time; but it usually stops without treatment. Then the patient usually sleeps deeply for about half an hour. When the patient wakes, he cannot remember anything about the convulsion. Sometimes he is confused and has a headache.

These symptoms and signs are caused by the patient losing control of all of his brain, i.e. 'generalised'. Without control, the brain makes the body act abnormally. You can easily see the loss of control and the abnormal working of the area of the brain which makes the muscles move. All the other parts of the brain are also without control and also working abnormally during a general convulsion (or fit).

Partial convulsions (fits) are different from these general convulsions. The patient may have a feeling which tells him that the fit is about to start. If only one part of the area of the brain which controls muscles is affected, only one part of the body may jerk (e.g. the face or one limb or one side of the body), and the patient may stay conscious. If only one part of the area of the brain which controls sensations is affected, the patient may only have abnormal sensation in one part of his body. If only another part of the brain is affected, the patient may have only abnormal (often violent) behaviour. These are 'partial' fits.

But any of these partial types of fit may develop into a general convulsion if the abnormal working of part of the brain spreads to all of the brain, including all the areas that control the muscles.

Sometimes convulsions do not stop but continue for hours or longer. This is a very dangerous condition that often results in death. This is called 'status epilepticus'.

The *causes* of convulsions or fits are the same as the causes for unconsciousness (see page 422).

> A convulsion (or a fit) is not a disease and is never the only diagnosis. A convulsion is caused by something which upsets the normal working of the brain. There is a disorder of the brain or the blood coming to the brain. The cause of the convulsion must always be diagnosed too and treated.

Epilepsy

Epilepsy is diagnosed if there are *repeated convulsions* over weeks, months or years. The *causes of epilepsy* are the same as the cause of a single fit (see above). Often it is not possible to find the cause of epilepsy. But this does not mean that there is no cause. It is common – 3 to 5 million people in Africa alone have epilepsy.

> Epilepsy is not a disease and is never the only diagnosis. Epilepsy is caused by something which affects the normal working of the brain. You must diagnose the cause of the epilepsy if possible. Epilepsy is not infectious.

Unfortunately, many people believe incorrectly that epilepsy is due to possession by evil spirits; or that people with it are insane (or psychotic); or sufferers are not able to learn and should not be educated; and people with epilepsy are not suitable to be friends or to marry or to employ. Many believe incorrectly that it can be passed on by contact with saliva. The problems these false beliefs cause patients with epilepsy are often far greater than the problems of the epilepsy itself, or the side effects of drug treatment.

Good control of epilepsy (by giving the correct drugs regularly all the time so that people have few (if any) fits) helps get rid of the false beliefs about epilepsy.

Health education to the general population as well as the family and the patient about the real cause of epilepsy (damage to the brain or occasionally abnormality of the blood going to the brain) is also very badly needed.

Management of a patient with convulsions (fits) or epilepsy

> Management includes six things:
> 1. When the patient is fitting, make sure that he cannot hurt himself.
> 2. When the patient is unconscious, give the nursing care for an unconscious patient.
> 3. Stop the fit with anti-convulsant drugs: give rectal or IV diazepam or IMI paraldehyde.
> 4. Find and treat the cause.
>   Take a full history from the patient's relatives or friends.
>   Do a full clinical examination.
>   Always check the BP, especially if pregnant.
>   Do blood glucose and give IV glucose if needed.
>   Make a malaria smear and give antimalarials.
>   Do a lumbar puncture. Treat for meningitis if necessary.
>   Test the urine.
> 5. Give phenobarbital or phenytoin when the patient can swallow, until you cure the cause of the fits (if possible).
> 6. Transfer if you cannot stop the fits or if you cannot find or treat the cause of the fits in the health centre.

1. *When the patient is fitting*

   Make sure he does not hurt himself, e.g. fall off a bed, fall into a fire, etc. Do not try to stop the movements as this is not possible and you may injure the patient. When the mouth is opening and closing, put something between the teeth so that the patient does not bite his tongue.

2. *If the patient is unconscious*

Give nursing care (see page 423). Check that the airway is clear (i.e. the patient can breathe) – keep on his side, keep his neck bent back, keep his jaw forward, clear his airway and suck out his throat if necessary.

3. *Give anti-convulsant drugs*

Give *diazepam* (10–)20 mg (2–)4 ml rectally using a small (5–10 ml) syringe (without a needle) pushed in 4–5 cm. Then hold the buttocks together or strap them together. If still fitting, repeat 10 mg (2 ml) in 10 minutes and again each hour up to a maximum of 50 mg. It would be better, if the fitting did not stop after the second dose, to give, if available, *paraldehyde* 0.2 ml/kg or 10 ml for the average adult in a glass syringe IMI, immediately, repeated in 5–10 minutes if the patient is still fitting.

After this give these drugs every 4–6 hours if necessary.

If paraldehyde not available, give *diazepam* by slow IVI. Dilute 10 mg (2 ml) with 8 ml saline and give at rate of no more than 1 ml, i.e. 1 mg/minute. Stop the injection as soon as the fitting stops or if the patient's breathing slows. Maximum dose is 15 mg. Give artificial ventilation if breathing stops. Repeat the dose after 20 minutes if the patient has not stopped fitting or starts again but it would be better to run a slow IV infusion 10 mg (2 ml) in 150 ml fluid each 6 hours.

Diazepam IMI is not good treatment to stop fitting as it is very slow acting.

4. *Find and treat the cause* (if the patient is not a known epileptic). (See page 425.)

(a) Always take a full medical *history* from the patient's relatives or friends (see Chapter 6). Ask about the possibility of drug overdose or poisons (including alcohol) or if he has had recent treatment for any illness (including insulin).

(b) Always do a full careful *physical examination* (see Chapter 6):
- smell the breath for alcohol;
- look for head injury;
- check the BP, especially if pregnant;
- check for shock and treat if present;
- check for severe infection (e.g. septicaemia) and treat if present;
- check for chronic conditions (e.g. cirrhosis, kidney failure, African trypanosomiasis).

(c) Always do a *lumbar puncture*. Treat for meningitis if:
- the CSF is cloudy, or
- the CSF is blood-stained, or

- the CSF looks clear but a rapid diagnostic test suggests meningitis, or
- the CSF is not obtained (failed LP).

(d) Always do a *malaria smear* and give *antimalarials* for cerebral malaria unless you are certain that the patient does not have malaria. (See page 413.) Give the patient artesunate 2.4 mg/kg (120–180 mg) by IVI or IMI or artemether 3.2 mg/kg (160–240 mg) or quinine 20 mg/kg (900–1200 mg) by IMI immediately.

(e) Always *test the urine* for protein, sugar and bile.

(f) Always check the *blood glucose* and give 50 ml 50% glucose if blood glucose low (less than 2.2 mmol/l or 40 mg/dl) or cannot be done.

(g) Always *check that the patient did have a fit* and does not have another condition, e.g. tetanus, rigor, rabies, or psychiatric condition ('acting out').

5. *Give phenobarbital or phenytoin*

Give phenobarbital 90 mg twice daily *or* 180 mg daily when the patient can swallow (and then stop diazepam or paraldehyde) until the cause of the fits is found, treated and cured (if possible). Reduce the dose each month if there are no more fits to the lowest dose which stops fitting occurring. Do not give phenobarbital if the patient is taking chloramphenicol; use phenytoin instead. The dose of phenytoin is about 300 mg daily – a little more if the fits are not controlled or less if there are side effects, especially dizziness, unsteadiness on the feet, swelling of the gums, anaemia, rashes, enlarged lymph nodes or encephalitis. Use other drugs if needed such as carbamazepine or valproic acid only if you have been taught to do so. Refer the patient to the Medical Officer for these drugs if you are unable to stop most or all of the fits.

6. *Transfer*

Transfer to Medical Officer care:

(a) if you cannot stop the fitting by treatment in the health centre (urgent);

(b) if the patient has his first fit or has only recently become epileptic and you cannot find and cure the cause (non-urgent);

(c) if patient has another abnormal sign in the nervous system which has recently developed or is getting worse (non-urgent);

(d) if phenobarbital or phenytoin alone will not control the fits (first check that the patient is taking the drug) (non-urgent).

Paralysis or difficulty walking

Paralysis is when the patient cannot make a muscle or group of muscles work.

The cause is not usually in the muscle, although check that the patient does not have a *muscle* injury or infection (pyomyositis) or a *bone* injury (fracture) or infection (osteomyelitis) or joint injury or infection (septic arthritis). Never forget both brucellosis (Chapter 18 page 174) and TB (Chapter 14 page 106), which make it too painful to move the muscle. The cause is usually a disease of the *nerves* which normally make the muscle move.

In the limbs:

- infections, especially leprosy, HIV, diphtheria, etc.,
- trauma, when a nerve is cut, hit or been pressed on (e.g. arm when sleep with arm over the back of the chair or foot when squatting during harvesting),
- nerve damage especially from diabetes; drugs (isoniazid without pyridoxine); lack of vitamin B.
- tick toxin can cause increasing paralysis (including swallowing and breathing) and death in a few days. **Always** look all over the body and in the hair immediately and remove any ticks. Do not squeeze them.

In the spinal cord:

- fracture of the spine,
- TB or bacterial infection of the spine,
- mass due to schistosomiasis or cysticercosis,
- osteoarthrosis or (especially if sudden onset) disc between vertebrae pressing on cord,
- poliomyelitis (if the legs are 'floppy', think of this; and urgently transfer to Medical Officer in case it is, and control of the infection needed or there is another cause which is treatable),
- encephalomyelitis,
- schistosomiasis,
- syphilis,
- vitamin B_{12} or folate deficiency.

In the brain:

- cerebrovascular disease (stroke),
- trauma,
- encephalitis and late meningitis,
- African trypanosomiasis,
- brain abscess or TB or schistosomiasis or cysticercosis, or tumour, etc.

Mental disturbance:

- acting out.

There are other causes in all of these places. See index of a specialist medical reference book if it is not one in this book. Normally, however, transfer the patient to the Medical Officer.

Paraplegia and quadriplegia

Paraplegia is paralysis of both legs.

Quadriplegia is paralysis of both legs and both arms. The usual *causes* are:

- injury to spinal bones, or
- TB or bacterial infection of the spine — pressing on the spinal cord
- schistosomiasis
- one of the causes of encephalomyelitis (see page 415).

Transfer all cases for Medical Officer investigation and treatment.

If the paralysis has started recently take great care not to make it worse. Do not bend or twist the patient's spine in any direction (especially the neck). Transfer the patient lying flat (e.g. on a board with sandbags or pillows packed around him so that he cannot bend or move the spine).

Headache

Headache is common. It occurs with many different kinds of illness.

Unless headache is the only symptom, use another symptom for *diagnosis*, e.g. headache and fever – find out and treat the cause of the fever, and the headache will probably go away.

If headache is the only symptom, think of all the structures in the head and neck. Take a history and do the examinations and tests to find if there is disease of one of them. Start with the structures on the inside of the head and neck, and work out towards the skin (see below).

If there is no evidence of disease, remember that anxiety and muscle tension are the most common causes of headache.

But do not miss the common curable causes – meningitis (especially the chronic meningitis of TB) and cerebral malaria.

Causes include diseases in the following structures:

1. *Brain* (*acute* diseases)
   - meningitis – bacterial (including syphilis and nocardia), TB, fungal (e.g. cryptococcus), toxoplasma (these unusual ones especially if HIV infection)
   - cerebral malaria
   - encephalitis including HIV infection.
   Do a lumbar puncture if necessary. Take a malaria slide and give antimalarials if necessary.
2. *Brain* (*chronic* infections/tumours)
   - African trypanosomiasis (sleeping sickness)
   - tuberculoma (a 'lump' of TB); abscess

- cysticercosis, schistosomiasis
- brain tumour (cancer).

Ask about epilepsy and other nervous symptoms. Look for weakness or change in reflexes or other nervous system signs. Are these getting worse? Look for other symptoms and signs of the above. Do these illnesses occur where patient is/was? *Do not* do a lumbar puncture. Transfer to the Medical Officer.

3. *Meninges*
   - meningitis – bacterial and tuberculous
   - cerebral haemorrhage.
   Do lumbar puncture if necessary
   See pages 409 and 414.

4. *Skull*
   - trauma.
   History of trauma
   Haematoma or tenderness under scalp.

5. *Muscles*
   - tension from work, worry or habit.
   Feel for tenderness of muscles.
   Move neck in all directions for stiffness and painful movements of muscles.

6. *Ears*
   - infection.
   Examine ears with auriscope.

7. *Nose*
   - sinusitis.
   Press over the sinuses for tenderness.
   Look for pus in nose.

8. *Mouth*
   - tooth decay and dental abscess.
   Tap each tooth gently for tenderness.

9. *Eyes*
   - doing close work if long sighted.
   Test eyesight with small print (see page 518).
   - iritis or glaucoma.
   Pupil too large; or small and irregular (see Chapter 31 pages 515 and 517).

10. *Blood vessels*
    - hypertension
    - pre-eclamptic toxaemia.
    Take blood pressure.
    Look for oedema.
    Test urine for protein.
    - migraine.
    Pain on only one side of the head.
    History of changes in sight and/or nausea and vomiting usually before headache.
    Treat with acetylsalicylic acid and metoclopramide.
    Ask Medical Officer about treatment with ergot-amine if above treatment not enough and prevention with propranolol or amitriptyline, etc. if numerous attacks.

11. *Blood coming to head*
    - other diseases especially those causing fever.
    Take temperature.
    Do examination of the rest of the body.

Neck stiffness

'Neck-stiffness' is a sign of meningeal inflammation or irritation.

The test for neck stiffness is done as follows.

Get the patient to lie supine (on his back looking upwards) on a flat comfortable surface and to relax. Tell him what you will do. Put your hand or both hands behind his head and gently pull his head forward. Normally the neck will bend forward until the chin touches the front of the chest.

If the patient has meningeal irritation, the above test will stretch the irritated meninges and cause pain and the patient will try to stop you doing this. He will not let the chin touch the chest. If you do keep lifting, often this will make the patient sit up as you lift the head forward, without the chin still touching the front of the chest. Sometimes the patient will lift up the knees to take the stretch off the meninges in the neck. This is called 'neck stiffness'.

If you are not sure if the neck is stiff (and it is if the chin will not touch the chest (unless the patient has bony or joint disease in his neck or torticollis)), try two other tests.

With the patient sitting up, try again to bend both the head and spine forward. If neither will bend forward normally this suggests meningeal irritation. The patient may sit with a straight neck and back and lean backwards using his two arms on the surface behind him to support himself – like the three legs of a tripod.

Kernig's sign, if positive, also suggests meningeal irritation. Get the patient to lie supine. Bend the knee to 90° (a right angle) and the hip to 90° (a right angle) and then try to straighten the knee (Figure 25.15). If there is meningeal irritation, this will cause pain and sometimes bending of the neck forward and the patient will stop you doing this. This is a positive Kernig's sign. Disease of the spine pressing on the nerves can also cause Kernig's sign to be positive.

If the patient has severe meningeal irritation, he may be on his side with his eyes closed and his head bent back on his neck (Figure 25.11 page 410).

Another sign of meningitis, but present only in infants, is a bulging fontanelle.

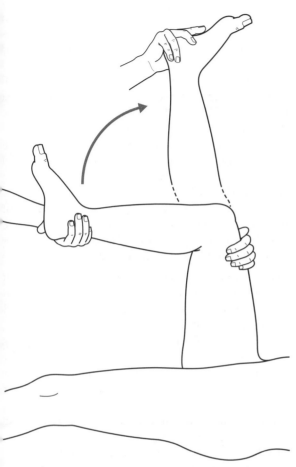

Figure 25.15 *Checking knee/hip flexion for Kernig's sign.*

There are four common causes of neck stiffness:

1. *Real 'neck stiffness'*, i.e. meningeal irritation
   Very important causes include:
   • acute bacterial (purulent) meningitis,
   • cerebral malaria,
   • tuberculous (and other chronic and subacute) meningitis, and
   • subarachnoid haemorrhage.
2. *'Meningism' or 'meningismus'*
   No organic disease of the meninges is present and the CSF is normal.
   This sometimes occurs with other infections, especially middle ear inflammation and pneumonia.
   You must always do a lumbar puncture and find clear CSF and if possible test for pus cells, protein and sugar *before* you make this diagnosis.
3. *Tetanus*
   See page 419.
4. *Torticollis and diseases of the muscles and bones of the neck*

The patient also cannot move his head from side to side. Causes include:
• muscle spasm,
• arthritis of the spine, and
• infections in the neck.
If you have any doubt about the diagnosis always do a lumbar puncture before you make this diagnosis.

Appendix 1   The proper method of doing a lumbar puncture

First you must understand the anatomy of the spine and the spinal canal. Look at Figure 25.16.

The front of the vertebra is a strong short cylinder of bone which is called 'the body' of the vertebra.

A

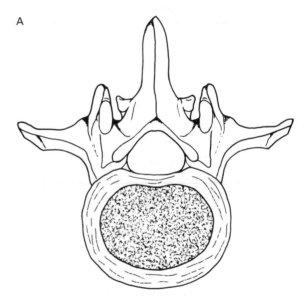

B

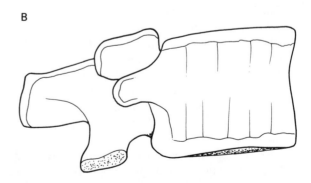

Figure 25.16 *Diagram to show a single lumbar vertebra (A) from above and (B) from the side.*

spinal cord

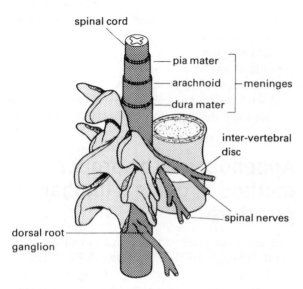

pia mater

arachnoid ⎤ meninges

dura mater ⎦

inter-vertebral disc

spinal nerves

dorsal root ganglion

Figure 25.17 *Diagram to show how vertebrae fit together and form the spine and spinal canal. The spinal cord goes through the canal, and nerves come through the holes in the spine.*

It is joined to similar bodies above and below it by 'intervertebral discs' (see Figure 25.17). This column of bone and discs is called the spine. It supports the weight of the body and allows the body to bend. (See Figure 25.18.)

Behind the body of a vertebra are thinner plates of bone which have several functions.

1. They form a hole surrounded by bone. The hole in each vertebra is lined with strong ligaments. These ligaments also go inside the hole in the next vertebrae, above and below. This makes a long cylindrical space surrounded by bone and strong ligaments, behind the vertebral bodies. This space is called the spinal *canal*. The spinal *cord* goes out of a hole at the bottom of the skull and down the spinal canal to the level of the first lumbar vertebra.

2. They have joints with the vertebrae above and below which make the spine stronger.

3. They have pieces of bone on each side and at the back called 'spinous processes'. These spinous processes are joined by strong ligaments and muscles to the spinous processes of vertebrae above and below them. These ligaments and muscles make the spine stronger and also move (bend and straighten, etc.) the spine.

4. They fit together with the vertebrae above and below leaving holes at the sides. Nerves pass through these holes from the spinal cord to the body. (See Figure 25.17.)

In the lumbar puncture you push a needle through the skin and ligaments between the posterior spinous process of the fourth and fifth (or the fourth and third) lumbar vertebrae, and then into the spinal canal (see Figures 25.19, 25.20 and 25.21). The needle will then go through the outer layer of the meninges (dura mater) and CSF will flow back through the needle. As the spinal cord ends at about the first lumbar vertebra (a little lower in infants) there are only some nerves in this area. You cannot damage the spinal cord here. You should not damage nerves; but if they are damaged, they will probably recover.

To do a lumbar puncture successfully, you must put the patient in the proper position and put the needle into the patient in the proper place and in the proper direction. **First see also 28 and 29 page 435.**

1. Before you start, sedate the patient with diazepam 5(–10) mg rectally (see Convulsions (fits) and epilepsy page 426) or paraldehyde 5–10 ml IMI if he is not likely to be cooperative.

2. Train an assistant to hold the patient properly. Good assistants often hold a patient well by putting one arm at the back of the patient's bent neck and the other arm behind the patient's bent knees, and then holding his own hands together.

3. Use a flat, hard surface such as a wooden bed, table or bench (a sagging bed is not good).

4. Put the patient with his head to your left.

5. The vertebral column (backbone) must be close to the edge of the bed.

6. The lumbar vertebral column must be parallel with the edge of the bed.

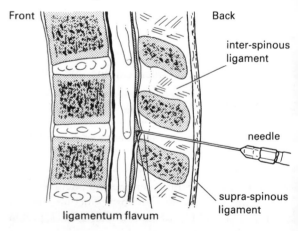

Front

Back

inter-spinous ligament

needle

supra-spinous ligament

ligamentum flavum

Figure 25.19 *Diagram to show the ligaments through which you must push the lumbar puncture needle to get into the spinal canal. The ligaments join the bones of the spine. The diagram shows the 2nd, 3rd and 4th lumbar vertebrae in section from the front to the back.*

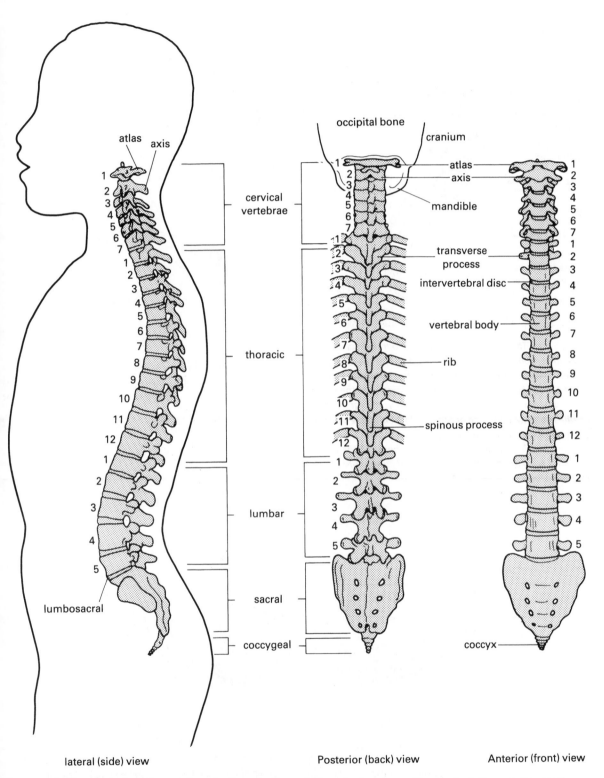

lateral (side) view   Posterior (back) view   Anterior (front) view

Figure 25.18 *Diagram to show the vertebrae (or the spinal bones). The spinal cord goes from the brain through the spinal canal and ends at about L1. Lumbar puncture is done at L3–4. Note how flexion (bending forward) of the spine will open up the space the lumbar puncture needle must go through into the spinal canal.*

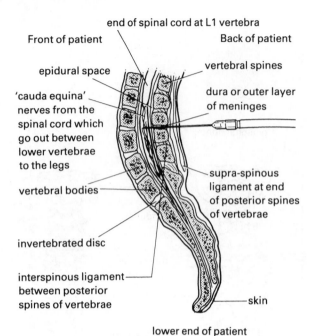

Figure 25.20 *This diagram shows the lumbar and sacral spine in section from the front to the back. Note the anatomy of the spine and spinal cord. Note the structures through which the lumbar puncture needle goes to get into the spinal canal between the third and fourth lumbar vertebrae. If the needle is directed too high or too low it will hit bone and not enter the spinal canal. Note that flexing (bending forward) the lumbar spine will open up the spaces between the lumbar vertebral posterior spinous processes and leave more space for the needle.*

7. The head must be bent forward, with the chin on the chest.
8. The knees and hips must be completely bent and the knees pushed up onto the chest.

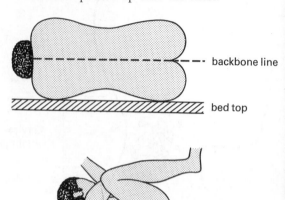

9. Check that the vertebral column is bent in a half circle.
10. Put a support (e.g. sandbag, folded towel) between the bed and the patient's waist, as the hips and shoulders are wider than the waist. (This is not necessary in children or very fat patients.)
   If you do not do this, the vertebral column will be twisted.

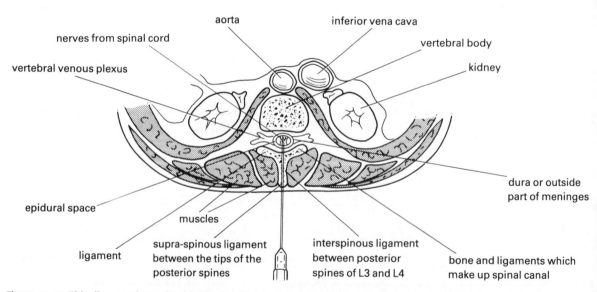

Figure 25.21 *This diagram shows the third lumbar intervertebral disc (in section from side to side). Note that a lumbar puncture needle must go straight in to reach the spinal canal. If it goes to one side it will miss the spinal canal.*

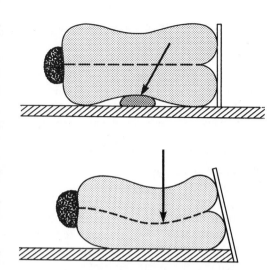

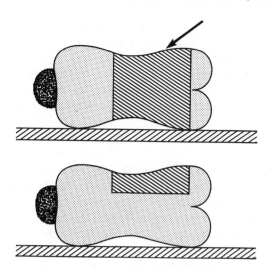

11. When looking from above the patient, check that the right shoulder is exactly above the left shoulder.

12. When looking from above the patient, the right iliac crest (hip) must also be exactly above the left one. Put the right knee on top of the left knee, with a pillow between them.

15. With your right hand, move a finger from the top of the right iliac crest straight down to the backbone. This will show you the position of the vertebral spine (bony lump) of the fourth lumbar vertebra.

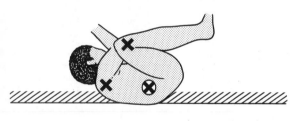

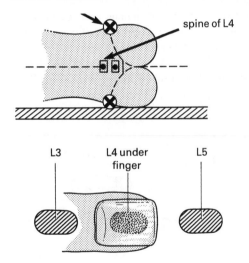

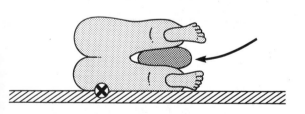

If you do all this properly the patient is now in the proper position for you to do the lumbar puncture. Do not attempt a lumbar puncture until the patient is in the proper position; or you will not get any CSF.

13. Wash your hands well. Then clean the patient's back with iodine in alcohol (or other antiseptic).

14. Put a drape on top of the right iliac crest and waist.

16. Move the finger which is on the spine of L4, straight down towards the patient's buttocks to find the space between L4 and L5 – this is where you will put the spinal needle in. Mark the skin vertically in the centre of this space by pressing firmly with your thumb-nail for half a minute.

17. Now you must find the centre line of the spine from the head to the buttocks. It is the line which joins the centre (highest parts) of the bony spines. It almost always is *not* the same place as the

hollow of the skin along the spine. You must feel the bony spines to find it. Mark this horizontally with your thumb-nail on the skin.

There will now be a cross on the skin between the vertebral spines and in the centre line of the spine. This is where you will put the lumbar puncture needle in.

Gently clean the area again with iodine (or other antiseptic).

18. In an older child or adult, give 2–5 ml of 1% lidocaine using a 26G needle. Put the needle through the skin exactly in the centre of the cross. First raise up a swelling *in* the skin (i.e. give an intradermal injection). Then inject deeper between the spines of L4 and L5. So that you do not lose the place after injecting the local anaesthetic, disconnect the syringe but leave the needle in the skin until you are ready to put the LP needle in. Wait 3 minutes for the local anesthetic to work.

19. Put the lumbar puncture needle in the gap between L4 and L5 where the needle for the local anaesthetic was, exactly in the centre of the cross. Check that the LP needle is in the proper position. *It must be at a right angle (90°) to the patient's back* at the L4 level *in both directions*. Check that this is so by looking *both* from above the patient and from the end of the patient along his spine. Then push the needle in, always checking that it is at right angles to the patient in both directions.

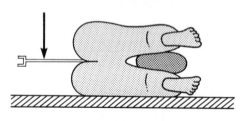

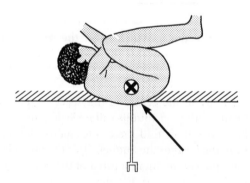

Check by looking from the end of the patient and from above the patient to see if the needle is straight.

20. In children you can use a needle from an IV drip set or a disposable needle.

In adults, use a size 20 or 18 spinal needle with the proper fitting inner part (stilette or trochar) (as the disposable and drip set needles are often not long enough for adults).

21. The layers you push the needle through are in order
(a) the skin
(b) subcutaneous fat
(c) spinal ligament
(d) meninges (dura mater) – this is the last layer and you often feel the needle suddenly go through into the space where the CSF is.

Push the needle in *very* slowly. Stop several times and remove the stilette and look to see if CSF comes out especially after you feel the needle has gone through something. Turn the needle round if you think the needle is in the proper position but no CSF comes out when you remove the stilette.

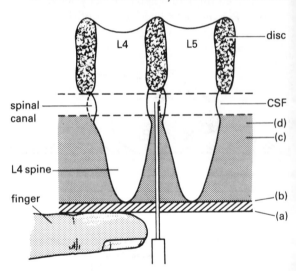

22. If you do not get CSF when you cannot push the needle in any further check that the needle:
(a) is exactly in between two vertebral spines; and that it
(b) is in the centre of the spine lengthways (and not in the centre of the skin fold in the back which often does not lie over the the centre of the spine); and that it
(c) has gone in the right direction (at right angles to the patient at L4 in both directions).

If all these are so, remove the stilette, continue to turn the needle around slowly, and slowly pull it out looking to see if CSF comes as you start to pull the needle out.

If you get no CSF put the needle in again in a slightly different direction – usually more towards the patient's head. Pull the needle right out to the surface of the skin before trying again.

If you still get no CSF after several changes of position (including pushing the needle towards the feet), take the needle right out.

23. Check that the needle was in fact in the centre line of the spine and in the middle of the space. Then try the LP again.

24. If you still do not get CSF repeat the whole process one space further up, towards the patient's head.

25. Collect the CSF in two sterile bottles, about 30 drops (2 ml) in each bottle.

26. If the CSF is blood-stained, do not remove the lumbar puncture needle. Allow the blood-stained CSF to continue to come out. Collect 2 or 3 ml in three or four bottles. Note if the CSF becomes clearer in each bottle (traumatic tap) or if the amount of blood stays the same in each bottle (subarachnoid haemorrhage).

27. Carefully remove the spinal needle, put on a small square of sterile gauze over the hole and lay the patient flat on his abdomen for 2–3 hours.

28. The whole procedure must be sterile. Wash or scrub the hands well, as for an operation. If possible, wear sterile gloves. Clean the patient well with an alcoholic solution of antiseptic. Only use a sterilised LP needle. *Never* touch the part of the needle which goes into the patient (especially the needle tip) with the fingers even after scrubbing up and putting on sterile gloves (i.e. use a 'no touch' technique).

29. See Chapter 19 page 257 for precautions to make sure you and your staff cannot be infected by HIV or HBV, etc. from any blood or CSF from the patient during this procedure.

Appendix 2   Examination of the CSF

Naked eye examination of the CSF
See page 408.

Urine 'dip sticks' used for measuring glucose and protein and pus cells in CSF
See pages 408–409.

Laboratory examination of the CSF
Always send the CSF for laboratory examination if possible. Ask for the first five of these tests on all CSF samples. Ask for a Medical Officer to send you a report on what the tests mean. (See Table 25.1 page 436.)

Tests on CSF samples:

1. Cells, total count. Normally fewer than 5/cubic mm are present.
2. Cells, differential count. Normally all are mono-nuclears (usually lymphocytes). (No red blood cells.)
3. Protein. Normally 15–45 mg% or 150–450 mg/l.
4. Sugar or glucose. Normally 45–100 mg% or 2.5–4 mmol/l (varies with blood glucose and is about two-thirds of blood glucose).
5. Gram stain for organisms. Normally negative (or no organisms seen).
6. Culture/sensitivity for bacteria. Normally negative (or no growth).
7. Ziehl–Neelsen (ZN) stain for AFB. Normally negative (or no AFB seen).
8. Culture for TB organisms. Normally negative (or no growth).
9. India ink stain for cryptococcus. Normally negative (no cryptococci seen).
10. Test for cryptococcal antigen. Normally negative.
11. Other tests if necessary.

Table 25.1 Typical CSF test results in the common conditions for which CSF tests are necessary.

	Cells		Gram stain	Protein	Sugar	ZN stain	Bacterial culture	TB culture
	Total	Differential						
Normal	0–5	All lymphocytes	No organisms	15–45 mg%	40–100 mg%	No AFB	No growth	No growth
Acute bacterial meningitis	Increased (up to thousands)	N > L	Often bacteria	Increased	< 40; usually none	No AFB	Often growth	No growth
Cerebral malaria	Normal	L > N	No organisms	Normal or increased	Normal	No AFB	No growth	No growth
Viral meningitis	Increased (tens or hundreds)	L > N	No organisms	Increased	Normal	No AFB	No growth	No growth
Encephalitis	Normal or increased (tens or hundreds)	L > N	No organisms	Increased or normal	Normal	No AFB	No growth	No growth
Tuberculous meningitis	Increased (up to hundreds)	L > N usually; N > L early	No organisms	Increased	Decreased or none	Some-times AFB	No growth	Often growth
Cerebral haemorrhage early	Many RBCs	Normal	No organisms	Increased	Normal	No AFB	No growth	No growth
Cerebral haemorrhage late	Normal or increased	L > N	No organisms	Increased	Normal	No AFB	No growth	No growth
Traumatic tap	Many RBCs	Normal	No organisms	Increased	Normal	No AFB	No growth	No growth
Cerebral tumour or tuberculoma or abscess	Normal or increased	Varies	No organisms	Increased or normal	Normal	No AFB	No growth	No growth

N = neutrophils L = lymphocytes

26 Disorders of the Urinary System

Anatomy and physiology

When the cells of the body do their work, they make several waste products, including urea, uric acid and carbon dioxide. The blood removes these waste products from the cells.

The carbon dioxide passes from the blood into the air in the lungs.

Each time the heart contracts (pumps), about one-fifth of the blood it pumps out goes through the kidneys. The kidneys remove most of the waste products from the blood which goes through them.

The kidneys remove the waste products from the blood so efficiently (well) that when this one-fifth of the blood mixes with the other four-fifths of the blood, which did not go through the kidneys (and still has waste products in it), the concentration (or amount) of waste products in the mixed blood is never high.

The waste products removed from the blood by the kidneys are dissolved in water, and this is called urine.

The urine goes down a tube, called a ureter, from each kidney, to the bladder. The bladder is a muscular storage bag in the pelvis. The bladder can hold about $\frac{1}{2}$ litre of urine before it must be emptied. The body passes the urine from the bladder out through the urethra. (See Figures 26.1, 26.2, 26.3.)

The urine also contains any salt or water which the body does not need. There is normally no protein and no sugar in the urine.

The body needs to pass about 800 ml of water in the urine every day, in order to remove the normal amount of waste products made each day.

Each kidney is made up of about one million separate little filters which do its work. The blood comes to the kidney in the renal artery which branches into more and more smaller vessels until it eventually ends up in little tufts (bunches or collections) of capillaries called 'glomeruli'. Water, salt and waste products are filtered out through these glomerular capillaries and red blood cells and protein are not allowed through. These tufts of capillaries are surrounded by the enlarged end of the

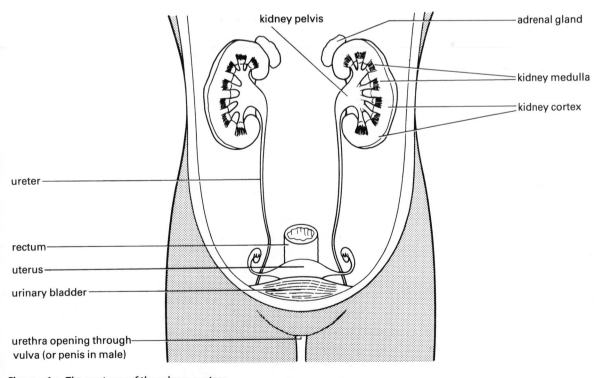

Figure 26.1 *The anatomy of the urinary system.*

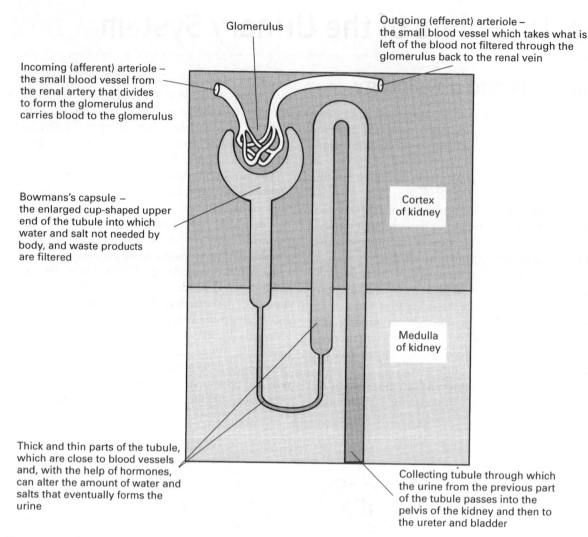

Glomerulus

Outgoing (efferent) arteriole –
the small blood vessel which takes what is
left of the blood not filtered through the
glomerulus back to the renal vein

Incoming (afferent) arteriole –
the small blood vessel from
the renal artery that divides
to form the glomerulus and
carries blood to the glomerulus

Bowmans's capsule –
the enlarged cup-shaped upper
end of the tubule into which
water and salt not needed by
body, and waste products
are filtered

Cortex
of kidney

Medulla
of kidney

Thick and thin parts of the tubule,
which are close to blood vessels
and, with the help of hormones,
can alter the amount of water and
salts that eventually forms the
urine

Collecting tubule through which
the urine from the previous part
of the tubule passes into the
pelvis of the kidney and then to
the ureter and bladder

Figure 26.2 *A diagram of one of the one million units in each kidney which take waste products and unwanted water and salt from the blood and put them into the urine.*

tubules (little tubes) which collect the water, salt and waste products filtered through the glomeruli and carry them to the ureter and bladder. However, the tubules can also get back some of the water or the salt if the body needs it. The message to the kidney tubules to do this comes through hormones (such as anti-diuretic hormone and aldosterone). (See Figure 26.2.)

Pathology

If the body is dehydrated, there is not enough water to make 800 ml of urine each day. So all the waste products in the urine are dissolved in only a little water. The urine is concentrated. The common causes of acute dehydration are gastroenteritis (when much fluid is lost from the body in vomiting or diarrhoea) and when the patient is too sick to drink enough. Chronic dehydration can occur in hot dry places in people who drink only a little water. In some of these people the waste products are not all dissolved in the water of the urine. The waste products then make small (or even large) stones in the kidneys or bladder. Infections in the urinary tract can make stones in the kidneys or bladder even when there is no dehydration.

If the body is very dehydrated, it will make very little urine. Then the body cannot remove the waste products and salt, and the concentration of the waste products and salt rises in the blood. This is called 'kidney failure' or 'renal failure'.

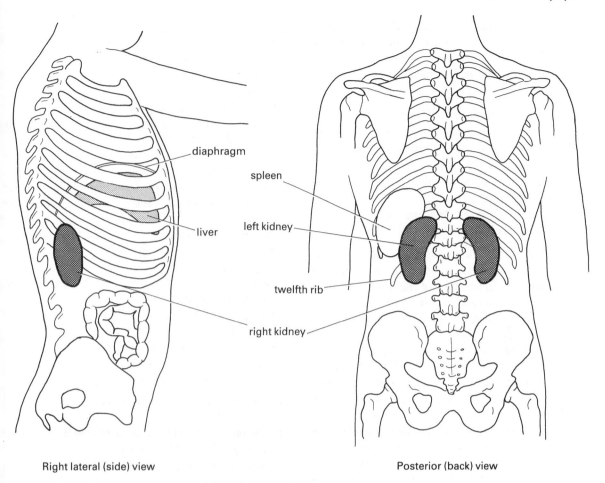

diaphragm

spleen

liver

left kidney

twelfth rib

right kidney

Right lateral (side) view

Posterior (back) view

Figure 26.3 *The position of the kidneys. Note that the kidneys are both posterior (at the back) and are also high in the abdomen, partly under the ribs.*

Some acute conditions can damage the kidney very quickly and severely – and stop the kidney working. The kidney cannot make urine, so the waste products and salt remain in the body and cause death in a few days. This is called 'acute kidney failure' (see page 453).

Some conditions damage the kidney so that it can still work; but it cannot work properly. It cannot dissolve all the waste products in only 800 ml of water. It needs much more water to remove all the waste products; but more waste products than normal remain in the blood. This is called 'chronic kidney failure' (see page 449). If a person with chronic kidney failure does not get enough fluid, then the concentration of waste products in his blood quickly rises, and he also gets acute kidney failure.

Infection is the most common pathological condition of the urinary tract. Infection in one part of the kidney tract easily spreads to another part (or all parts) of the urinary tract.

In the kidney itself the glomeruli are the parts most often damaged by disease. Other parts can, and are at times, damaged and you may hear such words as 'tubular necrosis', 'vasculitis', etc. Damage to the glomeruli, however, is called 'glomerulonephritis'. If the glomeruli (which you remember are made up of tufts of little capillaries through which water, salt and waste products are filtered but red cells and protein are not allowed through) are damaged, any of all of the following can occur:

1. Protein can leak through the glomeruli and cause protein in the urine (proteinuria) (see page 455).
2. A lot of protein can leak through the glomeruli and cause nephrotic syndrome (see page 447).
3. Red blood cells can leak through the glomeruli and cause blood in the urine or haematuria.
4. Acute inflammation of the glomeruli can occur and cause acute glomerulonephritis, also called acute nephritic syndrome (see page 446).

5. Acute kidney failure (see page 453) can occur if enough glomeruli are suddenly damaged and do not work.

6. Chronic renal failure (see page 449) can occur if more and more glomeruli are slowly damaged.

Conditions that cause glomerulonephritis are many, but in tropical countries most of them are due to abnormal reactions to infections including:

• hepatitis B virus and HIV infections;
• TB, leprosy and syphilis, streptococcal and other bacterial infections;
• malaria, especially *Plasmodium malariae,*
• schistosomiasis, onchocerciasis, *Loa loa* and filariasis.

Note that these infections do not infect the kidney. There is an abnormal immunological or body reaction to them. The appearance of the glomeruli under the microscope also can be quite different from one condition to another, although glomerulonephritis can produce only the above six conditions.

If for some reason there is not enough blood pressure at the glomeruli, cells near the glomeruli activate hormones including rennin and angiotensin which raise the blood pressure everywhere (to get more blood to the glomeruli). Kidney disease is one of the causes of high blood pressure. Drugs to reduce blood pressure include angiotensin converting enzyme (ACE) inhibitors (inhibit means to decrease the acting of or stop). ACE inhibitors stop the body converting or changing other chemicals into angiotensin.

Urea is the main waste product of the body and you can easily measure it in a laboratory. In the blood of a normal healthy person, there is less than 40 mg urea/100 ml of blood or less than 6.6 mmol urea/l (litre) of blood. If the blood urea is more than 100 mg/100 ml or more than 16 mmol/l, then the patient has kidney failure and may die unless you give him treatment. Creatinine gives an even better guide to kidney function but is a more difficult waste product to measure in the laboratory. The normal range is 15–35 mg/100 ml or 0.4–1.2 mmol/l.

Symptoms and signs of disease of urinary tract

Symptoms of urinary tract disease

1. *Urinary symptoms*
  • urethral discharge of pus, or white fluid, or watery fluid

• dysuria or pain on passing urine
• urinary frequency
• change in colour of urine
• blood in urine
• pain in
  – urethra (felt in the penis)
  – prostate (felt in the perineum in front of the anus)
  – bladder (felt in the lower central abdomen)
  – kidneys (felt in the loin (or back where the lower ribs join the spine))
  – ureter (felt anywhere from one loin to the iliac fossa or genitalia or inner upper leg on the same side).

2. *Symptoms of infection*
  • fever
  • rigors
  • malaise, etc.

3. *Symptoms of kidney failure*
  • see pages 449–450, 453.

4. *Symptoms of oedema*
  • swelling of ankles, back, face, etc.

Always ask all patients about these urinary symptoms:

1. pain or a burning feeling when passing urine (called dysuria),

2. passing urine more often than normal (called urinary frequency) and more than once at night (called nocturia),

3. abnormal colour of the urine, including blood in the urine.

Signs of urinary tract disease

1. *Urinary tract signs*
  (a) kidney
    • tenderness (see Figure 26.4)
    • enlargement (see Figure 26.5)
  (b) bladder
    • tenderness
    • enlargement
  (c) urethra
    • discharge (see Chapter 19 page 200)
    • tenderness
  (d) abnormalities of the external genitalia
  (e) prostate or uterine { enlargement lumpiness tenderness } on pelvic examination through the rectum ('PR')
    (See Figures 26.6, 26.7, 26.8 and 26.9.)
  (f) vaginal, urethral, bladder or uterine abnormalities on pelvic examination through the vagina ('PV')
    (See Figure 26.8 and an obstetrics and gynae-cology textbook.)

2. *Signs of infection*
   • raised temperature
   • fast pulse rate
3. *Signs of kidney failure*
   See pages 449, 453.
4. *Signs of oedema*
   Swelling of the ankles, back, face, etc. If you press gently with a finger you will make a hollow in the skin and underlying tissues which only returns to normal slowly.
   See Chapter 36 pages 588–590.
5. *High blood pressure*
   See Chapter 27 page 470.

Always look for these urinary tract signs on all patients during a general medical examination.

1. Kidney tenderness, during abdominal examination. (See Figures 26.4 and 26.5.)
2. Bladder tenderness ⎫ during abdominal
   bladder enlargement ⎬ examination
3. Abnormalities of external genitalia, during abdominal examination.

(See Chapter 19 page 200 and Figures 26.6, 26.7 and 26.8.)

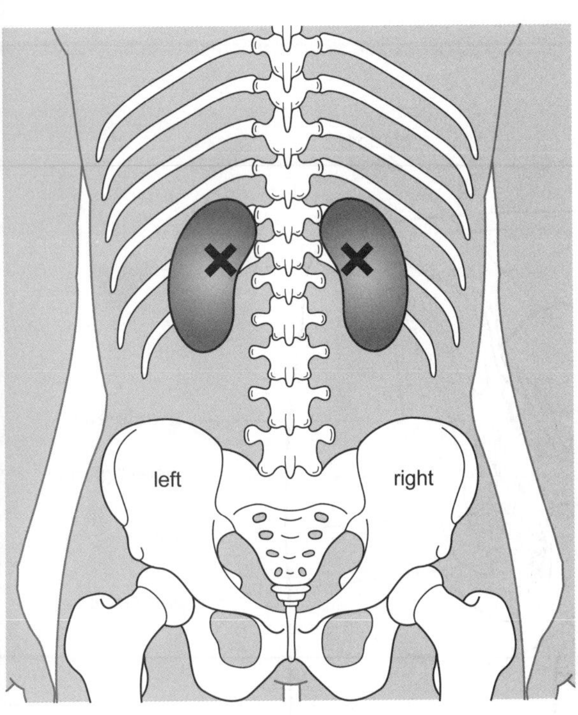

Tests

Urethral and cervical (if female) smear

Take smears only if you suspect urethritis and have a laboratory to do the tests and have been told to do them – see Chapter 19 pages 201 and 206.

Urine test

Test urine for:

• protein,
• sugar,
• blood,
• pus, and
• bile.

If you have no laboratory and no microscope, Figure 26.10 (see page 445) shows how you can still examine the urine and also what you may find.

Urine microscopy (examination of centrifuged urine under the microscope) normally shows fewer than 5 white cells (sometimes called pus cells) in each high power field (HPF) and fewer than 5 red blood cells (usually none) in each high power field (HPF). If you see more than 5 white cells/HPF this suggests

Posterior

Figure 26.4 *Diagram showing where (marked with a cross) you gently hit the patient with the side of your fist, to find out if the kidneys are tender.*

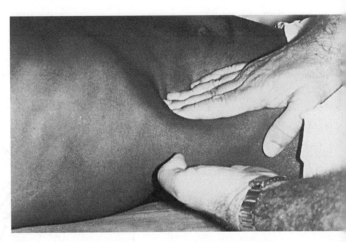

Figure 26.5 *Photograph showing the method of palpation of the kidneys. Use both hands. Put one hand flat on the abdomen beside the long central abdominal muscle and below the edge of the ribs. Put the other hand in the angle between the ribs and the spine and gently lift the kidney upwards. Ask the patient to take a deep breath. When the patient has nearly finished breathing in, press the front hand gently down and quickly bend the fingers of the back hand upwards. If the kidney is enlarged you will feel the kidney hit the top hand. Then feel the kidney slide back between the hands as the patient breathes out. In thin people you can often feel the lower part of a normal right kidney.*

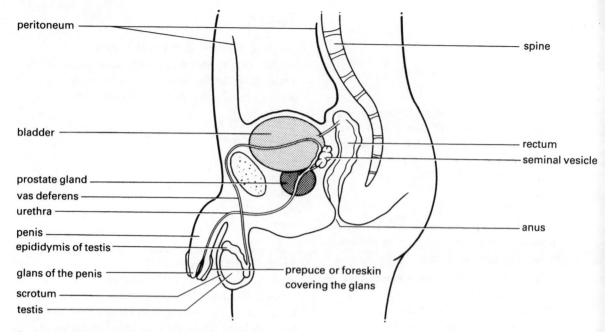

Figure 26.6 *The anatomy of the male pelvis. The pelvis is shown in section from front to back. Note the structures which you can feel anteriorly (in the front) on pelvic examination through the rectum (per rectum or 'PR') – anal sphincter (muscle), prostate, seminal vesicles and bladder.*

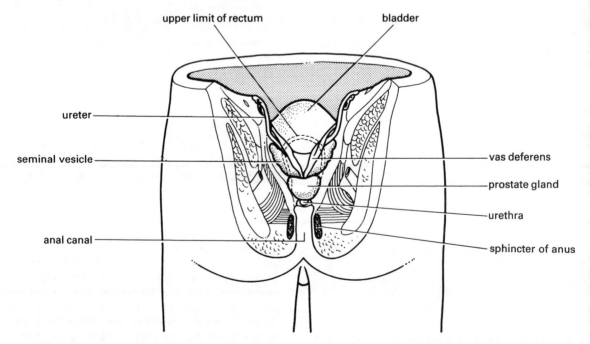

Figure 26.7 *The male pelvis from the back, as if the buttocks and bones and rectum at the back had been cut away. Note again the structures which you can feel on rectal examination 'PR' – anal sphincter, prostate, seminal vesicles and bladder.*

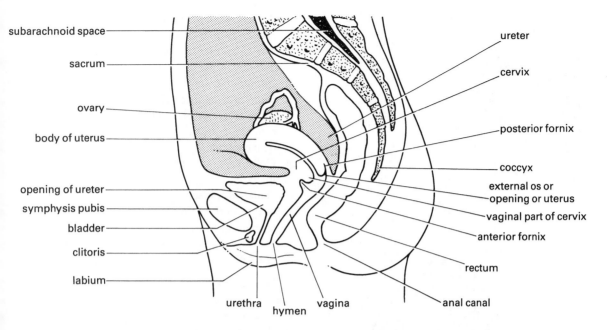

subarachnoid space

sacrum

ovary

body of uterus

opening of ureter

symphysis pubis

bladder

clitoris

labium

urethra

hymen

vagina

ureter

cervix

posterior fornix

coccyx

external os or
opening or uterus

vaginal part of cervix

anterior fornix

rectum

anal canal

Figure 26.8 *The anatomy of the female pelvis. The pelvis is shown in section from front to back. Note the structures which you can feel anteriorly (in the front). Through the rectum (per rectum or 'PR') you can feel the vagina and the cervix of the uterus. Through the vagina (per vaginum or 'PV') you can feel the urethra, bladder, cervix and uterus. For method of examination 'PV' see a specialist gynaecology/obstetrics book.*

inflammation of the urinary tract, which is most often caused by bacterial infection (see below) or glomerulonephritis. If you see more than 5 red cells/HPF, this is called 'haematuria'. Haematuria usually means a serious disease (see page 454).

Proteinuria is present if there is more than a trace of protein in the urine (see page 455).

There should be no sugar in the urine. If sugar is present, see page 455.

Blood urea and serum creatinine
See page 440.

Diseases of the urinary tract

Urinary tract infection

Definition
Urinary tract infection (UTI) is present if there is an acute or chronic inflammation of one or more parts of the urinary tract. It can have these special names:

1. Urethritis – urethra only inflamed.
2. Prostatitis – prostate only inflamed.
3. Cystitis – bladder only inflamed.

4. Pyelonephritis – kidney or kidneys inflamed (but all the other parts of the urinary tract are also affected as the infected urine runs through them).
5. Urinary tract infection – it is not known which parts of the urinary tract are inflamed, or all of the urinary tract is inflamed.

If one part of the urinary tract is infected, you should treat the patient as if all the urinary tract is infected.

Causes
These organisms can cause infection:

1. Ordinary bacteria – these cause infections which are usually acute but can also be chronic.
2. *Mycobacterium tuberculosis* – these usually cause chronic infections.
3. Schistosomiasis (*haematobium*) worms – there is usually chronic infestation. This only occurs in some countries. (See Chapter 18 page 187.)

Causes of bacterial urinary tract infection include:

1. Gonorrhoea or non-gonococcal urethritis (usually *Chlamydia*):
   Always ask about the possibility of these sexually transmitted diseases.

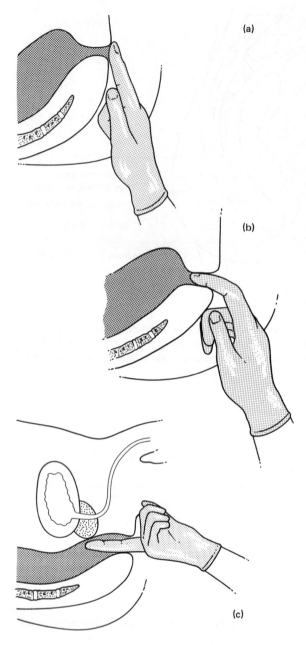

(a)

(b)

(c)

Figure 26.9 *Method of examination through the rectum ('PR'). Explain to the patient what you will do. Lay the patient on his left side with his back and hips bent forward. Wear a glove and put a lubricant on the index finger. First put the finger flat on the anus as shown (a). Then press gently backwards. The finger will then gently go into the rectum (b). Do not try to push the finger straight into the rectum. Then turn the finger round to the front of the patient (c). Gently examine the structures shown in Figures 26.7, 26.8 and 26.9 for tenderness, lumpiness or enlargement. At the end of the examination gently clean any lubricant remaining outside the anus.*

Always suspect these, even if the patient says he could not have a sexually transmitted infection.

2. Use of an urethral catheter, even if done correctly. Try not to use an urethral catheter.

3. Intercourse or pregnancy or no special cause in some normal females.

If the infection does not get better or if the infection returns often, look for an abnormality in the urinary tract.

4. Common abnormalities in the urinary tract include:
   • enlarged prostate gland,
   • stone in the bladder or kidney,
   • tuberculosis,
   • schistosomiasis (only in some countries), and
   • cancer.

Normal males do not get ordinary bacterial urinary tract infections, but normal females sometimes do. If a male gets urinary tract infection, always look for 1, 2 and 4 above.

Symptoms

Symptoms include:

1. Dysuria (pain or a burning feeling when passing urine).

2. Urinary frequency including at night.

3. Pain in the
   • back (loin) if the kidney is affected,
   • lower central abdomen if the bladder is affected.
   • rectal area and perineum if the prostate is affected.
   • penis if the urethra is infected.

4. Toxaemia (general symptoms of infection including fever, rigors, malaise, etc.) if the kidney is infected. (Toxaemia is not usually present if the infection does not involve the kidney.)

Signs

Signs include:

1. Tenderness over the affected area of the urinary tract (see above).

2. Toxaemia (fever, fast pulse, etc.) if the kidney is infected. (Toxaemia is not usually present if the kidney is not affected.)

Tests

Tests that you must do include:

1. Examination of a mid-stream specimen of urine for protein, sugar, pus cells and red blood cells (see Figure 26.10). If a laboratory is available, send for culture and sensitivity test also (see also pages 441 and 443).

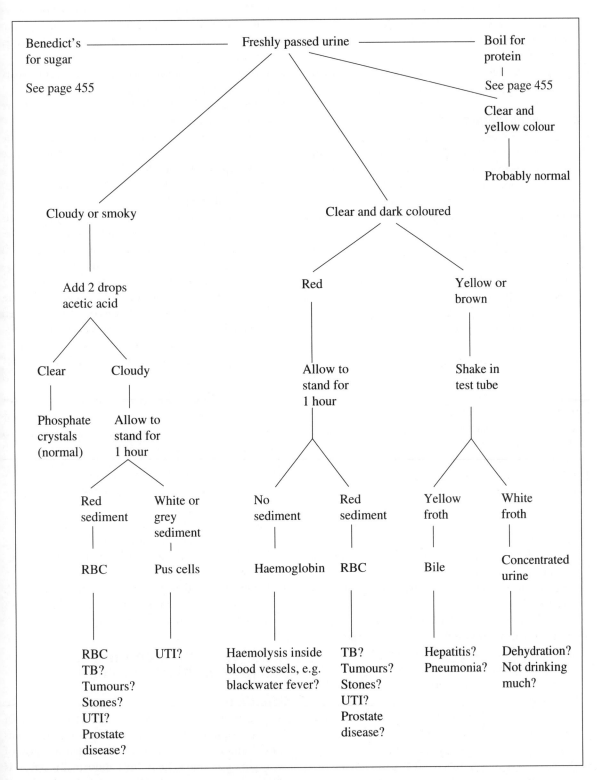

Figure 26.10 *Examination of the urine without a microscope.*
RBC, red blood cells; TB, tuberculosis; UTI, urinary tract infection

2. If urethritis is a possibility and if possible to do, take a urethral smear for gonococci and send it to the laboratory (see Chapter 19 page 206).

3. Test urine for schistosomiasis if patient from or in an area where this occurs. Look for miracidia (see Chapter 18 page 189). Send sample for ova or eggs to be looked for under the microscope.

Details of management

Examine a mid-stream specimen of urine for pus, blood, protein and sugar (if there is infection, pus and usually protein (trace to $\frac{1}{4}$) are present).

Ask if urethral or vaginal discharge is present and if a sexually transmitted disease is possible. Take an urethral and (in females) cervical smear for gonococci if a laboratory available; but treat for urethritis if the history or examination suggests it is possible (see Chapter 19 page 203).

Do an abdominal and pelvic examination (PV in women and PR in men) to check for genital tract disease (especially important if the infection is not quickly cured or it returns after treatment).

Check that the patient does not only have urinary frequency from normal pregnancy.

Treat as an outpatient. Admit for inpatient treatment only if sick.

1. *If* there is any possibility of urethritis:
Give drugs to treat urethritis (see Chapter 19 page 203).
Give treatment otherwise as follows.

2. Give one of the following in order of preference:
- Trimethoprim 300 mg daily (or 200 mg twice daily)
- Amoxicillin 500 mg and clavulanic acid 125 mg twice daily
- Trimethoprim 160 mg and sulfamethoxazole 800 mg twice daily
- Nitrofurantoin 50 mg four times a day (or 100 mg twice daily)
- Sulfadiazine or sulfadimidine 1 g four times a day (but only if no more effective drug available).

Give for 3(–5) days if cystitis in non-pregnant woman;
10 days if cystitis in pregnant woman;
14 days for all other people for all types of urinary tract infection.

3. Tell the patient to drink as much water as possible and empty the bladder completely each time he passes urine and do this often.

4. If the patient is very sick with pyelonephritis it is not safe in a health centre to give the usual hospital treatment of IV ampicillin and gentamicin without blood levels of the gentamicin; if available give IV or IM ceftriaxone 1 g daily for 14 days; or otherwise give chloramphenicol; if the patient does not improve, transfer to the Medical Officer urgently for treatment.

5. If there is the possibility of malaria, give antimalarial drugs (see Chapter 13 pages 79, 80).

6. If the infection comes back once in males or more often in females:
(a) check for possible sexually transmitted disease and treat patient and sexual partner/s (see Chapter 19 pages 203–204).
(b) check for schistosomiasis and treat if needed (see Chapter 18 page 190).
(c) if the patient is a woman, tell her to try the effects of passing urine immediately after intercourse; suggest she use other means of contraception if using a diaphragm; supply intra-vaginal oestrogen cream twice weekly if post-menopausal.
(d) if the patient has an urethral catheter, make sure the catheter is not partly or completely blocked and the patient drinks a lot of water and the catheter is changed regularly (do NOT give continuous prophylactic antibiotics which do not work).
(e) if the above are not effective refer all cases to the Medical Officer.

Examine a mid-stream specimen of urine (for pus and protein) after the treatment is finished to check that the infection has gone.

Transfer or *refer* to Medical Officer care:

1. if the patient is not clinically cured and the urine tests are not clear after this treatment (non-urgent);

2. if a male has more than one attack (non-urgent);

3. if a female has an infection that returns often (e.g. three or more infections in less than 1 year) (non-urgent); or

4. if there is blood in the urine at any time which is not caused by schistosomiasis (see Chapter 18 pages 187–191) (non-urgent).

Acute glomerulonephritis (acute nephritic syndrome)

Definition

Acute glomerulonephritis is an acute inflammation of the glomeruli. It is not caused by infecting organisms in the kidney. It is caused by an abnormal reaction of the body's immune system. This abnormal reaction is often to a streptococcal infection of the throat and skin (impetigo or infected scabies, etc.), which the atient had some weeks before, but also to numerous other causes. See pages 439–440.

Clinical features

A respiratory or skin infection (usually caused by a *Streptococcus* organism) or other infection occurs 2–3 weeks before the start of the illness in many, but not all, cases. Then there is suddenly:

- malaise,
- swelling (oedema) of the face and legs,
- only a small volume of urine, which looks like black tea and has positive tests for red blood cells and protein, and
- high blood pressure (developing over a day or two).

See a specialist book for details of diagnosis and management.

Transfer such cases to the Medical Officer for exact diagnosis and treatment unless the patient starts to get better within a couple of days, as the treatment could be difficult, especially if very high blood pressure and especially if acute renal failure develops.

Treatment would include:

1. Penicillin in case any infection of skin or respiratory tract is still present. Treat any underlying skin condition.
2. Rest in bed.
3. Measure fluid intake and output and give each day only 500 ml as well as the volume of the previous day's urine output. Daily weighing of the patient at the same time and remembering that 1 litre of fluid weighs 1 kg is usually the best way to do this.
4. Give a low salt and low potassium diet.
5. Give diuretics, e.g. furosemide/frusemide 40 mg and double this dose each 1–2 days to try to reduce oedema and get the body weight back to normal and reduce the blood pressure.
6. Treatment of high blood pressure if above 160/100 (see page 471).
7. Treatment of acute kidney failure (see page 453).

Nephrotic syndrome

Definition

Nephrotic syndrome is a condition in which a patient has glomerular damage and enough protein leaks out of the capillaries in the glomeruli into the kidney tubules and then into the urine to cause the following.

1. There is much protein in the urine (more than $\frac{1}{8}$ or 1+ on the boiling test of the urine or more than 3 grams protein per 24-hour output of urine).

2. There is oedema of the whole body (swelling because of an abnormal amount of fluid in the whole body) because not enough protein (albumin) is left in the blood to hold the water and salt part of the blood inside the blood vessels.
3. You can find no other cause for the oedema (such as malnutrition, severe anaemia, heart failure, chronic liver disease, toxaemia of pregnancy, acute nephritic syndrome, filariasis, etc. (see Chapter 36 page 588).

Causes

Many conditions damage the glomeruli in the kidney and lead to nephrotic syndrome including the following:

- diabetes mellitus,
- the end result of some cases of acute glomerulo-nephritis,
- autoimmune diseases,
- a reaction to certain infections such as *Plasmodium malariae*,
- damage to the kidney (and other parts of the body) by amyloid protein collecting in them caused by chronic infections and chronic inflammations which have lasted for a long time such as lepromatous leprosy and severe bronchiectasis,
- some drugs,
- some cancers especially lymphomas,
- and many others.

In many cases it is not possible to find out what condition has led to nephrotic syndrome but this does not affect your management of the disease. However, check to see that your patient does not have a cause (including the above) you can stop.

Symptoms

Usually swelling caused by oedema is the only symptom (see Figure 26.11). Malaise may be present.

Signs

Usually oedema is the only sign.

Complications

High fats in the blood develop and can cause atheroma (Chapter 27 page 472).

Low proteins in the blood can allow infections, especially malaria and pneumococcus, to occur.

At times, clots of blood occur in the veins.

Chronic kidney failure may develop.

Tests

The urine has much protein in it (more than $\frac{1}{8}$ or 1+). You must test the urine in all patients who have oedema.

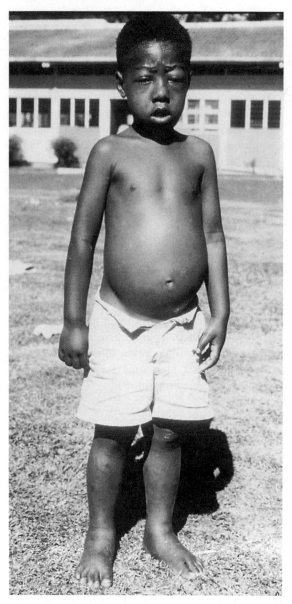

Figure 26.11 *A child with nephrotic syndrome. Note that he has swelling of all of his body including his face. Swelling of the face suggests (but does not prove) a kidney cause for oedema of the whole body. General oedema (though often with a different distribution) can be caused by: (1) kidney disease (especially nephrotic syndrome), (2) malnutrition, (3) chronic liver disease (cirrhosis), (4) severe anaemia, (5) heart failure, (6) filariasis (usually only the limbs affected), (7) other conditions (see text). Swelling of the face alone may be caused by an allergic reaction and needs urgent treatment with adrenaline and antihistamine, if the allergic swelling starts to block breathing.*

Differential diagnosis

See Chapter 36 page 588 for causes of oedema of the whole body. Very important causes include:

1. other kidney diseases, including nephrotic syndrome
2. malnutrition,
3. heart failure,
4. severe anaemia, especially if caused by hookworm and
5. chronic liver disease (cirrhosis).

Details of management

Do not diagnose nephrotic syndrome unless there is generalised oedema and much protein in the urine (more than 1+ or $\frac{1}{8}$).

Admit for inpatient treatment to check the effect of treatment and the progress of the disease (but you can treat as an outpatient if necessary).

Give the following *treatment*:

1. No salt in the diet, i.e. no salty food, no salt added when cooking food and no salt added after food is cooked.
2. Routine diuretics.
   Hydrochlorothiazide 50–100 mg each morning.
3. Normal protein diet with no added salt. High protein diet does not help as most of this protein is lost by the kidney. (Tinned fish and meat are not satisfactory as they contain much salt. Give fresh foods if possible.)
4. Antimalarial drugs as indicated, a curative course then prophylactic antimalarials. (See Chapter 13 pages 79, 80 and 88–89.)
5. Treatment for intestinal worms.
   See Chapter 23 page 355 (to stop any protein loss from worms in bowel).
6. Test the urine for protein every day and weigh the patient to check if he is improving.
7. Give powerful diuretics if the patient is not improving. Start with a small dose.
   Furosemide/frusemide 40–160 mg daily. If this is not successful give 20–60 mg IVI daily for a few days.
8. Special diuretics such as spironolactone or amiloride or triamterene would be helpful if added to the above if ordinary diuretics and furosemide/frusemide are not enough to control the oedema.
9. Potassium chloride 1200 mg (2 tabs) three times a day if you give furosemide/frusemide and/or the patient is not on a tuber diet, but do not give potassium chloride if the patient is also taking spironolactone or amiloride or triamterene.

10. Look carefully for acute bacterial infections and malaria. Give proper treatment quickly if they occur. If pneumococcal vaccination is possible, vaccinate the patient.

Transfer the patient to Medical Officer care, but only after discussion with the Medical Officer:

1. if you cannot remove the oedema after 3–6 weeks; or
2. if the proteinuria has not gone after 3–6 weeks; or
3. if a micro-urine examination shows more than the normal number of red blood cells or white blood (pus) cells;

as special tests may show a cause that can be treated; and as other drugs (e.g. prednisolone) can sometimes help treatment of special cases; and other drugs such as ACE inhibitors and NSAIDs may improve the kidney function.

Schistosomiasis

Schistosoma haematobium is a very important cause of disease of the urinary tract.

Schistosomiasis of this type only occurs in parts of Africa and the Middle East. (See Figure 18.13 page 188.)

Find out if you are in an area where schistosomiasis occurs. If so, see Chapter 18 pages 187–191 for details of schistosomiasis.

Chronic kidney (renal) failure (CRF)

Chronic kidney failure is present when the kidneys are permanently damaged and cannot excrete (put) all the waste products made by the body into the urine. The amount of waste products in the body increases and damages many functions of the body. There are many causes of chronic kidney failure. You can treat very few of these causes successfully in the health centre. (See below.)

Think of chronic kidney failure in any patient who has:

- anaemia (especially if it does not improve with treatment),
- blood pressure higher than 160/100,
- loss of appetite, nausea, and often vomiting (for no obvious reason),
- wasting of muscles (for no obvious reason),
- breath that smells like urine smells,
- deep breaths, even though the patient does not feel short of breath (usually late in the disease), or
- bleeding into the skin (usually only late in the disease).

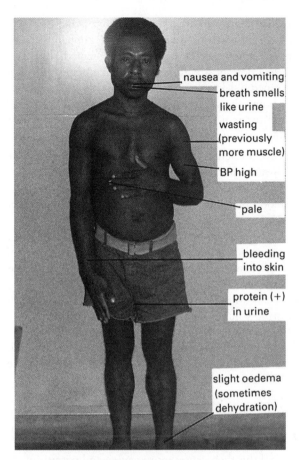

nausea and vomiting
breath smells like urine
wasting (previously more muscle)
BP high
pale
bleeding into skin
protein (+) in urine
slight oedema (sometimes dehydration)

Figure 26.12 *A patient with chronic kidney failure. The patient came to the health centre because he had the symptoms of anaemia. Routine treatment of the anaemia did not make him any better. The signs of kidney failure were then looked for and found. The diagnosis was confirmed by a blood urea test.*

A history of previous kidney disease or vascular disease (atheroma) elsewhere makes the diagnosis more likely.

Test the urine for protein. Protein in the urine makes the diagnosis very likely if the other signs are present.

Send blood to the laboratory to confirm the diagnosis; ask for a blood urea and creatinine test (and, if available, electrolytes). (See page 440.)

Causes of chronic renal failure that can be treated need to be looked for in all patients. These causes include high blood pressure, urinary tract infection (including with TB and schistosomiasis), urinary tract obstruction (including from an enlarged prostate and schistosomiasis), diabetes mellitus, HIV infection, dehydration, infections, drugs or chemicals which cause kidney damage (diuretics, ACE inhibitors and NSAIDs, especially when used together but if stopped the kidneys improve; or herbal traditional remedies; or too high a dose of streptomycin or gentamicin, and if not stopped quickly the kidneys will not improve), etc.

Some things may help the patient's symptoms and slow the rate at which the kidney failure gets worse. These include the following:

- Give a calcium channel blocker such as amlodipine or verapamil or if unavailable methyl-dopa and hydralazine (not other blood pressure drugs) to keep the blood pressure down to about 140/90. See Chapter 27 pages 470–471.
- Good diet with plenty of carbohydrate but just a normal (and not increased) amount of protein; or if high quality protein available a small amount of this protein.
- A large fluid intake of about 3 litres a day so that urine volume is at least 2–3 litres (each day).
- Control of salt intake according to blood and urine tests, although it is more likely a large amount of salt is needed, but this may need to be reduced if the blood pressure becomes too high.
- Early treatment of any nausea and vomiting (common in CRF) with anti-nausea drugs and if needed intravenous fluid; as mild dehydration can cause kidney failure to quickly become much worse (and this then causes more nausea and vomiting).
- Blood electrolyte tests which include calcium and phosphate, to see if the patient would be helped by calcium carbonate or aluminium hydroxide or sodium bicarbonate.

In view of these things, *refer* the patient to the next visiting Medical Officer or discuss with him about non-urgent transfer about the above.

Acute kidney failure

See page 453.

Ureteric (renal) colic

Ureteric colic is a pain caused by something (usually a stone formed in the kidney) going down the ureter from the kidney to the bladder.

Ureteric colic is a very severe pain. It usually begins in the loin (one side of the back, where the lowest ribs join the spine) and then spreads to the iliac fossa (lower outer front of the abdomen), labia or penis or testes or inner leg on the same side. It is a constant pain which may slowly get much worse. It is not a true colic (see Figure 36.1 page 593).

The attack may continue for only a few minutes; but sometimes it continues for hours. Passing urine is often painful. Blood is often passed in the urine. Tests may show protein and blood in the urine.

Stones never dissolve themselves. But if they are small, they may be passed in the urine. If stones remain in the urinary tract for a long time, infection often occurs.

Treatment includes the following:

1. Treat any ureteric colic with IMI pethidine 100 mg or morphine 10–15 mg and atropine 0.6 mg every 4 hours or more often if necessary.
2. Treat any urinary infection present. Do not use sulfonamides. See page 446.
3. Keep any stone that is passed. Give it to the Medical Officer for analysis in the laboratory.
4. Give 3–4 litres of fluid daily (to make a large urine volume).

Transfer the patient to a Medical Officer within 2 days to check if there is an obstruction of the ureter which can destroy the kidney. This is especially important if there is continuous pain and tenderness over one kidney. The Medical Officer will do special tests and X-rays to make sure the ureter is not blocked and to find out the cause for the stone and work out what treatment is needed to stop more stones forming. He will also check for other causes of colic, including infections with TB or schistosomiasis or tumours.

Some common diagnostic problems and their management

Urinary frequency (Passing urine more often than normal)

Do a full history and examination (see Chapter 6 and pages 440–444).

Do a pelvic examination PR and PV (see pages 442–444).

Test the urine (see pages 441 and 445). If needed test the urine for schistosomiasis.

Find out if the patient is passing large volumes (amounts) of urine often or if he is passing only small amounts of urine often.

Large amounts of urine passed often
Look for:

1. *Diabetes mellitus*
   - sugar (glucose) in the urine
   - drinking a lot

• eating a lot
• losing weight if young; or overweight if old.
See Chapter 30 pages 499–504.
Treat dehydration if present (see Chapter 23 page 364).
Diet low in animal fat and refined sugars.
Oral hypoglycaemic drugs or insulin (see Chapter 30 pages 499–504).
Refer or transfer to Medical Officer.

2. *Chronic kidney failure*
   • protein in the urine
   • anaemia that does not get better with routine treatment
   • blood pressure higher than normal
   • wasting.
   See page 449.

3. *Taking of diuretic drugs*

4. *Neurotic disorder – acting out (drinking more than is necessary)*
   • no other abnormalities found on examination
   • urine tests all normal
   • the patient has a mental problem
   If you find and solve the problem, and the patient drinks less, the frequency stops.

5. *Rare medical conditions*
   If you cannot find the cause, refer or transfer to Medical Officer.
   Do not allow the patient to become dehydrated.

Small amounts of urine passed often

1. *Urinary tract infection*
   • dysuria (pain on passing urine) also
   • urethral discharge if there is urethritis
   • fever if the kidney is infected
   • tenderness over urethra, prostate, bladder or kidney/s if these are infected.
   See pages 443–446.

2. *Schistosomiasis*
   • patient in or from an area where schistosomiasis occurs
   • blood in urine, especially at the end of passing urine – worse after exercise
   • eggs or miracidia in urine on examination.
   See Chapter 18 pages 187–191.

3. *Obstruction of the urethra by an enlarged prostate gland or a urethral stricture*
   • older man if there is an enlarged prostate; or middle-aged or older man who has a history of gonorrhoea or NGU if there is a stricture
   • for months or years it has been difficult to pass urine – difficult to start, then a thin stream and difficult to pass all the urine

• sometimes you can feel an enlarged or lumpy prostate on pelvic examination PR
• no pus or protein in the urine unless there is also a urinary tract infection.
If there is pus and protein in the urine, treat for urinary tract infection (see page 446).
If patient is not cured, refer or transfer non-urgently to the Medical Officer (probably for an operation).

4. *Normal pregnancy* pressing on the bladder
   • the patient is well, but is in either early pregnancy (1 or 2 periods missed) or late pregnancy
   • the urine tests are normal.
   No treatment except explanation is necessary.

5. *Pelvic disease* such as pelvic inflammatory disease or schistosomiasis, or amoebiasis or cancer of the female genital tract pressing on the bladder.
   • vaginal discharge or bleeding
   • abnormal tenderness or enlargement of organs or lumps on pelvic examination PR and PV.
   Treat pelvic inflammatory disease (see Chapter 19 page 204) and amoebic infections (see Chapter 23 page 372 and schistosomiasis, see above).
   Refer or transfer most cases non-urgently to the Medical Officer.

6. *Blood in the urine* when schistosomiasis is not present (no eggs or miracidia in the urine), and you cannot find other disease.
   Refer or transfer to the Medical Officer all patients who have blood in the urine with no obvious cause. It may be disease, especially cancer, which can be cured if treated early, but may cause death if not treated until late.

7. *Chronic disease of the bladder* such as a stone or late schistosomiasis or TB or cancer.
   • long history of urinary symptoms
   • urinary symptoms getting worse
   • blood or protein or pus in the urine.
   Refer or transfer non-urgently to a Medical Officer.

Dysuria (pain on passing urine)

Do a full history and examination (See Chapter 6 and pages 440–444).
Test the urine (see pages 441 and 445).
Do a pelvic examination PR and PV (see pages 442–444).
Pull back the foreskin of the penis and look under it and on the glans of the penis.

Look for:

1. *Sores on, or inflammation of, the penis, vulva or vagina*
   • Urinary frequency may not be present.
   • The urine tests are usually normal.

If sore, see Chapter 19 pages 198 and 204.
If discharge, see Chapter 19 page 203.

2. *Urethral infection*
   - Urine frequency is present.
   - Ask if there is urethral or vaginal discharge of pus or of white or watery material.
   - Ask about the possibility of a sexually transmitted disease.
   - Still suspect a sexually transmitted disease, even if the patient says it is not possible.
   - Look for urethral discharge.
   - The urine tests may not have much pus or protein in a mid-stream specimen.

   If urethritis is likely, see Chapter 19 page 203.

3. *Prostatitis*
   - Urinary frequency is usually present.
   - Ask about the possibility of a sexually transmitted disease in younger men.
   - Ask about symptoms of an enlarged prostate (increasing difficulty in passing urine, etc.) in older men.
   - Examine for tenderness of the prostate, on pelvic examination PR.
   - The urine test may not have much pus or protein in a mid-stream specimen.

   Treat as for urethritis and urinary tract infection. See pages 203 and 446.

4. *Cystitis due to bacteria*
   - Urinary frequency is present.
   - Tenderness over the bladder may be present.
   - Symptoms and signs of pyelonephritis may be present.
   - Urine tests show pus and protein.

   Treat for urinary tract infection (see page 446).

5. *Cystitis due to schistosomiasis*
   - Patient from or in an area where schistosomiasis occurs.
   - Blood in the urine, especially at the end of passing urine and after exercise.
   - Severe pain if clots of blood are passed.

   Treatment – see Chapter 18 page 190.

6. *Pelvic disease* irritating the bladder, especially pelvic inflammatory disease.
   - Vaginal discharge or bleeding.
   - Abnormal tenderness, lumps, or enlarged organs on pelvic examination PR or PV.
   - Urine tests normal, unless urine has vaginal secretions in it.

   Treat for pelvic inflammatory disease (see Chapter 19 page 204) and amoebic infections (see Chapter 23 page 372).

7. *Pyelonephritis*
   - Urinary frequency.
   - Fever, fast pulse, toxaemia.
   - Tenderness in the loin/s over the kidneys.
   - Urine tests show pus and protein.

   Treatment – see page 446.

8. *Note* that people often complain of dysuria when they have pain all over or a fever, and pass concentrated urine. The dysuria improves as the person gets better. There is no disease of the urinary tract.

Incontinence of urine (the patient cannot control when urine is passed)

Do a full history and examination (see Chapter 6).

Examine the urine (see pages 441 and 445).

Do a pelvic examination PR and PV (see pages 442–444).

Look for:

1. *No proper control of the body and bladder by the brain*
   - Young children
   - Old people with dementia – do not diagnose this until you have done all the examinations below with normal results *and* you find that the patient has a chronic organic psychosis (see Chapter 35 pages 568–569 and 573).
   - During fitting (convulsions).
   - Unconsciousness from any cause.
   - Some psychoses.

   Treat the cause if possible.

2. *Damage to parts of the spinal cord which control the bladder*
   - Injury to or infection of the spine pressing on the cord; pain in the back, often with a tender lump in the spine.
   - Tuberculosis or schistosomiasis or HIV infection or other cause of cord inflammation.
   - Difficulty in walking or paralysis of the legs.
   - Loss of sensation in the legs.
   - Anus not closed or tight when pelvic examination PR done.

   Transfer the patient urgently to Medical Officer care, unless the condition has been present for many months or for years.

3. *Vesicovaginal fistula or damage to the bladder during labour*
   - Present soon after difficult childbirth.
   - Continuous leak of urine.

   Transfer non-urgently to Medical Officer for operation.

4. *Infection in the bladder*
   - Dysuria and frequency.
   - Pus and protein in the urine.

   Treatment – see page 446.

5. *Obstruction of the urethra* causing the bladder to be too full. A little urine goes through the narrow urethra constantly.

- Older man if there is an enlarged prostate; or middle aged or older man who has a history of urethritis if there is a stricture.
- For months or years it has been difficult to pass urine – difficult to start, then a thin stream and difficult to pass all the urine.
- Sometimes you can feel an enlarged or lumpy prostate on pelvic examination PR.

If there is pus and protein in the urine, treat for urinary tract infection (see page 446).

If the incontinence is not cured refer or transfer the patient non-urgently to a Medical Officer (probably for an operation).

Anuria and oliguria (the patient does not pass urine or passes little urine)

There is usually one of these causes of anuria.
Look for:

1. *The urine is made by the kidneys but the bladder cannot empty* ('acute retention of urine')

- You can feel or percuss the bladder in the lower abdomen (see Chapter 36 pages 598–601).
- The bladder is tender as well as enlarged.

Find out why the bladder cannot empty.

- There is a history and signs of an enlarged prostate gland or an urethral stricture (see above), *or*
- There are signs and a history of damage to the spinal cord, usually trauma or TB. (See Chapter 29 pages 490–492 and Chapter 25 page 427), *or*
- There are signs of loss of control of the bladder by the brain, such as unconsciousness (see Chapter 25 pages 422–424).

Empty the bladder by *gentle*, continuous pressure over the bladder with your hand.

If this is not possible, insert an urethral catheter with all the special care necessary to avoid infection of the bladder.

2. *The kidneys do not make urine* ('acute kidney or renal failure') (ARF)

- You cannot feel or percuss the bladder because it is not enlarged (it is usually empty).
- The patient is usually very sick with the condition that caused the acute kidney failure.

Look for the cause of the acute kidney failure

- Any condition that caused dehydration or shock that continued for more than a short time before being controlled: external or internal bleeding, and especially antepartum or postpartum haemorrhage; burns; severe gastroenteritis; septicaemia; malaria.
- Acute haemolysis (see Chapter 21 page 315) and especially blood which was wrongly crossmatched or malaria with 'blackwater fever' or some snakebites or certain drugs.
- Complete ureteric obstruction, especially if has past history of kidney stones or schistosomiasis or recent ureteric colic or blood clots in the urine.
- Some drug treatment especially
  (a) one, or especially more than one, of the ACE inhibitors (e.g. enalapril, captopril, trandolopril, etc.); NSAIDs, e.g. ibuprofen; and diuretics e.g. furosemide/frusemide.
  (b) amino-glycosides (especially overdose), e.g. streptomycin, gentamicin;
  (c) sometimes cloxacillin, sulfonamides, trimethoprim, rifampicin.
- Acute glomerulonephritis.
- Many other causes (see a specialist book).

Manage as follows as emergency.

- Immediately treat the condition that caused the acute kidney failure, especially if it is dehydration, shock or infection (see Chapter 27 pages 466–470)
- Insert an indwelling catheter into the bladder if still no urine passed to make sure there is not a full bladder which cannot be felt.
- If no increase in urine volume when certain patient is fully hydrated and especially if oedema developing or signs of heart failure, then reduce IV fluids to 5% dextrose 500 ml, but increase the 500 ml by the volume of any urine passed or other fluids lost, each 24 hours.
- Try the effect of large dose of IV furosemide/frusemide 80–160 mg once.
- Arrange urgent (emergency) transfer to Medical Officer care if no urine passed or less than 400 ml in 24 hours after what treatment possible has been given.
- If, before transfer, the patient develops severe muscular weakness, or paralytic ileus or an irregular pulse, it is likely that the potassium in the blood has become so high it will soon stop his heart. Treat immediately with IV 25 g glucose (50 ml of 50% or 100 ml of 25%) and 5 units of soluble insulin slowly (over 5–10 minutes). This is likely to keep the potassium lower for 4–6 hours and allow time for transfer. Check the blood glucose each hour and if low (less than 2.2 mmol/l or 40 mg/100 ml) give more IV glucose. Repeat treatment if needed.

3. *The patient is not telling the truth*
- The bladder is not enlarged or tender.
- The patient has no serious symptoms or signs, and looks well.
- The patient usually has a big mental problem.

Admit and observe the patient for 24 hours to see if he is telling the truth or not.

Abnormal colour of the urine

Normally the colour of the urine shows how much waste product is in the urine.

If the person is dehydrated or has no extra water to pass, the concentration of waste product in the urine is high. The urine is 'concentrated'. The colour of the urine is yellow (although the patient may say it is red).

If the person has much water to pass the concentration of waste product in the urine is low. The urine is 'dilute'. The urine colour is clear or like water.

If a person says his urine is an abnormal colour, always look at the urine yourself to see what colour it is and if it is abnormal. Do all the tests for urine (see pages 441 and 445).

Yellow urine

Look for causes of:

1. normally concentrated urine (see above);
2. abnormally concentrated urine, from dehydration (see Chapter 23 page 362);
3. bile in the urine – but this usually makes the urine dark (see Chapter 24 page 392).

Clear urine (like water)

Look for causes of:

1. normally dilute urine (see above);
2. dilute urine because the patient has kidney failure and cannot concentrate the urine (see page 449).

Cloudy urine

Look for causes of:

1. pus from a urinary tract infection (see page 443);
2. phosphate crystals – these do not mean any disease at all and they dissolve if acid is added to the urine; the urine then becomes clear.

Red urine

Look for causes of:

1. red blood cells in the urine ('haematuria') (see below);
2. haemoglobin in the urine (although then the urine is usually brown or black, not red) (no red blood cells are in the urine) – causes for this include malaria with 'blackwater fever', some snakebites, wrongly crossmatched blood, some drugs in some people (e.g. primaquine in people with G6PD deficiency); the patient is very sick;
3. bile in the urine (the urine is really brown or black, not red) (see Chapter 24 page 392);
4. food, e.g. beetroot, or sweets (lollies) with red colour in them;
5. normally concentrated urine (the urine is really a yellow colour, not red).

Black urine (like tea or coffee without milk)

Look for causes of:

1. bile in the urine (see Chapter 24 page 392), or
2. haemoglobin in the urine (see above).

See page 445 for ways to test urine for pus, blood, bile, haemoglobin, etc. without laboratory help. If a laboratory is available, you can examine the urine for pus cells and red blood cells under the microscope, and for bile, blood, protein, sugar and haemoglobin with test tablets or paper strips.

Blood in the urine (haematuria)

Check that the patient does have blood from the urinary tract and not either:

1. menstrual blood in the urine, *or*
2. red urine not caused by red blood cells (see above).

If there is blood in the urine, look for:

1. *Trauma to the urinary tract*
   - History and signs of trauma are present.
   Transfer all cases to Medical Officer care urgently.
2. *Urinary tract infection*
   - Dysuria and urinary frequency.
   - Pus and protein with the blood in the urine.
   - Treatment removes the blood from the urine and it does not appear in the urine again.
   Treatment – see page 446.
3. *Schistosomiasis*
   - Patient is from or in an area where schistosomiasis occurs and is usually a boy.
   - There is more blood at the end when passing urine, and more after exercise.
   - Eggs or miracidia are in the urine, on examination (see Chapter 18 pages 187–191).
   Management – see Chapter 18 page 190.

4. *Acute nephritic syndrome/glomerulonephritis*
- Throat or skin infection 1–3 weeks before, but not always.
- Oedema (puffy face, etc.).
- Blood pressure high.
- Urine has protein and blood in it and the volume is small.

See page 446 and refer to Medical Officer.

5. *Stone in the urinary tract*
- Ureteric colic (see page 450).
- Persistent urinary tract infection. See page 443.

6. *Causes that you cannot diagnose at the health centre but must be diagnosed* (because some conditions, such as early cancer and TB, can be cured, but kill if not diagnosed and treated).

Refer or transfer all patients who have blood in the urine for which you cannot find the cause.

Pus in the urine (pyuria)

Look for:

1. urinary tract infection (see pages 443–446); or
2. acute glomerulonephritis (see pages 446–447).

If these conditions are not present, or if treatment is not effective, refer or transfer the patient to Medical Officer care.

There may be other conditions, such as TB or stone, which must be diagnosed and treated.

Sugar in the urine

You can diagnose sugar in the urine with a positive Benedict's test. There are only two common conditions which cause sugar in the urine:

1. Diabetes mellitus – glucose in the urine
- Benedict's test and tablet test for sugar positive.
- Stick test for glucose test also positive.

See Chapter 30 pages 499–504 for management.

2. Pregnancy and lactation – lactose from breast milk in the blood and urine.
- Benedict's and tablet tests for glucose positive.
- Stick tests, test *negative.*

No treatment necessary.

Protein in the urine (proteinuria or albuminuria)

Protein in the urine is shown by using a dip stick as directed on the bottle or by the boiling test as follows.

Put 2.5 cm clear urine into 2 test tubes. Heat one to boiling over a flame. (1) If cloudy add 2 drops of 4.5% acetic acid. The cloudiness disappears if due to phosphates but remains if due to protein. (2) If clear after boiling add the acetic acid. If cloudiness appears there is protein in the urine. If the urine stays clear, there is no protein. (The second tube is used to compare appearance of the urine with the urine in heated tube.)

If you find more than a very little protein in the urine, there is usually a serious disease of the kidneys. Look for the causes:

1. urinary tract infection (see page 443),
2. haematuria (see page 454),
3. pre-eclamptic toxaemia of pregnancy and eclampsia (see an obstetrics book),
4. nephrotic syndrome (see page 447),
5. acute nephritic syndrome (see page 446) or
6. chronic kidney failure (see page 449).

You may find small amounts of protein in the urine of people who have other conditions that do not affect the kidneys directly:

1. heart failure,
2. fever of any cause,
3. operation.

Bile in the urine

See Chapter 24 page 392.

27 Disorders of the Heart and Blood Vessels

Anatomy and physiology

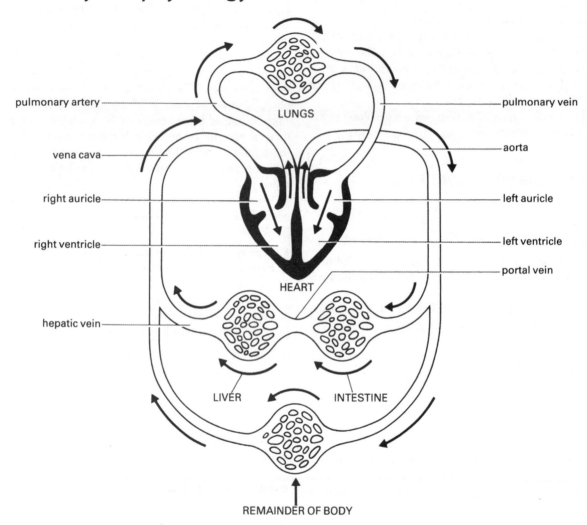

pulmonary artery

LUNGS

pulmonary vein

aorta

vena cava

right auricle

left auricle

right ventricle

left ventricle

portal vein

HEART

hepatic vein

LIVER

INTESTINE

REMAINDER OF BODY

Figure 27.1 *Diagram showing circulation of the blood. The blood goes from the lungs to the left side of the heart. This blood contains much oxygen and little carbon dioxide. The left side of the heart pumps the blood through the arteries to the capillaries in the body, and the intestine. Through the walls of these capillaries the blood gives food and oxygen to the cells and removes carbon dioxide and waste products. The blood then goes from the capillaries into veins. The blood in the capillaries of the intestine also takes food from the intestine and it then goes through the portal vein to the liver. In the liver the blood goes into capillaries which put most of the food from the intestine into the liver for storage. The blood from the liver, which contains enough food for the rest of the body, then goes into veins again and travels to the right side of the heart. The blood from the capillaries in the rest of the body travels in veins straight to the right side of the heart. The right side of the heart pumps the blood to the lungs through the pulmonary artery and then into capillaries again. The lungs remove carbon dioxide from the blood and put in oxygen. The capillaries in the lung then join to form the vein which goes to the left side of the heart. The circulation of the blood then starts again.*

The body is made of many cells. All these cells need food from the intestine and liver and oxygen from the lungs. Waste products and carbon dioxide must also be removed from the cells. The blood takes all things to and from the cells. Many other important things also go from one part of the body to another in the blood (see Chapter 21 page 312). The body, therefore, moves the blood in a big circle through the parts of the body in a special order. The blood moves round this circle in the blood vessels – arteries, capillaries and veins. The heart pumps the blood through the blood vessels. This is called the 'circulation' of the blood (see Figure 27.1). The system of the heart and blood vessels is called the 'cardiovascular' system. (See Figures 27.2, 27.3, 27.4, 27.5 and 27.6.)

The heart normally pumps about 70 ml of blood into the blood vessels of the lungs and of the body with every contraction or beat. The heart normally contracts about 70 times every minute.

The blood cannot go backwards into the heart because of the one-way valves (aortic and pulmonary) where the heart is joined to the blood vessels.

The small arteries (arterioles) let the blood go into the capillaries slowly. When the heart beats, the big

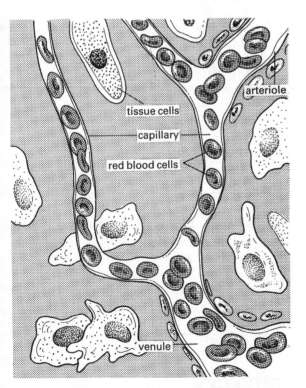

Figure 27.2 *Diagram of the smallest arteries (arterioles) and the smallest veins (venules) of the capillaries as seen through the microscope.*

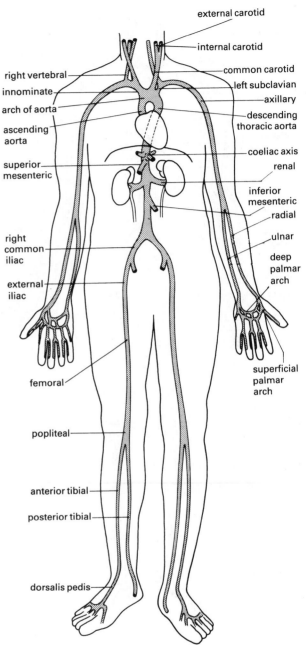

Figure 27.3 *Diagram showing the main arteries of the body. The names of the arteries are not important.*

arteries stretch to let all the blood into them. These stretched big arteries then slowly push the blood through the small arteries and arterioles into the capillaries before the next heart beat. Some blood remains in the arteries before the heart beats again, so there is always pressure in the arteries. When the heart pumps more blood into the arteries the pressure is

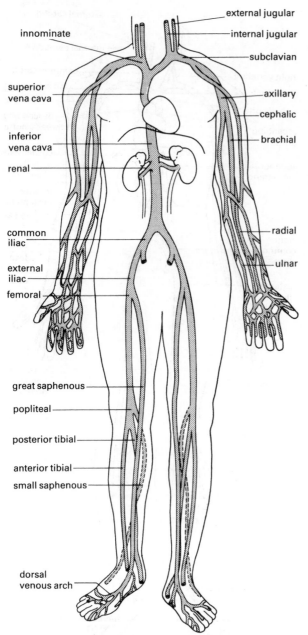

innominate

external jugular

internal jugular

subclavian

superior vena cava

axillary

cephalic

inferior vena cava

brachial

renal

common iliac

radial

external iliac

ulnar

femoral

great saphenous

popliteal

posterior tibial

anterior tibial

small saphenous

dorsal venous arch

Figure 27.4 *Diagram showing the main veins of the body. The names of the veins are not important.*

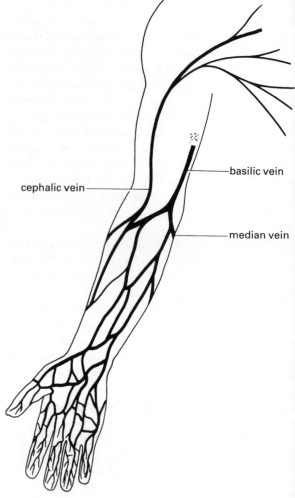

cephalic vein

basilic vein

median vein

Figure 27.5 *Diagram showing the veins of the arm.*

highest – called the 'systolic blood pressure'. The systolic pressure is normally between 100 and 120 mm mercury when measured with a sphygmomanometer. The pressure in the arteries is lowest just before the heart pumps more blood into the arteries – called the 'diastolic blood pressure'. The diastolic pressure is normally between 70 and 80 mm mercury. The blood

pressure (BP) is written with the systolic pressure (e.g. 120) first and the diastolic pressure (e.g. 80) second, like this: BP 120/80.

One special set of arteries is the coronary arteries. These are two small arteries which come out of the large blood vessel into which the left ventricle pumps all the blood (the aorta), just above the heart. These arteries then run back to supply the muscle of the heart from the outside. (The muscle of the heart wall is too thick for oxygen and food to spread into it from the blood inside the heart, and needs its own blood vessels.) See Figure 27.7.

Pathology

If the blood does not circulate (go round the body), then the body cells cannot work properly. If the cir-

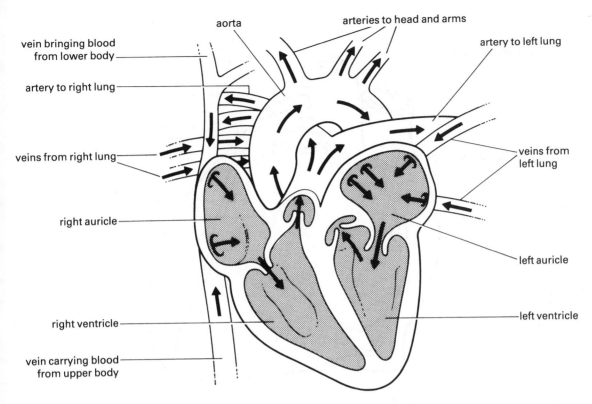

aorta

arteries to head and arms

vein bringing blood
from lower body

artery to left lung

artery to right lung

veins from
left lung

veins from right lung

right auricle

left auricle

right ventricle

left ventricle

vein carrying blood
from upper body

Figure 27.6 *Diagram showing the internal anatomy of the heart. The arrows show the direction the blood goes. Note the 'one way' valves which make the blood go in one direction only when the heart muscle contracts (gets smaller) and squeezes the blood out of the heart.*

culation of the blood stops, the body cells start to die. If the circulation of the blood to the brain stops for more than 3 or 4 minutes, many of the brain cells die or can never work properly again – even if the circulation starts again.

The blood does not circulate properly if either of the following things happen.

1. *Heart failure*. If the heart cannot pump enough blood round the body quickly enough, then heart failure is present.

   For details about heart failure see pages 461–466.

2. *Shock*. If there is not enough blood in the blood vessels for the heart to pump around the body, then shock is present.

   For details about shock see pages 466–470.

If the blood pressure remains much higher than the normal blood pressure, this condition is called *hypertension* or high blood pressure. Hypertension can damage the arteries and the organs they go to. For details about hypertension see pages 470–472.

If the blood pressure remains lower than normal blood pressure and so low that not enough blood is circulated this condition is called *hypotension* or low blood pressure.

Hypertension is one of many causes of heart failure. Heart failure after it occurs and shock are two of the many causes of hypotension.

Vasculitis is said to be present if the blood vessels are inflamed and damaged. *Atherosclerosis* is the most important blood vessel disease. Blood vessels can also be damaged by syphilis, infection in nearby tissues and in the blood, autoimmune diseases, hypertension and other conditions.

Symptoms and signs of cardiovascular disease

Symptoms of cardiovascular disease

Abnormal shortness of breath (dyspnoea)

With mild disease, shortness of breath occurs only after exercise (i.e. walking fast, carrying heavy things, working hard, etc.).

459

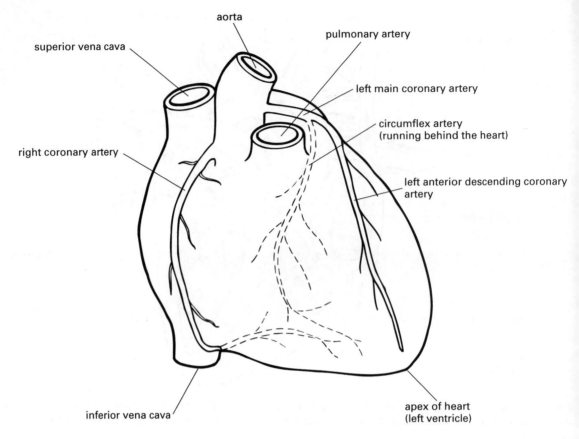

Figure 27.7 *The heart (like the abdominal organs outside the peritoneum, see Chapter 23 page 348) in most parts is surrounded by, but is not inside, an empty bag called the pericardium. Diagram showing the coronary arteries of the heart from the front.*

With worse disease, shortness of breath also occurs when the patient is walking slowly and later just sitting.

With severe disease, lying down makes the shortness of breath even worse (called 'orthopnoea') and sitting up makes it a little better.

There are many causes of shortness of breath other than heart disease. (See Chapter 20 pages 305–307.)

Oedema

Oedema (swelling caused by fluid) of the ankles occurs if the patient usually walks around. Oedema of the back occurs if the patient spends most of the time lying down. Gravity causes this excess fluid not held in any vessels, etc. to go to the lowest part of the body.

There are many causes of oedema other than heart disease. See Chapter 36 pages 588–591.

Chest pain

Chest pain is not usually caused by heart disease in most developing countries. If pain is from the heart, it is in the centre of the front of the chest but may also be felt in the arms or jaw. It is of only a few types. Angina pectoris comes only when the heart is doing more work pumping more blood, e.g. on exertion (see page 473). Myocardial infarction pain is when no blood gets to part of the heart muscle and it starts to die. The pain is constant (see page 473). Pericarditis pain may be constant but may be worse on breathing or swallowing. Heart pain is usually like a tight band around the chest or a heavy weight on the chest. See page 473.

Palpitations

Palpitations are present when the patient feels his heart beating faster or harder than normal or irregularly (i.e. out of time). See 3 on page 473 and 9 on page 474.

Signs of cardiovascular disease

Pulse rate (PR) and pulse regularity and pulse volume

The normal PR for adults is 60–80/minute. The normal pulse is regular in time.

The normal pulse has a good volume – you can feel it lift your finger as it beats strongly. This means that each contraction of the heart pumps the normal amount of blood into the arteries.

In cardiovascular disease the pulse may be

- fast (more than 100/minute), *or*
- slow (less than 60/minute), *or*
- small volume (or 'weak') (this means that each contraction of the heart pumps less blood than normal into the arteries), *or*
- irregular in time.

If the pulse is irregular or has small volume, listen to the heart beat with a stethoscope on the chest to find out the true heart rate. Sometimes the heart beats more quickly than is counted at the pulse at the wrist, because you cannot feel some of the small volume beats.

Blood pressure (BP)

The normal BP is

- 100–140 systolic (*but* it can be lower),
- 70–80 diastolic (*but* it can be lower).

Many subsistence farmers and rural people have a BP lower than 100/70. If they feel well, the pulse is not fast, the systolic BP is over 70, they are not dizzy on standing and they do pass urine, there is no problem.

If the patient has a low BP caused by shock, he will also have the other symptoms and signs of shock – pulse fast (over 100) and of small volume (weak); dizziness and further drop of blood pressure if he sits up; shortness of breath; pallor; skin usually cold and moist; etc.

If the BP is higher than 140 systolic or 90 diastolic the patient has high blood pressure or hypertension.

Signs of heart failure (see this page)

1. raised jugular venous pressure
2. enlarged liver (almost always)
3. oedema
4. fast pulse (usually)
5. cyanosis (often)
6. crackles in the lungs (sometimes).

Signs of shock (see pages 466–469)

1. The patient is dizzy, faint, restless or even unconscious.
2. The pulse is fast (over 100) and small volume (sometimes you cannot feel it at all).
3. The blood pressure is low (less than 100 and often less than 70 systolic) (sometimes you cannot record it at all). If you sit the patient up it will go lower.

4. Shortness of breath (usually deep breaths).
5. Pallor, or paleness.
6. Skin cold and moist (occasionally warm and dry; but only in *some* severe infections).
7. The patient makes little or no urine.

Disorders of cardiovascular structure and function

Heart failure

Definitions and diagnosis

Heart failure is present if the heart cannot pump enough blood around the body quickly enough for the body's need of blood. Heart failure may be acute or chronic, severe or mild.

You can check the amount of blood the heart is pumping round the body by examining these things.

1. *The pulse* – in heart failure it is usually faster than normal (more than 100/minute) and has a small volume (it feels weak). But the pulse could be slower than normal (less than 40/minute). An irregular pulse can also occur in heart failure.
2. *The blood pressure* – in heart failure it is usually normal or low. But high BP for a long time may cause heart failure and when heart failure develops it could therefore still be high.
3. *The colour and temperature of the body tissues, especially the skin* – in heart failure the skin is often cool or even cyanosed (blue).
4. Only a little or no urine made.

Acute severe heart failure can cause shock if the heart can only pump a very little blood round the body (see pages 466–469).

In heart failure blood can return to the right side of the heart from the body more quickly than the right ventricle can pump it out again. This causes the veins behind the heart to become overfilled and they distend (or stretch). Some fluid from the blood leaks (goes out) of the distended veins and causes oedema (swelling) of the organs nearby. You can check for overfilling of the veins by looking for these things:

1. oedema of legs and sacral area (lower part of back),
2. enlargement of the liver (tenderness also if it happened quickly),
3. distension of the veins in the neck (raised jugular venous pressure) (see Figures 27.8 and 27.9).

If the blood returns to the left side of the heart more quickly than the left ventricle can pump it out, then the veins behind the left side of the heart (i.e. the pulmonary veins or the veins in the lungs) are overfilled and distended. Some fluid will leak out causing oedema of the lungs. You can tell if there is pulmonary oedema by listening with the stethoscope for crackles in the lower parts of the lungs.

It is also possible to examine the heart for signs of heart failure (change in LV and RV apex beats; third and fourth heart sounds). But this is difficult and you should not try to do it unless you have been taught. (Heart murmurs are not signs of heart failure.)

- Raised jugular venous pressure ⎫
- Enlarged liver   ⎬ if right heart failure
- Oedema of legs or sacral areas ⎭
- Crackles in the lung bases   – if left heart failure
- Pulse often too fast or too slow ⎫
- Blood pressure often too low or too high ⎬ decrease in blood pumped out and blood circulation
- Skin pale and cool or even cyanosed
- Decreased or no urine output   ⎭

When you diagnose heart failure, always look for the cause.

Unfortunately, it is not possible to treat many of the causes of heart failure. But you can cure or help some of the causes of heart failure. It is important that you quickly diagnose and treat causes that will result in death unless treated. If you cannot diagnose the cause or if you cannot treat the cause in the health centre, then refer or transfer the patient for the Medical Officer to diagnose and treat. However, if you can diagnose the cause and there is no treatment possible for the cause, then do not transfer the patient.

Common causes of heart failure which you can diagnose and some of which you can treat include:

1. *Severe acute pneumonia.* The toxins from the organisms damage the heart muscles. Also the heart does not get enough oxygen from the blood which has gone through the diseased lung. But the heart must pump faster and do more work

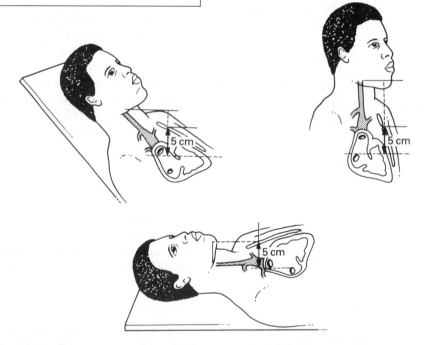

Figure 27.8 *Diagrams showing jugular venous pressure. (1) Note that in all positions in all persons (as in this patient), the vertical height of the sternal angle remains 5 cm above the level of the middle of the right atrium or auricle. (2) Note that the jugular venous pressure is normally not higher than the level of the sternal angle. (3) Therefore, in a normal person, the jugular veins are full when he is lying flat. You can see the top of the pulsation of the jugular veins of a normal person best when the patient is lying at 45° (i.e. half way up). If he is lying lower the veins are normally full. If he is lying higher the top of the pulsation is behind the clavicle, and too deep in the neck to see. (4) So, as the jugular venous pressure rises, the patient must sit further upright for you to see the upper level of the pulsation (otherwise the upper level is in the head). But you can see the venous pulsations of the neck at a higher level than normal (the sternal angle level).*

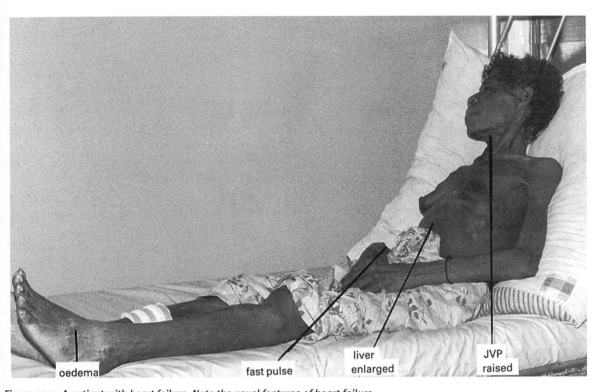

Figure 27.9 *A patient with heart failure. Note the usual features of heart failure.*

because of the infection. These things can cause heart failure.

2. *Chronic lung disease* usually caused by chronic obstructive lung disease (COLD) (but in some countries caused by schistosomiasis). Chronic lung disease destroys not only alveoli but also many blood vessels in the lungs. The remaining blood vessels (because of low oxygen in the lungs) contract and become narrow (unlike blood vessels anywhere else). The heart tries to pump the normal amount of blood through these few narrow vessels. The pressure therefore rises and makes the heart work harder. Finally, the heart cannot do all this work, and it fails. Little blood then goes through the lungs. Much blood distends the veins behind the heart. This causes congestion (overfilling of the veins) including raised JVP and oedema of the organs behind the heart.

If acute lung infection (acute bronchitis or pneumonia) then occurs, the toxins damage the heart, less oxygen goes to the heart and the heart failure gets worse. The heart failure may start or get worse during an acute chest infection (acute bronchitis or pneumonia) in a patient with COLD (chronic obstructive lung disease).

> A common cause of heart failure is an acute chest infection in a person with chronic lung disease.

3. *Other infections* which affect the heart, include:
   • typhus fever,
   • trypanosomiasis both acute and chronic (Chagas' disease in South America and East African trypanosomiasis in Africa),
   • typhoid fever,
   • relapsing fever,
   • septicaemia.

4. *Severe anaemia*
   The blood contains a small amount of haemoglobin, so the heart must pump it around the body more quickly to take enough oxygen to the body. But while it does this extra work, the heart gets less oxygen. This can cause heart failure.

5. If you give a *large volume of intravenous fluid* (or a smaller volume too quickly) to someone who already has a condition (such as anaemia) which can cause heart failure, the extra work of pumping this extra fluid can make the heart fail.

6. *Beriberi.* If diet is poor and there is not enough vitamin B_1 (also called aneurine or thiamine) in it, the

heart muscle cannot get enough energy to pump properly. The lack of vitamin B_1 also makes the blood vessels dilate (get bigger) and so the heart must pump more blood to fill the blood vessels. These cause heart failure with a fast pulse and increased difference between systolic and diastolic BP, warm hands and feet, but cold when later the heart failure becomes severe. Sometimes lack of vitamin B_1 also stops the nerves in the legs working properly, and this causes pain and weakness in the legs. Beriberi occurs most often in poor people, during a famine or in alcoholics (Chapter 23 page 380).

7. *Acute rheumatic fever* (see page 475)
8. *Hypertension* (see page 470)
9. *Coronary heart disease* (see page 472)
10. *Thyrotoxicosis* (see Chapter 30 page 498)
    Often the pulse is fast and irregular; the patient has lost weight despite eating well; the eyes are staring or the patient has exophthalmos; and the skin feels warm.
11. *A patient with heart failure stops his treatment.*
12. *'Epidemic dropsy'*
    If a group of people eat food that contains mustard oil or another poison and then develop heart failure and other symptoms and signs, notify the Medical Officer immediately (and tell the people not to eat mustard oil or that other food until the Medical Officer has it tested for poison).

You can diagnose or treat most of the above conditions at the health centre.

Refer or non-urgently transfer all other cases as there are conditions that the Medical Officer:

1. may be able to diagnose and possibly treat, e.g.
   • thyrotoxic heart disease,
   • hypertension,
   • coronary heart disease,
   • pericarditis (especially due to infection with bacteria, TB or HIV),
   • infective endocarditis,
   • syphilitic heart disease,
   • arrhythmias (abnormal heart rate or rhythm),
   • diastolic heart failure,
   • pregnancy (with the extra work the heart has to do) in a woman with other heart disease.
2. may diagnose, but as expensive surgery or other treatment is needed, may not be able to treat:
   • congenital heart disease,
   • coronary heart disease,
   • hypertension with a curable cause,
   • valvular heart disease from rheumatic fever and other causes.

3. may diagnose, but there is no specific known treatment at present:
   • endomyocardial fibrosis,
   • cardiomyopathies of various sorts including:
     – 'dilated cardiomyopathy' and
     – 'peri-partum cardiac failure',
   • Chagas' disease.

Differential diagnosis

Check that the patient does not have another cause for the symptoms or signs of heart failure:

• *Oedema* – toxaemia of pregnancy, acute glomerulo-nephritis, chronic liver disease or filariasis, etc. See Chapter 36 pages 588–590.
• *Enlarged tender liver* – especially liver abscess. See Chapter 24 pages 401, then 398–400.
• *Shortness of breath* – especially pneumonia, acute bronchitis, asthma or TB. See Chapter 20 pages 305–307.

If you think the patient could have heart failure always look for raised jugular venous pressure (almost always raised if there is heart failure).

Treatment

1. Treat the heart failure itself.
2. Look for and treat the cause of the heart failure.

Treat the heart failure itself.

---

1. Rest
2. Oxygen if acute and severe
3. Diuretics
4. No salt in food
5. Potassium chloride if necessary
6. Stop any drugs which decrease the pumping of the heart
7. Consider vasodilator treatment
8. Digoxin
9. Transfer if needed
10. Consider aminophylline treatment

---

1. *Rest*
   Sit the patient up in bed if he is in an acute stage and short of breath. When sleeping or lying tilt the bed 20° (head end up and foot end down). The patient must rest for some weeks if he is in a chronic stage; but do not stop him walking around.
2. *Oxygen if acute and severe*
   Give intranasal oxygen 1–2 litres/minute. Give only in acute heart failure. *Do not* give more than

2 litres/minute if he has COLD. There is not usually enough oxygen available for treatment of chronic heart failure from COLD.

3. *Diuretics*

Give furosemide/frusemide 40 mg IVI immediately for acute heart failure. You can repeat this in $\frac{1}{2}$–1 hour if necessary and increase the dose to 60–80 mg if necessary.

Give hydrochlorothiazide 50–100 mg every morning in the acute and chronic stage.

Give furosemide/frusemide 40–160 mg also every morning if the hydrochlorothiazide tabs are not effective.

Diuretics are the most effective and important treatment in most cases

---

However, do not give a diuretic if the patient has shock. If the patient has shock, give digoxin.

4. *No salt in food*

Tell the patient not to eat salty foods or put any salt in food when it is being cooked or when he is eating it.

5. *Potassium chloride if necessary*

Give potassium chloride 1200 mg (2 tabs) three times a day if on diuretics *and if*

(a) the patient is taking furosemide/frusemide *and* hydrochlorothiazide; or

(b) he is *not* on a tuber diet (e.g. sweet potato, yam, taro, etc.); *or*

(c) he *is* taking digoxin.

6. Stop any drugs which decrease the pumping of the heart, e.g. calcium channel blockers (e.g. amlodipine, verapamil, nifedipine); or could damage kidney function or keep fluid in the body, e.g. NSAIDs (e.g. ibuprofen).

7. Vasodilators help almost all people in almost all types of heart failure.

In acute heart failure the only ones on the WHO list at present you can try are sublingual (dissolved under the tongue) glyceryl trinitrate 500 mg tablet or isosorbide dinitrate 5 mg. These can be repeated in 30 minutes and then each 2–4 hours. Do not give more of these if the systolic BP less than 90 mmHg until it is above 90 mmHg.

In acute and chronic heart failure and especially if the BP is above 140/90 an angiotensin converting enzyme (ACE) inhibitor should be given. At present, the only one on the WHO list is enalapril. Start with a low dose 1.25 mg (or at the most 2.5 mg). After 12 hours the dose can be repeated. After 24 hours the dose can be increased by 2.5 mg each 2 days to 10 mg twice daily. However, do not give enough that the systolic BP falls to 90 systolic. Also, these drugs cause the serum potassium to rise and at times the kidney function to decrease. The patient therefore needs to be transferred to the Medical Officer at the hospital for the urea, creatinine and electrolytes to be checked within a week of starting enalapril. By that time, it would be best to stop any potassium chloride being given until the blood results were known. If transfer was delayed, stop also digoxin.

8. *Digoxin*

Give digoxin if

(a) there is heart failure in a previously healthy person *or*

(b) the patient has shock. (Do not give diuretics if the patient has shock. Use digoxin instead.) *or*

(c) the pulse and heart rate is fast and irregular (atrial fibrillation) *or*

(d) all the other treatment for heart failure (above) and treatment of the cause (below) does not control the heart failure.

Digoxin is not given often in health centres.

The signs of too much digoxin are:

(a) loss of appetite or vomiting or

(b) pulse slow (<60) or irregular (if the pulse was not slow or irregular before starting digoxin).

If the signs of too much digoxin develop *then*:

(a) *stop the digoxin* for 48 hours,

(b) *after 48 hours* start the digoxin again at *only half of the previous dose.*

Digoxin dose

- 0.5 mg or $\frac{1}{2}$ mg or 500 micrograms once and repeat one more time only in 6 hours, i.e. 2 doses *for large and young adult* IMI or orally
- 0.5 mg ($\frac{1}{2}$ mg) or 500 micrograms once only *for small or old adult* by IMI or orally *then*
- 0.25 mg ($\frac{1}{4}$ mg) or 250 micrograms daily *for large young adult* orally
- 0.125 mg ($\frac{1}{8}$ mg) or 125 micrograms daily *for small or old adult* orally.

You must always give potassium chloride 1200 mg (2 tablets tid) if you are giving diuretics with the digoxin.

If a patient on digoxin loses his appetite or vomits or his pulse is slow or irregular, **stop the digoxin** for 48 hours and **then** give it at only **half of the previous daily dose.**

9. After transfer and tests the Medical Officer may continue or change some of your treatment and add other drugs including
   (a) small doses of beta blockers
   (b) hydralazine and a nitrate
   (c) spironolactone.
   Do not yourself, without doing and understanding the results of the blood tests, continue an ACE inhibitor or add these other drugs (as incorrect combinations may kill the patient).
10. *Aminophylline or theophylline if* all other treatment fails and transfer of the patient to the Medical Officer delayed, may sometimes help.
    Give aminophylline by *slow* IVI:
    • For a large adult (>50 kg), give 375 mg (15 ml)
    • For a small adult (<50 kg), give 250 mg (10 ml)
    • Give it by *slow* IVI (take 10 minutes by the clock).
    Give aminophylline for acute severe heart failure after the frusemide/furosemide and for acute heart failure that is not responding to all the other treatment.
    Also try it for chronic heart failure that is not responding to all other treatment.
    After this large starting dose, give only a small dose, 100 mg (1 tab) twice daily for a small adult or 100 mg (1 tab) three times a day for a large adult (i.e. about half ($\frac{1}{2}$) of the dose for asthma).
    Stop if there is nausea or vomiting not caused by digoxin. Increase the dose every 2–3 days until the heart failure is controlled or nausea or vomiting occurs. Do not give more than 400 mg daily if heart failure.

Look for and treat the underlying cause

1. Chest infections – give antibiotics, etc. See pneumonia (Chapter 20 pages 289–291).

> Antibiotics are an essential part of the treatment in many cases of heart failure as chest infection is a common cause.

2. Chronic obstructive lung disease. See Chapter 20 page 297.
3. Other infections. Septicaemia. See Chapter 12 page 64. Typhus. See Chapter 17 page 164. Trypanosomiasis. See Chapter 18 pages 181, 184.
4. Anaemia. See Chapter 21 pages 316–319.
5. Beriberi – thiamine (aneurine or vitamin B_1) 50 mg (1 tab) immediately and daily for 2 weeks. (If available, 50 mg (1 ml) IMI immediately.)

Give a good mixed diet.

Give aneurine to all patients who have no obvious underlying cause for heart failure; especially if the patient is on a poor diet (famine, old, drinks a lot of alcohol or has bad dietary habits), or is anaemic, or has weak or painful legs.

6. IV saline or blood given too fast – stop or slow down the drip.
7. Acute rheumatic fever – start prophylactic treatment with benzathine penicillin and treat any streptococcal infection with benzylpenicillin.
8. Hypertension – start a tablet to lower the blood pressure as well as all the above treatment.
9. Coronary heart disease – start acetylsalicylic acid and start all the lifestyle changes needed.
10. Thyrotoxicosis – transfer for treatment with special drugs
11. A patient on treatment who has stopped his drugs – start treatment again.

Refer or transfer to Medical Officer

1. All cases of heart failure who do **not** have a lower respiratory tract infection or COLD or anaemia or another cause you can treat (for diagnosis – because they may have a curable cause) (non-urgent).
2. All cases of heart failure with an irregular pulse (urgent if acute heart failure).
3. All cases of heart failure which are not controlled until vasodilators added.

Shock

The medical term 'shock' means collapse because not enough blood is circulating through the body. Shock is always acute and very serious. (Shock, in the medical sense, has nothing to do with the 'shock' people are said to have when they get a big surprise or very bad news and are mentally upset.)

There are two main causes of shock:
(see page 467 also for a third cause)

1. There is not enough volume of blood. This can be caused by loss of blood itself through bleeding from broken blood vessels, or loss of just the water and salt from the blood through blood vessel walls (as in dehydration, burns, septicaemia, etc.) or not enough water and salt absorbed into the blood vessels (as in late stages of dehydration especially from gastroenteritis).
2. There is dilation or widening of some of the venous and capillary blood vessels. Blood collects in these blood vessels and does not return to the heart. This is often caused by toxins from infections

or anaphylaxis (acute allergy) or a change in the nervous system control of the blood vessels.

In either case, there is not enough blood for the heart to pump around the body and fill the arteries, and so the blood pressure falls.

The body then tries to keep the blood going to the most important parts of the body (brain, heart and liver) by closing down the blood vessels to the less important parts (skin, muscles, gastrointestinal tract and later kidneys). These parts then become pale and do not work properly. Also the heart pumps all the blood to the important parts as fast as it can, i.e. the pulse rate is fast.

If, after this, there is still not enough blood for the heart to pump round to the brain, liver and heart, these organs also do not work properly. If the blood volume is not quickly increased the patient soon dies.

3. A third cause for shock occurs when the heart itself is weak and cannot pump the blood around the body even when there is enough blood (severe heart failure).

Diagnosis

The diagnosis of shock is usually obvious from the symptoms and signs (see Figure 27.10).

1. The patient feels weak, faint and dizzy (especially when he stands up, but often also when sitting). In severe cases, he is restless or unconscious. This is because not enough blood is going to the brain.
2. The pulse is fast (over 100/minute) and has a small volume.
3. The blood pressure is low (less than 100 and usually less than 70 systolic) and lower if the patient sits up.
4. There is shortness of breath (deep breaths).
5. There is pallor or paleness.
6. The skin is cold and moist (sometimes in *some* infections the skin may be warm and dry).
7. Little or no urine is made.

Cause

The cause of shock is usually obvious. If it is not, find out from the history and examination of the patient

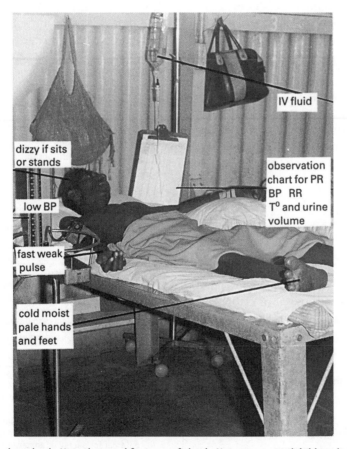

Figure 27.10 *A patient who has shock. Note the usual features of shock. Note two essential things in treatment.*

(see Chapter 6). *Do this while you are starting treatment* for the shock. The cause is usually one of these things:

1. Loss of blood or fluid from the blood vessels.
   - external bleeding
   - internal bleeding (e.g. from ruptured spleen or ectopic pregnancy or fractured leg or hip)
   - burns
   - gastroenteritis
   - malaria
   - severe infections (peritonitis, septicaemia, typhus fever, relapsing fever, etc.)
   - allergic reactions.
2. Dilation of blood vessels.
   - infections
   - allergic reaction
   - severe pain
   - fright or fear
   - standing still for a long time
   } 'fainting' – usually a *slow* pulse
3. The heart not pumping properly.
   - severe infections with toxaemia and low oxygen, e.g. severe pneumonia, malaria, acute trypanosomiasis, typhus fever, relapsing fever
   - chronic trypanosomiasis (Chagas' disease)
   - coronary heart disease with myocardial infarction 'heart attack'.

Management of a patient with shock

Immediately put up an intravenous drip of 0.9% sodium chloride (even before you diagnose the cause).

Diagnose the cause. The cause is usually obvious. If it is not, diagnose it from the history and examination of the patient (or from a history given by the patient's relatives or friends). *Do this while you are putting up the drip.*

Shock is usually caused by:

1. loss of fluid
2. loss of blood (common)
3. septicaemia or infection
4. allergy (uncommon)
5. heart not pumping properly (very uncommon).

If no cause is obvious, look carefully for internal bleeding (especially ruptured spleen or ectopic pregnancy). If you cannot find the cause, treat for shock from septicaemia.

> Management
> 1. Keep the airway clear. Give artificial ventilation if necessary.
> 2. Give oxygen.
> 3. Give analgesics, if severe pain.
> 4. Keep the patient lying down and warm.

5. Diagnose and treat the cause:
   (a) If loss of fluids – give IV fluids.
   (b) If loss of blood – stop bleeding.
   - give IV fluids and/or plasma volume expander[1] and/or blood.
   (c) If septicaemia – Give IV chloramphenicol, artesunate (or infusion of quinine), fluids, digoxin.
   (d) If acute allergic reaction:
   - give IM (or IV) adrenaline,
   - give IV antihistamine,
   - give IV fluids.
6. Look for signs of heart failure. Treat heart failure if it occurs.
7. Transfer patient if necessary.

Treatment depends on the cause (see below). But do the following in all cases,

1. Make sure the *airway* is clear. If the patient is unconscious, give routine care of the airway for an unconscious patient (see Chapter 25 pages 423–424). If he is not breathing enough, give artificial ventilation (see Chapter 37 pages 607–612).
2. Give *intranasal oxygen*, 4 litres/minute.
3. *If there is severe pain give morphine* 7.5 mg for small adult or 10 mg for large adult *slowly* over 5 minutes by IVI.
4. *Keep the patient lying down flat.* Keep the legs raised. Keep the patient warm but not hot.
5. *Treat the cause* (see below).

> (a) When loss of fluid (dehydration) is the cause (usually from gastroenteritis) treat as described below.

- IV 0.9% *sodium chloride* as fast as possible until signs of shock go. Check the patient after each litre. Give up to 4 litres. If the patient is still shocked

---

[1] *Plasma volume expanders*
These, by themselves, can very occasionally cause allergic reactions, anaphylaxis and shock (with low BP). Some now think that as IV 0.9% saline may be as effective and does not have these reactions, plasma volume expanders should not be used. Therefore:
1. If plasma volume expanders are not available just use 0.9% saline in their place.
2. Do not change from 0.9% saline to plasma volume expander unless the saline is not being successful – just continue 0.9% saline.
3. If using plasma volume expanders and an allergic reaction occurs or the BP falls even more
   (a) stop the plasma volume expander
   (b) give 0.9% sodium chloride in its place
   (c) treat for allergy or anaphylaxis with IV adrenaline and antihistamine etc. (See pages 469–470.)

after 3–4 litres, consider changing to IV plasma volume expander.

- IV *plasma volume expander* (polygeline 3.5% (Haemaccel) or dextran 70, 6% (Macrodex or Gentran 70) or SPPS (stable plasma protein solution) or albumin 4–5% or alternative). But see note on page 468 before using. If use, give as fast as possible until the signs of shock disappear. Give 0.5–1.5 litres (1–3 bottles).
- When the signs of shock go, finish that bottle of plasma volume expander, then change back to 0.9% sodium chloride.
- IV 0.9% *sodium chloride* 1 litre every hour until the signs of dehydration go.
- See gastroenteritis (Chapter 23 page 364) for details of replacement of continuing fluid losses and maintenance fluids.
- If the 3–4 litres of 0.9% sodium chloride and the 1.5 litres of plasma volume expander do not cure the patient's shock, there is probably also another cause of the shock, e.g. septicaemia *or* hidden blood loss. See below for treatment.

(b) When loss of blood is the cause (e.g. bleeding peptic ulcer, obstetric bleeding, trauma, etc.) treat as described below.

- Stop the bleeding if possible. If you cannot be certain you can stop the bleeding arrange an urgent blood transfusion and emergency transfer.
- Give IV 0.9% *sodium chloride* as fast as possible. Give up to 1500 ml. If the signs of shock go, finish off that bag of saline and then change to maintenance fluids (0.18% sodium chloride in 4.3% dextrose, 1 litre every 8 hours – see Chapter 23 page 364).
- If the signs of shock are still present after 1500 ml 0.9% sodium chloride, continue 0.9% sodium chloride as fast as possible but consider changing to plasma volume expander. See, however, note on page 468 first. If change give: IV *plasma volume expander* (polygeline 3.5% (Haemaccel) or dextran 70, 6% (Macrodex or Gentran 70) or SPPS (stable plasma protein solution) or albumin 4%) as fast as possible. If the signs of shock go, finish that bottle of plasma volume expander and change to maintenance fluids (see above or Chapter 23 page 364).
- If the signs of shock have not gone when you are giving the third bottle of IV plasma volume expander, i.e. 1000–1500 ml, the patient needs *blood*.

- If possible transfer the patient to the Medical Officer before blood is necessary. If you cannot transfer the patient quickly, see a reference book for details of how to crossmatch and give blood.

(c) When septicaemia or other acute severe infection is the cause treat as described below.

Treat for septicaemia if:
- the history, symptoms or signs suggest septicaemia; *or*
- there is no obvious cause for shock.
- Give IV *chloramphenicol* 2 g immediately then 1 g every 6 hours.
- If *immediate* IVI is not possible, give 1 g by IMI. Then give an IV 1 g dose also as soon as an IVI possible.
  If an IV dose is still not possible 1 hour after the first IM dose, then give another 1 g by IMI.
- Give 1 g by IVI (or by IMI) every 6 hours after the first dose.
  Give by IVI if:
  – shock is still present or
  – a drip is necessary.
- For details about antibiotics, see acute severe bacterial infections (Chapter 12 page 64 and Chapter 11 pages 55–61).
- Give IVI artesunate 2.4 mg/kg (120–180 mg) or other IV artemisinin drug immediately. If not available give instead *quinine* not by IVI but by IV infusion 20 mg/kg (800 mg for small adult or 1200 mg for a large adult) in 500 ml of 5% dextrose slowly over the first 4 hours in another (a second) drip. Give IMI artesunate (dose as above) or artemether 3.2 mg/kg (160–240 mg) or IMI quinine (dose as above) only if IV drip is not possible. Complete the treatment course. (See malaria Chapter 13 pages 79–81.)
- Give IV *fluids* as in 'Loss of fluids' (page 468). But do not give more than the least fluid necessary to correct the shock. Look carefully for heart failure; treat it, if it occurs (stop IV fluids and see pages 464–466).

(d) When acute allergic reaction is the cause (anaphylactic reaction) treat as described below.

- Give IMI *epinephrine/adrenaline* tart. 1:1000 solution 0.5 ml ($\frac{1}{2}$ ml) immediately. If the patient is about to die, you can give the epinephrine/adrenaline intravenously slowly at 0.1 ml (or $\frac{1}{10}$ ml) every minute, i.e. 0.5 ml (or $\frac{1}{2}$ ml) in 5 minutes. The best way to do this is to mix 0.5 ml ($\frac{1}{2}$ ml) of epinephrine/adrenaline with 4.5 ml of 0.9% saline and give 1 ml each minute.

- Give IVI *promethazine* 50 mg (2 ml) immediately.
- If available, give IVI hydrocortisone 200–300 mg.
- Give IV *fluids* as in 'Loss of fluids' (page 468). Watch carefully for heart failure; treat it if it occurs (pages 464–466).
- *Repeat the antihistamine and adrenaline* after 10 minutes if necessary.

6. When you give intravenous fluids, look carefully for signs of heart failure.
- Signs of heart failure are high jugular venous pressure or shortness of breath and crackles in the lungs that were not present before the IV fluids started. Later the liver enlarges and becomes tender and oedema develops.
- Heart failure is not likely in shock from dehydration or blood loss until after the fluid or blood loss is replaced; and then more fluid given.

(a) When mild heart failure occurs:
- Change to 0.18% sodium chloride in 4.3% dextrose and slow the drip to 1 litre every 12 hours.
- Give digoxin 0.5 mg or 500 micrograms IV slowly over 2 minutes immediately *or* 0.5 mg orally immediately. See page 465 before you give further doses.

(b) When severe heart failure occurs (patient becomes very breathless or has a lot of crackles in his chest)
- Stop the IV fluids.
- Give furosemide/frusemide 40 mg IVI immediately once and repeat in $\frac{1}{2}$ to 1 hour if necessary.
- Then see pages 464–466.

Transfer to Medical Officer care

1. Any case which needs blood transfusion (urgent – emergency).
2. Any case which does not greatly improve with treatment in 3 hours (urgent – emergency).
3. Any case for which you cannot find or treat the underlying cause successfully in a health centre (urgent – emergency).

Prevention

Prevention is by carefully observing and giving proper treatment early to all patients who have a condition that can cause shock.

Systemic vascular hypertension

The systemic circulation is the system of blood vessels which supplies all parts of the body except the lungs (which is the pulmonary circulation) (although the liver has a second supply of veins from the intestine (the portal vein system)). It includes the aorta and all its branches and the veins which drain back into the right atrium. The blood pressure in it depends on the volume of blood pumped out by the left ventricular contraction, how easy it is for the large arteries to stretch to hold this extra volume, the contraction or dilatation of the small blood vessels (arterioles) letting the blood quickly or slowly out of the arteries into the capillaries, as well as blood volume, etc.

Systemic hypertension, often just called hypertension or high blood pressure, is said to be present when the blood pressure is 140 systolic or higher and/or 90 diastolic or higher on three separate blood pressure measurements on two separate examinations. However, it would not be treated in some developing countries unless it was 160/95 or higher. It is most often discovered when a patient has a stroke or another condition and the blood pressure is then taken.

In some parts of Africa up to 20% of adults suffer from hypertension, with blood pressure above 160/95. Causes include kidney disease and abnormalities of many other organs. However, few hospitals are able to do the tests to find these causes and even fewer able to treat any causes found. Even if patients do have lots of tests in hospital, most cases have no cause found and are called 'essential hypertension' (essential meaning no cause is found). However, we know that there are a number of things which make it more likely for people to get hypertension and for any hypertension they have to be worse; and these include urbanisation, drinking more alcohol than is healthy (more than one (to two) standard drinks for a woman or two (to three) standard drinks for a man daily), having a lot of salt in the diet, having body weight above the ideal, smoking tobacco and not exercising.

If blood pressure is higher than normal, it can cause damage to the blood vessels (as damage would happen to any hose or tube or pipe which had a pressure in it greater than it was made for). The types of blood vessel damage caused include atheroma (see page 472) and actual bursting of the artery. These abnormalities in arteries can cause cerebrovascular disease or stroke, damage to the retina of the eye with loss of vision, kidney failure and also coronary heart disease with angina or myocardial infarction (see page 473). As well as this, the heart may not be able to pump all the blood through the narrowed vessels at such a high pressure and blood may collect behind the heart and heart failure develop. Most patients with high blood pressure have no symptoms until one of the above complications occurs.

Treatment

If a patient has high blood pressure you should do the following:

1. Tell him the above risks of hypertension even though he may have no symptoms from the hypertension.
2. Tell him that if he corrects any of the risk factors (above) that he has, over the next 6 months, his blood pressure may fall and the risks from hypertension will be less. He should therefore avoid excess alcohol, not eat salty foods or add salt to cooking or when he is eating food, diet to get his weight to the ideal for his height, stop smoking if he smokes tobacco and start doing regular exercise for at least 20–30 minutes at least four to five times a week (even walking quickly without stopping is enough).
3. Start drug treatment only if
   - the blood pressure at first is dangerously high (i.e. 220/120 or above on three readings or 210/110 or above for 1–2 weeks). Immediate treatment is needed.
   - after 6 months of lifestyle changes (in 2 above) the blood pressure is still abnormally high.
   - there are in fact drugs available to treat him now and for the rest of his life.
   - he agrees to take tablets every day for the rest of his life and is likely to do so.
4. Before starting treatment, send blood for a full blood count, electrolytes, urea and creatinine and also send urine for examination for protein, glucose and microscopy.
   Ask your Medical Officer to review the results and the case before starting treatment if treatment is not urgent or after starting treatment if the blood pressure is dangerously high, to make sure there is no underlying cause which is easily treated and that he is suitable for treatment.
5. Use the lowest dose of the cheapest, once daily treatments available. This will be from one of the following groups:
   - Thiazide diuretics, e.g. hydrochlorothiazide 12.5–50 mg daily.
   - Centrally acting alpha agonist, e.g. reserpine 0.1–0.25 mg (no more) or methyldopa (but this needs twice daily treatment and is expensive),

Table 27.1 Some side effects of antihypertensive drugs. (from *Manson's Tropical Diseases*, ed. G. G. Cook and A. Zumla, 21st ed. reproduced by permission of Elsevier © 2003)

Common side effect	Diuretic	β-blocker	ACE inhibitor	Angiotensin receptor antagonist	Calcium antagonist	α-blocker
Headache	–	–	–	–	+	–
Flushing	–	–	–	–	+	–
Shortness of breath	–	+	–	–	–	–
Tiredness	–	+	–	–	–	–
Impotence	+	+	–	–	–	–
Cough	–	–	+	–	–	–
Gout	+	–	–	–	–	–
Oedema	–	–	–	–	+	–
Low BP on standing	–	–	–	–	–	+
Cold hands and feet	–	+	–	–	–	–
Urinary incontinence on exertion	–	–	–	–	–	+
Swelling of tissues under the skin	–	–	+	+	–	–
Constipation	–	–	–	–	+	–

250–750 mg twice daily. These drugs can cause tiredness or depression.

- Beta blockers including propranolol 40–160 mg twice daily or atenolol 25–100 mg daily.
- Alpha blockers, e.g. prazozin 0.5–5 mg twice daily.
- Angiotensin converting enzyme (ACE) inhibitors, e.g. captopril 12.5–100 mg daily and enalapril 2.5–40 mg daily and trandolapril 0.5–4 mg daily (and the newer related angiotensin II receptor antagonists, e.g. losartan and irbesarten).
- Calcium-channel blockers, including nifedipine 30–60 mg daily, verapamil 120–240 mg daily and amlodipine 2.5–10 mg daily.
- Vasodilators including hydralazine which needs to be used together with a beta blocker (or diuretic) and WHO does not recommend normally.

Black Africans tend not to get the BP lowered by beta blockers and ACE inhibitors as much as other races.

Advise salt restriction as this may be very important. Try thiazides and calcium channel blockers (but hydro-chlorothiazide and methyldopa together have been reported as very effective). In South Asia try a diuretic and ACE inhibitor. In Oriental patients salt restriction also may be very important. In Pacific Islanders the changes in life style are very important, as well as drugs. In the elderly start with just a diuretic.

If drugs are given, the patient needs to be started with a low dose of one and seen each month and the blood pressure taken and the dose very slowly increased, as long as he does not have any serious side effects from the drugs until the normal highest dose of that drug is reached. If by then the BP has not improved, stop the drug and try another. If the BP has improved, but is still too high, add another drug and increase the dose slowly. If it is possible, the urea, creatinine and electrolytes should be checked at each visit as sometimes these drugs stop the kidney working properly. The aim is to have have a BP of less than 140/90 without significant side effects and no loss of kidney function and electrolytes normal.

Hydrochlorothiazide 25 mg is a good drug to give first or if another drug is started first to add to that drug if that drug alone does not control the blood pressure.

Prevention

The patient should avoid those things which make hypertension more likely, as mentioned on pages 470–471, and good treatment should be given for any conditions which cause kidney disease.

Atherosclerotic vascular disease

Atherosclerosis is a gradually increasing disease which affects all the arteries of the body. Plaques or lumps slowly form and get larger within the inside lining of the arteries. These plaques are full of fatty material. After many years these plaques can get so big that they nearly block the artery and the blood flow becomes so slow through the artery that the blood clots and blocks the artery. At times the plaques rupture (break open) and the fatty material is carried down the artery (which of course gets smaller and smaller as it gets nearer the organ it supplies) until the artery is small enough to get blocked by the fatty material. The part of the body supplied by the artery blocked in either of these two ways can cause pain or not work properly or die.

If the arteries which become partly or completely blocked, supply

- the heart – coronary heart disease (angina pectoris or myocardial infarction (heart attack)) follows,
- the brain – cerebrovascular disease (stroke) follows,
- the legs – peripheral vascular disease (intermittent claudication or gangrene) follows,
- the kidneys – reno-vascular disease (high blood pressure or kidney failure) follows, etc.

Things which are known to lead to atherosclerosis include:

- getting older,
- being male,
- others in the family with the condition.

Nothing can be done about these things.

They also include:

- smoking tobacco,
- having high blood pressure not controlled by treatment,
- having high levels of fat (cholesterol and triglycerides) in the blood,
- diabetes mellitus not controlled by diet and drugs,
- not exercising,
- diet lacking fruit, vegetables, fish and vitamins but being high in animal fat or a lot of alcohol (a small amount of alcohol may help),
- being overweight.

People can of course change all of these things and then their risk of atherosclerosis and the diseases it causes will be much less.

Atherosclerosis used to be very uncommon in developing countries. It is now becoming much more common, especially in people living in towns and cities.

Health Education so that people know what the risks for atherosclerosis are, so that they have the chance to avoid it, is obviously essential.

Coronary heart disease or ischaemic heart disease

Coronary heart disease is caused by any condition that narrows the coronary arteries which take blood from the aorta to the heart muscle. The commonest cause of narrowing is patches of atheroma which can partly block the artery, or if a clot forms on top of one of them or the plaque ruptures, can completely block the artery suddenly. Another cause of narrowed arteries is syphilis. There are other uncommon causes.

Frequency, cause, pathology, symptoms, signs and complications

This condition is uncommon in village people in non-industrialised countries who still live in their traditional ways; but it occurs in middle-aged and elderly town people who have changed to some of the western ways of living, eating, smoking, working and not exercising. (See atherosclerosis page 472 for more details.) It is common in middle-aged and old people in industrialised countries.

If the coronary arteries are partly blocked, not much blood can get to the heart muscle. When the heart does not have a lot of work to do, such as sitting or sleeping, there is enough blood for the heart muscle. When the heart has a lot of work to do, such as exercising or after a large meal or if the patient becomes excited or cross, then there is not enough blood for the heart muscle. This lack of blood causes pain – like pain in any other part of the body if this part of the body is repeatedly exercised, doing something it is not able to keep on doing. This pain is called 'angina pectoris' or just 'angina'. Angina comes on exertion (and after the above things) and goes once the exertion is stopped within a minute or so; but will come back again when the same amount of exertion is done again. The pain is in the centre of the front of the chest, but as well as that can sometimes also be felt in the arms or jaw. It is like a crushing weight or tight band. Sometimes this partly blocked artery can also cause the heart to beat irregularly. Sometimes it can cause the muscle to work so poorly that heart failure develops.

If the artery becomes completely blocked, then the part of the heart muscle which it normally supplied will die and eventually be replaced by scar tissue which cannot pump blood. Meanwhile, the patient will have pain like angina, except that it will be there all the time for hours and not go away. Occasionally, people do not feel the pain, especially if the nerves to the heart are damaged by diabetes mellitus. The patient with a blocked coronary artery is at risk of dying from the pulse being too fast or too slow or heart failure or shock. This is called a 'myocardial infarction' or a 'heart attack'.

Differential diagnosis

Check that there is not another cause of:

- chest pain (see Chapter 20 pages 307–308) or
- heart failure (see pages 462–464) or
- shock (see pages 467–468) or
- irregular heart rate, e.g. thyrotoxicosis.

Treatment

Treatment of all patients

On diagnosis, make sure the patient starts correcting any of those things which caused the condition if they apply to him;

1. reduce body weight to the ideal,
2. do not eat a lot of animal fat but more cereals, vegetables and fruit,
3. control any diabetes well,
4. treat any hypertension present by lifestyle changes, especially reducing salt in the food and if needed drugs to get the blood pressure if possible down to 140/90 or less,
5. stop any tobacco smoking,
6. exercise regularly for at least 20–30 minutes at least four or five times a week (walking quickly without stopping will do),
7. send blood for serological test for syphilis.

Treat any other condition which may be making the patient worse:

1. Carefully look for and treat any anaemia present.
2. Look for and treat any heart failure present.
3. Look for a fast or irregular pulse and discuss any such patient with your Medical Officer about tests for thyrotoxicosis and other tests and if the patient should have digoxin.
4. Look very carefully for thyrotoxicosis in all patients and if possible arrange for tests for this or get your Medical Officer to see the patient.

Further treatment of angina pectoris

1. Acetylsalicylic acid 100–150 mg daily (to try to stop blood clots forming in the artery).
2. Glyceryl trinitrate (0.5 or 0.6 mg tablet) to be dissolved under the tongue slowly if angina occurs. Repeat the dose every five minutes if pain contin-

ues, up to 3 doses. Also take glyceryl nitrate before doing things known to usually cause angina. Side effects include flushing, headaches and dizziness. If the pain comes back after 1–2 hours further doses can be taken. Isosorbide dinitrate (5 mg or 10 mg tablets) can be used instead. If the pain occurs often, isosorbide dinitrate 5 (up to 40) mg may be given regularly to prevent pain coming, e.g. on waking and about 4 p.m. (not every 12 hours as a nitrate free period of 12 hours is needed for the drug to continue to work). Long acting tablets and creams and patches of nitrates do exist.

3. If the patient still continues to have problems refer him to your Medical Officer for consideration for further treatment which could include beta-blocker drugs or calcium channel blocker drugs. Cholesterol lowering drugs, coronary artery dilatation then stenting, or bypass grafting surgery, are not normally available.

Treatment of myocardial infarction

1. Make the patient rest and sit or lie down.
2. Give oxygen 2–4 litres by nasal prongs.
3. Get the patient to swallow 300–500 mg of acetyl-salicylic acid immediately (to help stop more blood clotting). Continue 100–150 mg daily.
4. Put glyceryl trinitrate 0.5 or 0.6 mg or isosorbide dinitrate 10 mg under the tongue and let it dissolve slowly. If the pain is still present and the blood pressure over 100, at 5 to 10 minutes give a further 1–2 doses.
5. Insert an intravenous cannula.
6. If the pain is still present, give morphine 10–15 mg (1–1.5 ml) by IVI slowly over 5–10 minutes rather than by IMI.
7. Give metoclopramide 10 mg by IVI or IMI and repeat later if any nausea or vomiting.
8. Treat any heart failure present in the usual way, including oxygen, diuretics and digoxin (see pages 464–466).
9. If the pulse rate and heart rate (listening at the heart apex with the stethoscope) is 40 beats per minute or less, then (a) lift up the legs (feet above hips) and tilt the head end of the bed down and (b) give atropine 0.6 mg (1 ml) IVI then repeat if still needed in 5 minutes and can be repeated in 1 hour and then each few hours to a maximum of 3 mg in 24 hours to try, if possible, to get the heart rate above 60.
10. If the pulse is irregular and fast (over 140) start digoxin (see page 465) and propranolol 40 mg or atenolol 25 mg.

11. A beta blocker, e.g atenolol 50 mg daily as long as the patient does not have severe heart failure or any asthma even if the pulse is normal, improves the chances of survival.
12. If shock develops most patients die.
    Do not give any more nitrate.
    Make sure all of the above otherwise are done especially that treatment for fast or slow heart rate is given.
    If the patient is taking a beta blocker or calcium channel blocker drug stop these. Stop also any drugs the patient was already taking for an irregular or slow or fast heart rate.
    If the patient does not improve it is just possible he could be short of fluid, especially if he was on treatment with a diuretic or had vomiting or for other reasons needs a higher venous pressure. Give 250 ml of 0.9% sodium chloride IV quickly and see what happens. If the patient improves give further doses of 250 ml until the blood pressure is 70–90 and then slow the rate to enough to keep the blood pressure at this level. Watch closely for heart failure with crackles in the lungs and high jugular venous pressure; if these occur, or if the patient gets worse, stop the IV fluids.
13. If the patient stops breathing or his heart stops give cardiopulmonary resuscitation (see Chapter 37 pages 607–612).
14. Start an ACE inhibitor, e.g enalapril 2.5 mg bd after 24 hours to help the heart recover as long as the patient has no shock or very low blood pressure. Start even if the blood pressure is not high. Increase the dose, aiming for a blood pressure no higher than 120/80.
15. Keep the patient moving around in the bed; and after the first day, as long as there is no shock or pulse rate problem, get him out of bed to do short walks. This is to try to stop blood clots forming.

Most deaths occur soon after the myocardial infarction, most in the first hour and most of the rest in the first day. If, therefore, the patient survives this time, there is a good chance he will slowly get better and you can slowly get him to do more and more activity. Many other treatments including thrombolysis (to dissolve the blood clot in the artery), dilatation and stenting, pacemakers to keep the heart beat normal, even surgery of the blocked artery and numerous drugs are possible, but are not usually available. Talk to your Medical Officer about what facilities are available at the hospital and what you should do about such cases and their treatment, and if you should transfer such cases as an emergency as soon as you start the above treatment, etc.

Prevention

People should not eat too much animal fat or refined carbohydrates (such as white sugar); not get fat; not smoke; exercise regularly; and get proper treatment for hypertension, diabetes mellitus, etc.

Deep venous thrombosis and pulmonary embolism

See Chapter 23 pages 301–302.

Rheumatic fever

Rheumatic fever is an acute non-infectious inflammatory disease of the joints and heart and other parts of the body.

It is caused by an abnormal reaction of the immune system of the body to a streptococcal infection (usually a throat infection) the patient had about 2 weeks before.

It affects children but also young adults mainly where there is poverty, overcrowding in houses and usually in the dry season.

Symptoms and signs

1. Usually fever is present, with one or more of the other signs and symptoms.
2. Acute arthritis; but at times just joint pain:
   - starts quickly,
   - affects a large joint,
   - affects only one or two joints at a time,
   - can be a typical acute arthritis but at times joint pain only,
   - gets completely better in the affected joint after a few days,
   - then affects another joint or joints,
   - lasts for 1–5 weeks moving from joint to joint.
3. Carditis (inflammation of the heart). This causes:
   - fast pulse (more than expected from the temperature) and at times other signs of heart failure (these can get better),
   - damage to the heart valves (this does not cause immediate trouble, but may not get better, and

especially if further attacks can slowly get worse and cause heart failure a few to many years later).
4. Chorea or abnormal twisting movements of the body which the patient cannot stop. This occurs only occasionally.
5. Skin rash only occasionally.
6. Nodules under the skin only occasionally.

Treatment

1. Rest if there is acute arthritis or heart failure.
2. Acetylsalicylic acid 60–120 mg/kg/day in 4–6 doses regularly (see Chapter 7 pages 32–33) starting with 600–1000 mg 6 hourly.
3. Usual treatment of heart failure if this develops (see pages 464–466). If it does not quickly improve, transfer to Medical Officer in case prednisolone or other treatment needed.
4. Procaine benzylpenicillin 1 g or 1,000,000 units IMI for 10 days to kill any of the bacteria left from the infection which caused the abnormal reaction.
5. Routine antimalarial treatment if in a malarious area (see Chapter 13 pages 79, 80).

The arthritis usually gets better very quickly with treatment; but may need 4–6 weeks treatment if it comes back.

Prevention of further attacks is necessary so that the heart is not damaged again. Give long acting penicillin injections, e.g. benzathine penicillin, 1.2 million units, every month for 10 years or until the age of 20–25 years (whichever is longer).

Get a Medical Officer to see non-urgently after recovery, to find out if heart valve damage has been done.

If a patient has damaged heart valves from any cause and if bacteria get into the blood (during operations or dental extractions, etc.) they can start to grow on the damaged heart valves before the body can destroy them (infective endocarditis). To stop this happening give all patients with damaged heart valves one dose of (1) amoxicillin 3 g orally or benzyl (crystalline) penicillin 1.2 g, i.e. 2,000,000 units IMI and (2) streptomycin 1 g or gentamicin 120 mg IMI and (3) procaine benzylpenicillin 900,000 units IMI all 1 hour before the operation or dental extraction.

28 Disorders of the Bones and Muscles

Anatomy

See Figure 28.1.

Osteomyelitis

Osteomyelitis is an infection of the bone.

Acute osteomyelitis is caused by bacteria, usually staphylococci (which may be resistant to penicillin), and, in some parts of the world, salmonellae (which are usually resistant to penicillin).

Chronic osteomyelitis can develop from acute osteomyelitis that is not treated properly. Chronic osteomyelitis can also be a chronic infection from the start and is then often caused by *Mycobacterium tuberculosis*, usually in the spine. Chronic osteomyelitis in the other bones is usually caused by ordinary bacteria.

Acute osteomyelitis

The organism causing the bone infection may get to the bone through the blood or by direct spread.

The *history* from the patient may include:

1. A recent skin infection which may be still present.
2. A recent injury to the bone.
3. The sudden start of symptoms and signs.

or:

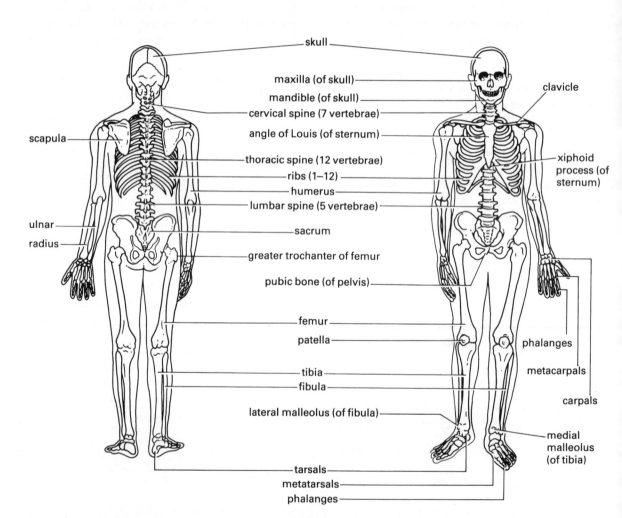

Figure 28.1 *Diagram showing the skeleton (or bones of the body).*

skull

maxilla (of skull)
mandible (of skull)
cervical spine (7 vertebrae)
angle of Louis (of sternum)

thoracic spine (12 vertebrae)
ribs (1–12)
humerus
lumbar spine (5 vertebrae)

sacrum

greater trochanter of femur

pubic bone (of pelvis)

femur
patella

tibia
fibula

lateral malleolus (of fibula)

tarsals
metatarsals
phalanges

scapula

ulnar
radius

clavicle

xiphoid process (of sternum)

phalanges
metacarpals
carpals

medial malleolus (of tibia)

1. A patient with sickle cell disease.
2. The sudden onset of symptoms and signs in a bone (often the fingers or toes, but it can be any bone) which have not improved in 2 days and have not settled within 7–9 days after the usual treatment for an infarction crisis (see Chapter 21 page 322)

or

1. The patient has a puncture wound; or bite; or other penetrating injury; or septic arthritis; or a limb (usually foot) affected by diabetes or leprosy with loss of sensation and the formation of ulcers over bone.
2. The original wound or infection does not heal as expected as the nearby bone has become infected.

Symptoms usually include:

1. Fever, rigors, etc. (especially if spread to the bone from the blood).
2. Severe pain where the bone infection is, which gets worse quickly (except in anaesthetic limbs).
3. The patient cannot use the affected limb.

On examination you will usually find these signs:

1. Fever, fast pulse, etc.
2. Severe tenderness, swelling, heat and other signs of acute inflammation where the bone infection is.
3. Muscle spasm (the patient cannot use the affected limb).

Complications include:

1. Septicaemia.
2. Acute bacterial arthritis of a nearby joint.
3. Damage to the bone, so that it does not grow properly later.
4. Chronic osteomyelitis, usually with a sinus which discharges pus.

Treatment includes:

1. Rest the affected part by splinting it, and putting the patient to bed.
2. Give dicloxacillin (or flucloxacillin or cloxacillin) 1–2 g 6-hourly, preferably by IV infusion but orally if mild infection. You can reduce the dose when the patient appears to be cured; but you must still continue the antibiotic until at least 4–6 weeks. If you at first use penicillin and it does not work quickly, change to, e.g. dicloxacillin, except if the patient has sickle cell anaemia or HIV infection, when change to chloramphenicol (as these infections are often due to salmonellae).
3. Analgesics (see Chapter 7 pages 32–34).

Transfer the patient for antibiotic treatment or operation if:

1. the affected area is not much improved in 2–4 days (urgent), or
2. it does not appear to be completely cured in 2–3 weeks (but continue the antibiotics for 4–6 weeks) or
3. you do not have enough antibiotic (urgent – emergency).

Chronic osteomyelitis

Symptoms may include continuous or repeated discharge of pus from a sinus over the affected bone.

On examination the bone is usually thickened. There are usually scars or sinuses in the skin over the bone. There is usually tenderness over the affected bone.

Repeated acute attacks of acute osteomyelitis occur.

Transfer such cases for treatment. Treatment includes antibiotics and rest in the acute stage; but importantly later, an operation by the Medical Officer.

Osteomyelitis of the spine

Osteomyelitis of the vertebrae causes a continuous neck or back ache which gets slowly worse, and also stiffness and tenderness of that part of the spine.

If the condition is acute and the patient also has a fever, the osteomyelitis may be caused by ordinary bacteria (especially staphylococci). If the condition is chronic, then TB or brucellosis are more likely causes (see Chapter 14 page 105 and Chapter 18 page 174).

Transfer all suspected cases of osteomyelitis of the spine to the Medical Officer for diagnosis and treatment. This is very important, as if treatment is not given quickly, enough of the bone may collapse (squash) and press on the spinal cord and this could cause paralysis. If transfer is not immediately possible, start treatment for an acute case with chloramphenicol or (di)cloxacillin or a chronic case with both chloramphenicol or (di)cloxacillin and anti-TB drugs; but the courses of treatment must be given until completed.

Osteomalacia

Osteomalacia is a condition of adults where there is not enough calcium in the bones and also the blood. This causes:

1. Bone pain and tenderness, especially ribs, pelvis and femurs.

2. 'Pathological' fractures of the bones, where for little or no injury small breaks (which are painful) occur in the bones.
3. Obstructed labour in women due to the deformed bones narrowing the pelvis.
4. Muscle weakness which makes the patient waddle (walk like a duck), have problems climbing stairs or getting up from a chair without also pushing with the hands, etc.
5. Muscle spasms.
6. Malaise.
7. Often associated anaemia.

Causes include:

1. Lack of sunlight, which the body uses to make vitamin D and which helps calcium absorption from the bowel. This occurs in Muslim women who cover all their skin when outside, children and old people who stay in the house all the time, places where it is always cloudy or people who live in deep dark valleys and there is little sun.
2. Lack of vitamin D in the food eaten.
3. Gastrointestinal conditions where vitamin D is not absorbed (malabsorption syndrome).
4. Some conditions of the kidney, liver, etc. and if some particular drugs are taken.

If the above causes affect children, they get rickets. If they affect adults, they get osteomalacia.

If this condition occurs in your area you should be told about this and what is the best treatment for the people there.

Treatment usually consists of:

1. Vitamin D in the form of ergocalciferol 1.25 mg (50,000 IU) tablet or capsule 1 daily for 2–4 weeks or 6 weekly for 2–4 weeks; then weekly for 3 months; then 1 monthly for a year and probably continue this monthly for life.
2. Calcium at least 500 mg daily or 500 ml milk daily for the first 2-4 weeks.
3. Attempt to stop the cause if possible.

Neoplasms (cancer) in bone

Neoplasms in bone may be either primary (benign or malignant) or secondary (malignant).

Symptoms and signs can include:

1. Pain and/or tenderness in a bone which does not improve, and keeps the patient awake at night.
2. A deformity of a bone – most often a lump.
3. A pathological fracture (a fracture after only a small injury or no injury, because the bone was weak because it had been partly replaced by cancer cells).

4. Compression of the spinal cord, if vertebrae were affected by the cancer and then collapse.
5. Anaemia.

Transfer to or consult the Medical Officer in case it is due to an infection which could be treated.

Radiotherapy is usually helpful; but it is usually not available. Chemotherapy may be possible.

Pyomyositis or tropical myositis

Pyomyositis is an acute bacterial infection of one or more of the large skeletal muscles. This is most often the thigh or trunk muscles, but occasionally the psoas muscle which is inside the abdomen in front of the spine and which moves the hip. The organism is usually *Staphylococcus aureus*. The muscle may be hard and woody for some days or weeks. Then an abscess usually forms in the muscle and general symptoms and signs of infection develop.

Pyomyositis is common only in developing and tropical countries, most often in young men.

Symptoms and *signs* include:

1. General symptoms and signs of infection – malaise, fever, fast pulse, etc. If a large abscess or septicaemia develop, these become severe.
2. Pain in the affected muscle, which is present at rest and much worse when the patient moves the muscle. The affected muscle is firm and tender and painful if stretched during examination.
3. The general and local symptoms and signs of infection get much worse in the next few days. The muscle may become fluctuant; but only if it is just under the skin.
4. If it is not treated, the affected muscle becomes a bag of pus, and the patient becomes wasted, with anaemia, etc. Septicaemia and death can occur.

Differential diagnosis of painful muscles:

1. generalised illness, e.g. malaria, influenza.
2. unusual exercise.
3. trauma to muscles with haematoma.
4. parasitic diseases of the muscle (e.g. trichinosis, cysticercosis).
5. pain in nearby structures:
   • joints,
   • bones (osteomyelitis or fracture),
   • tendons.
6. referred pain.
7. others – see a medical reference book.

If the diagnosis is not certain, put a needle into the affected muscle. You can usually aspirate pus if the condition is pyomyositis.

Treatment is simple, if you make the diagnosis.
1. Antibiotics.

    If possible use no IM injections. Give IV or oral (di)cloxacillin or, if unavailable, erythromycin or tetracycline. Penicillin may be effective, but needs repeated injections. Chloramphenicol may be needed. Do not continue with tetracycline or penicillin if the patient is not quickly getting better. (See Chapter 11 pages 56–61.)

2. Incision and drainage, if pus has formed.

    This is best done under general anaesthetic by the Medical Officer. Bleeding is sometimes severe and may need packing of the abscess cavity and local pressure to stop it. Incision and drainage is essential once pus has formed, for the patient to get better.

    If the abscess is large or the patient very sick or if the patient does not quickly improve, it would be best to *transfer* such cases as soon as possible to your Medical Officer.

29 Disorders of Joints (Arthritis)

Anatomy

There are three types of joints in the body (see Figure 29.1).

Pathology, symptoms and signs

Arthritis is inflammation of a joint. Arthritis may be acute or chronic.

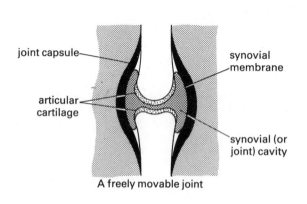

A freely movable joint

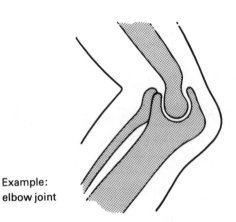

Example: elbow joint

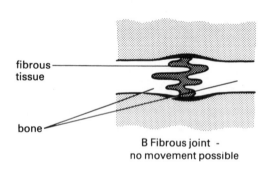

B Fibrous joint - no movement possible

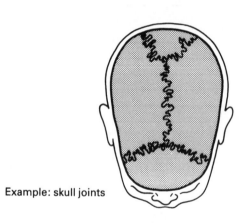

Example: skull joints

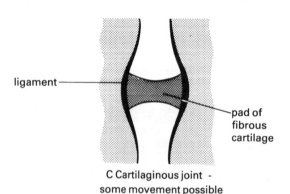

C Cartilaginous joint - some movement possible

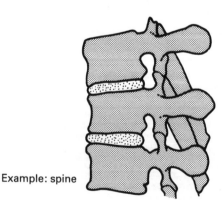

Example: spine

Figure 29.1 *Diagram to show three types of joint. Note that in the freely movable type joint the articular cartilage is often not present. (For details of the anatomy of the spine see Chapter 25 pages 429–432.)*

Symptoms and signs in the affected joint itself

The joint can have any of the usual symptoms and signs of inflammation.

1. Pain – acute and chronic cases.
2. Tenderness – acute cases only.
3. Swelling – acute and chronic cases.
4. Heat – acute cases only.
5. Redness and shininess – acute cases only.
6. Loss of function – i.e. the joint cannot be moved properly (both active movement, i.e. when the patient moves it and passive movement, i.e. when the patient relaxes or rests and the examiner moves it), and the joint cannot work properly or bear weight – acute and chronic cases.
7. Abnormal fluid in the joint itself (called 'effusion') – acute and chronic cases.

The patient complains of:

• pain,
• swelling, and
• loss of function (cannot move or use the joint).

On examination (depending on the type of arthritis);

1. *Inspection*
   • swelling
   • redness
   • deformity.
2. *Palpation*
   • swelling caused by
     – fluid in the joint
     – bone overgrowth at edges of joint
     – soft tissue swelling around the joint
   • tenderness
   • heat
   • movement
     – passive, less than normal, painful, sometimes with crepitus (a grating feeling or noise)
     – active, less than normal, painful, sometimes with crepitus.
3. *Work or weight bearing*
   • less than normal or not possible at all.

Symptoms and signs in the muscles which move the affected joint

In acute arthritis the muscles go into spasm so that the joint cannot be moved normally (movement causes pain). Later, and in chronic arthritis, the muscles waste and become thin and weak.

Even later, if the patient does not have physiotherapy, the muscles and tendons become shortened and changed into bands of fibrous tissue or scar tissue and cannot be stretched. These hold the joint in abnormal positions. These muscle and tendon changes are called contractures.

General symptoms and signs

These can include fever, fast pulse, malaise, wasting, etc.

1. Some may be the result of the cause of the arthritis, e.g. rheumatic fever.
2. Some may be caused by the effect of the arthritis, e.g. toxins from the bacteria causing acute bacterial arthritis.

Disease in other parts of the body may be present and cause symptoms and signs

An example is tuberculosis of the lungs in a patient with tuberculous arthritis.

Note on examination of the spine

Check for:

• deformity (lump or twisting) of the spine,
• tender areas on palpation or percussion of the spine,
• movement of the spine in all directions,
• legs – movement and sensation,
• abdomen – bladder enlargement or incontinence of urine.

See also Chapter 14 pages 105–106.

Tests

The only important test you must do at a health centre is *the aspiration of a joint if the joint may be infected with bacteria (septic arthritis).* (Put a needle into the joint and suck out any fluid with a syringe.) If pus is present, you must give antibiotics in high doses.

Always use careful aseptic procedure when you aspirate a joint. Do not introduce bacteria into the joint and cause acute bacterial (septic) arthritis. Scrub up. Use mask gown and gloves. Prepare the skin carefully with iodine in spirit or another suitable antiseptic. Use sterile needles and syringes. Always give a local anaesthetic before putting the large needle into the joint. Suck out all of the fluid that is in the joint. Put a sterile dressing over the needle hole.

Method of aspirating joints

These diagrams show where you can put a needle into the various joints (see Figures 29.2, 29.3, 29.4, 29.5, 29.6 and 29.7). But do *not* try to aspirate a hip joint unless you have had special training. Transfer a patient who needs aspiration of the hip joint to the Medical Officer.

Details of joint conditions

Traumatic arthritis

Traumatic arthritis is an acute arthritis caused by an injury to the joint. There is usually a *history* of an injury.

On examination you will find:

1. acute arthritis with tenderness over the damaged area of the joint or of the ligaments around the joint; and usually an effusion;
2. no general symptoms and signs of infection.

Aspiration shows clear yellow fluid or blood.
   Treatment includes:

1. aspiration to remove all the blood or fluid from the joint;

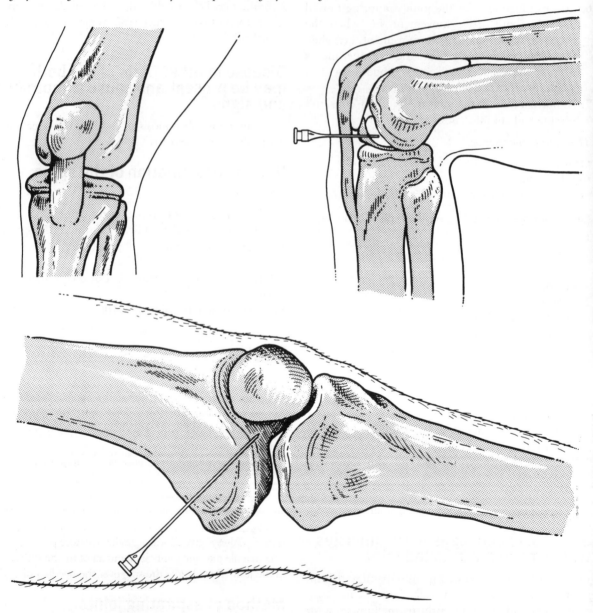

Figure 29.2 *Methods of aspirating the knee joint. The top diagrams show an anterior method you can use when the knee is flexed (bent). The lower diagram shows a lateral method you can use when the knee is extended (straight). Usually you will use the lower method as a patient with acute arthritis usually cannot flex (bend) the knee.*

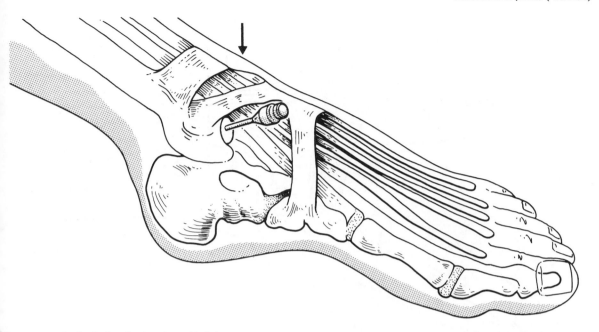

Figure 29.3 *Method of aspirating the ankle joint.*

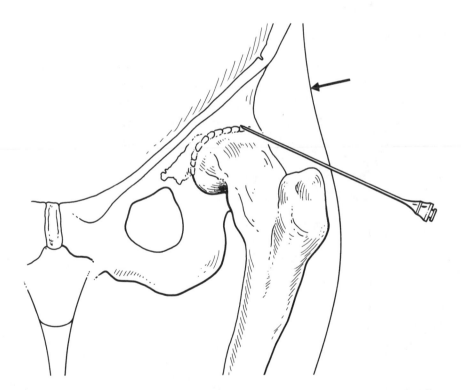

Figure 29.4 *Method of aspirating the hip joint. Do not try to aspirate the hip joint unless you have had proper training.*

2. splint so that the joint cannot move until the acute stage is finished;
3. exercise muscles in the splint – 30 contractions of the muscles which move the joint in the splint, four times a day but without letting the joint bend (doing this every hour is even better);
4. paracetamol if necessary.

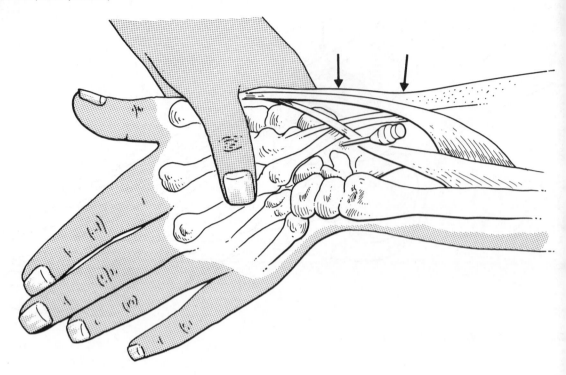

Figure 29.5 *Method of aspirating the wrist (radio-carpal) joint.*

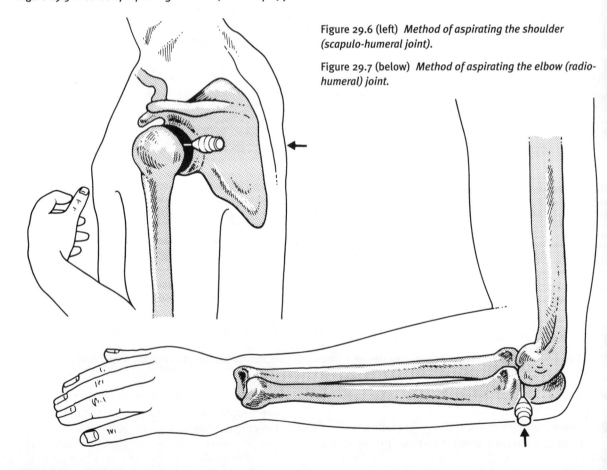

Figure 29.6 (left) *Method of aspirating the shoulder (scapulo-humeral joint).*

Figure 29.7 (below) *Method of aspirating the elbow (radio-humeral) joint.*

Table 29.1   The common causes of acute and chronic arthritis.

Acute		Chronic
1. Traumatic	The most common	1. Osteo-
2. Acute bacterial (septic)	The most important as (1) treatment cures (2) joint destroyed if not treated	2. Chronic bacterial (septic) 3. TB 4. Brucellosis
5. Rheumatoid 6. Spondyloarthritis 7. Tropical arthritis	Usually chronic Acute, recurrent, but mostly chronic Acute, recurrent or chronic	5. Rheumatoid 6. Spondyloarthritis 7. Tropical arthritis
8. Rheumatic fever		
9. Others See page 492 and Rheumatology reference book	See page 492 and Rheumatology reference book	9. Others See page 492 and Rheumatology reference book

Transfer to Medical Officer if:

1. there are signs which may be caused by a fracture; *or*
2. the joint is unstable (ligaments are torn and it bends more than normal in any direction).

Acute bacterial (septic) arthritis

Acute bacterial arthritis is not common; but it is very important. Treatment will cure it. If it is not treated, it will destroy the joint.

Symptoms, signs and tests

Symptoms and signs of infection in another part of the body (especially skin infection but also urethral or lung or other infection, etc.) have often been present *before* the arthritis. The infection was carried to the joint by the blood. Sometimes there has been a wound that entered the joint. Sometimes there was a soft tissue or bone infection that got bigger and went into the joint. Sometimes there was an aspiration of the joint with an unsterile needle.

Symptoms and signs of HIV infection must always be looked for, as HIV infection makes it more likely the patient can get this infection.

Symptoms in the joint are usually extreme pain and swelling of the affected joint, which the patient cannot move.

Signs in the joint (see Figure 29.8) are usually:

• swelling, caused by an 'effusion' made of pus,
• tenderness,
• heat,
• redness or shininess, and
• severe pain on moving the joint with guarding of

the muscles which move that joint. This is usually so severe that the patient will not allow any movement of the joint.

General symptoms and signs of infection caused by the toxins from the arthritis are usually severe – fever, rigors, fast pulse, etc.

Look for evidence of HIV infection. Send a blood test for HIV after counselling if HIV infection possible.

Aspiration of the joint shows pus.

Treatment

1. Aspirate all the pus from the joint. Use strict aseptic precautions. Send pus for Gram stain, culture and sensitivity if possible. Repeat the aspiration when more pus forms (daily or more often if necessary).
2. Give antibiotics as for any acute severe bacterial infection (see Chapter 12). Give chloramphenicol 1 g orally immediately and repeat every 6 hours. Give 1 g by IMI or IVI if necessary. Continue the antibiotic for at least 2 weeks. Reduce dose when the patient improves. Dicloxacillin (or cloxacillin or flucloxacillin) would be a suitable drug if the infection came from the skin.
3. Splint the joint (usually with a well padded plaster-of-Paris (POP) back-slab). Elevate (raise up) the affected limb.
4. Give acetylsalicylic acid or paracetamol 1 g every 6 hours if needed for pain.
5. Give antimalarial drugs if indicated (see Chapter 13 pages 79, 80).
6. When the acute inflammation starts to improve, begin physiotherapy. Supervise the patient doing active exercises four times a day in the splint (the

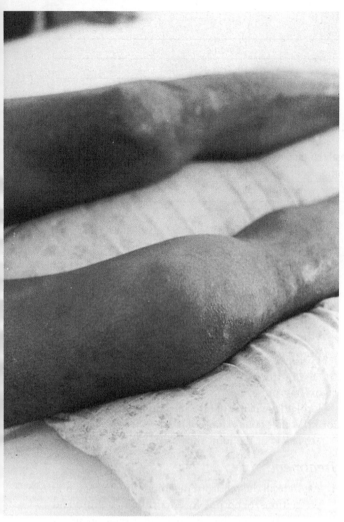

Figure 29.8 *Acute bacterial ('septic') arthritis of the right knee. Note the large amount of swelling. Note that because of severe pain the patient is lying with the knee slightly bent over a pillow and would not allow the examiner to bend it during examination. This joint needs immediate aspiration. The patient needs immediate large doses of antibiotics.*

patient should contract all the muscles which normally move the joint 20–30 times; but without bending the joint). The health worker should move the joint through all its movements out of the splint, once daily. Remove the splint and start active exercises of the joint when all the signs of acute inflammation have gone.

Transfer to Medical Officer care:

1. all severe cases (urgent – but not emergency);
2. all cases of acute arthritis of the hip joint (urgent – but not emergency);
3. any case not much improved in 2 days (urgent – but not emergency);
4. any case where you have not aspirated all the pus for 2 days running (urgent – but not emergency) and
5. any case not cured in 2 weeks (non-urgent).

Rheumatic fever

Rheumatic fever is an acute non-infectious inflammatory disease of the joints and heart, and other parts of the body.

The arthritis usually:

• starts quickly,
• affects a large joint,
• affects only one or two joints at a time,
• is usually a typical acute arthritis but can also be just pain in the joints,
• gets completely better in the affected joint after a few days,
• then affects another joint or joints,
• lasts for 1–5 weeks moving from joint to joint.

See Chapter 27 page 475 for other details.

Rheumatoid disease

Rheumatoid disease is a chronic disease that affects the whole body but especially the joints. The cause is not known. Often patients are middle-aged adults; but it can affect people of any age.

First, general symptoms and signs of ill health are present for some weeks – malaise, fever, aches and paints, etc. Then there can be anaemia, weight loss, etc. The arthritis can start at any time during or after (or even before) these symptoms and signs.

The arthritis usually:

1. is chronic, but it can start with an acute attack and become acute from time to time;
2. is roughly symmetrical (i.e. same joints on both sides of body);
3. starts in the small joints of hands and feet (especially the first joints of the fingers) (see Figure 29.9); and the hands are almost always involved.
4. then spreads to larger joints (wrists, ankles, knees, etc. and sometimes the spine);
5. has symptoms of pain and stiffness, worse in the morning or after rest and a little improved by use or exercise;
6. has, at first, signs of:
   • swelling of soft tissues around the joint,
   • effusion, and
   • inflammation;

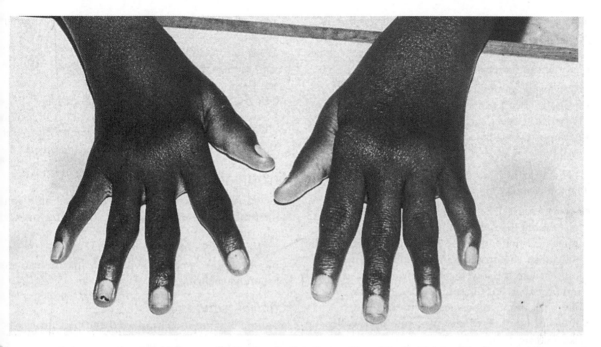

Figure 29.9 *Late severe rheumatoid disease affecting hands. Note the swelling of the first joints of the fingers, which suggests rheumatoid disease.*

7. has, later, severe joint destruction with deformity, stiffness and loss of use of the joint, especially if not treated properly.

Aspiration is usually not necessary for diagnosis (as many joints are involved and the arthritis is not very acute); but aspirated fluid is yellow and cloudy if you do this.

Sometimes acute bacterial arthritis can develop in a joint affected by rheumatoid arthritis.

Rheumatoid disease causes inflammation of much of the rest of the body. Nodules are typical. They occur under the skin at places where there is often pressure, e.g. the back of the forearms, sacrum and feet. They can be small to several cm in size. They sometimes ulcerate. Other inflammation causes fever, weight loss, enlarged spleen, bleeding, anaemia, block of small arteries, peripheral neuropathy, pleural effusions, dry inflamed conjunctivae and sclera and many other symptoms and signs.

A blood test called rheumatoid factor is usually positive but some normal people can have a positive test too.

Treatment in the health centre includes:

1. Drugs
   (a) Non-steroidal anti-inflammatory drugs (NSAIDs)
   Acetylsalicylic acid 500–1000 mg each 6 hours, or

Ibuprofen 200–400 mg each 6–8 hours but only if more effective for this patient, and also
   (b) Paracetamol 500–1000 mg four times a day if needed for pain (not anti-inflammatory).
2. Physiotherapy to keep the joints and muscles working.
3. Splints worn at night to hold the joints in their proper positions to stop deformities developing.

Ask your Medical Officer to see the patient non-urgently, as although he will not have supplies of 'anti-tumour necrosis factor' drugs which are the latest addition to treatment to decrease the inflammation, he may have
(a) methotrexate and
(b) sulfasalazine and
(c) chloroquine
which, especially if used together, can often control the inflammation.

It is usually best not to give the patient long term corticosteroid treatment.

Spondyloarthritis

This is the overall name given to a group of non-infectious but inflammatory arthritic conditions which share some common clinical features and occur in people most of whom have a particular (HLA-B27) genetic make-up.

The special names for some of these (which are not important to remember) are:

• Ankylosing spondylitis
• Psoriatic arthritis
• Reactive arthritis, including Reiter's syndrome
• Arthropathy associated with non-infective inflammatory bowel disease.

The arthritis is different from rheumatoid disease. The joints are:

• not symmetrical, i.e. not the same ones on both sides
• lower more than upper limb but
• joints near the end of the limb rather than near the body (like rheumatoid) but include the sacro–iliac joint (where the lower spine joins on to the pelvis) and other parts of the spine
• often have the tendons near them inflamed
• often include the whole finger or toe (swollen up like a sausage).

The inflammation involves the tissues near the joints more than the joints themselves and when this occurs the joints eventually become fixed – including the spine which does not bend.

The tissues other than the joints involved include:

• mucous membranes causing conjunctivitis, mouth ulcers, urethritis, prostatitis, bowel ulcers, etc.
• skin and nails
• eyes with iritis.

There are none of the typical nodules of rheumatoid disease or the other features of rheumatoid disease mentioned.

The rheumatoid test is negative.

The one often best known is reactive arthritis or Reiter's syndrome.

• It occurs 1–3 weeks after:
gastrointestinal infections with *Salmonella, Shigella, Campylobacter,* etc., or
sexually transmitted disease, especially *Chlamydia,* or streptococcal infections.
• It is most common in young men.
• It causes:
arthritis as above and at times
conjunctivitis and at times
urethritis.
• The first attack usually goes after 2–4 months, but in many the arthritis returns and can become chronic.

The other features of spondyloarthritis can then develop.

• Treatment includes:
aspiration of the joint,
acetylsalicylic acid or other NSAID,
tetracycline or doxycycline if also urethritis.
• If problems develop, especially acute iritis, the patient needs treatment for the iritis and referral to the Medical Officer about possible other treatment.

'Tropical arthritis'

Tropical arthritis is an unusual type of chronic (but sometimes acute) arthritis that occurs in some tropical countries.

The cause is sometimes infection with filaria. Most times the cause is not known. Many may be variants of spondyloarthritis.

Clinical features

Young adults are usually affected; but patients can be any age.

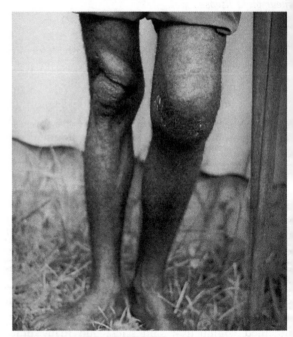

Figure 29.10 *Tropical arthritis affecting the left knee. The patient was treated first with chloramphemicol in the correct large dose for 2 weeks (but joint fluid aspirated and examined in the laboratory did not confirm the diagnosis of bacterial infection). He was then treated with diethylcarbamazine for 3 weeks. He had large doses of acetylsalicylic acid during this time, and a splint and physiotherapy. At 6 weeks he still has arthritis with a lot of swelling but not much pain. This is common in 'tropical arthritis'.*

It affects one or two (only sometimes more) joints, usually the knees or ankles.

Symptoms include swelling or pain of the joint.

Signs include marked swelling (caused by effusion) and painful movement of the joint (see Figure 29.10). Tenderness and heat may occur in acute cases. Limited movement and deformity may occur in late severe cases. Usually no general signs are present.

Aspiration gives fluid which is green or yellow and clear or cloudy; but the fluid is usually different from pus.

Do ICT test or *send* a serology test for filariasis or *thick smears for microfilaria* to laboratory (see Chapter 22 page 336).

Sometimes the arthritis goes away without treatment. Sometimes it returns later. Sometimes chronic pain and swelling continue for months or years. In severe or prolonged cases, the joint is destroyed.

Management of a case of tropical arthritis
Always check that it is not:

1. acute infective arthritis, by aspirating the joint;
2. traumatic arthritis and rheumatic fever and rheumatoid arthritis, by history and examination;
3. tuberculous arthritis, if possible, by history and examination (if this is not possible, transfer the patient for investigation).

Admit all suspected cases. Do tests for filariasis.

Treatment
1. Aspirate all the fluid from the joint. Use strict aseptic precautions. Send the fluid for Gram stain, culture and sensitivity (if possible). If you think the fluid may be pus, treat as for acute bacterial (septic) arthritis (see page 485).
2. Splint the joint (usually in a well padded POP back-slab) until the acute stage finishes. When you are certain that no further improvement will occur (e.g. after 6 weeks), remove the splint.
3. Physiotherapy.
   Make the patient do active exercises four times a day in the splint. Show the patient how to contract all the muscles which normally move the joint but without moving the joint itself. Tell the patient to do this 20–40 times four times every day.
   Move the joint through all its movements out of the splint once daily; but only after the acute inflammation has started to improve (if it was present).
   Make the patient do active exercises with movement of the joint after all the signs of acute inflammation have gone.
4. Acetylsalicylic acid 1 g four times a day.

5. Antimalarial drug if indicated. (See Chapter 13 pages 79, 80.)
6. Albendazole and either diethylcarbamazine or ivermectin if the patient is in (or has been in) an area where filariasis occurs. See Chapter 22 page 337 for details.

Transfer to Medical Officer care if:

1. the arthritis may be acute bacterial (septic) arthritis which is not improving with antibiotics (urgent); or
2. the arthritis may be tuberculous arthritis (non-urgent).
3. the arthritis does not settle on the above treatment (non-urgent).

Tuberculous arthritis
Tuberculous arthritis is a chronic inflammatory arthritis caused by infection of the joint with tuberculosis bacteria.

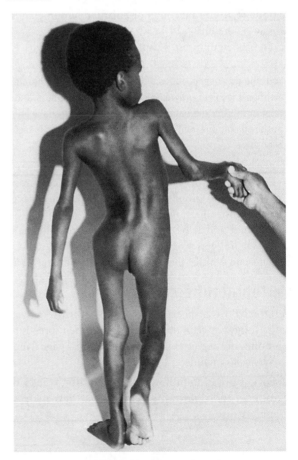

Figure 29.11 *Tuberculous arthritis of the left hip. Note that any patient with chronic arthritis of one joint must be transferred for test. Note the typical severe wasting of the muscles of the left thigh.*

Tuberculous arthritis is not common; but it is important. Treatment will cure it. If it is not treated, it will destroy the joint.

Most often if affects the hip or knee (see Figure 29.11); but it can affect any joint.

Most often the patient is a child or young adult; but it can affect people of any age.

Symptoms include pain and stiffness of the joint, or a limp.

Signs include:

1. *Chronic arthritis which slowly gets worse* (swelling, tenderness, warmth, pain on moving joint; limited movement of joint, the patient cannot use joint properly, etc.).
2. *Severe wasting of the muscles* which move the joint.
3. Nearby lymph glands usually enlarged.
4. A sinus discharging pus near the joint late in the disease.
5. Symptoms and signs of TB in other parts of the body (e.g. chronic cough or enlarged lymph glands) may be present.
6. The tuberculin test is usually positive.

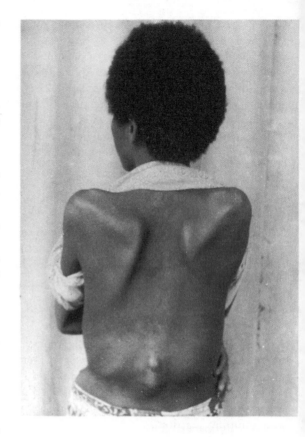

> You should suspect tuberculous arthritis in any chronic arthritis that gets progressively worse over months and refer or transfer the patient for tests. This is especially important if only one joint is affected and if the tuberculin test is positive.

Do not diagnose a case of arthritis as osteoarthrosis if there are signs of *inflammation* which *get slowly worse*. Osteoarthrosis does not usually have inflammation of the joint and it has times when it gets better and times when it gets worse. Think instead of tuberculous arthritis and transfer the patient for tests and treatment.

Vertebral tuberculosis

Vertebral TB is a special type of TB arthritis. It starts in the joints between the vertebrae and then spreads to the bones of the vertebrae. See Chapter 14 page 105.

Symptoms include:

1. Back pain and stiffness which lasts for weeks or months and does not get better but gets increasingly worse.

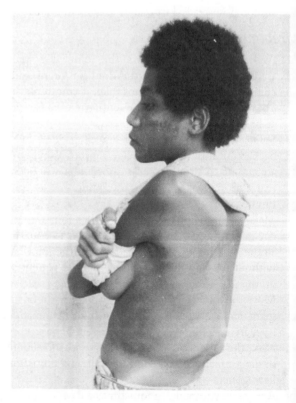

Figure 29.12 *Tuberculosis of the spine. Note the deformity of the spine (often called a 'gibbus'). TB of the spine is often called Pott's disease. This patient needs urgent transfer before she becomes paraplegic.*

2. Later, a lump or deformity in the spine (if some infected bones collapse).
3. Sometimes, weakness or paralysis and loss of sensation in the legs and the patient cannot pass urine properly (if there is spinal cord pressure).

Signs include:

1. Tenderness and stiffness of part of the spine.
2. Later, a lump or deformity of the spine.
3. Sometimes, weakness or paralysis and loss of sensation in the legs and an enlarged bladder or urinary incontinence (if there is spinal cord pressure).
4. There may be symptoms or signs of TB in other parts of the body, e.g. chronic cough or enlarged lymph glands.
5. The tuberculin test is usually positive.

Transfer the patient for diagnosis by X-ray, if you suspect vertebral TB or bacterial infection (see below). Transfer urgently for treatment, if cord pressure occurs. Start anti-TB drugs if there is delay in transfer; or immediately if any suspicion of cord pressure develops.

Suspect vertebral tuberculosis at the stage of chronic, constant, increasing backache with stiffness and tenderness of the spine, before a lump forms or the spinal cord is damaged. (See Figure 29.12.)

Anti-TB treatment is often very effective in stopping pain and even allowing paralyses to recover even without surgery as long as the treatment is given quickly.

Drugs cannot take away the deformity.

Bacterial infection of the spine

Bacteria and especially *Staphylococci* can cause an infection in the spine which looks like vertebral TB except:

1. Quickly becomes severe if *Staphylococci*; but less quickly if brucellosis.
2. There may be more general symptoms and signs of infection.
3. There is not necessarily any evidence of TB (but of course there may be HIV infection).

Transfer all such cases urgently to the Medical Officer for diagnosis and treatment. If there is any delay, start the patient on chloramphenicol (Chapter 12). See Chapter 28 page 477 for more details.

Osteoarthrosis (osteoarthritis)

Osteoarthrosis is a degeneration or 'wearing out' of joints.

It occurs in older adults in the joints they use most – hips, knees, spine, etc. *or* in younger persons in a joint which has previously been seriously injured.

Osteoarthrosis is not an *arthritis*. There is no inflammation of the joint (unless it has been injured again or used a lot, just before examination). There are no general symptoms or signs of inflammation or infection.

Clinical features

Symptoms are usually of pain in a joint during and after use. The pain is improved by rest.

Signs include:

1. Swelling caused by overgrowth of the ends of the bone at the 'worn out' joint.
2. Crepitus (a 'crackling' you can feel or hear) when the joint is moved.
3. Full movement of the joint is not possible.
4. Some wasting of muscles which move the joint is present.
5. *If recent injury or hard work* by the joint, there may be some tenderness and sometimes an effusion.

If you aspirate any effusion present the fluid will be clear yellow. It is not pus.

Usually there is a slow start of the symptoms and signs. Very slowly the condition gets worse. Usually there are times when there is little or no pain and times when the symptoms are much worse.

Always check that the condition is not tuberculous arthritis. If there is inflammation of the joint, and if the arthritis gets worse and worse over weeks or months, and if there is severe muscle wasting, and especially if only one joint is affected, then suspect tuberculous arthritis.

Other diseases you should check for include chronic infective (bacterial) arthritis, spondyloarthritis, 'tropical' arthritis and rheumatoid arthritis.

Outpatient or inpatient treatment is possible.

Treatment

1. Rest. The patient should use the affected joint as little as possible. Tell the patient how to lose weight if his weight is above ideal.
2. The patient should do exercise to strengthen the muscles which move the joint without putting weight on the joint during the exercises. *Show* the patient how to contract the muscles which move the joint without letting the joint move, or how to move the joint without putting weight on it. *Tell* the patient to do 20–40 of these exercises three to four times every day.
3. Give acetylsalicylic acid 500–1000 mg four times a day when pain is present.

Transfer to Medical Officer care is not necessary unless tuberculous arthritis is a possibility (see page 489).

Osteoarthrosis of spine

Osteoarthrosis of the spine is the same as osteoarthrosis of other joints, except that it affects the spinal joints. The nerves that go from the spinal cord to the body may *sometimes* be pressed on. This can *sometimes* give pain radiating to the arms, trunk or legs and/or weakness of the muscles of the arms or legs.

Symptoms include:

1. Pain and stiffness in the neck or back, often worse after exercise and improved by rest.
2. Pain radiating to the trunk or the limbs (sometimes), often worse in a particular body position.
3. Weakness of some muscles (sometimes).

Signs include:

1. Stiffness of the neck or back (which will not bend properly in all directions); pain on some movements of the spine; and sometimes tenderness on percussion of the spine.
2. Loss of sensation of part of a limb (sometimes).
3. Muscle weakness of part of a limb (sometimes).

The symptoms and signs may be severe, then greatly improve only to return again (i.e. there are good and bad times).

Treatment is as for osteoarthrosis of other joints, and especially 'extension exercises' to strengthen muscles along spine. The patient should lie prone (face down) and relaxed on the floor. He should then contract (tighten) the muscles along the back of the spine to lift the head and legs backwards off the floor – and bend his trunk (rest of body) backwards. After a few seconds he then relaxes. The number of times this is done should be slowly increased as he is able until 20–40 are done twice daily.

Check that the patient has no weakness of the legs, loss of control of the bladder, signs of inflammation of the spine, increasing worsening of the disease, or symptoms and signs of TB in other parts of the body. If the patient has any of these things, *transfer* the patient for the Medical Officer to check that it is not TB or bacterial infection of the spine.

Deformity of spine

Causes include:

1. fracture,
2. TB or bacterial infection,
3. cancer of spine,
4. idiopathic developmental scoliosis. (This starts in childhood or adolescence and continues until growth stops. There is a gradually increasing sideways curve to the thoracic and lumbar spine, which can look very bad and stop the lungs working properly. It is important to refer such children to the Medical Officer before the deformity becomes bad.)
5. others – see a specialist orthopaedic reference book.

Acute arthritis of many joints from other causes

The causes of rheumatoid disease with arthritis (see page 486) and 'Reactive arthritis' (see pages 487–488) are not known in most cases. But both of these diseases have characteristic clinical features. Even if you are not certain that the patient has one of these when you first see him, the characteristic clinical course usually makes you certain after some weeks.

Sometimes also you will suspect rheumatoid disease or reactive arthritis; but the arthritis gets better quickly or has a course not typical of these diseases.

There are a large number of other conditions which can cause arthritis similar to rheumatoid disease or one of the types of spondyloarthritis; and these are often hard to diagnose in a health centre.

Whenever you see a case of arthritis first *check that it is not acute bacterial arthritis* or *tuberculous arthritis;* although these usually affect only one joint. Other conditions which the patient may have are:

1. *Virus infections such as hepatitis and rubella* can cause an arthritis that affects several joints. The arthritis is usually not severe. Other signs of the virus infection are present.
2. *Virus infection carried by mosquitoes and other insects* (arboviruses) can cause both single cases and epidemics of arthritis of several joints. Fever and rashes of various types are often present at first; but the disease gets better after some weeks or months. See Chapter 17 page 166.
3. *Allergic reactions of various types* (see Chapter 10 page 44), especially the 'serum sickness' type and those caused by drugs (including intravenous iron infusions) can cause acute and chronic arthritis of many joints which finally gets better. Reactions in leprosy (Chapter 15 page 138) can also cause arthritis.
4. There are also a large number of *other causes.*

If the patient has arthritis which you cannot diagnose and which continues to get worse, refer or transfer to a Medical Officer for diagnosis.

Diagnosis and management of joint problems

Acute arthritis of one or a few joints

Admit all cases for inpatient treatment.

Find cause by history and examination (see Chapter 6 and pages 480–485 of this chapter and Table 29.1 page 485):

- acute bacterial infection
- trauma
- rheumatic fever
- rheumatoid disease (usually chronic and many joints affected)
- spondyloarthritis
- tropical
- virus
- allergic.

Do a diagnostic joint aspiration on all cases of acute arthritis unless you are certain that the diagnosis is *not* bacterial infection.

Treatment

1. Aspirate any joint which has fluid in it. Use proper aseptic precautions (see page 485). Aspirate (suck out) any fluid in the joint until no more fluid remains. If you find pus, repeat the aspiration whenever more pus is formed (daily or more often if necessary).
2. If aspiration shows pus, or if aspiration does not get any fluid out, give chloramphenicol 1 g orally immediately and repeat every 6 hours. Continue chloramphenicol for at least 2 weeks. (See Chapter 12 page 64.)
3. Splint the joint (usually with a well padded POP back-slab). Elevate (raise up) the affected limb.
4. Acetylsalicylic acid 500–1000 mg every 6 hours or ibuprofen 200–400 mg every 6–8 hours.
5. Antimalarial drugs if indicated (see Chapter 13 pages 79, 80).
6. Give treatment for filariasis if the patient is in (or has been in) an area where filarasis occurs. Give doxycycline or tetracycline if the patient has had or then has urethritis and the aspirated fluid is yellow or green but does not look like pus. See Chapter 26 page 448 first and Chapter 19 page 203.
7. When the acute inflammation improves, start physiotherapy. Make the patient do active exercises four times a day in the splint. Show the patient how to contract all the muscles which normally move the joint without moving the joint itself. Tell the patient to do this 20–40 times four times each day. Move the joint through all its movements out of the splint once daily. Remove the splint and start active exercises (with the patient moving the joint) when all the signs of acute inflammation have gone.

Transfer to Medical Officer if:

1. It is a severe case (urgent – but not emergency).
2. The hip joint is affected (urgent – but not emergency).
3. The patient is not greatly improved in 2 days (urgent – but not emergency).
4. Pus is present but you cannot aspirate it for 2 days (urgent – but not emergency).
5. The patient is not cured in 2 weeks (non-urgent).

Chronic arthritis of one or a few joints

Do a history and examination. See Chapter 6 and pages 480–485 of this chapter to find the cause.

Outpatient or inpatient treatment is possible.

Treatment

If:

- there are signs of inflammation of the joint (warm, shiny, tender, not able to be used properly etc.) *or*
- there is a sinus near the joint *or*
- the joint does not improve much with treatment, or later the joint gets slowly worse *or*
- muscle wasting is or becomes severe –

then the arthritis may be caused by TB or chronic bacterial infection.

Transfer these patients to Medical Officer care.

If

- none of the above are present

then:

1. Rest. (The patient should do things which put weight on the joint, or make it work, as little as possible.) The patient should use the affected joint as little as possible. Tell the patient how to lose weight if his weight is above ideal.
2. The patient should do exercises to strengthen the muscles which move the joint without putting weight on the joint. *Show* the patient how to contract the muscles which move the joint without moving the joint, or how to move the joint without putting weight on it. *Tell* the patient to do 20–40 of these exercises four times a day.

3. Acetylsalicylic acid 500–1000 mg four times a day when pain is present.

If the joint improves with this treatment and there are no important signs of inflammation of the joint (not warm, red or shiny, tender, etc.), then the condition is probably osteoarthrosis. Repeat the treatment whenever it is necessary.

Arthritis of many joints

Do a history and examination (see Chapter 6 page 21 and pages 480–485 of this chapter) to find the cause:

- rheumatoid disease,
- spondyloarthritis,
- viral infection,
- serum or drug or allergic reaction,
- rheumatic fever, usually only 1–2 joints,
- leprosy reaction.

Give treatment for any cause.

Give acetylsalicylic acid 500–1000 mg four times a day or ibuprofen 200–400 mg each 6–8 hours.

Add paracetamol 500–1000 mg four times a day if needed.

Increase physiotherapy.

Make splints if needed.

Look carefully for signs and symptoms of acute bacterial arthritis – aspirate any joint which may have bacterial infection (see page 485).

If the patient is not cured in 1 month transfer to Medical Officer non-urgently for diagnosis and treatment.

Backache

Look for a disease in the organs listed below.

Do a full history and examination (see Chapter 6). Test the urine for pus, protein and blood.

> Examine the spine for tenderness and movement. Do a pelvic examination PV if necessary.

1. Spine
  (a) *Direct traumatic injury.*
  (b) *Acute back strain* (muscle or joint damage from lifting something heavy):
    - sudden start during lifting,
    - pain, tenderness and stiffness of part of the spine,
    - acetylsalicylic acid or other NSAID (ibuprofen), if needed with paracetamol (and if needed with codeine) and avoidance of lifting or heavy work for some days is all that is usually needed; if severe pain continues, refer to the Medical Officer.
  (c) *Chronic back strain:*
    - the patient is often a student or a clerical worker or a woman,
    - chronic ache,
    - usually lower back or neck,
    - often worse after the back is used,
    - no abnormalities on examination of spine,
    - often improves if patient improves posture and strengthens muscles by 'extension exercises' (see page 492).
  (d) *Osteoarthrosis of spine* (see page 492):
    - pain, stiffness and tenderness varies with time.
  (e) *TB of spine* (see page 490):
    - slow start; but constant and increasing pain and tenderness and stiffness of part of the spine,
    - may have other evidence of TB.
  (f) *Acute bacterial infection of the spine* (see page 491):
    - quickly increasing pain, tenderness and stiffness of the spine,
    - often fever and symptoms and signs of infection.
  (g) *Chronic infections, especially brucellosis.*
2. Kidney
  (a) *Ureteric colic* (see Chapter 26 page 450):
    - pain from where lowest rib joints spine to genitalia,
    - kidney often tender,
    - blood in urine often.
  (b) *Pyelonephritis* (urinary tract infection) (see Chapter 26 page 443):
    - fever,
    - urinary pain and frequency,
    - kidney tender,
    - urine shows pus and protein.
3. Reproductive system
  (a) *Pregnancy.*
  (b) *Labour or miscarriage.*
  (c) *Painful menstrual period (dysmenorrhoea):*
    - on examination, no abnormalities found.
  (d) *Pelvic inflammatory disease:*
    - pelvic examination PV shows pus in vagina, tenderness on moving cervix and tenderness or masses in pelvis.
4. Gastrointestinal diseases
    - peptic ulcer penetrating backwards into pancreas, etc.
5. Generalised infections
  (a) *Malaria* (see Chapter 13).
  (b) *Viral diseases, especially influenza.*

Deformity of the spine

See page 492.

30 Disorders of the Endocrine Glands

Anatomy and physiology of the endocrine glands

Glands that make secretions that flow into the blood (and not to outside the body or into one of the mucous membrane lined tubes, such as the gastrointestinal tract) are called endocrine glands.

The secretions of the endocrine glands are called 'hormones'. Hormone means 'messenger'.

Endocrine glands find out if something needs changing in the body. They usually do this from finding changes in the blood. The endocrine gland then puts more or less of its hormone into the blood and this hormone goes to other parts of the body with a message for those parts of the body to change their function (and occasionally their structure). See Figure 30.1.

Pathology of the endocrine glands

Diseases of endocrine glands cause symptoms and signs in three ways.

1. More hormone is secreted than is needed.
2. Less hormone is secreted than is needed.
3. Effects of the disease in the gland – the most common effects are (a) swelling of the gland and (b) spread of any malignant cancer cells from the gland to another part of the body.

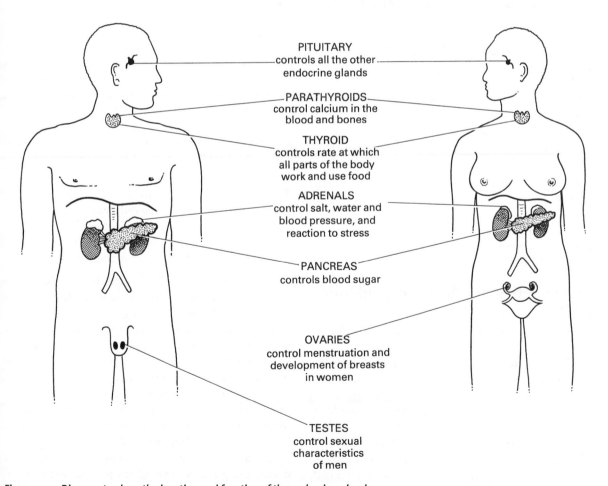

PITUITARY
controls all the other
endocrine glands

PARATHYROIDS
control calcium in the
blood and bones

THYROID
controls rate at which
all parts of the body
work and use food

ADRENALS
control salt, water and
blood pressure, and
reaction to stress

PANCREAS
controls blood sugar

OVARIES
control menstruation and
development of breasts
in women

TESTES
control sexual
characteristics
of men

Figure 30.1 *Diagram to show the location and function of the endocrine glands.*

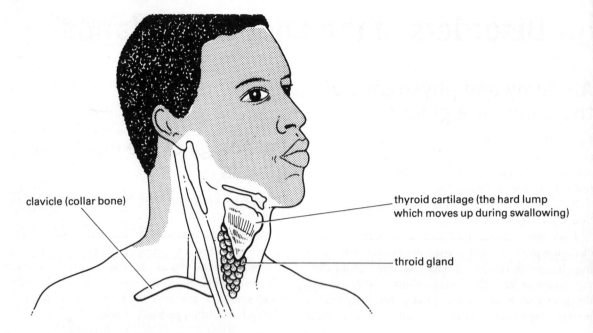

clavicle (collar bone)

thyroid cartilage (the hard lump which moves up during swallowing)

throid gland

Figure 30.2 *Diagram to show the position of the thyroid gland in the neck.*

Diseases of the thyroid glands

The thyroid gland normally makes the right amount of thyroid hormone to allow all the cells of the body to work normally. (See Figure 30.2.)

Diseases of the thyroid gland which you may see in a health centre include:

1. iodine deficiency disorder in adult (endemic goitre),
2. children born to women with iodine deficiency disorder (endemic cretinism),
3. hypothyroidism or myxoedema, and
4. hyperthyroidism or thyrotoxicosis.

Iodine deficiency disorder (endemic goitre)

A goitre is an enlargement of the thyroid gland from any cause.

There are many causes of goitres including thyrotoxicosis (page 498), cancer of the thyroid, and inflammation or infection of the thyroid. But if there are several people in the community with goitres, the most likely cause is iodine deficiency disorder or endemic goitre, caused by a shortage of iodine in the blood.

Endemic goitre occurs when there is not enough iodine in the food and so there is also not enough iodine in the blood. The thyroid gland grows bigger (i.e. a goitre forms) to try to take more iodine from the blood. This shortage of iodine usually occurs in areas which are mountainous or far from the sea as there is iodine in sea water; but the iodine in the soil in mountains has been washed away by rain or snow.

Usually it affects girls at puberty and women during pregnancy more than others (as this is when more iodine is needed).

Symptoms and *signs* include:

1. swelling in the neck caused by a goitre (see Figure 30.3) – this is usually the only symptom and sign;
2. difficulty in breathing – but not usually;
3. difficulty in speaking – hoarse voice – but not usually
4. difficulty in swallowing – but not usually.

Some textbooks and many Medical Officers say you should not treat patients with endemic goitre with iodine. But in some parts of the world, iodine makes many endemic goitres get smaller. You must find out the Health Department policy for your area and follow this policy. Do not give iodine if the goitre goes from the neck into the chest or if the patient has difficulty in breathing. Refer or non-urgently transfer these patients to the Medical Officer. (Iodine treatment could make the goitre swell at first and block breathing before it became smaller.)

Endemic goitre can be prevented by the government passing laws so that all salt sold has iodine in it. If goitres are common in a community, it is possible

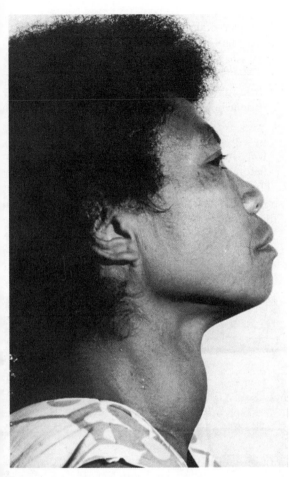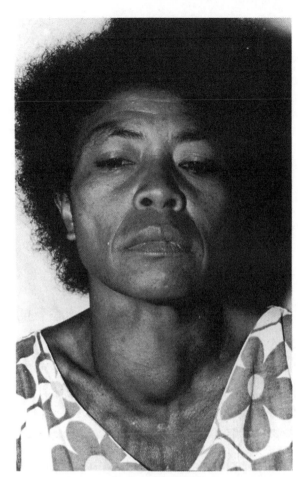

Figure 30.3 *An enlarged thyroid gland. This is called a 'goitre'. See Figure 30.2 for normal position and size of the thyroid gland. A normal gland is not usually visible except in some females at puberty and in the child-bearing years; but even then it should not be very large.*

to treat the whole community (or at least the women and girls) with prophylactic iodised oil fluid injection. The main reason for giving iodine is to stop endemic cretinism occuring in the children of affected women (see below).

If you find a few people with endemic goitre, or if you find only one patient with endemic cretinism (see below) in the community, then notify the Medical Officer so that he can arrange a survey and if needed iodine prophylaxis.

Goitres causing difficulty in breathing or swallowing can be surgically removed.

Endemic cretinism

A patient has endemic cretinism if he has:

1. deafness from birth and cannot speak;
2. spastic (stiff, difficult to bend) legs and was slower than normal children in learning to sit, walk, etc.;

3. mental subnormality;
4. squint (eyes look in different directions).

Not all patients with endemic cretinism have all these symptoms and signs – deafness and lack of speech are the most common (see Figure 30.4).

Endemic cretinism is caused by a shortage of iodine in the mother's blood before the child was born. So endemic cretins are born only in areas where adults have goitres.

Notify the Medical Officer if you find any case of endemic cretinism or if you find several adults with a goitre in an area. The Medical Officer will arrange a survey and, if necessary, mass treatment with iodine, to prevent more endemic cretinism.

No treatment is possible for cases of cretinism.

Prevention is by everyone eating salt with iodine in it; or, if this is not possible, by giving all girls and women prophylactic iodised oil fluid injections.

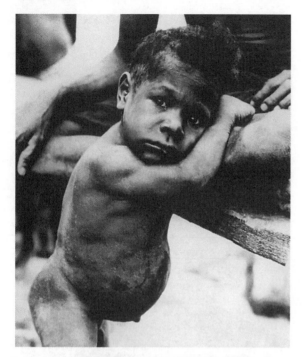

Figure 30.4 *Endemic cretinism. Note that the child cannot walk (he has 'spastic' legs). He is deaf, cannot talk and is mentally dull. He has a large abdomen and an umbilical hernia, which are also common in cretinism.*

Thyrotoxicosis or hyperthyroidism

Thyrotoxicosis or hyperthyroidism is present when too much thyroid hormone is made by the thyroid gland. The most common cause of this is an abnormal reaction of the immune cells of the body which affects the thyroid gland and the eyes and is called 'Graves' disease'.

Thyrotoxicosis is not common, but it is important. It usually affects adults, especially women.

Thyrotoxicosis may cause any of these three groups of conditions (all of them need not be present).

1. All parts of the body work faster than normal but not as well as normal. (This is caused by too much thyroid hormone.) Look for:
   - weight loss and weakness of the muscles, although the patient eats well;
   - pulse fast, even while the patient is at rest or asleep;
   - pulse irregular (sometimes with some weak beats so that the heart rate counted with the stethoscope on the chest is more than the pulse rate felt at the wrist);
   - heart failure for no other obvious cause;

> Always think of thyrotoxicosis in anyone (especially older adults) who have heart failure and you cannot find the cause, especially if pulse is irregular.

   - shaking of the hands (look for this when the patient holds his hands out straight ahead of him with the fingers apart);
   - nervousness or mental illness;
   - feels hot and sweaty all the time (more than before).

2. The eyes may seem to be staring (i.e. the patient does not blink often; and when he looks up and then down, the whites of the eyes show above the brown or blue). (See Figure 30.5.) The eye or eyes may be pushed out (exophthalmos).

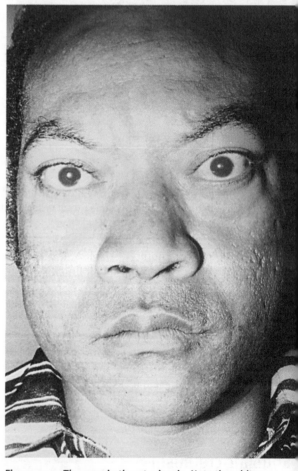

Figure 30.5 *The eyes in thyrotoxicosis. Note the whites of the eyes above the corneas. The patient appears to be staring and does not blink often (lid retraction). When you look from the side, you can see that the eyes are pushed out (exophthalmos).*

3. A goitre (swelling of the thyroid gland) is present or comes. (But only if there are also some of the other signs.) (See Figure 30.3.)

It is possible to cure thyrotoxicosis. But if it is not treated, it can cause death from heart failure or blindness from exophthalmos.

If you suspect a patient has thyrotoxicosis because of any the above features, refer or non-urgently transfer the patient to the Medical Officer for diagnosis and treatment (urgent if corneal damage).

Hypothyroidism (myxoedema)

Hypothyroidism is present when not enough thyroid hormone is made by the thyroid gland. Again, the most common cause is an abnormal immunological reaction. It can, however, be from iodine deficiency when even the large (goitrous) thyroid cannot get enough iodine from the blood to make enough thyroid hormone. It can follow hyperthyroidism. There are many other causes. Most of the effects of low thyroid hormone are the opposite to the effects of hyperthyroidism.

1. All parts of the body work slower than normal and not as well as normal:
   • weight gain,
   • slow pulse,
   • aches and pains and all muscular action slower than normal,
   • mentally dull,
   • tired all the time,
   • depressed and eventually even psychosis,
   • feels the cold weather more,
   • hoarse voice,
   • skin dry and flaky,
   • hair dry and can start to fall out,
   • the patient can slow down so much that he eventually goes into a coma and dies.
2. The eyes are not particularly affected but may seem to be puffed up and the tissues around them swollen or oedematous.
3. A goitre may or may not be present.

It is possible to cure hypothyroidism by giving thyroid hormone tablets, called (levo)thyroxine. If it is not treated it will cause death. The patient must take these regularly for the rest of his life or the condition will return.

If you suspect the patient has hypothyroidism because of any of the above features refer, or non-urgently transfer, the patient to the Medical Officer for diagnosis and treatment.

Diabetes mellitus

Diabetes mellitus occurs when there is more glucose (sugar) in the blood than is normal and the blood glucose stays at these abnormally high levels. Rising or high blood glucose would normally make the pancreas make and release insulin into the blood, which would cause the body cells to take the glucose out of the blood into themselves, lowering the blood sugar. Diabetes occurs when there is an *abnormality of the pancreas* so that it cannot make enough insulin. It can also occur if there is an *abnormality in the body cells* so that they are partially resistant to the action of insulin and need large amounts of insulin in the blood to make them take the sugar out of the blood. If the pancreas has to make these large amounts of insulin for a long time, it can become exhausted (worn out) and not able to continue to make this amount of insulin.

Lack of insulin affects not only glucose in the body, but also other sugars and carbohydrates, fats, protein, water and electrolytes. Sudden changes in these may cause acute disease or death. After some years these changes cause permanent damage in other parts of the body and in particular the arteries, especially the arteries in the eyes, kidneys, nervous system and feet. These changes are called the 'complications' of diabetes.

Three types of diabetes are recognised in tropical countries.

1. Type 1 diabetes, or insulin-dependent diabetes mellitus (IDDM), is not as common as other types. It is due to inherited factors, viral infections, immunological abnormalities (autoimmune disease) and other things. As a result of these causes, all the cells of the pancreas that usually make insulin are destroyed, and the body then has no insulin. This type of diabetes occurs in younger people and is not as common as NIDDM because (a) it occurs less often, and (b) the patients often die soon after the disease develops.
2. Type 2, or non-insulin-dependent diabetes mellitus (NIDDM), is more common and is again due to inherited factors. It is often associated with obesity, high blood pressure, gout, abnormal fats in the blood, etc. (called 'metabolic syndrome') and is due to resistance of the body cells to the effects of insulin. In NIDDM the pancreas still makes some insulin. This type affects 1–4% of the population; but in some areas it is much higher, even up to 50%. It was thought to be relatively rare in Africans and the Chinese; but rates are now rising. Obesity is the main thing that brings on Type 2 DM. Now that obesity occurs in children as well as older people, even children are getting Type 2 DM.

Table 30.1 Features of the two main types of diabetes mellitus.

Factors	Type 1 insulin-dependent diabetes mellitus (IDDM)	Type 2 non-insulin-dependent diabetes mellitus (NIDDM)
Age of onset	Younger	Older (but now young children)
Family history of diabetes mellitus	Not often	Usually
Duration of symptoms	Weeks	Months to years
Body weight	Normal or low	Obese
Ketones in urine	Yes	No
Rapid death without treatment with insulin	Yes	No
Diabetic complications present at diagnosis	No	Sometimes

3. Malnutrition–related diabetes mellitus (MRDM) is more like Type 1 or IDDM, except that a serious complication called 'ketoacidosis', which occurs in IDDM, does not occur in MRDM. It is thought that some patients have had a history of malnutrition, which may have damaged cells in the pancreas, and that others have 'chronic fibrocalculus pancreatitis' or 'tropical calcific pancreatitis' where all of the pancreas as well as the insulin producing cells are damaged and healing was by fibrous scar tissue and calcium. Attacks of abdominal pain often occur (page 401).

Diabetes can also occur in a number of other less common situations.

Table 30.1 shows the features of the two common types of diabetes.

If the blood glucose is high, glucose gets through the glomeruli into the urine and holds water with it. This leads to large urine volumes, dehydration and thirst.

When there is no insulin to enable the body cells to use glucose, as in IDDM (though not as expected in MRDM and not in NIDDM), large amounts of fat (instead of glucose) have to be broken down to supply energy. This causes weight loss (as this fat can be only partly broken down without insulin and glucose metabolism) and ketones and acids from the fat are left in the blood. This 'ketoacidosis' (unless treated with rehydration and insulin) quickly leads to unconsciousness and death.

Some infecting organisms grow better in the body if the glucose is high.

Complications occur in all types of diabetes and include the following:

1. Kidney damage with proteinuria or nephrotic syndrome or kidney failure.
2. Damage to the blood vessels in the retina of the eye with progressive loss of vision and blindness (called diabetic retinopathy). Cataracts are also more common.
3. Damage to the nervous system with:
   - peripheral neuritis, sometimes with pain but with permanent loss of sensation in the legs (similar to leprosy); and ulcers and infections due to loss of sensation (like leprosy);
   - sudden loss of function of any nerves, including those which control eye movement which may recover;
   - permanent loss of function of nerves to the internal organs of the body which causes low blood pressure on standing, abdominal fullness, constipation or diarrhoea, impotence (not able to have penile erection to have sexual intercourse) etc.
4. More infections of all sorts – some difficult to treat.
5. Damage to blood vessels in the legs when no pulses may be noted above the affected area and often with death of toes (dry gangrene) (although in developing countries, feet problems in diabetics are most often due to loss of sensation and infection).

Think, therefore, of diabetes in anyone who:

1. is thirsty, drinking a lot of fluid and passing a lot of urine; *or*
2. has weight loss even though he is eating well; *or*
3. is obese; *or*
4. has infections:
   - not expected – especially thrush in the mouth or vagina or on the penis or skin, and
   - all cases of TB.

Also think of diabetes if you see patients with complications that can be caused by diabetes including:

1. Loss of vision for no obvious reason.
2. Kidney problems including proteinuria, nephrotic syndrome and kidney failure.
3. High blood pressure.
4. All sorts of abnormalities of the nervous system.

5. Ulcers on the feet from loss of sensation when the patient does not have leprosy.

6. Gangrene of the toes or feet with poor circulation and loss of pulses.

In all the cases, test for glucose in the urine. If Benedict's solution or many of the tablet tests are used these are positive for other sugars as well as glucose. If the patient is pregnant or breastfeeding a baby, the sugar (lactose) from the breast milk can get into the blood and urine (and give a positive test for sugar with Benedict's solution and many of the tablet tests), even when the patient has no glucose in the urine and does not have diabetes. Test patients who are pregnant or breastfeeding a baby with a stick or paper test, which is positive for glucose only. If there is sugar in the urine do a blood test for blood glucose.

Diagnosis of diabetes is made by:

1. Symptoms of diabetes and a blood glucose of 11 mmol/l (200 mg/dl) or above,

2. fasting blood glucose of 7 mmol/l or 126 mg/dl or above,

3. 2 hour blood glucose of 11 mmol/l or above during a glucose tolerance test.

If the patient has diabetes, if possible, transfer the patient to Medical Officer care for confirmation of the diagnosis and starting treatment.

The treatment for diabetes includes seven things:

1. Diet and having normal body weight.

2. Daily exercise which also helps to have a normal body weight.

3. No symptoms from diabetes or from treatment of diabetes and satisfactory blood glucose levels.

4. If Type 1 (IDDM), insulin.

5. If Type 2 (NIDDM), tablets; but only if 1 and 2 not effective.

6. Health education.

7. Proper prevention and treatment of
   (a) hypoglycaemia,
   (b) hyperglycaemia,
   (c) other possible complications.

---

1. The patient should have a diet containing as little refined sugar and fat and salt as possible, be high in starchy carbohydrates and fibres with good protein. This should be eaten at regular times each day. Most traditional village diets, except for sugar cane and sweet fruits, are usually all right. The patient should eat enough food to get to the normal weight for his height and age. (See Chapter 23 pages 381–382.) Then the patient should eat only enough to remain at this normal weight.

2. The patient should have daily physical exercise (at least 30 minutes of walking quickly daily).

3. The aim of treatment should be to keep the blood glucose between 4 and 8 mmol/l all the time and not above 6 mmol/l on waking in the morning. However, as testing of blood or urine at home is not usually possible or affordable in most developing countries, a more realistic aim, especially in rural areas, may be:
   (a) near normal blood glucose levels if these tests are done at any time;
   (b) no symptoms of high blood sugar;
   (c) no episodes where the blood sugar is low;
   (d) no other treatment side effects;
   (e) good quality of life.

4. Type 1 or insulin-dependent diabetes will need insulin injections every day. This will be either:
   (a) Soluble insulin, also called unmodified or clear or short acting insulin – these injections last for 4 to 6 hours; *or*
   (b) Depot-insulin, also called modified, cloudy or intermediate or long acting insulin – these last for hours to more than a day. The usual ones available are either insulin zinc suspension or isophane insulin and they are intermediate acting insulins lasting for up to 12 to 18 hours.
   (c) Many other kinds of insulin are available. Find out which ones are being used where you work and find out all about their actions.
   (d) Make sure you know the strength of insulin in your area. Insulin available should now be just 100 units/ml; but this is not so in all areas.
   (e) Insulin can be given by ordinary subcutaneous injection using a syringe or special 'pens', although there are other ways including a 'jet' injection.
   (f) The Medical Officer will work out the best type and dose of insulin for the patient. This may be:
   • soluble short acting insulin 20% (1/5) of the total daily dose 20–30 minutes before **each** meal, and
   • intermediate acting depot insulin 40% (2/5) of the total daily dose before bedtime,
   or
   • a mixture of 33% (1/3) of the total daily dose as a short acting insulin and 66% (2/3) of the total daily dose as an intermediate depot

insulin given in 2 doses a day, 66% (2/3) before breakfast and 33% (1/3) before the evening meal.

These and other regimes keep changing depending on the amount and type of food the patient is about to eat, and the amount of activity the patient is about to do, and the development of any illness the patient gets, and the results of any blood or urine test.

Insulin is best kept in the refrigerator; but as long as it is not left in the sun or in a very hot place, it stays effective even in the tropics, out of a refrigerator, for many months.

Keep some soluble short acting insulin in the health centre always and learn how to use it as it can be used for all diabetic problems you will see; and can be given by subcutaneous, intramuscular and intravenous injections (do not give depot insulins by intravenous injection).

Do not stop insulin if the patient gets sick in any way or has vomiting or is not eating, as this may well lead to very high blood glucose levels and ketoacidosis with dehydration. If sick or vomiting, start intravenous 4.3% dextrose in 0.18% sodium chloride and see section on Hyperglycaemia/ketoacidosis on page 503 for when to do blood glucose tests and what dose of insulin to give depending on the blood glucose levels, until the patient improves. During this time any depot or long acting insulin should be stopped.

5. Type 2 non-insulin-dependent diabetes mellitus patients may need tablets as well as exercise and diet, if they are severely affected when first seen, or if 3 months of exercise and diet does not control the diabetes (if they had mild diabetes when first seen). Metformin is the first drug used, especially in obese patients. It can cause gastrointestinal upsets, but if started in a small dose and gradually increased these usually are not a problem. It should not be given to people with kidney failure as it can cause dangerous side effects. The first dose is usually 0.5 g daily and after a month increase to 0.5 g twice daily and after another month 0.5 g three times a day. However, if control of the diabetes or side effects occur, the dose is not increased any further from that level. The tablets should always be taken with meals. Glibenclamide is the drug usually used out of a group of drugs called sulfonylureas. Glibenclamide is a short acting one (and chlorpropramide is a long acting one and should now no longer be used as this long action causes a lot of side effects from low

blood sugar). Low blood sugar is the most dangerous side effect of all of these drugs. Glibenclamide is used first in Type 2 diabetic patients who are not obese and especially if they have a poor appetite. Unfortunately, for most diabetics they tend to make people eat more and put on weight. The dose of glibenclamide is 2.5 mg in the morning; and after a month 2.5 mg twice daily; the next month 2.5 mg three times a day; and increased monthly to a maximum dose of 5 mg three times a day. It is taken in these divided doses with meals. It is not increased once diabetes control is obtained or if side effects, especially hypoglycaemia, occur. Some patients need both drugs if the first one chosen is itself unable to control the diabetes.

6. Health education is essential. The patient must know and be convinced by the health worker to carry out the following:
(a) eat a proper diet;
(b) exercise every day;
(c) get his body weight into the normal range and keep it there;
(d) always take drugs, food and exercise (and any tests done) regularly at approximately the same time every day;
(e) care for his feet in the same way a patient with leprosy does (see Chapter 15 pages 146–147) from the time of diagnosis, even if at that time there is not then noticeable loss of sensation, as there will already be some changes there. Shoes or sandals should always be worn;
(f) if he gets sick do not stop the tablets or insulin but immediately come to the health centre for treatment.

7. Treat any complications quickly and properly, especially infections, gastroenteritis, high blood sugars (hyperglycaemia) or low blood sugars (hypoglycaemia).

Hypoglycaemia

If a patient with diabetes develops any of these – weakness, sweating, shaking, mental abnormality, vomiting, unconsciousness – do a blood glucose estimation immediately as these suggest low blood glucose near to 2.5 mmol/l. If the blood glucose is low (even below 3.5) or if you have no way of doing blood glucose tests, then immediately give two large dessertspoonfuls of sugar in water by mouth or intragastric tube. If the patient cannot swallow or is unconscious, give 50 ml of a 50% dextrose solution by IV injection. If the patient is hypoglycaemic this should improve him within minutes. If the patient is not hypoglycae-mic, it will not do any harm. Always find out the cause for the hypoglycaemia, e.g. overdose of tablets, meal missed, more exercise than normal, etc. and tell the patient how to avoid more hypoglycaemic attacks.

Hyperglycaemia/ketoacidosis

If the patient is seriously ill in any way and the blood glucose is high (above 15 mmol/l) it is likely that the patient has developed ketoacidosis and dehydration. Start intravenous 0.9% sodium chloride for dehydra-tion. Give 500 ml–1 litre quickly, then 500 ml each hour for 4–6 hours. The patient may well need 4–6 litres of fluid. Give 20 units of soluble insulin by SCI immediately or by IVI if shocked, followed by 5 units subcutaneously every hour. Do the blood glu-cose test every 2 hours.

Once the glucose in the blood starts to go into the body cells, it takes a lot of potassium with it and the potassium in the blood and serum can become low. Low serum potassium can stop the heart. (High serum potassium is even more likely to stop the heart.) If available, 1 hour *after both* IV saline (1–1.5 l) and insulin 20 units have been given, add potassium chloride solution to the IV fluid. Thirty (30) mmol which is 20 ml (or one of the 20 ml ampoules) of potassium chloride solution 11.2% (equivalent to K+ 1.5 mmol/ml Cl 1.5 mmol/ml) is drawn up into a syringe and put into each 1 litre of saline and mixed into it BEFORE the bottle of saline is put up for infusion. Run the bottle of 1 litre of 0.9% sodium chloride with 30 mmol (20 ml) of potassium chloride in it over 2 hours.

Stop the potassium if the patient does not pass urine after 2 hours (? acute kidney failure and potassium would then be dangerous) until urine is passed. Stop the potas-sium after 60–90 mmol (i.e. after 2–3 ampoules of 20 ml in 2–3 litres of IV saline has been given over 4–6 hours (as all the potassium needed should have been given)). If no IV potassium is available, still treat the patient as above without potassium, as without rehydration and insulin treatment most patients will quickly die. Transfer the patient as an emergency to the Medical Officer as soon as possible; although if the patient survives the first 12 hours the danger of low potassium should be over as the patient by then should be eating and drinking and be given oral rehydration fluid and some foods con-taining potassium (e.g. tubers, bananas, citrus fruit, etc.). If no IV potassium is available, as soon as the patient has improved and can safely swallow, start oral rehydra-tion fluid which contains 20 mmol potassium in each

litre; but unfortunately, until the patient significantly improves, oral fluids are not well absorbed.

> 1. *Never ever* give an intravenous injection of potassium.
> 2. *Never* put potassium into a small volume of solution for infusion.
> 3. *Never* give potassium more quickly than 30–40 mmol in 2 hours.
>
> Each of these things could stop the heart and cause death.

When the blood glucose falls below 15 mmol/l and the clinical dehydration is gone, any intravenous solu-tion can usually be changed to 1/5 normal saline and 4% dextrose and the insulin be given every 4 hours depending on the blood glucose level (in mmol/l) as follows.
- If blood glucose is above 15, give 12 units of soluble insulin.
- If blood glucose 10–15 give 8 units of soluble insulin.
- If blood glucose 5–10 give 4 units of soluble insulin.
- If blood glucose less than 5, do not give any insulin.

At the same time as starting treatment for keto-acidosis, look for and treat the cause of the ketoacido-sis. The cause is almost always an infection somewhere. If the cause is not clear give IV or IM antibiotics as for septicaemia (see Chapter 12) and IV or IM drugs for malaria. (See Chapter 13 page 81.)

Once the patient is eating, drinking and able to get up and walk again, and the condition which caused the ketoacidosis has been treated, the patient can then be changed back to regular insulin, and later, if they were previously on tablets, onto their regular tablets. It is always essential to fully treat any infection such as pneumonia, urinary infection, skin infection, malaria, etc. and treat any gastroenteritis or other thing which brought on the attack of ketoacidosis.

If blood glucose test not available

If at any time a diabetic patient becomes very sick or unconscious and you do not have the equipment to do blood glucose tests, as well as treating any obvious infection, malaria or obvious cause, try the effect of 50 ml of 50% intravenous glucose. The patient will be 'cured' if he was hypoglycaemic. If this is not effective, put up a drip and give fluids as for dehydration from ketoacidosis (above); but do not give extra insulin or potassium, although it is likely he has hyperglycae-mia and ketoacidosis. In this case, the patient would have to be transferred as an emergency to the Medical Officer for tests and treatment.

If transfer of newly diagnosed diabetic to the Medical Officer not possible

If it is not possible for you to transfer a newly diagnosed diabetic to the Medical Officer for confirmation of the diagnosis and treatment, manage as follows.

1. Give all the required health education (as above) about diabetes.
2. If a Type 2 non-insulin-dependent diabetes case, start on diet and exercise if mild, and then review in 3 months about the need to add tablets; although if it is severe and the patient has symptoms, start metformin if obese or glibenclamide if not obese and increase the doses as above. If, when on the maximum dose of one drug, control is not obtained, then add the other drug, increasing the dose slowly until both are given at maximum doses. If the diabetes is still not controlled, the patient will obviously need insulin but would be best seen by the Medical Officer.
3. If the patient has Type 1 insulin-dependent diabetes mellitus, the patient will need admission, diet, exercise and a dose of insulin according to the blood glucose levels done 4 hourly until the blood sugars return to near normal (see page 501); and then changed to a home maintenance dose according to blood glucose tests and clinical progress.

Prevention

Prevention of diabetes (NIDDM) is by not eating too much (especially refined carbohydrate foods) and not having weight above ideal.

Acute adrenal insufficiency

The adrenal gland of the body normally makes a small amount of cortisone each day to keep the body working properly; and a large amount of cortisone at a time of stress (e.g. acute infection or accident or operation) needed to get the body over this stress.

Cortisone or cortisone-like drugs called adrenocorticosteroid drugs including hydrocortisone, prednisone, prednisolone and dexamethasone and others are given to try to stop some very dangerous inflammatory conditions, e.g. severe asthma, leprosy reactions, etc. Do not start these drugs unless you have been taught when and how to do so, as they are normally started only by a Medical Officer.

Once a patient starts taking a large dose of cortisone-like drugs (and possibly any more than 7.5 mg of prednisolone), the adrenal glands of the body stop making cortisone. After a couple of weeks of not making cortisone, it takes some days or weeks for the adrenal glands to be able to make a normal amount of cortisone again, and especially the large amounts needed at times of stress. If the patient suddenly stops taking his drug, he will have no cortisone in his body and may develop gastrointestinal symptoms, weakness, low blood pressure and then shock and die (called acute adrenal failure). At a time of stress such as a severe illness, if the patient does not take an extra dose of the cortisone-like drug, he is even more likely to develop this and die.

Also, the high dose of cortisone makes the patient more likely to get diseases from infections, especially malaria, TB, amoebae in the bowel; and *Strongyloides* may spread out of the bowel into the rest of the body.

If you have a patient who is taking a cortisone-like drug, see a specialist reference book for further details. Remember, however, these rules:

1. The patient must take the drug as directed and not stop it (unless the Medical Officer stops it, and he would usually just slowly reduce the dose to allow the adrenal glands time to start making cortisone again).
2. If there is a time of stress the patient must take 3–4 times the normal dose of the drug immediately (up to 50 mg prednisolone) and then daily. You must consult the Medical Officer urgently about what to do.
3. The patient must take prophylactic antimalarials and prophylactic isoniazid, if he is in an area where malaria occurs or if TB is common (but make sure first he does not have TB disease and need DOTS).
4. Treat any infection quickly and well with antibiotics and antimalarials.
5. If a patient taking one of these drugs develops any severe illness or gastroenteritis or becomes shocked or unconscious, as well as treating these new medical problems as usual, give also oral prednisolone 50 mg immediately and each morning (or if unable to take oral drugs IV hydrocortisone 200–300 mg immediately and then 100 mg 8 hourly) until the patient is transferred to the Medical Officer.

31 Disorders of the Eye

Dr John Sandford-Smith has published an excellent book *Eye Diseases in Hot Climates* (fourth edition, 2003, Elsevier, India), which clearly explains in 420 pages all that needs to be known about eye diseases. If you can, get and use a copy of this book.

Do not have this 'blind spot'

One of the worst things that can happen to any of us is to be blind. It is even worse if we know that this blindness need not have happened – it could have been easily prevented but was not, or could be easily treated and is not.

The WHO estimates that there are 45 million blind people in the world and 135 million others with problems with their eyesight. Ninety per cent of these people live in developing countries. Three-quarters of this blindness could have been easily prevented (but was not) or could be easily treated (but is not).

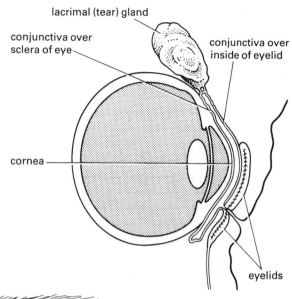

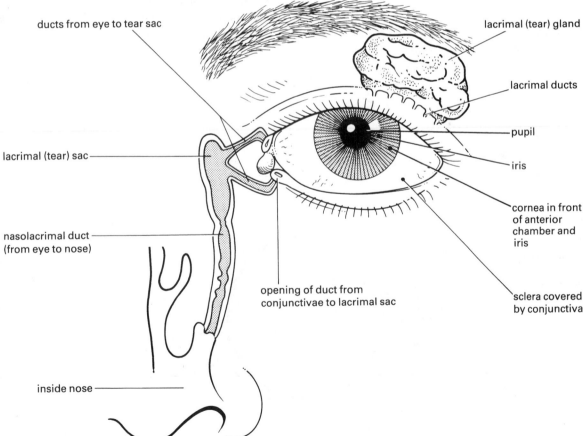

Figure 31.1 *Diagrams to show the structure of the eye and the tear gland and ducts.*

The common causes of this blindness are:

- trachoma
- xerophthalmia
- onchocerciasis
- glaucoma
- cataract
- uncorrected refraction error
- diabetic retinopathy.

Prevention of some of these and treatment for others (although treatment is too late to help those which should have been prevented) is, however, simple and cheap.

Dr Sandford-Smith points out that many health workers have a 'blind spot' about eye diseases and blindness – they do not realise and act on the above facts. Make sure you do not have a blind spot about blindness. Make sure you know about these eye diseases. Make sure you do all you can, so as few people as possible in your area develop preventable blindness or live with blindness if this is treatable.

Anatomy

(See Figures 31.1, 31.2 and 31.3.)

History and examination

Symptoms of eye diseases

1. loss of vision
2. pain in the eye
3. eye red; watering; or sticky (from pus).

Signs of eye diseases

Examine structures of the eye from the outside ones to the inside ones to find any signs present.

1. *Look at the site, shape and size, etc. of the eyes*
   - exophthalmos (eye pushed out, e.g. hyperthyroidism)? (See Chapter 30 page 498.)
   - orbital cellulitis (infection all around the eye)?
2. *Look at the eyelids*
   - 'stye' or cyst (page 509)?
   - entropion (page 513)?
   - oedema?
   - haematoma?
   Ask the patient to open and close his eyes.
   - ptosis (drooping of upper eyelid)?
   - lagophthalmos (eyelid cannot be closed) (see Chapter 15 page 137)?

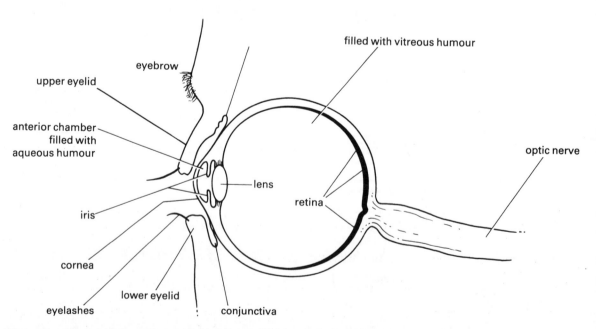

Figure 31.2 *Diagram of the eye in section from front to back, to show the structure of the eye in more detail.*

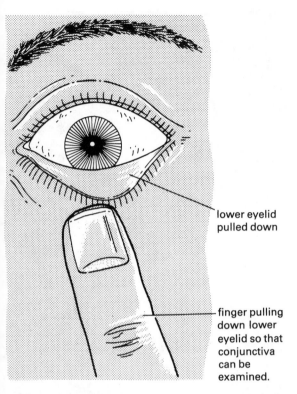

lower eyelid pulled down

finger pulling down lower eyelid so that conjunctiva can be examined.

Figure 31.3 *Examination of the conjunctiva of the lower lid.*

3. *Look at the conjunctiva*
   (a) over the sclera,
   (b) inside the lower lids (see Figure 31.3),
   (c) inside upper lids (turn upper lid inside out) (see Figure 31.4).
      • foreign body?
      • inflammation of all conjunctiva or just around cornea?
      • pus?
      • nodules?
      • pterygium?

4. *Look at the cornea*
   (a) Anaesthetise with amethocaine 2% or tetracaine 0.5% sterile eye drops, 1 drop into the outer side of the eye every minute for 2–3 minutes, as necessary (see Figure 31.5) Note that local anaesthetic is only needed if the patient has pain.
   (b) Stain with fluorescein. Put one drop of sterile solution, or lay the end of a sterile ophthalmic strip on the conjunctiva of the sclera (white part of the eye) on the lateral (outer) side of the eye for a few seconds. Then get the patient to blink. Corneal ulcers will show as green areas.
   (c) Shine a light in from side and ask the patient to look up, down, right and left.

(d) Use a torch and a loupe (magnifying glasses) if available. Otherwise use an auriscope without a speculum (see Figure 31.6).
   • foreign body?
   • ulcer?
   • clear or cloudy?
   • scar?

5. *Look at the anterior chamber by shining a light into it*
   • clear?
   • cloudy?
   • pus or blood at the lower part?

6. *Look at the iris and the pupil*
   • pupil shape round or irregular?
   • pupil size normal, large or small?
   Shine a light into the pupil
   • pupil constricts (gets smaller) when light goes in and dilates (gets bigger) when light goes away, or not?

7. *Look at the lens*
   • cataract?

8. *Test eye movements*
   Ask the patient to follow with his eyes one of your fingers, which you move up, then down, then to the right and then to the left;
   • double vision (noticed by the patient)?
   • squint (both eyes do not look in the same direction noticed by you)?

9. *Visual acuity*
   • check vision with a special eye chart at 6 metres (6/6 or less) *or* count fingers *or* see light;
   • read a special eye chart or small print for close vision.

Check for symptoms and signs of disease in the rest of the body, if the eye condition is not just an eye injury.

Using these symptoms and signs, you can easily diagnose the most important eye diseases. See Table 31.1.

Treatment of eye diseases

Many of the important eye diseases are infective or traumatic (and traumatic injuries often get infected), so it is important always to do certain things if a patient has an eye condition.

1. Always look for foreign bodies in the eye. (This is especially important if the eye is red and painful.) Carefully look all over all surfaces of the conjunctiva. Carefully look all over the cornea.

2. Always look for corneal ulcers. Always stain the eye with fluorescein. Then shine a light into the eye from each side, and above and below.

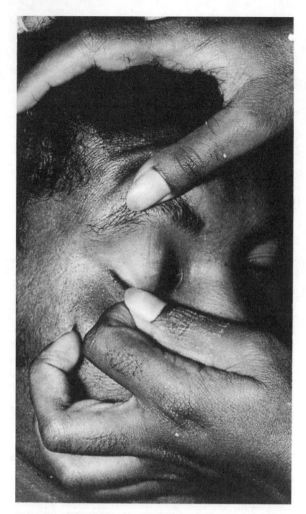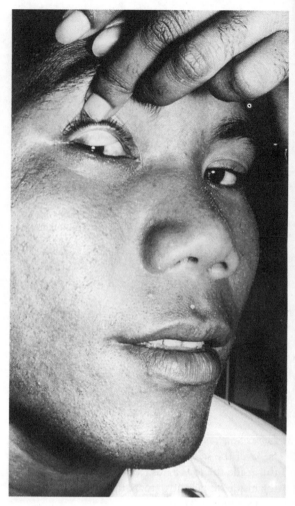

Figure 31.4 *Examining the conjunctiva of the upper eyelid. Left photograph, first step. Right photograph, second step. See text for details. The conjunctivae may be red and inflamed all over with or without the formation of pus (conjunctivitis). They may be inflamed just around the cornea (acute iritis). A vascular fleshy growth may be growing across it to the cornea (pterygium). A foreign body may be present.*

3. If an infection or injury is present, use an antibiotic ointment in the eye. Any anti-infective eye ointment is usually safe and soothing.

4. If an eye infection is serious, chloramphenicol eye drops or ointment is the most powerful antibiotic usually available. It should be put into the eye at least every 3 hours. If the infection is inside the eye, give also chloramphenicol capsules (or injections, if vomiting is present). (Penicillin alone is not very effective for most infections inside the eye.) Gentamicin drops or tetracycline ointment may be all that is available.

5. If there is any injury or infection inside the eye or a severe injury or infection on the cornea, always dilate the pupil with atropine eye ointment or drops. Use atropine 3–4 times daily until the pupil dilates. The pupil will stay dilated for a week, sometimes more (even after the atropine is stopped). If necessary, continue the atropine once daily. Injuries or infections in the eye may fix the iris, so that the pupil cannot get bigger or smaller. It is better for sight and for other reasons if the iris is fixed with the pupil big rather than small. This is the reason for using atropine.

6. Always put a pad on an eye with a serious injury or infection in it or on the cornea. But a pad is not good treatment for conjunctivitis. Hold the pad on the eye with strip of adhesive cellulose tape or sticking plaster. Put the strips diagonally across the corners of the eye (and not across the

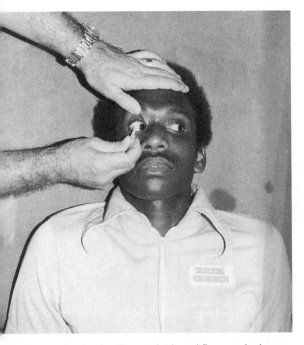

Figure 31.5 *Putting local anaesthetic and fluorescein drops into the eye. Local anaesthetic is only necessary if the patient has pain. Fluorescein is necessary in all patients. Note that the drops are put in the outer side of the eye while the patient looks towards the other side.*

centre of the eye, i.e. do not press the dressing onto the eye).

7. If a patient has only one eye, the patient and you must take great care of this good eye. If the patient develops injury or disease in his one good eye, transfer him quickly, if you are not certain of the diagnosis and treatment.

8. Before transferring any non-emergency eye case, first check that the Medical Officer at the hospital will take the case. He may prefer a non-urgent case to wait until the ophthalmologist (eye specialist) is visiting the hospital.

Some common eye diseases

The common stye and Meibonian cyst

The eyelid at the edge of the eye (usually the hair in eyelid) may become infected and cause a pimple or abscess or 'stye'. The Meibonian gland in the hard part of the eyelid with its opening also at the edge of the eyelid can become blocked, and the secretions then cause a *swelling* in the eyelid which can become in-

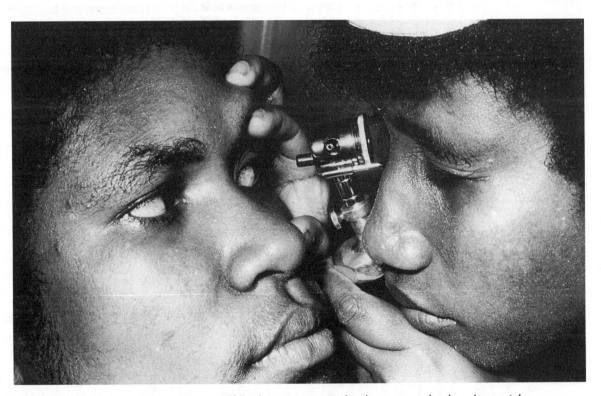

Figure 31.6 *If you use an auriscope with a magnifying lens you can examine the eye more closely and accurately.*

Table 31.1 Clinical findings of the common eye disorders.

History and examination	Acute conjunctivitis	Foreign body in cornea	Corneal ulcer	Acute iritis (infection from outside)	Acute iritis (from other diseases)	Acute glaucoma	Cataract
History of injury	No	Often	At times	Corneal ulcer or penetrating injury	No	No, sometimes yes	Sometimes
Red discharging eye	Yes, pus	Yes, watery	Yes, watery	Yes, varies	Yes, watery	Yes, watery	No
Pain in eye	No	Yes	Yes	Yes	Yes	Yes	No
Loss of vision	No	Often	Often	Yes	Yes	Yes	Yes
Conjunctiva	All inflamed, pus	Inflamed	Inflamed	Inflamed – only around cornea or all	Inflamed only around cornea	Inflamed around cornea only	Normal
Cornea	Normal	Foreign body	Ulcer	Ulcer or injury often	Normal	Cloudy	Normal
Anterior chamber	Normal	Normal	Normal	Cloudy or hypopyon	Cloudy or hypopyon	Not easily seen	Normal
Pupil	Normal	Normal	Normal	Small irregular, will not dilate	Small irregular, will not dilate	Large, oval, will not constrict	Normal
Lens	Normal	Normal	Normal	Normal	Normal	Normal	White
Other disease present	At times	No	No	No	Often yes	No	Not usually

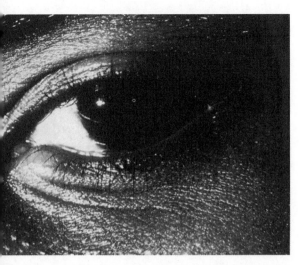

Figure 31.7 *A common stye affecting the medial (centre) part of the lower lid.*

fected and cause an abscess. The stye is smaller and at the edge of the lid and after a few days discharges pus at the edge of the eyelid and goes away; but new ones may form. The Meibonian cyst may just get larger, but if infected the abscess is painful and can burst out through the skin or in through the conjunctiva.

Treat infection with hot bathing 3–4 times a day and antibiotic eye ointment 3–4 times daily. Treat a Meibonian abscess with also oral antibiotics, e.g. doxycycline. If the abscess does not settle or a cyst gets big enough to block vision or press on the eye, send the patient to the Medical Officer for excision and curettage.

Conjunctival foreign bodies

Conjunctival foreign bodies cause pain, redness and watering of the eye.

Remove foreign bodies from under the lower eyelid with the patient looking up. See Figure 31.3.

Remove them from under the upper lid with the patient looking down. Turn the upper lid inside out over swab stick or a finger. See Figure 31.4.

Chemicals in the eye

Lime is a common and dangerous chemical in the eye. Chemicals can quickly cause damage to the eye. Give immediate proper first aid.

1. Hold the affected eye open and pour large amounts of water across it for 10–15 minutes, even though this causes pain. (Isotonic 0.9% sodium chloride solution or even oral rehydrating solution would be better if available.)

2. Then anaesthetise the eye with a local anaesthetic, see pages 507, 509.
3. Stain the cornea with fluorescein, see page 509.
4. Remove any foreign bodies very carefully.
5. Wash the eye with water again if necessary.
6. If the cornea is clear, treat with antibiotic eye ointment three or four times a day.
7. If the cornea is not clear, treat as for iritis (see page 515), but the oral chloramphenicol is not necessary.
8. Transfer the patient to Medical Officer care if he is not much better in 1–2 days.

Acute conjunctivitis

Conjunctivitis is inflammation of the conjunctiva of the eye with or without the formation of pus.

Causes include:

- gonorrhoea or chlamydia in infants at birth (from the mother's cervix or vagina),
- trachoma, acute stage (see page 512),
- infection with (other kinds of) bacteria,
- viral infections,
- allergic reactions,
- a mild chronic conjunctivitis with swelling of the conjunctivae which does not respond to the usual treatment for conjunctivitis can occur from onchocerciasis,
- vitamin A deficiency, especially in children, can cause dry conjunctivae with dry corneas and this can result in painful conjunctivitis. (See pages 514–515.)

Spread of most infectious types of conjunctivitis is by direct contact, or by a vehicle (e.g. towel), or by vectors (especially flies).

Symptoms include:

- red watering eyes,
- eyelids stuck together with pus in the morning, and
- some discomfort (but no pain).

> If there is pain, another serious disease is present as well as conjunctivitis.

Signs include:

- inflammation of the conjunctivae, over the sclera and under the eyelids of both eyes; and
- discharge, which may be watery, or pus.

Treatment

1. *Show* the patient how to put antibiotic eye ointment or drops under the lower eyelids. *Tell* the

patient to do this four times daily to both eyes. *Give the patient antibiotic eye ointment or drops to take home.* Treat for 5 days. Do not pad the eye.

2. If possible, admit the patient for hourly treatment with drops for the first 8–12 hours by a member of your staff. This is usually much more effective than the patient giving himself the treatment. The patient can then continue the treatment at home.
3. If infant/newborn. See Chapter 19 pages 207–208.
4. Treat also for trachoma, vitamin A deficiency, onchocerciasis, etc., if these could be present.

Explain how the infection usually spreads, and how to stop this spread.

If the patient is not cured, look carefully for foreign bodies, iritis, vitamin A deficiency, onchocerciasis and trachoma and urgently treat any of these found or transfer the patient.

You must always stain the cornea with fluorescein and examine it for any corneal foreign body or corneal ulcer. Examine the anterior chamber and pupil for iritis.

(These things are especially important if the conjunctivitis is only on one side because infective conjunctivitis almost always spreads to both eyes. If conjunctivitis is only in one eye there is usually a local cause in that eye, such as foreign body, entropion (rolling in of the eyelid) or blocked tear duct, etc.)

These things are especially important if the inflammation is only around the cornea, because conjunctivitis causes inflammation of all of the conjunctivae. If the inflammation is only around the cornea, then a corneal ulcer or foreign body or iritis or glaucoma is probably present.

Trachoma

Trachoma is a chronic inflammation of the conjunctivae and cornea caused by *Chlamydia trachomatis*. About 150 million people have the infection. About 5 million people are blind from it.

Trachoma is common all over the world. But it is much more common, and causes much more severe disease, in areas that are hot, dry and dusty; where there are many more flies and there is rubbish or faeces or cattle which increase their breeding; and where there is not enough water for people to wash regularly.

Infected people are much more infectious early in the infection. Spread of the trachoma organisms happens when the eye discharge from infected people is passed directly to other people on fingers, towels, anything used to wipe the face, clothes, bedclothes,

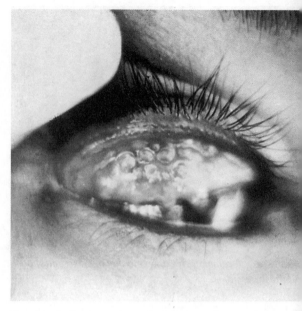

Figure 31.8 *Trachoma. Note the follicles on the conjunctiva of the upper eyelid.*

etc. Flies are also important in spreading the disease. Trachoma can also be caused by the chlamydia STD organism at birth. It is usually children who have active infection. Older children and adults usually have the results of the infection, which is often blindness.

There are four stages in the development of trachoma.

1. *Early trachoma*
   First the eyes are uncomfortable and watery, and the conjunctivae inflamed, like any other conjunctivitis. However, the condition continues. After about a month, small pink-grey lumps, called 'follicles', develop under the upper eyelid (see Figure 31.8). There is little pus in the eye, unless there is secondary infection by other bacteria.
2. *Pannus formation*
   Small blood vessels start to grow into the top of the cornea. This is called 'pannus'. Use a loupe or magnifying glass to look for the grey colour of *early* pannus at the top of the cornea.
3. *After some months to years*, especially if there are not repeated reinfections and it is not hot and dusty, *the lesions may heal without treatment.*
   The follicles leave white scars on the inside of the upper eyelid. The pannus (which may spread over much of the cornea) leaves a whitish colour and small pits on the cornea (the cornea is normally completely clear).

4. *Entropion and trichiasis occurs*

The scarred tissue inside the eyelid, like any scar tissue, becomes smaller over the years. This pulls or turns the edge of the eyelid in, and this is called 'entropion'. This makes the eyelashes scrape over the cornea every time the patient blinks. This is called 'trichiasis'. The entropion and trichiasis causes more and more corneal damage, and finally blindness.

At any stage the patient may get an acute bacterial infection in the eye, which can cause a lot more damage to the cornea.

Treatment

In the early stages, before entropion and trichiasis
Treat the patient with tetracycline or sulfonamide or both.
The usual method is:

1. For individual patients give tetracycline or oxytetracycline 1% eye ointment or oily drops at least twice daily (better 4 times daily) for 6 weeks.
2. For supervised treatment of groups of patients, put into each eye tetracycline or oxytetracycline 3% eye ointment (not the usual 1% which does not sting) at least once every day (better if twice daily) for 1 week in each month for 6 months.
3. For severe cases or cases when genital infection as well, tetracycline or doxycycline if not pregnant or a child (otherwise SMX/TMP or even sulfadimidine or erythromycin) orally for 2 weeks as well as the topical treatment. (For adult doses, see Chapter 11 pages 56–61.)
4. The best treatment is an oral macrolide drug, azithromycin, 1 g for adults and 20 mg/kg for children once only – although it may be best repeated in 6 months or more often. But it is expensive.
5. Treat also for vitamin A deficiency and onchocerciasis if these could be present

In the late stages of entropion and trichiasis

1. Remove any eyelashes that are scraping over the cornea. Pull them out with a pair of forceps. Do not cut them as this leaves a sharp end to scrape over the cornea.
2. Transfer the patient to a Medical Officer for an operation for the entropion, and other operations if necessary.

If there is acute bacterial infection at any stage
Treat quickly, as for corneal ulcer (see page 514).

Control and prevention

1. Kill the organism in the reservoir.
   Treat all infected cases early, when they are most infectious. School surveys may be necessary every 6 months, to find cases early. If trachoma is very common, give the teacher enough 3% tetracycline eye ointment to treat all the children once daily for 5 days, every month for 6 months. If more than 20% of the population is affected, it is worth considering treating all of the population.
2. Stop the means of spread.
   It is very important that there is enough water for regular washing of the hands and face. Give education about personal hygiene. Control of flies will help.
3. Immunisation is not yet possible.
4. Prophylactic treatment (see 1 above).

Corneal or scleral foreign bodies

Usually, there is a *history* of something going into the eye.
   Symptoms include:

1. pain in the eye,
2. the patient cannot open the eye properly, and
3. red, watering eye.

   Examination shows:

1. inflammation of the conjunctiva, and
2. foreign body on the cornea if you anaesthetise the cornea and stain it with fluorescein and examine with a light and loupe or an auriscope.

Treatment

1. Anaesthetise the eye with local anaesthetic or sterile eye drops (see pages 507, 509).
2. Stain the cornea with fluorescein (see page 507).
3. If the foreign body does not penetrate (go right through) the cornea into the eye, remove it. Remove the foreign body with the point of a large hypodermic needle. Hold the needle parallel to the surface of the eye with your hand resting on the patient's face. If the foreign body is iron, also remove any rust stain surrounding it.
4. Then treat as for corneal ulcer (see page 514).
5. Look for signs of infection inside the eye (pus in the anterior chamber, or the pupil small or irregular). If either of these are present, also treat for acute iritis (see pages 515–516).

Transfer to Medical Officer care

1. If the foreign body penetrates through into the eye. Do not try to remove it (urgent – emergency). Mean-

while treat for acute iritis — see pages 515–516 and give tetanus prophylaxis – see Chapter 25 page 420).
2. If you cannot remove the foreign body (urgent).
3. If you cannot see a foreign body but it may have gone right into the eye and still be there. This is especially important if the foreign body is made of iron (as it can destroy the sight).

> Always look for a foreign body in anyone who has a painful or red eye.

Corneal ulcer

A corneal ulcer is present when there is loss of part of the outside surface of the cornea (see Figure 31.9).

Corneal ulcers are caused by foreign bodies, abrasions (scraping types of injuries), drying (when the eyelids will not close, e.g. leprosy), ingrowing eyelashes (e.g. trachoma), other injuries, bacterial infections, herpes virus infections, fungal infections, onchocerciasis, vitamin A deficiency, chemicals especially lime, etc.

Symptoms include:

1. pain in the eye,
2. red watery eye, and
3. some loss of vision.

Signs:

1. The conjunctiva is inflamed.
2. You can see the ulcer on the cornea, but often only if you give a local anaesthetic and stain with fluorescein and use a torch and loupe or an auriscope. In areas where onchocerciasis occurs you

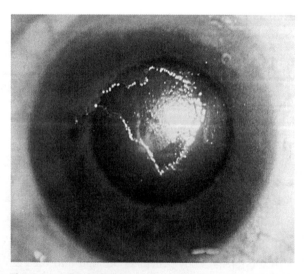

Figure 31.9 *Corneal ulcer.*

may find white areas deep in the cornea (but no surface ulcer); these slowly become bigger.
3. There is some loss of vision, if the ulcer is central.
4. Iritis (small pupil and pus in the anterior chamber) may be present if the ulcer penetrates (goes through) the cornea.
5. Foreign body or trichiasis or other cause may sometimes be found.

Treatment

Admit for inpatient treatment, unless the ulcer is very small.

1. Give antibiotic eye drops hourly during the day and 2 hourly in the night. Drops are more effective than ointment. In many places, only gentamicin drops are available. If drops containing several antibiotics (antibiotic compound eye drops) or chloramphenicol are available, use these instead.
2. If no drops are available or you cannot get anyone to put them in hourly and 2 hourly, use antibiotic ointment. If possible, use antibiotic compound eye ointment or chloramphenicol eye ointment four times a day. (Do not use any ointment or drops which contain hydrocortisone or prednisolone or cortisone-like drug.)
3. Keep a firm pad on the eye all the time. But do not pad the eye if there is a discharge from the eye.
4. Examine the eye (after staining with fluorescein) every day.
5. If the ulcer gets worse or iritis develops, treat for iritis – see pages 515–516.
6. If there is any possibility of vitamin A deficiency, give vitamin A immediately (see below); or if onchocerciasis treat for onchocerciasis (see page 516).

Transfer to Medical Officer care

1. if the ulcer gets worse (urgent);
2. if the ulcer does not improve within 2 days of the start of treatment (urgent);
3. if the ulcer has not almost healed after 5 days of treatment (non-urgent).

Note – There may be a scar for which no treatment is possible. Do not transfer if there is only a scar.

> Always look for a corneal ulcer in anyone with a red painful eye.

Vitamin A deficiency

Vitamin A deficiency, affecting the eyes, is common between the ages of 6 months and 6 years. It is uncommon in adults but can occur in pregnant or breastfeeding women or in adults of both sexes in times of famine or war. Other nutritional deficiencies are often present also and should be looked for and treated (see Chapter 23 page 379).

The earliest symptom or sign (not helpful in young children) is often not being able to see properly at night – night blindness.

Dryness of the conjunctiva and cornea (called 'xerophthalmia') is an important sign. The conjunctiva looks dry, roughened and wrinkled. Patches of dry non-wettable conjunctiva can be seen when the child stops crying. Bitot's spots are spots of white material often in groups on the conjunctiva near the cornea.

The eyelids can be red and swollen.

The eye can become painful and there is pain on looking into the light.

The cornea is then not clear and colourless as normal, but looks dry and a little dull and hazy.

In severe disease, a spreading white spot appears on the cornea. A large corneal ulcer may form. The cornea may break open. This can occur suddenly, especially if the patient gets measles. Blindness follows.

Prevention is by eating a diet with enough vitamin A, especially fruits and vegetables with orange or dark green colouring, red palm oil and if available, liver, meat, fish and eggs. If a good diet is not possible, a single oral dose of a capsule of 200,000 IU of vitamin A every 6 months will prevent the condition.

Treatment is by oral synthetic vitamin A or retinol 100,000 IU (55 mg) for those under 1 year old and 200,000 IU (110 mg) for those over 1 year old, immediately and repeated the next day and again in 2 (1–4) weeks later. If vomiting give 100,000 IU (55 mg) of a water soluble vitamin A (retinol) IMI instead. Pregnant women should be given lower doses, as high doses may cause abnormalities in unborn babies – 5000 IU or 5.5 mg orally or IMI daily for 2 weeks. If any involvement of the cornea, apply antibiotic ointment, carefully close the lid and pad the eye; but do not bandage tightly or press the pad onto the eye. If a white area in the cornea or a corneal ulcer, give also an oral antibiotic.

If you see an eye affected by vitamin A deficiency, do not forget that you must not only treat 'first the eye' as above, but also 'second the child' (for vitamin and other nutritional problems), 'third the kitchen' (so that a better diet stops this and other nutritional conditions occurring in the patient and the family in the future) and 'fourth the community' (to improve nutrition and prevent others getting this and other nutritional problems).

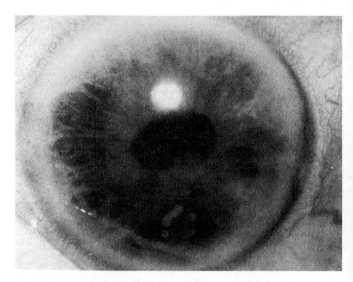

Figure 31.10 *Acute iritis. Note that: (1) There are dilated blood vessels in the conjunctiva around the cornea (not present all over the conjunctiva). (2) The anterior chamber is not clear. (3) The pupil is small and irregular – it does not dilate in a dark place.*

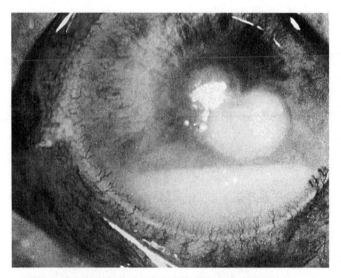

Figure 31.11 *Acute iritis with hypopyon. Note that: (1) The circum-corneal conjunctival vessels are enlarged. (2) A corneal ulcer is present (the cause of the iritis). (3) The pus has settled to the bottom of the anterior chamber (called hypopyon). (4) The anterior chamber is all cloudy, so that you cannot see the small irregular pupil clearly.*

Acute iritis (or iridocyclitis or anterior uveitis)

Acute iritis is an acute inflammation of the eye, including the anterior chamber and iris.

Causes include:

1. infection from outside the eye (e.g. after injuries or corneal ulcer);
2. infection which started inside the eye, i.e. taken there by the blood (e.g. leprosy, TB, syphilis, toxoplasmosis, septicaemia, onchocerciasis, herpes, etc. – especially in HIV infected patients);
3. non-infective causes (e.g. autoimmune diseases (rheumatoid disease and spondyloarthritis), leprosy reaction; etc.); and
4. no cause diagnosed (many cases if it is not infection).

Symptoms include:

1. severe pain in the eye, made worse by light, and
2. loss of some vision.

Signs include:

1. inflammation of the conjunctiva around the edge of the cornea only (not under the eyelids);
2. pus in the anterior chamber (cloudy anterior chamber called a 'flare' or hypopyon, see Figure 13.11);
3. collections of pus cells like white dots on the back of the cornea;
4. pupil irregular and small and does not contract and dilate normally;
5. eye tender when touched through the eyelid;
6. loss of some vision;
7. you may find the cause of the iritis (see above).
   See Figures 31.10 and 31.11.

Treatment

Try to find the cause. Always stain the cornea with fluorescein, and look for foreign body and ulcer and vitamin A deficiency – see page 514. Always think of infection and if this could be because the patient has also an HIV infection. Always look for leprosy, and especially a leprosy reaction (see Chapter 15 page 138); always look for onchocerciasis (see Chapter 32 pages 542–544).

If the cause is obvious, e.g. corneal injury or ulcer or vitamin A deficiency, treat as usual and as below.

If the patient could have onchocerciasis treat for this and as below.

If the cause is leprosy or you cannot find the cause, treat as below *and* also transfer to Medical Officer care (urgent).

1. Antibiotic eye ointment – use antibiotic compound ointment or chloramphenicol put under the lower lid every 3 hours.
2. Atropine sulfate 1% eye ointment – put under the lower lid four times a day, until the pupil is widely dilated, and then once daily.

3. Keep a firm pad on the eye all the time. But do not pad the eye if it is discharging.
4. Chloramphenicol 1 g every 6 hours – give by IMI if necessary. Reduce the dose to 750 mg four times a day when the patient improves.
5. Acetylsalicylic acid 500–1000 mg with, if needed codeine 30 mg should be given every 6 hours for pain, if necessary.

Continue the treatment for 10 days, or until all the redness goes and the eye is completely better (up to 3 weeks), whichever is the longer.

Transfer to Medical Officer care:

1. All cases urgently (unless the cause is a corneal injury or ulcer you can treat and the condition does quickly (in 2 days) improve on treatment) as most cases will need:
   (a) special tests to tell what is the cause,
   (b) special antibiotics for some of the infections,
   (c) systemic or topical corticosteroids, as well as
   (d) treatment of any cause found.
2. Any case you treat which is not greatly improved in 2 days and cured in 2 weeks.

Always look for acute iritis in anyone with a painful red eye.

Onchocerciasis (river blindness)

See Chapter 32 pages 542–544 for description and treatment of this disease.

See also 'Conjunctivitis' (page 511), 'Corneal ulcer' (page 514) and 'Acute iritis' (page 515).

The eye damage is caused by the very many microfilaria which get into all parts of the eye.

The cornea can gradually develop white scarring in it (not due to an ulcer), which starts at the edges of the lower half of the cornea and slowly spreads inwards and upwards and eventually the whole cornea can be scarred.

A chronic iritis (iridocyclitis or anterior uveitis) (see page 515) can develop.

Glaucoma (see page 517) is not common but can develop.

Cataract (see page 517) can occur.

Retinopathy (damage to the retina) occurs, but an opthalmoscope or slit lamp would be needed to see these changes in the retina.

The optic nerve carrying sight to the brain from the eye can also be damaged.

The loss of vision can be of any type; but once it has occurred, treatment usually does not bring sight back.

The way to prevent blindness, therefore, is to give treatment for onchocerciasis with ivermectin *before* significant problems with sight are present. (Ivermectin kills the microfilaria (without producing a dangerous reaction as diethylcarbamazine can) and for many months stops the females producing microfilaria). If any patient in an area where onchocerciasis occurs, develops any problem with his eyes, it would be best to treat him with ivermectin immediately and then at least every year (see Chapter 32 page 543). Better, all people in such areas should be treated with ivermectin. The best thing would be to eliminate (get rid of) onchocerciasis completely. Some countries are already doing this. However, of the 100 million at risk from this disease only 5 million have been treated regularly with ivermectin. New drugs such as moxidectin, which may kill the adult worms, may become available. Nodules containing adult worms near the eyes may be best surgically removed.

Glaucoma

Glaucoma occurs when the fluid produced in the eye is not absorbed properly and the pressure inside the eye becomes high.

If this happens quickly, as in *closed angle glaucoma*, the eye becomes inflamed with:
• red conjunctivae around the cornea,
• cloudiness of the cornea,
• the anterior chamber difficult to see,
• the pupils large, oval and dilated,
• the eye is hard in comparison to the normal eye and tender to touch, and
• there is great loss of sight.

Transfer all such cases (emergency) to the Medical Officer for possible operation.

If this happens slowly it causes *open angle glaucoma*. There are three symptoms and signs:
1. gradual loss of vision – the normal blind spot all people have gradually gets larger and the things at the edge of what can be seen get less – but this happens so slowly over years that many people do not notice it until a lot of the sight is lost.
2. changes in the appearance of the optic disc of the retina; but these need an ophthalmoscope or slit lamp to see.
3. a rise in the pressure of the fluid inside the eye, but this needs a special instrument to measure.

Anyone can get open angle glaucoma; but it is more common:

1. as people get older,
2. in certain families,
3. in people from Africa and the Caribbean (especially West Africa, where even young people can be affected).

Treatment is usually by surgery as medical treatment would be with pilocarpine or timolol or other eye drops regularly for the rest of the patient's life (and this is expensive, may not be used regularly, may have side effects, needs regular checks to see if it is still working properly, etc.).

This condition is a large problem as 1% of the population of the world suffers from it and diagnosis is difficult without special equipment. Find out what is available for diagnosis and treatment where you work. If anyone has any loss of sight, especially if they are from one of the above groups, refer them to the Medical Officer or any ophthalmologist who is available for diagnosis and possible treatment.

Cataract

A cataract has formed if the clear lens of the eye becomes cloudy and will not allow the light to get through into the eye.

Causes include:
1. rubella infection of fetus during pregnancy;
2. a large number of illnesses including diabetes and kidney failure and drugs including alcohol and tobacco and adrenocorticosteroids if given for a long time;
3. a large number of eye infections, injuries and conditions;
4. old age;
5. living in a hot/tropical country with a lot of sunlight;
6. others.

Symptoms: Slow loss of vision, which continues to get worse, is usually the only symptom.

Signs include:
1. The pupil is white not black when you shine a light into it. At first, this may be only in the centre or the edge, but gradually the white areas get larger until the whole lens is white.
2. There is loss of vision which varies from little to total.

Treatment
The only thing which can help is an operation to remove the lens, which will allow the light through and to put a new plastic lens in. (If a new lens is not

put in the patient would have to wear very thick glasses which are hard to use and expensive.) Ophthalmologists (eye doctors) may visit your area at special times to do these operations. Medical Officers and now some paramedical workers are being trained to do this operation. Special help is available in many developing countries to get very cheap lenses. The treatment is very successful and patients can usually see very well again (almost back to normal). Find out what is available in your country.

In most places, the operation is done only when cataracts are in both eyes and the patient is not able to see well enough to continue normal living. Usually, only one eye has the surgery at one time.

Make a list of all patients with cataracts you see, so when cataract surgery is being done in your area, you can send all these people for possible surgery.

Diabetic retinopathy

Diabetic retinopathy is damage to the retina caused by weakness of or leak from or block of the blood vessels in the retina caused by diabetes mellitus (see Chapter 30 page 499) that has been present for years.

After 20 years, almost all Type 1 IDDM and a half of the Type 2 NIDDM patients will have diabetic retinopathy. Diabetic retinopathy will be less bad in patients who have good control of their diabetes with blood sugars near to normal.

There may be loss of vision.

It can be diagnosed only with the use of an ophthalmoscope and only after training to be able to recognise it.

It can be treated only with the use of a laser.

If an ophthalmologist (eye doctor) is available or regularly visits and has a laser, then all diabetic patients should be sent to him regularly as he directs, e.g. each year, to see if their diabetic retinopathy has got worse and if it needs treatment to stop blindness developing.

Prevention is by diet and exercise and if needed insulin or oral drugs to keep the blood sugars as close to normal as possible.

Macular degeneration

The macular is the place on the retina which is most sensitive to light and where the eye focuses the light from the thing we look directly at.

In older people new blood vessels can form here, leak and cause scar tissue to form, which decreases sight in days to weeks. Much more often, the scar tissue is just slowly formed without leaks from blood vessels

and sight decreases over months to years. Usually, both eyes are affected. This is called 'age related macular degeneration' (ARMD). Occasional cases occur for different reasons in younger people.

The patient loses central vision and sees things that he looks at less clearly than things seen out of the 'side of his eye or vision.

The condition cannot be diagnosed and treated in the health centre without an ophthalmoscope. Treatment is not usually possible even in the hospital.

Retinal detachment

The retina can occasionally detach (or peel off) the back of the eye.

Affected patients are usually myopic (short-sighted) or have had a cataract operation or have had an eye injury.

The patient may have noted black spots floating around in his eye ('floaters') for years and 'flashing lights' recently and then loss of sight from one side of his eye (like a curtain being pulled across the eye). The loss of sight can stop or keep going until a lot or all of the sight in that eye is gone.

The condition cannot be diagnosed in a health centre without an ophthalmoscope.

In some hospitals an eye doctor can put the retina back on again as long as the patient is seen soon after the detachment occurred – not weeks later. If you have a patient who may have this condition, transfer the patient urgently to the Medical Officer; but only if he says he can help.

Long sight and short sight

Short sight (or myopia) is present when a patient cannot see things a long way away but can see things well if they are close.

The diagnosis is almost certain if you get the person to look at things in the distance through a small hole (pinhole) in a card and he can then see them much better.

This condition usually develops slowly during childhood until early adult life. It is due to the eyeball growing too long or the lens being too strong or the curvature of the cornea being too much.

Long sight (hypermetropia) is the opposite – people may see things well at a distance but cannot see things well if they are close, e.g are unable to read a book. Try the pinhole test. Long sight usually develops in middle-aged and older people.

Presbyopia (presby means old) occurs as people get older. The lens becomes harder and will not change shape to focus the light on the retina when things close or far away are looked at — both long sight and short sight develop.

Astigmatism occurs when the cornea is not symmetrical (the same shape on all sides) and when light comes into the eye some is focused in front of, some on and some behind the retina (instead of all on the retina). The patient has blurred sight, which he tries to help by changing the focus of the eyes repeatedly. He may seem to be frowning and may complain of tired eyes. He can see much better looking through the pinhole.

These patients may have no other abnormality of the eye.

Examination shows all these patients cannot see the small part of the eye chart if he has short sight, or small print held at normal reading distance from the eyes if he has long sight. There is no other abnormality.

If the patient cannot see enough for normal living, refer or transfer him non-urgently to the ophthalmologist (eye specialist), who will give him glasses to wear. Some paramedical workers have been taught how to give the correct glasses to people with these problems.

If this is not possible, the patient may be able to buy spectacles (glasses) in the market or shop to help him see better.

Strabismus (squint)

The two eyes do not look in the same direction at the same time.

Causes include:

1. abnormal development in a child (unknown cause),
2. trauma, and
3. disease of brain or the nerves (e.g. diabetes) to the eye.

Treatment

If a child has a squint, refer or non-urgently transfer the patient to the eye specialist. It is essential that this is done before he is 5–7 years old, as otherwise the patient may become blind in one of the eyes.

Eye injuries

Bruising of eyelids

No treatment is necessary.

Sub-conjunctival haemorrhage

If you can see all of the edges of the haemorrhage (even if part of the edge goes right up to the cornea or the eyelid edge), then the haemorrhage is probably not serious and probably no treatment is needed.

It will go away by itself.

However, if the haemorrhage extends towards the back of the eye and you cannot see where it ends, then the bleeding may be from behind the eye as a result of a skull fracture. This could be serious, so the patient should be transferred to a Medical Officer for care.

Corneal abrasions

Treat as for a corneal ulcer (see page 514).

Hyphaema (blood in the anterior chamber)

Order complete rest in bed and an eye pad until all the blood goes.

Transfer urgently to Medical Officer care if most of the anterior chamber is filled with blood (for urgent surgery).

Iris damage

Treatment does not help. Treat other conditions present.

Cataract after injury

No curative treatment is possible. If there is severe pain or loss of sight, transfer urgently for surgery.

Wounds of the eyelids

Carefully suture to make the edges of the eyelids level.

All penetrating wounds of cornea and sclera

Urgent transfer to Medical Officer care is necessary. Meanwhile, treat as acute iritis and give tetanus prophylaxis.

Eye conditions in patients with HIV infection

Ophthalmic herpes zoster (eye affected by shingles)

This may occur early in the HIV infection. Suspect HIV in any otherwise healthy adult with this condition (but not all have HIV infection) (see page 153).

Complications are common and 30% become blind in that eye.

Transfer such cases quickly.

Conjunctival carcinoma (cancer of the conjunctiva)

This also may come early in HIV infection and may be due to the papilloma virus and HIV together.

If a slow growing tumour appears on the conjunctiva, transfer such patients quickly for surgery.

Molluscum contagiosum

This needs treatment if it occurs on the eyelid and causes conjunctivitis (see Chapter 32 page 546).

Kaposi's sarcoma

This causes a black lump on the eyelids or a bright red lump on the conjunctiva.

No eye treatment is usually possible; but see Chapter 19 page 232.

Dilated conjunctival vessels

Due to the HIV virus usually. Make sure it is not one of the other causes of conjunctivitis.

No treatment is needed.

Lymphoma of orbit

Tumour of lymphatic system in the eye – socket behind the eye, pushing the eye out (exophthalmos).

Think of thyrotoxicosis (page 498). Transfer suspected cases for diagnosis and possible treatment.

Corneal ulcers

These are often due to herpes simplex virus and are at the edge of the cornea (see page 514).

Transfer such cases for special treatment.

Acute iritis or uveitis

See page 515. This is much more common if HIV infection.

Transfer all such patients.

Damage to the retina

Damage can be done by the HIV virus itself or other infections but cannot be seen without an ophthalmoscope.

These can cause gradual or fairly rapid loss of sight.

Transfer patients for diagnosis and treatment.

Problems of diagnosis and management

Painful or red eye

Take a history of the present illness and also about the loss of sight, pain, redness and discharge.

Do a full examination of the eye, see pages 506–507.

1. *Find out where the redness is*

    If it is all over the conjunctiva (on the undersurface of the eyelids as well as around the cornea) then diagnose:
    • conjunctivitis (see page 511), or
    • foreign body or chemical in eye (see page 511).

If it is mainly around the cornea, then diagnose:
    • corneal ulcer, or
    • corneal foreign body, or
    • iritis, or   } (see 2 below)
    • acute glaucoma.

2. *Put fluorescein into the eye* (see pages 507 and 509)

    If the cornea stains green in some parts, then diagnose:
    • corneal ulcer (see page 514), or
    • corneal foreign body (see page 513).

    If the cornea is normal, then diagnose:
    • iritis, or   } (see 3 below)
    • glaucoma.

3. *Find out the size of the pupil*

    If the pupil is small, then diagnose iritis. See page 515.

    If the pupil is large, then diagnose glaucoma (see page 517). Transfer to Medical Officer (urgent if there is still some sight in the eye).

Loss of vision/sight

1. Eye painful or red:
    • foreign body or chemical in eye,
    • corneal ulcer,
    • acute iritis,
    • acute glaucoma.

    See painful red eye and causes and treatment of these (see this page).

    Urgent treatment essential.

    Urgent referral often needed.

2. Eye painless and quiet/white (not red):
    • Refractive errors (long- and short-sightedness, etc.).
    Vision improves with pinhole test.
    Spectacles needed non-urgently.
    • Opacities in cornea (scars), lens (cataracts), other parts.
    Opacities seen with light shone into eye.
    Surgery by eye doctor needed non-urgently.
    • Diseases of the retina or optic nerve, etc.
    Diabetic retinopathy – diabetic for many years.
    Open angle glaucoma – see page 517.
    Macular degeneration – old person with gradual loss of sight in both eyes (see page 518).
    Detachment of retina – sudden progressive loss of vision in eye in predisposed person (see page 518).

    Not able to be diagnosed in health centre without ophthalmoscope.

    Referral to eye doctor needed.

    Non-urgent except retinal detachment, when urgent if doctor can do the needed surgery.

32 Disorders of the Skin

Anatomy and physiology

The skin has a number of functions:

1. protection of the body from things outside the body – mechanical injury, heat, cold, light, chemicals, organisms, etc;
2. keeping salt, water, tissue fluid, tissues, organs and other things inside the body;
3. keeping the temperature of the body normal, e.g. by sweating when the body is too hot; and
4. taking sensations into the body, e.g. touch, pain, heat, cold, etc.

Pathology

There are many different types of lesions of the skin. See Figure 32.2 for illustrations of these.

1. *Macule* (or macular lesion)
   A macule is an area of skin which is different from the surrounding skin. It is not raised above the level of the skin surface. You can see (e.g. different colour) and/or feel it in the skin.
2. *Papule* (or papular lesion)
   A papule is like a macule, but it is raised above the level of the skin surface.
3. *Nodule* (or nodular lesion)
   A nodule is an area of skin which is different but is raised above the surface, but larger than a papule (> 1 cm in diameter).
4. *Vesicle* (or vesicular lesion)
   A vesicle is like a papule, but there is clear fluid under the surface of the lesion.
5. *Pustule* (or pustular lesion)
   A pustule is like a vesicle, but the fluid contains pus.

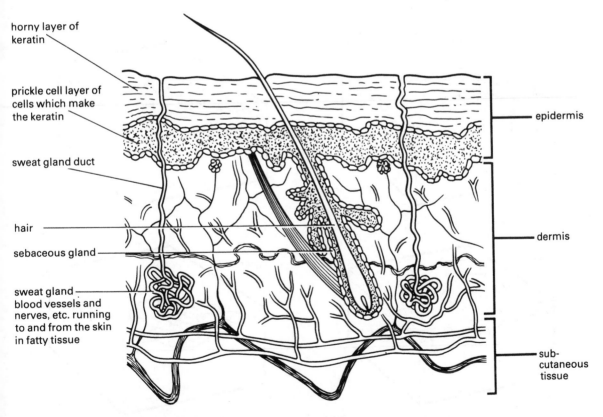

horny layer of keratin

prickle cell layer of cells which make the keratin

sweat gland duct

hair

sebaceous gland

sweat gland blood vessels and nerves, etc. running to and from the skin in fatty tissue

epidermis

dermis

sub-cutaneous tissue

Figure 32.1 *Diagram to show the structure of the skin under the microscope. In some parts of the body certain parts of the structure of the skin are more marked than usual (e.g. thick horny layer on the soles of the feet).*

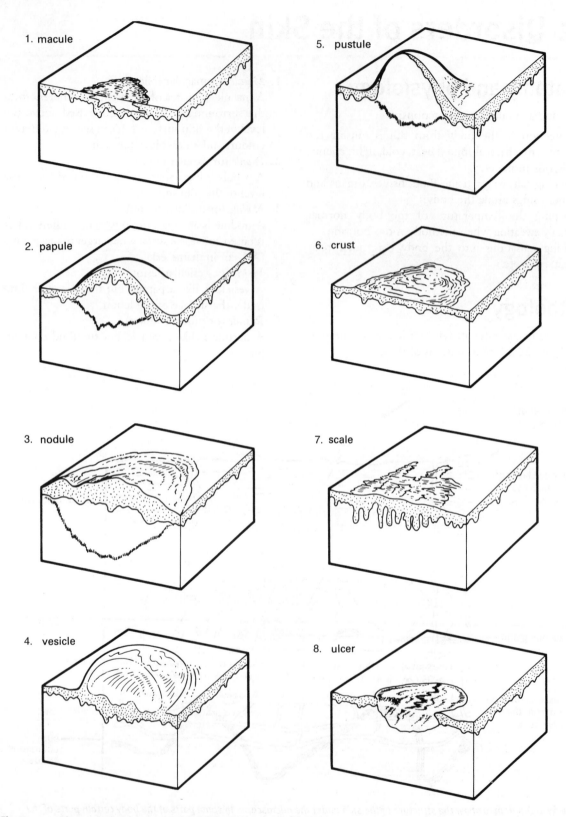

Figure 32.2 *Diagrams showing some of the different types of skin lesion.*

6. *Crust*

A crust is dried exudate (fluid which comes from the lesion) and may consist of:
• serum (yellow),
• blood (red or brown),
• pus (yellow, grey, green), or
• mixtures of these.

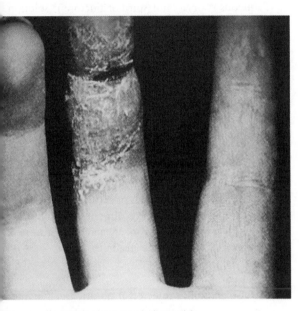

Figure 32.3 *Acute eczematous dermatitis.*

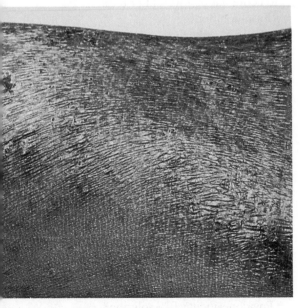

Figure 32.4 *Chronic eczematous dermatitis. The area has become 'lichenified' – the skin is thick and dry and the normal creases are deep.*

7. *Scales* are built up surface layers of the skin. They may be:
• yellow and greasy (e.g. seborrhoeic dermatitis),
• silvery (e.g. psoriasis), or
• grey (e.g. eczema).

8. *Ulcers* are areas where the skin has been destroyed.

9. *Dermatitis* is any inflammation of the skin. There are many different types of dermatitis.

10. *Eczema* (or eczematous reaction or eczematous dermatitis).

Eczema is the most common type of dermatitis (see Figures 32.3 and 32.4). In the acute stage the affected area gets red, shiny and warm because the blood vessels widen. Then small vesicles appear on the surface of the skin. These vesicles soon burst. The exudate dries and forms a crust. Secondary bacterial infection may occur. After some time chronic eczema develops. The affected area may be thick, dry, scaly and the normal lines in the skin become very deep (called lichenification). Cracks can develop deep into the flesh underneath.

Diagnosis and treatment of skin conditions

Sometimes you can easily recognise the symptoms and signs of a certain disease. If you cannot, then do a full history and examination and test the urine (see Chapter 6). Look at the skin *all over* the body. Decide which of the two main groups of skin conditions your patient is in:

1. *Generalised illness with a skin condition*, e.g. chickenpox, measles, syphilis, yaws, leprosy or other infections; malnutrition; allergic reaction to a drug; etc.

2. *Localised skin conditions*, i.e. conditions affecting only the skin.

Important causes include:
(a) external parasites, e.g. scabies, lice;
(b) fungal infections, e.g. tinea;
(c) bacterial infections, e.g. impetigo;
(d) eczematous dermatitis which has many causes;
(e) itching which causes scratching which causes damage to the skin (i.e. dermatitis) which causes more itching …

Localised skin conditions are very common and important, and so you should know about:

1. the preparations that are available to treat localised skin conditions; and

2. how to use these skin preparations.

Preparations NOT to use

Vaseline and mineral oil are often used in many places to try to soften the skin, keep it moist, and make it look healthy and shiny. These, however, cover and block the small holes in the skin through which sweat glands and sebaceous glands bring the secretions they make onto the surface of the skin (to keep the skin moisturised, healthy and shiny). The secretions then have to collect in the glands, which swell up and cause irritation and inflammation of the skin. Organisms find this a good place to grow and bacterial and fungal infection often follows. *Ask patients who have skin problems if they put vaseline or mineral oil on their skin. If they do, advise them to stop. Aqueous cream or emulsifying ointment can be used instead* and can be bought in shops and pharmacies. Vegetable oils, put on when the skin is still wet, keep the skin moist.

Preparations to use

Lotions or creams are used if the skin condition the patient has is acutely inflamed and is moist or weeping (fluid coming through the skin or the abnormality in the skin).

Ointments or pastes are used if the skin condition is chronic and dry and lichenified (see page 523).

Preparations often available for treatment of skin conditions

Those on the WHO list of essential drugs are marked with an asterisk (*). Those you need to prepare or make yourself are marked with a superscript number [1]; and directions on how to make them up are on pages 525–526. You may find other preparations are supplied and common ones of these are included.

You do not need all of these preparations.

1. *Antibacterial preparations*
   - Eusol[1] solution
     – use for dressings if there is a lot of pus or dead tissue in the lesion
     – stop when the lesion is clean
   - Antiseptics
     – hexachlorophene 3% emulsion – use with water to clean the skin or a lesion
     – chlorhexidine compound solution in either water or spirit (alcoholic) solution – use to clean the skin or a lesion
   - Antibiotics
     – antibiotic compound ointment (e.g. neomycin 5 mg and bacitracin 500 IU/g ointment)*
     – antibiotic compound powder
     – powder from inside a tetracycline capsule (use no other antibiotics in this way)
     – silver sulfasalazine 1% or silver sulfadiazine 1% (usually with chlorhexidine) cream* (often kept just for patients with burns)
   - Methylrosanilinium chloride, usually called crystal violet or gentian violet, 0.5% in either water ('aqueous')* or alcohol (spirit or 'tincture')* solution. Use only the water solution and never the alcohol solution on mucous membranes
   - Iodine 2.5% solution in spirit (alcohol) – use to clean a lesion of the skin
   - Povidone-iodine (polyvidone-iodine) 10% solution*
   - Povidone-iodine 7.5-10% in alcohol or water preparation
   - Acriflavine emulsion (use only with strong 3% saline[1] dressing); stop when infection goes or the acriflavine will stop the skin healing
   - Potassium permanganate (Condy's crystals) 1:10,000 solution[1] in water*, a pinch of crystals in a bucket of water (a pink not purple colour); needs to be made up freshly as it does not work after an hour or so; soak dressing in it or bathe the area in it
   - Honey[1]
   - Sugar paste[1]

   Give also an oral or injected antibiotic (see Chapter 11 pages 56–61) if there is a severe infection.

2. Preparations for dressings to get dead tissue and pus to come out of a wound or ulcer
   - Eusol solution[1]
   - Strong 3% saline[1]
   - Honey[1]
   - Sugar paste[1]
   - Acriflavine emulsion with 3% saline

   Stop once wound is clean.

3. *Antifungal preparations*
   - Benzoic acid 6% and salicylic acid 3% cream or ointment* or benzoic acid compound ointment (Whitfield's ointment) (also helps thick skin soften and peel off)
   - Salicylic acid 10% paint
   - Methylrosanilinium chloride (gentian violet) 0.5% solution in water* or spirit (alcohol), but is useful for only *Candida* ('thrush') (see above)
   - Potassium permanganate (Condy's crystals) 1:10,000 solution[1] in water* (see above)
   - Iodine 2.5% solution in spirit (alcohol)
   - Povidone-iodine 10% solution*
   - Povidone-iodine 7.5-10% in spirit (alcohol) or water preparations

---

1 For details of how to make this, see pages 525–526.

- Sodium thiosulfate 15% solution* (for tinea versicolor only)
- Miconazole 2% ointment or cream*
- Selenium sulfide detergent based suspension 2%*
- Honey[1]

4. Anti-inflammatory preparations

These are used for eczema and other dermatitis and to help healing.

- Potassium permanganate (Condy's crystals) 1:10,000 solution[1] in water* (see above)
- Aluminium diacetate 5%* or 10% or 13% solution (Burow's solution) in water – dilute before using
- Weak 1% saline[1] solution
- Calamine lotion*
- Zinc cream
- Glycerine and ichthammol
- Cod liver oil ointment
- Wool fat anhydrous (lanoline)
- Ammoniated mercury ointment 2.5% (Ung. HAD)
- Hydrocortisone 1% cream or ointment* for use on face, genitalia and other places and babies; but only if any infection is being controlled
- Betamethasone 0.1% (or other fluorinated corticosteroid cream and ointment*; more powerful than hydrocortisone but never to be used on the face, genitalia or babies or if infection not controlled).

5. Anti-itch preparations

- Anti-inflammatory preparations but especially
Weak 1% saline[1] solution
Potassium permanganate (Condy's crystals) 1:10,000 solution[1] in water* (see above)
Calamine lotion*
Anti-inflammatory steroid preparations (see above)
- Give also an antihistamine orally or by injection or small dose (10 mg) of amitriptyline if required

6. Anti-external parasite preparations

- Benzyl benzoate 25% solution*
- Iodine solution 2.5% – dilute immediately before use with an equal volume of water
- Carbaryl 0.5% or 1% lotion and 1% shampoo
- Malathion 0.5% lotion and 1% shampoo
- Permethrin 5% (50 mg/g) cream*
- Permethrin 1% (10 mg/g) lotion*
- Gamma benzene hexachloride (lindane 1% solution) no longer recommended
- DDT 2% emulsion – not recommended and usually not available
- DDT 10% powder – not recommended and usually not available

7. *Skin structure changing preparations (on WHO essential medicines list but some often not obtainable)*

- Benzyl peroxide 25% lotion* or cream
- Coal tar 5% solution* (usually used as a paste or ointment) – has anti-inflammatory and anti-itch actions and often used instead of corticosteroids; usually put on at night and wash off in the morning as sunlight can cause irritation
- Dithramol 0.1–2% ointment*
- Fluorouracil 5% ointment*
- Podophyllum resin 10–25% solution*
- Salicylic acid 5% solution
- Urea 10% ointment or cream; a strong moisturiser and also softens dry thick skin

8. *A number of preparations have more than one function and can be very useful if the diagnosis is not certain, or if two or more conditions are present, e.g.:*

- Potassium permanganate solution
  - anti-inflammatory
  - anti-itch
  - antifungal
  - antibacterial
- Methylrosanilinium chloride (crystal violet)
  - antibacterial
  - antifungal (for *Candida* ('thrush') only)
- Iodine solution
  - antibacterial
  - antifungal
  - antiscabies
  - (but iodine can itself cause a rash in some people)

How to make simple useful skin preparations

Eusol solution

Mix chlorinated lime 12.5 g (20 ml) with enough water to make a paste. Add a little more water and shake. Add boric acid 12.5 g (20 ml) and shake. Add enough water to make 1 litre. Shake well. Leave overnight. Filter. Store in a dark coloured bottle. Note that Eusol is a clear solution with the smell of chlorine. It does not store well and you should use it within a week. If the solution is more than a week old, or does not smell of chlorine, throw it away.

Potassium permanganate 1:10,000 solution

Dissolve $1\frac{1}{4}$ ml or $\frac{1}{4}$ of a teaspoonful (not heaped) of potassium permanganate (Condy's crystals) in 10 litres ($\frac{1}{2}$ bucketful) of clean water. It is a dark pink but not a purple colour.

Strong (3%) saline

Dissolve $7\frac{1}{2}$ ml ($1\frac{1}{2}$ teaspoonful, not heaped) of salt in 200 ml (1 cup) of clean water.

Weak (1%) saline

Dissolve $2\frac{1}{2}$ ml ($\frac{1}{2}$ teaspoonful, not heaped) of salt in 200 ml (1 cup) of clean water.

Honey

Most ordinary honey is suitable but some are much better than others. A hospital laboratory may test various kinds for you on an agar plate with bacteria to see which is best. Otherwise, put the same amount of the different kinds of honey you can get into similar little containers of milk and see which one takes the longest for the milk to go sour. Use this kind of honey for dressings.

To keep flies away when using a honey dressing on a patient, use a dressing able to absorb quite a lot of honey but also later some pus, etc. Then cover this with a piece of plastic sheeting (or plastic bag or food wrap) and seal the edges of this with adhesive tape). Stand the legs of the patient's bed in cans containing water or oil if there is a problem in keeping ants away.

Honey kills most bacteria and some fungi and cleans wounds quickly.

Sugar paste

This is less messy than honey and may be nearly as effective.

- Hydrogen peroxide 30% (100 vol) (take care as this can burn until diluted) 7.5 ml is added to:
- Glycerine 480 ml and stirred, then add and mix
- Caster sugar 400 mg
- Icing sugar 500 mg

or if unavailable, ordinary white sugar 1 kg crushed (with a mortar and pestle or rolling pin on board, etc.).

Dressings

Use a *wet gauze bandage* for all painful conditions on legs, arms, feet, hands, and head, especially if you think they will heal slowly.

Use *adhesive plaster* for all small painless conditions on rounded parts of the body, joints, etc.

Use *crepe bandages* for all painful conditions on joints and thighs, and for large deep ulcers, wounds, etc. anywhere.

Use *elastic plaster bandage* on soles, palms and early boils.

Use dry *gauze bandages* only for tinea of the feet. (See Table 32.1.)

Note these things about treatment

1. Do not make a dermatitis worse by treatment which irritates the already damaged skin. (For example, do not immediately use Whitfield's ointment on an acutely inflamed fungal infection. It is better to use potassium permanganate solution wet dressings to start with until the condition is not acute. Then you can use the Whitfield's ointment (see Figure 32.7).)
2. You must treat any bacterial infection.
3. Always look for signs of scabies and lice if there is (a) an itch or (b) skin infection, especially (c) more than one area is affected and especially (d) it returns after treatment.
4. Always treat an itch which causes scratching. If you do not treat the itch, the scratching causes dermatitis and the dermatitis causes more itch and more scratching …
5. Always think of the possibility that drugs or skin treatment have caused the skin problem – especially skin in the sun. Treatment for a condition, which has gone, may have caused a new skin condition.

The common skin conditions

For the common skin conditions due to:

- fungi, see pages 527–531,
- bacteria, see pages 532–538,
- insects, see pages 538–540,
- worms, see pages 542–546,

Table 32.1 Dressings for skin conditions.

		Cost	Pain relief?	Helps healing?	Stays on?	Pain when removed?
Gauze bandage (WOW)	Wet	Cheap	Good	Good	Good	No pain
	Dry	Cheap	Some	Some	Poor	No pain
Adhesive plaster		Very cheap	None	None	Good in dry weather	A little painful
Elastic plaster bandage		Expensive	Some	Some	Good	Very painful
Crepe bandage		Expensive	Very good	Very good	Good	No pain

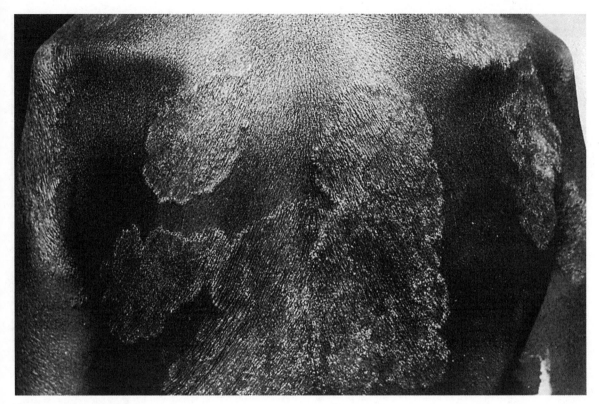

Figure 32.5 *Tinea of the body.*

- viruses, see pages 546–547,
- protozoa, see page 538 and see other chapters,
- diet, see page 547 and see other chapters,
- eczematous reactions, see pages 548–549,
- other causes, see pages 549–551.

Tinea

Tinea is an infection of the skin with one of many fungal organisms.

Complaints include itching and worry about the appearance of the skin.

Examination usually shows affected areas of skin that are roughly circular. The edges are often a little raised and a little inflamed. Sometimes there are small papules, vesicles or pustules at the edge. The skin in the rest of the lesion is often peeling. Hairs are usually broken off at scalp level leaving a black dot in the hair follicle. The centre of the lesion may appear to be healing. (This is why it is sometimes called 'ring worm' (see Figure 32.5).)

Tinea may infect the main parts of the body (trunk or limbs); or only the scalp, the groin, the feet, or the nails. The appearances are a little different in each place. Tinea imbricata is a little different in appearance and more difficult to treat. (See Figures 32.6, 32.7 and 32.8.)

Make sure the lesion is not caused by leprosy. Do tests for loss of sensation, etc. If you have real doubts, do a biopsy (but not on face). Scrapings of skin and cut off pieces of nail can be sent to the laboratory (if it does these tests) with a request for examination for tinea or fungal organisms.

If the tinea is severe or widespread or comes back after successful treatment or is unusual in any way, or if there is tinea of the scalp on anyone older than a child, always check for HIV infection.

Routine treatment (but not for an acutely inflamed area)

Treat as an outpatient.

1. Remove any hair from the affected area.
2. Wash the affected area with soap and water every day. Rub off any scales. Dry the skin well after washing. Keep the skin as dry as possible.
3. Put benzoic acid and salicylic acid ointment (Whitfield's ointment) (or salicylic acid paint or other benzoic acid and salicylic acid paint, cream or ointment) on the affected area twice daily. Put it on the normal skin for

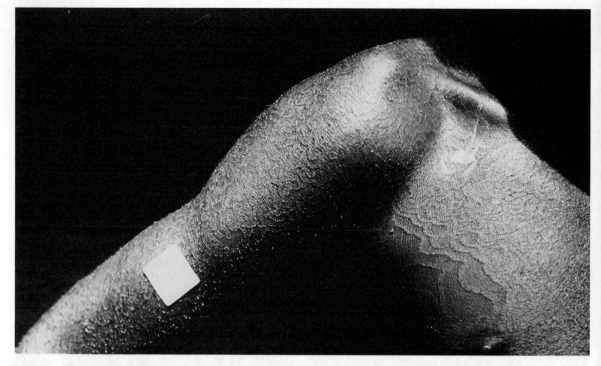

Figure 32.6 *Tinea imbricata. There is an abnormality in the immunity of many of these patients. This is probably inherited, because the disease is common in certain families. The disease usually returns, even after successful treatment.*

2 cm round the edge of the affected area also. Do not cover more than one quarter of the body every day (covering the whole body can cause death).

4. Change and wash the clothes every day (if possible).
5. Continue the treatment every day until all the tinea goes and then for 2–4 weeks after this.

Treatment of an acutely inflamed area of tinea

1. Do not treat with Whitfield's ointment or salicylic acid paint at first.
2. Bathe the area with potassium permanganate 1:10,000 solution and then put on a *little* acriflavine emulsion on a dressing soaked in strong 3% saline.
3. Also give SMX 800 mg/TMP 160 mg orally twice daily or tetracycline 250 mg four times a day or doxycycline 100 mg daily for at least 5 days for infection if necessary.
4. Give routine treatment (as above) only when the acute inflammation improves.

> The above treatment by itself will not cure:
> - tinea of the nails,
> - most cases of tinea of the scalp or
> - some cases of tinea of the skin.

There are now many new more effective, but much more expensive, antifungal skin drugs which are put on to the skin. These include the 'imidazoles' – miconazole, ketoconazole, clotrimazole, econazole, bifonazole and others. Terbinafine 1% cream or gel is even more expensive and effective. If the above routine treatment is not effective and if you do not have a supply of miconazole cream, the patient may decide to purchase one of these; but make sure the diagnosis of fungus infection is correct before he spends the money.

None of the above will cure tinea of the nails or almost all cases of tinea of the scalp. Ciclopirox olamine and amorolfine nail laquer applied for 6 months for fingernails and 12 months for toenails *may* cure this condition.

Most cases of tinea of the nails and of the scalp and beard (and also any of the body not cured by even the above new drugs) need systemic oral treatment.

Terbinafine 250 mg daily is effective but expensive and would have to be used for 24 weeks for tinea of the nail of the big toe, 12 weeks for other toe nails, 6 weeks for fingernails, 6 weeks for the scalp or beard and 2–6 weeks for other skin infections. Side effects are rare but can cause death. They include loss of white

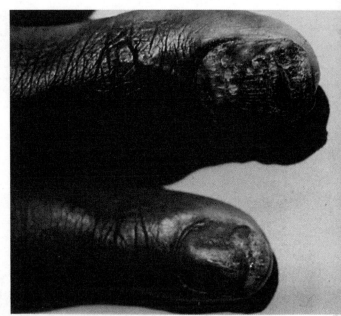

Figure 32.8 *Tinea of the nails.*

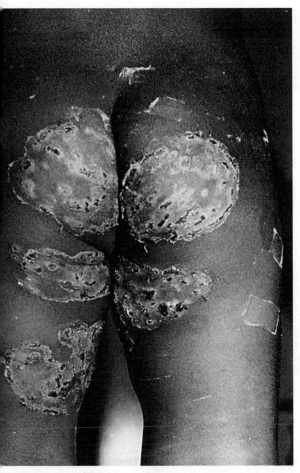

Figure 32.7 *Tinea of the body, with secondary bacterial infection. You must treat the bacterial infection and the skin inflammation before you treat the tinea infection.*

blood cells then infections, skin reactions and hepatitis.

Itraconazole 200 mg once daily for 3 months (or 200 mg twice daily for a week and then none for three weeks and repeat this cycle for the same number of months as terbinafine is recommended, is an alternative). It must be taken immediately after a meal.

Griseofulvin (preferably the ultra microsize preparation) 330–375 mg once daily, or, if unavailable, the less effective microsize griseofulvin 500 mg once daily) with the main meal of the day can be tried; but does not work at all for tinea versicolor.

Tinea versicolor (white spot)

Tinea versicolor is a different fungus infection which causes many small lesions which are pale and covered with powdery skin (see Figure 32.9). The patient may complain of the appearance or of the itch.

Treat with 10–20% sodium thiosulfate solution ('hypo' or X-ray fixer) on the whole body daily for 3 weeks; or Whitfield's ointment (benzoic acid and salicylic acid) daily on the affected areas (but not more than $\frac{1}{4}$ of the body daily); or selenium sulfide 2.5% solution shampoo but use it as a skin preparation, putting it on at night and not washing it off until the next morning, but being careful not to get it in the mouth, as it is a poison. The imidazole and terbinafine topical preparations are effective but more expensive.

Griseofulvin tablets do not help. Itraconazole and terbinafine should not be needed (but should cure in a week).

Candidiasis

Candida (*Monilia*) organisms are normally present in and on the body. They can grow more than normal and cause disease if:

1. there is more sugar in the area, e.g. diabetes mellitus;
2. something has killed off other organisms competing for food, etc., e.g. use of antibiotics for a long time which kill bacteria (but not *Monilia*);
3. the area is warm and moist, e.g. under babies' nappies; or under breasts or in the groin;
4. hormone changes, e.g. pregnancy or oral contraceptive use;
5. immunity decreased, especially in HIV infection, but also with cancer, anti-cancer drugs, corticosteroid drug treatment.

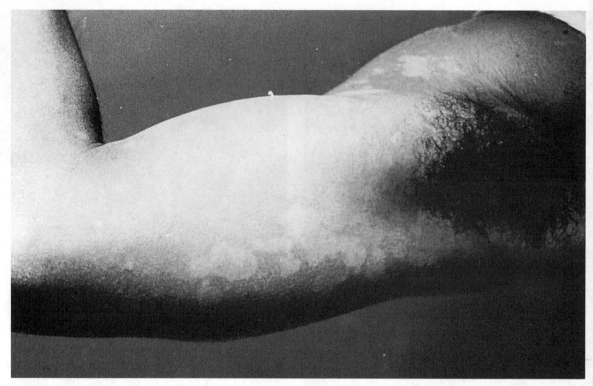

Figure 32.9 *Tinea versicolor.*

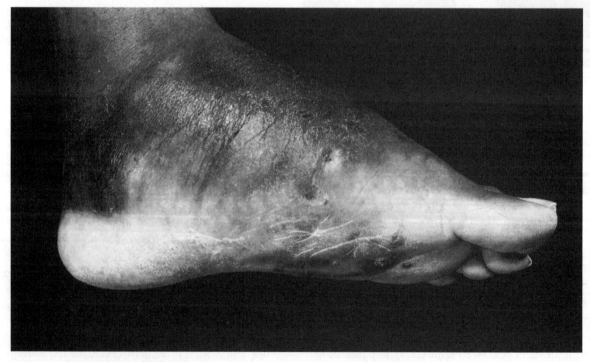

Figure 32.10 *Foot affected by mycetoma.*

If *Candida* grows more than usual it produces red raw macules or patches with small pustules at the edge. The patches spread outwards. Especially in the mouth or vagina, white plaques are stuck on the top of the macules or patches. The lesions can be itchy and painful.

Treatment includes the following.

1. Find what is the cause of this overgrowth (1–5 above) and treat the cause if possible.
2. Treat large wet skin lesions with potassium permanganate dressings or baths twice daily.
3. At other times try to keep the skin area dry.
4. Put nystatin cream, *or*
   imidazole cream, *or* if not available
   crystal violet 1% in water solution
   onto the lesion twice daily
   using the appropriate (see page 526) lotion, cream or ointment preparation for the area.
5. If the condition is severe give an oral imidazole tablet (see pages 528–529) (not griseofulvin which is not effective).

Mycetoma ('madura foot')

Mycetoma is a fungus infection which spreads to deep structures (such as the bones). It is common in dry areas of Africa, the Middle East and parts of Asia. It is common in people who do not wear shoes, especially farmers. Most often it affects the patient's foot but can affect the hand, scalp or back, etc.

First there is a painless swelling of the area. The area affected slowly becomes larger. Lumps may appear on the swollen area. The lumps may burst and sinuses may form. Pus, with little lumps of coloured material (e.g. black, red, yellow), comes out of the sinuses. There is still no pain or fever, and the patient can still use the affected area. But over months or years the affected area becomes larger. The infection does not often spread to the lymph glands or to other parts of the body.

After many years, the infected area (usually the foot) is so badly affected that the patient cannot use it. (See Figure 32.10.)

Treatment of some of these infections with drugs is possible. However, surgery is usually necessary. Refer or non-urgently transfer affected patients to the Medical Officer.

Prevention may be possible if you can get people in the areas where the disease is common to wear shoes.

A similar condition may affect the hand.

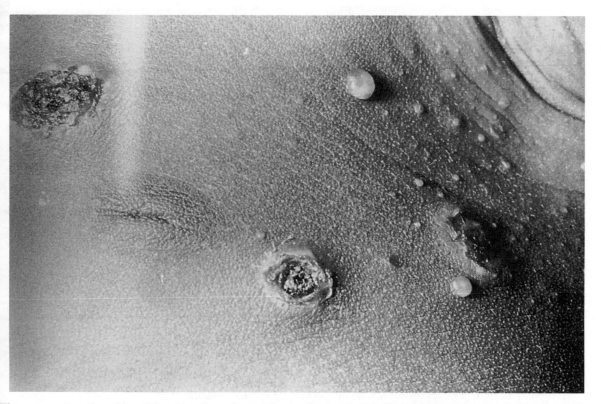

Figure 32.11 *Impetigo with vesicles. Sometimes the vesicles develop into large bulbous lesions.*

Impetigo

Impetigo is a bacterial infection of the skin, usually caused by staphylococci or streptococci. It is very infectious and spreads to others by direct contact or by vehicles, such as towels.

First a blister forms. This bursts to leave a red wet surface. A thick yellow crust forms. Then new blisters form. There are other types of impetigo (Figure 32.11).

Management

1 to 5 and 8 are the most important treatments. Antibiotics are not usually needed.

1. Gently rub off the scabs and crusts with antiseptic solution (see 2 below.).
2. Wash the whole area with antiseptic solution (water, not alcohol) 2–3 times a day, and then daily, when it improves.
   Suitable antiseptics include chlorhexidine compound antiseptic or hexachlorophene emulsion or povidone-iodine 7.5% body wash or potassium permanganate solution.
3. Put a dressing over the affected area, especially if it is large or has pus coming from it.
4. Put antibiotic compound ointment under a dry dressing or put a *little* acriflavine emulsion on a dressing wet with strong 3% saline onto the affected area; or paint the area with crystal violet solution (but this is messy). Do this 2–3 times a day at first; and then daily, when it improves.
5. Change and wash the clothes daily (if possible).
6. Give antibiotics for 5–10 days only *if*
   - the patient develops general symptoms and signs of infection, *or*
   - the skin lesions are very large or inflamed, *or*
   - the condition does not respond to the above treatment, *or*
   - the condition repeatedly returns see 8 first, *or*
   - you are not certain that the patient will do the treatment properly.
   Give SMX 800 mg/TMP 160 mg twice daily or tetracycline 250 mg (1 cap) four times a day or doxycycline 100 mg daily (but not if pregnant, when give erythromycin 500 mg three to four times a day or if not available, penicillin). If the condition is very severe and does not improve with the above the best antibiotic is dicloxacillin (or cloxacillin or flucloxacillin) 500 mg qid.
7. Look very carefully for scabies and lice, especially if there is an itch. (The lesions of scabies and lice are not always typical.) Treat if present (see pages 538–540).
8. If the condition appears in new areas, or returns after it was cured and treatment was stopped, then wash the *whole body* (including the perineum and inside the nose) with the antiseptic solution daily. Then give all the above treatment, especially 6 and 7.
9. If the condition is difficult to cure or keeps on returning, counsel and do test for HIV infection.
10. Tell the patient that the infection spreads by pus from the infected areas taking germs to new areas. He should not touch the infected areas. He should wash his hands often. He should not allow others to touch his towel and clothes until he is cured.

Furuncle or boil

A boil is an infection (usually caused by staphylococci or streptococci) of the skin in the place where a hair grows. A boil starts as a small tender lump in the skin. It becomes bigger over some days, and has all the signs of acute inflammation. It then 'points' – softens in the centre as pus forms. The skin bursts and the pus comes out. A day or two later the 'core' comes out – the dead part of the skin which made the hair. (See Figure 32.12.)

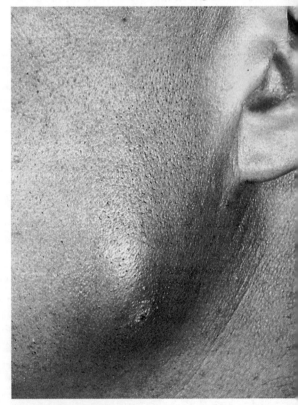

Figure 32.12 *Furuncle or boil.*

In an area where myiasis occurs, check that any slowly developing 'boil' is not caused by the myiasis (see page 540).

Treatment

At early stage (only inflamed swelling)

1. Paint the lesion (and several cm all round it) with iodine solution 2.5% or povidone-iodine 10% alcohol solution.
2. Cover the area with a large square of elastic plaster bandage. Stretch the elastic plaster as you stick it on to the skin. (This will 'splint' the area.)
3. Give paracetamol or acetylsalicylic acid 500–1000 mg four times a day for pain, if necessary.
4. Test the lesion under the elastic plaster for fluctuation every day.
5. If the lesion goes, remove the plaster; but only when it has *completely* gone.
6. If *definite* fluctuation develops, remove the elastic plaster with one quick pull. This will probably also pull off the thin skin over the surface of the boil and allow it to drain – incision will then not be necessary.

At other stages

See Chapter 11 about antibiotics and a surgery book about incision (cutting open) to drain the pus. Antibiotics alone will not cure the condition once pus has formed. The lesion needs also incision to let the pus drain out.

If repeated boils

Treat and test as for repeated impetigo (see page 532).

Tropical ulcer

Tropical ulcer is a skin infection with special types of bacteria (*Bacillus fusiformis* and spirochaetes), which cause an acute severe infective ulcer, which may become a chronic ulcer.

The special bacteria that cause tropical ulcer may be spread by direct contact and by flies or other insects.

A tropical ulcer usually comes on exposed areas, usually below the knee. First a painful vesicle (blister) forms. This bursts and leaves an ulcerating, dirty surface. The ulcer spreads very quickly. It is painful and itchy. The edge is slightly raised but not undermined. The surface is covered with a smelly grey-green or bloody membrane. (See Figure 32.13.)

The patient has no general symptoms and signs of infection. After about a month, the ulcer stops spreading. It may heal. If it does not heal, the base slowly becomes scarred and skin cannot then grow over the surface as there are no blood vessels from underneath to keep it alive. The patient may then have the ulcer for life. If at any time it does heal, it has a very thin skin over it which is easily and often broken by minor injury and an ulcer forms again.

Treatment

If the ulcer is severe or large, or has been present for more than 2 months admit for inpatient treatment. If it is small, treat as an outpatient.

1. Give procaine benzylpenicillin 1 g or 1,000,000 units IMI daily until the ulcer is healing well or at least 7 days (this is very important if it is a true tropical ulcer). After a month or if penicillin is not effective SMX/TMP or tetracycline and metronidazole may be needed. But antibiotics alone will not cure it.
2. Give tetanus toxoid if needed.
3. If possible, rest the affected area. Keep the leg with the ulcer on it higher than the rest of the body. If this is not possible, firmly bandage a cotton wool pad over the dressing, using (if possible) a crepe bandage.
4. Dress the ulcer twice daily (or more often if necessary) with Eusol, or strong (3%) saline solution, or honey or sugar paste or pawpaw until the ulcer is clean. The dressing should stay wet. Cover it with a sheet of plastic if needed.

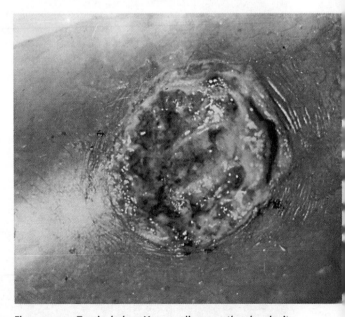

Figure 32.13 *Tropical ulcer. You can diagnose the ulcer by its very quick growth, its typical appearance (raised edge, a grey bloody membrane on the surface). There are very few general symptoms and signs.*

5. When the ulcer is clean, dress with any non-irritating non-sticky dressing, e.g. cod liver oil ointment or antibiotic compound ointment or vaseline or even something such as coconut oil or palm oil on gauze, as long as it will come off without sticking to the underlying healing ulcer. Change the dressing only when it is really necessary. You must not make the ulcer bleed when you take the dressing off. Keep the ulcer covered until it is completely healed.

6. Skin graft the ulcer if it is larger than 3 cm in diameter, and does not heal with treatment.

7. The resultant scar may always need protection from injury with a dry dressing.

Transfer to Medical Officer care non-urgently if:

1. The ulcer has not healed with treatment in 6 weeks.

2. You cannot do a skin graft, if needed.

3. The ulcer is very large, or there is bone at the base (bottom) of the ulcer.

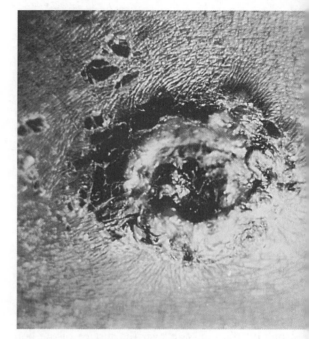

Figure 32.14 *An early yaws skin lesion.*

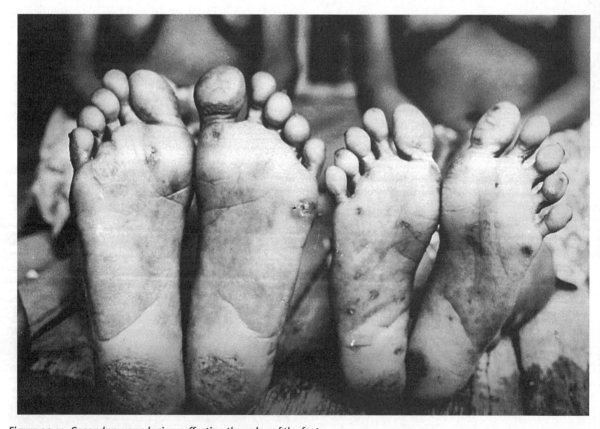

Figure 32.15 *Secondary yaws lesions affecting the soles of the feet.*

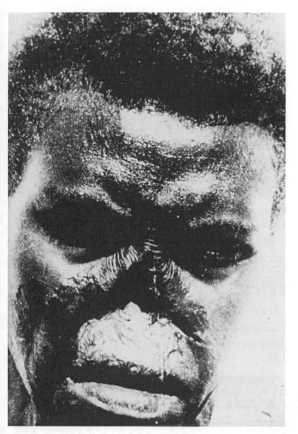

Figure 32.16 *Late yaws affecting the face.*

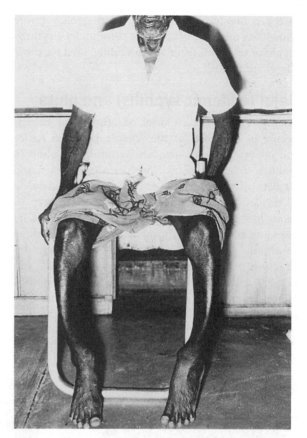

Figure 32.17 *Late yaws affecting the bones.*

Yaws

Yaws is a bacterial (a spirochaete, *Treponema pertenue*) infection spread by direct contact or possibly by flies. It occurs in humid moist warm tropical areas of the world.

It affects children much more often than adults. The first (or primary) lesion is a sore, on an exposed area, often on the leg (see Figure 32.14) (but also can be arm and face). It begins as a macule and becomes a papule. It is not painful but it is itchy and usually becomes an ulcer 1–5 cm wide and is raised at the edge. It has an irregular white-yellow crust; and if you remove the crust, it leaves a bleeding surface with yellow spots. After 3–6 months it heals. The nearby lymph nodes are enlarged but not tender.

Secondary skin lesions appear when the primary lesion is getting better or has gone. They are similar to the primary lesions but many shapes (see Figure 32.15). There may be many of them all over the body. If a lesion appears on the sole of the foot, it is painful and the patient limps. Lesions in moist areas of the body may look like condylomata lata. Skin on the hands and feet may become thick and crack. Bones and joints may become painful, tender and thickened at this stage. The forearm and lower legs and especially the fingers, may become swollen and tender. Fever may be present. After some weeks or months, all these things may go; but they may often return again and again for some years.

Late yaws develops in some patients. This can cause deep large skin ulcers (gumma); thickening and cracking of the skin of the feet; large fibrous nodules under the skin near joints; curving of the long bones; and destruction of the bones of the nose and face (see Figures 32.16 and 32.17).

Syphilis serology becomes positive in yaws.

Benzathine benzylpenicillin 2.4 g for adults and 1.2 g for older children cures yaws. But if you find a case, arrange for a survey to find out if control measures are necessary. If a survey shows only a low frequency (less than 5% of the population), you need to treat only the family and obvious contacts of a case. If there is medium frequency (5–9%), treat all children in the community. If there is high frequency (more than 10%), treat everyone in the community. Erythromycin or tetracycline for 15 days can be used for those allergic to penicillin.

Bejel (endemic syphilis) and pinta

Endemic syphilis (called bejel or other local names) occurs in dry areas of the Middle East and Africa and is caused by non-sexually transmitted syphilis in childhood. Spread is by close personal contact, and by utensils such as cups, etc. Children can develop all the lesions of secondary syphilis (see Chapter 19 pages 208–210) and sometimes skin lesions, which are the same as yaws (see above). After some years these conditions go; but after some more years, severe destruction of the skin and the bones of the face can occur as in late yaws. Late cardiovascular and neurological lesions as in syphilis do not occur. The serological test for syphilis is positive. (See Figure 32.18.)

Treatment is with penicillin, as for syphilis (see Chapter 19 pages 204 and 210).

Pinta (which has other local names) occurs in Central and South America and perhaps the Middle East. It is caused by an organism related to the syphilis and yaws bacteria. Spread is by non-sexual transmission, like yaws. First there is an itchy scaly papule. This slowly enlarges and joins with new papules which continue to appear around its edge. The papule becomes up to 10 cm in diameter. Nearby lymph nodes are enlarged. This lesion often remains, but later many other lesions appear on the exposed parts of the skin. These lesions are most often dark. After many years, the lesions on the limbs become symmetrical (i.e. the same on both sides) depigmented (pale) and thin. The serological test for syphilis is positive. (See Figure 32.19.)

Treatment is with penicillin, as for syphilis (see Chapter 19 pages 204 and 210).

Anthrax

Anthrax is a bacterium whose spores can live in the soil for many years and causes an infection of cattle and sheep, etc.

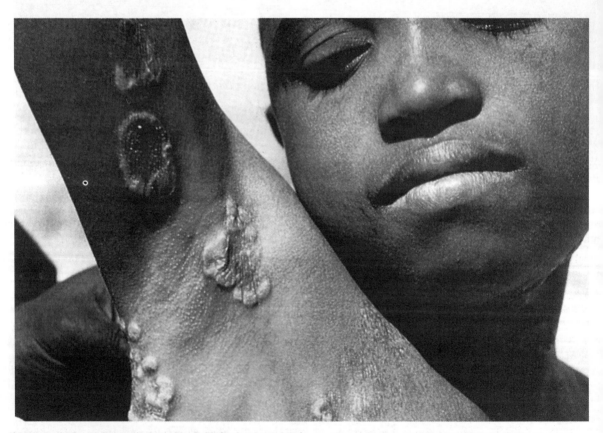

Figure 32.18 *Secondary rash caused by bejel (endemic syphilis).*
(Source: W. Peters and H.M. Gilles. A Colour Atlas of Tropical Medicine and Parasitology. London, Wolfe Medical Publications, 1981) (Dr A. Buck)

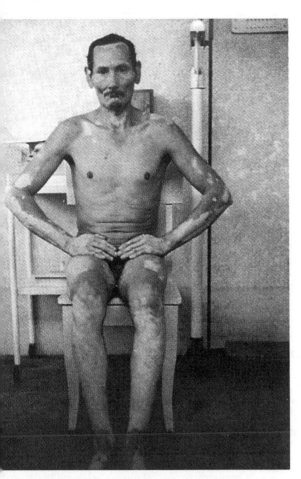

Figure 32.19 *Depigmented lesions caused by pinta.*
(Source: W. Peters and H.M. Gilles, A Colour Atlas of
Tropical Medicine and Parasitology, London, Wolfe Medical
Publications, 1981)

It can infect people on exposed parts of their skin, most often on the face if they are in contact with infected animal skins. A papule forms quickly. This soon becomes a vesicle filled with blood-stained fluid. Small vesicles appear around the original vesicle. The area around the lesion becomes very swollen, and looks inflamed; but it does not pit on pressure, and it is not very tender. After some days the vesicle dries, becomes black, and starts to heal. Usually, there is some enlargement of the nearby lymph glands, but few general symptoms and signs of infection. But the infection can spread from this skin lesion and cause septicaemia and death.

Other severe forms of the disease can occur. If the spores are inhaled this can cause severe pneumonia. If infected meat is eaten, gastroenteritis, often with dysentery, can occur.

If you suspect a patient has anthrax, immediately start treatment with penicillin (as it is resistant to chloramphenicol), and check with your Medical Officer for methods of control and prevention.

Mycobacterium tuberculosis *infection of the skin*

Occasionally, this causes an ulcer on the face or neck, which slowly over months gets bigger (often under the nose and destroys the lip and nose). It can be diagnosed by a smear for AFB, but if negative refer to Medical Officer for biopsy (do not yourself biopsy face). Treatment with anti-TB triple therapy cures the infection but needs to be done before a lot of the face is destroyed.

Mycobacterium ulcerans *ulcer*

Mycobacterium ulcerans is a bacterium which can cause a chronic undermined skin ulcer. The reservoir is probably soil and water and infection occurs when minor injuries let the organism into the skin. It is common in children.

The lesion usually starts as a firm papule, nodule or plaque, up to 2 cm in diameter or just oedema of the skin. As it grows it bursts to form an ulcer. The ulcer grows slowly over weeks or months. It goes down to the muscle, and sideways underneath the skin. This causes a very typical appearance, where the skin overhangs the edge of the ulcer, sometimes by several centimetres (see Figure 32.20). Surrounding ulcers may

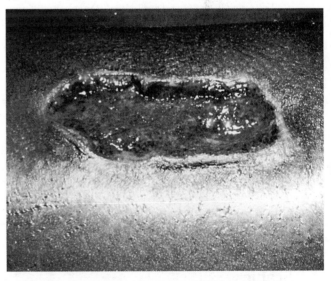

Figure 32.20 *A* Mycobacterium ulcerans *infection. A probe can go several centimetres under the apparently normal skin at the edge of the ulcer.*

start and soon be joined under the skin. It remains painless. It stops eventually after months or years; but by then may have caused severe scarring or even loss of all the skin of an arm or leg.

Osteomyelitis or other local complications or tetanus can occur.

Diagnosis is by the typical appearance of the ulcer/s and AFB seen on a smear or by a biopsy sent for examination in the laboratory.

If you suspect this condition, non-urgently *transfer* the patient for surgery to make flaps out of remaining skin, clean under these flaps and in the base of the ulcer with antiseptic such as silver nitrate 0.5%, do skin grafts if needed and consider special drugs. (Clofazimine and rifampicin may sometimes help, but only if the above surgery is also done.) Heat treatment may help.

Cellulitis

Cellulitis is an inflammation of the cellular and other tissues underneath the skin. These tissues normally hold the structures under the skin together. It may complicate any infection of the skin. The inflammation in cellulitis usually spreads along the divisions between the organs under the skin. If cellulitis is not cured quickly, pus can form. Abscesses can then form and even gangrene of the skin can occur.

There is usually pain in the area, but not at one small definite place. There is swelling, redness and tenderness of the affected part of the body, but again it is not usually in one small particular place. Blisters can form on the skin. There is usually malaise, fever, fast pulse, etc.

Treatment is by rest and antibiotics. Benzyl (crystalline) penicillin, 1,000,000 units by IMI every 6 hours until the condition improves and then procaine benzylpenicillin 900,000 units daily by IMI is usually enough. If the condition gets worse, the antibiotic should be changed to chloramphenicol 1 g orally every 6 hours. If pus has collected in any area, and it can be drained easily without risk of damaging any important structure, incision should be made over the area. Should pus be deep, however, or should the inflammation be in an area where there are many important structures, such as the neck or hand, *transfer* the patient urgently to the Medical Officer.

Cutaneous leishmaniasis ('oriental sore' and 'espundia')

See Chapter 18 pages 175–181.

Scabies

Scabies is an infestation of the surface layer of the skin by an insect, the scabies mite (*Sarcoptes scabiei*). The sca-

bies mite spreads from one person to another during close personal contact. It usually infests all people who live in the same house as a person with scabies.

The patient usually complains of an itch in part of the body, often worst at night, about 4–6 weeks after infestation; or of repeated sores in part of the body.

The usual lesion of scabies is a dark papule, several mm in diameter (Figure 32.21). You can sometimes see the path the mite made through the skin. The patient scratches the lesions and often causes a bacterial infection (such as impetigo) or an eczematous reaction in the area. A generalised allergic reaction with urticaria can develop.

Most often it affects the areas between the fingers, the front of the wrists, the elbows, the breast, the penis, the pubic region and, in babies, the sides of the feet (Figure 32.22).

> Because of scratching infection, eczema and allergic reactions, the appearance of scabies lesions may be unusual. Always suspect scabies in anyone with an itchy rash, or even a rash all over.

The skin can become thick or scaly or crusted (and not be as itchy) in some chronic cases. This also occurs in people with HIV infection and lepromatous leprosy. It is sometimes then called 'Norwegian scabies' or 'crusted scabies'.

Treat as an outpatient.

1. Apply permethrin 5% (50 mg/g), *or* benzyl benzoate 25% *or* tetmosol 5% *or* malathion 0.5% *or* sulfur 6% ointment (*or* if none of the other treatments is available, gamma benzene hexachloride 1% emulsion, but *not* for babies) lotion or cream like this:
   (a) The previous recommendations to wash all the body with soap, rubbing it with a cloth, rinsing, and drying the skin are now not thought to be essential; and may make absorption of the chemical more likely to cause side effects.
   (b) Shake the bottle of lotion very well, and rub the lotion or cream on all the body, especially in the folds of the skin. Scabies does not often affect the skin of the face; but if it does use treatment on the face too, but make sure the treatment does not get in the eyes, nose or mouth. The usual amount needed for an adult is 50 ml of lotion or 30 g of cream. The medicine must remain on the skin for 24 hours.
   (c) After 24 hours, wash the lotion off and preferably put on clean clothes.
   (d) Four days later, repeat the treatment as in (a), (b) and (c).

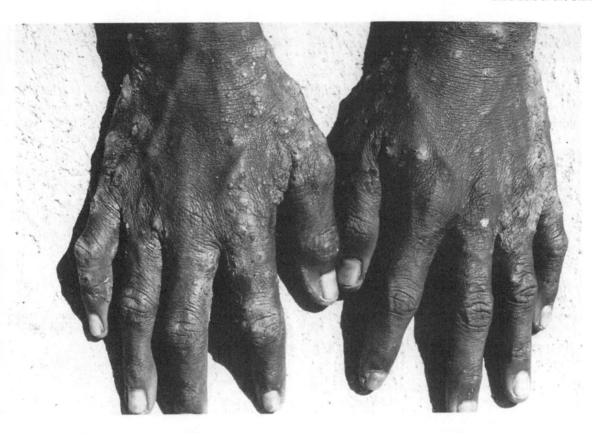

Figure 32.21 *Scabies.*

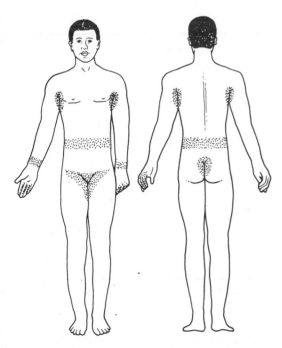

Figure 32.22 *Diagram to show the usual distribution of scabies lesions.*

Give the patient a private room where he can completely undress. The patient can wash himself. **But a health worker must apply the lotion** to all the skin of the patient (except usually the face). The patient without help cannot do it well enough.

If the patient is a mother, wash the breasts before breastfeeding. After breastfeeding, put the application on again. If the medicine is washed off the hands, immediately put more on.

2. If the lesions are infected, give procaine benzylpenicillin 1 g or 1,000,000 units IMI, or SMX 800 mg/TMP 160 mg twice daily or if not pregnant tetracycline 250 mg four times a day or doxycycline 100 mg daily starting on the day of the first permethrin or other lotion treatment until the infection goes. If impetigo is present, treat this first (see page 532) before giving the insecticide treatment.

3. Treat (or show the patient how to treat) all members of the patient's family, and anyone else who

lives with him. Other people with early infection may not know they have it as the itch may take 1 month or so to start.

4. The previous recommendation to change and wash the clothes and bedclothes, and put them in the sun, at the end of every 24 hour treatment is probably not needed as the scabies organism dies soon if not actually in a person's skin.

5. Itch may continue for up to a couple of weeks. Anti-itch preparations can be used. If available, crotamiton 10% cream helps itch (and is a weak scabies treatment).

6. Educate the patient about the cause and prevention of the disease. Encourage the patient and his family to wash regularly with soap (if it contains 5% tetraethyl thiuram monosulfide (tetmosol) it is even more effective). Encourage the patient to keep clean and regularly wash his clothes, bedclothes, and house.

7. Tell the patient to come for treatment when any new lesions appear (before they are bad or there are many).

In 'crusted scabies' thick crusts may need to be removed by salicylic acid 5–10% ointment or urea 10% ointment (as well as all of the usual treatment). In these cases and also cases not responding to other treatment, talk to your Medical Officer about other treatment, including ivermectin.

Lice (pediculosis)

Lice are insects that can live on people. They can carry dangerous disease (e.g. typhus, relapsing fever, etc.). But usually they cause only itching and skin rash. There are three types of lice.

Head lice live *on the scalp* and put their eggs on the hair ('nits'). Lice cause severe itching of the scalp. Scratching often causes eczema or results in bacterial infection of the scalp. The glands in the neck are often enlarged. You can diagnose lice by finding them or their eggs on the scalp or hair.

Body lice live *in the clothes* except when biting which causes itching, scratching and eczema or bacterial infections of the body, especially around the waist. You will find the lice and eggs in the clothes (especially under the edges).

Pubic lice affect the pubic area, and also the eyelashes and *live on the hair.*

Treatment is with one of the following preparations that the lice are not resistant to in your area – melathion 1% or permethrin 1–5% or benzyl benzoate 25% or gamma benzene hexachloride 1% or carbaryl 0.5–1% or phenothrin 0.2–0.5% cream, lotion or emulsion.

For head lice put one of these insecticides on the hair and scalp. Cover the hair with a cloth for some hours. The next day wash and carefully comb the hair to remove all the eggs. Repeat the treatment a week later. In some countries, some (not all) ordinary shampoos and hair conditioners seem to suffocate and kill head lice.

For body lice, boil or iron the clothes and bedclothes or treat them with insecticide. This should be enough; but often the patient is also treated with insecticide, i.e. treat the patient and his clothes with insecticide. See Chapter 17 page 165 for methods of mass treatment in epidemics.

Treat pubic lice with insecticide; if needed also shave off hair. Do not cut or shave eyelashes or eyebrows; apply petroleum jelly twice daily for 2 weeks.

Control and prevention is by treatment of cases, good personal hygiene, and using repellents in epidemics of typhus, relapsing fever, etc.

In resistant cases, talk to your Medical Officer about treatment with temephos or ivermectin.

Tungiasis

Tungiasis occurs in South America, Africa and Asia. It is an infestation with the chigoe or jigger flea, which affects man and pigs.

Most often it affects the feet. The flea gets into the skin, and grows to the size of a small pea. It then pushes eggs out through the skin lesion. First there is itching. Later there can be secondary bacterial infection. Tetanus can occur.

In treatment you must remove the whole flea in one piece with a sterile needle and prevent and treat secondary bacterial infection and give tetanus prevention. If there are very many lesions, soak the affected area in a 5% solution of benzene hexachloride.

Prevention is helped by wearing shoes.

Myiasis

Myiasis is an infestation with the larvae (maggots) of flies. The larvae can go into the skin and make a lesion like a furuncle or boil, although usually with less inflammation and pain. In areas in Africa and Central and South America where myiasis occurs, always think of this condition when a patient has an inflamed swelling of the skin.

Treat by putting oil (such as liquid paraffin or vaseline) on the lesion so that the larvae cannot breathe and start to come out of the skin to get air. If you

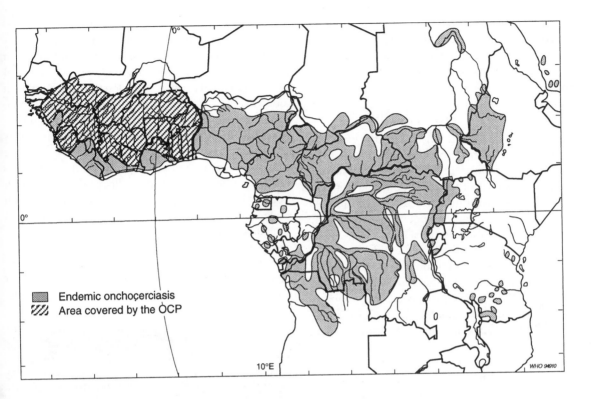

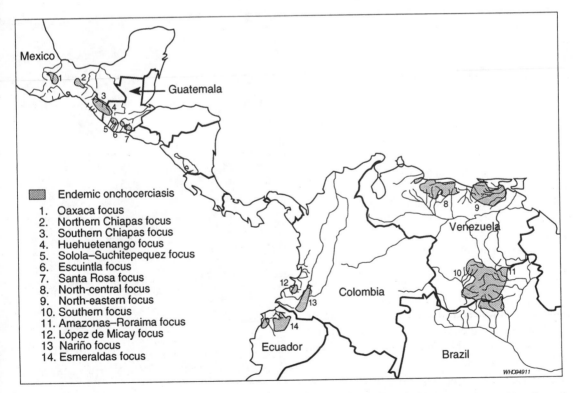

Endemic onchocerciasis

1. Oaxaca focus
2. Northern Chiapas focus
3. Southern Chiapas focus
4. Huehuetenango focus
5. Solola–Suchitepequez focus
6. Escuintla focus
7. Santa Rosa focus
8. North-central focus
9. North-eastern focus
10. Southern focus
11. Amazonas–Roraima focus
12. López de Micay focus
13. Nariño focus
14. Esmeraldas focus

Figure 32.23 *The distribution of onchocerciasis. (Source: WHO Technical Report Series No. 852, 1995; Report of a WHO Expert Committee on Onchocerciasis Control)*

then put more oil on and press the sides of the lesion this will usually remove the larvae. Sometimes surgery is necessary, especially in America. Try not to damage the insect during removal as this may cause severe inflammation. Treat any secondary infection with antibiotics.

Onchocerciasis ('river blindness')

Onchocerciasis is a chronic disease of the skin and the eyes. It is caused by an infestation with a filarial worm (*Onchocera volvulus*) of the tissues just under the skin. The adult worm may cause nodules in the skin. The larvae of the worm (microfilaria) travel through the skin and the eyes. Immunological reactions of the body to the microfilaria (especially to them when they die there) cause dermatitis and blindness.

Onchocerciasis is common only in parts of Africa, the Middle East and in Central and South America. (See Figure 32.23.) Eighty to 120 million people are at risk of this disease, 18 million infected, half a million have damaged sight and one quarter of a million are blind.

The vector is *Simulium* (a small black fly) which breeds mostly in fast flowing rivers, etc; but some types can fly many kilometres from rivers; and may be blown further by the wind. The fly is infected when biting a person with microfilaria in their tissues; and after about a week can pass on the infection to people it bites.

The symptoms and signs in people are almost all due to immunological ('allergic') reactions they have to the microfilaria. These reactions are at their worst when the microfilaria dies. Some people can have many microfilaria and no disease. Others may have fewer microfilaria and severe disease. Eye disease may be more common where there are more adult filaria (and more nodules) in the upper part of the patient's body. Hot dry climate or hot humid climate may also help determine how much eye and how much skin disease occurs.

Once a person is infected the filarial worms develop and travel around in the tissues of and under the skin. At times they stop travelling and painless nodules may develop under the skin at these points. These may become large lumps and are most common where bones are just under the skin (e.g. around joints, hips, ribs, back of head). If the adults travel to the brain epilepsy may be caused.

The adults make many embryos (called microfilaria) which travel around the body in the tissues of the skin and eye (but not in the blood).

At first, the microfilaria cause a very severe itch present all the time and stopping sleep at night, although the skin can look quite normal. Later, they cause dermatitis with severe itching and then form macules and papules (and the skin looks something like the peel of an orange). The skin later loses its elasticity and looks like an old person's skin. The skin can become lichenified (or thickened) and wrinkled. This is sometimes called 'lizard' or 'elephant' skin. After some years of severe itching and scratching, the skin can become thin and loose (called 'tissue paper' skin) and patches of the skin become pale (called 'leopard' skin). Lymph nodes become enlarged. Folds of skin and lymph nodes can form in the groin or axilla ('hanging' groin or axilla). (See Figures 32.24, 32.25 and 32.26.)

The microfilaria can cause many sorts of damage to the eyes, which can lead to blindness ('river blindness'). See Chapter 31 page 516. They can causes conjunctivitis or a chronic oedema of the conjuncti-

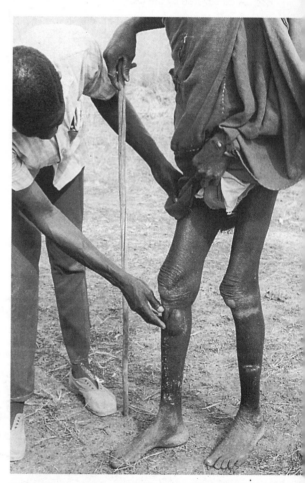

Figure 32.24 *Nodules of onchocerciasis. If you remove and cut a nodule you can see the adult worms lying inside.*

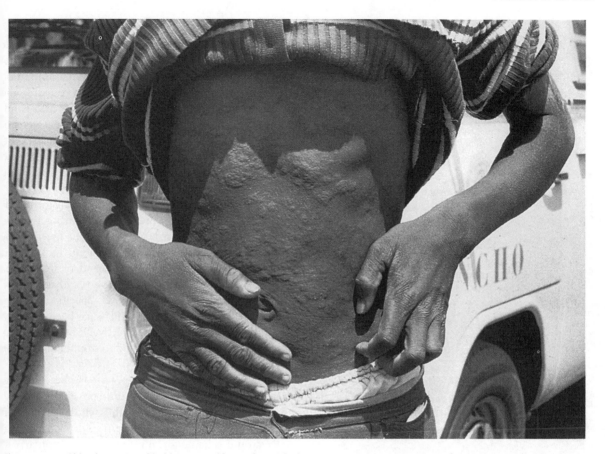

Figure 32.25 *Skin changes and itching caused by onchocerciasis.*

vae and eyelids. They can also cause whitish spots on the cornea and later a thickening and loss of clearness of the cornea, often with blood vessels growing in the affected area. This change starts at the bottom of the cornea and grows up over the cornea so that the patient cannot see through it. Microfilaria can also cause iritis and later glaucoma and cataract. The retina of the eye and the optic nerve may also be damaged. From any one or more of these things the patient often becomes blind.

Children with onchocerciasis may not grow to normal size.

You can *diagnose* onchocerciasis like this:

Take a 'skin snip'. Clean the skin with alcohol; lift up a small piece of skin on a sharp sterile needle; use a scalpel or sterilised razor blade to slice off 1–2 mm of skin in width and length deep enough to show the white material under it and to just cause blood to ooze; take six samples from different areas but none near the nodules; put them into saline, then look at the saline under the microscope half an hour later for moving microfilaria and 24 hours later for dead microfilaria.

Treatment is with a drug called ivermectin given each year. Ivermectin kills all the microfilaria which would normally live for about 1 year and makes the adult worm not able to produce more microfilaria for 6–12 months. It does not kill the adult worms, so treatment may need to be continued until they die (5–20 years). The dose is 150–200 micrograms (0.15–2 mg)/kg body weight which usually means two of the 6 mg tablets for an adult. It is not given to small children (e.g. <90 cm tall) or to pregnant women. The drug manufacturers supply this drug free to any government who uses it in an onchocerciasis control programme. It has been found that distribution by properly organised community programmes is the best way of getting it to all of the population.

Treatment may not be necessary in patients who do not have symptoms or signs other than lumps. As eye disease may develop at any time, however, it is best to treat all infected persons.

Treatment is essential if there are any eye symptoms or signs or severe dermatitis, or many nodules.

Other treatment, which may at times be done by the Medical Officer, may include:

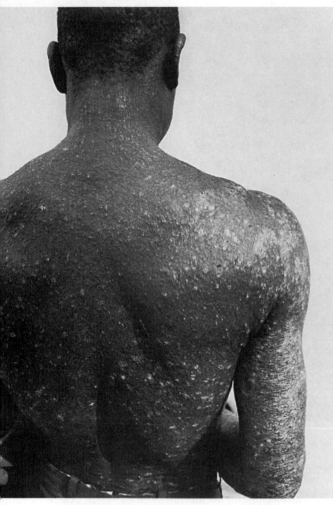

Figure 32.26 *Onchocerciasis. Characteristic pale patches on the skin caused by scratching. Early in the disease the itchy skin may look normal.*

1. surgical removal of the nodules which contain adult worms especially those that are on the head near the eyes and whose microfilaria may damage the eyes;
   or
2. treatment with diethylcarbamazine and an anti-histamine, but with careful small doses of diethyl-carbamazine first (otherwise severe dangerous allergic type reactions can occur).

The only present treatment which will kill the adult worm is suramin. However, it is an extremely toxic drug but is not given now that ivermectin is available. A safe drug to kill the adult worms is badly needed.

If there are eye lesions, see Chapter 31 page 516.

Control and *prevention* is by the following:

1. Kill the microfilaria in the bodies of all the people in affected areas with ivermectin so that they cannot infect *Simulium* flies. This is now the major method of control. If onchocerciasis occurs in your area and if regular treatment of all people in the area is not being given, see what you can do to help get this started. The drugs have been donated (at no cost) to all countries who will carry out the programme. All that is needed is government agreement and community organisations to do it.
2. Stop the means of transmission by stopping the breeding of flies. This was previously the major method of control. Flies can be stopped from breeding by spraying things into the river systems to kill their larvae. This has been done by hand or from aeroplanes. Insecticides such as temephos, carbamates and pyrethroids were used; but now a specific microbial larvacide *Bacillus thuringiensis* H14 has been found to be the cheapest and most effective. Protective clothing and repellents can be used to stop the flies biting people.
3. Raising the resistance of potential new hosts by immunisation is not at this time possible.
4. Prophylactic treatment of the whole population is being done with ivermectin (although the real reason it is being given is to kill the microfilaria so that the flies cannot be infected and continue to spread the infection).

Loiasis

Loiasis is an infestation of the subcutaneous tissue with a filarial worm *Loa loa*. It occurs in Africa.

The adult worms are up to 7 cm long. They can cause areas of oedema, and often pain, in the skin ('Calabar swellings'). The swellings are often many centimetres in diameter and may last for a number of days. Sometimes the adult worms are seen wriggling under the skin or crossing the conjunctiva of the eye.

The adult produces microfilaria which circulate in the blood. These infect *Chrysops* ('mango' or 'softly-softly' flies) which then give the infection back to man.

Treat people who have repeated swellings as for onchocerciasis with ivermectin (see above). Diethyl-carbamazine may be more effective but must be used with care in case a severe allergic reaction is caused. Albendazole may also be effective treatment.

Prevention, by fly control and stopping the *Chrysops* fly biting people, is difficult. Mass treatment of the population with diethylcarbamazine is usually not warranted, especially as the people may also have onchocerciasis and may develop side effects to large doses of diethylcarbamazine. Ivermectin should be effective and safe given as for onchocerciasis.

Guinea worm

Guinea worm infestation occurs in parts of Africa, the Middle East, India and South America.

The Guinea worm is a long (e.g. 1 metre) worm which lives under the skin of people and dogs and cats. Adult worms cause irritation of the skin in one area, usually a leg. A painful blister forms. The blister bursts and a very itchy ulcer forms, see Figure 32.27. The itch is helped by putting the leg in water. When the patient puts the leg in water, the end of the worm comes out through the ulcer and passes its larvae into the water. The worm larvae go into water fleas, and

develop into larvae which are then infective for people. If people drink water with these infective larvae in it, the larvae develop into new worms under their skin; and the cycle starts again.

Symptoms and *signs* include:

1. There may be allergic reactions, e.g. fever or vomiting or asthma as the worm starts to go through the skin.
2. A painful blister forms where the worm goes out through the skin. This is usually on the foot or leg or part of the body that is cool and often wet. The blister bursts and an itchy ulcer forms. You can see the end of the worm passing white larvae when the ulcer is in water.
3. After 3–4 weeks the worm dies or leaves the body.
4. If the worm goes into another part of the body, or if it dies, or if other infections go into the ulcer, the patient may develop
   (a) abscess,
   (b) arthritis, or
   (c) tetanus.

Treatment includes:

1. Treat any bacterial infection with antibiotics (see Chapter 11 pages 56–61).
2. Give metronidazole 400 mg three times a day. This helps symptoms but does not kill the worm or stop it producing larvae. However, metronidazole weakens the worm's attachment to the patient's tissues so that it is easier to pull out. Mebendazole can also be used.
3. Prevent tetanus (see Chapter 25 page 420).
4. Put the affected part into cold clean water for half an hour daily for a few days, so that the worm will pass all its larvae. Then tie the end of the worm to a sterile stick with sterile cotton. Slowly wind the worm out of the ulcer round the stick until it becomes tight. Do only a little each day, and take care not to break the worm. Cover with antiseptic and a sterile dressing.

Control and *prevention* is by supplying safe drinking water; or if this is not possible, by boiling drinking water; or if this not possible, filtering all drinking water through two layers of fine clothing material (such as is used for making shirts), to remove the infected water fleas.

Skin rashes due to worms – including cutaneous larva migrans

Human hookworm and other worms can cause a mild itch or rash when they enter through the skin; but are then carried from the skin to other parts of

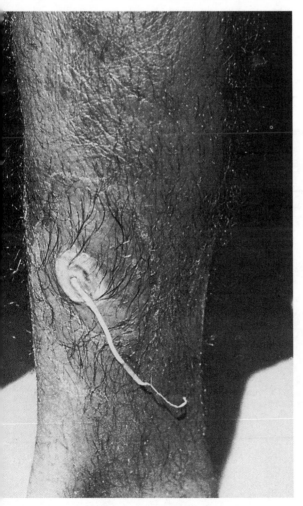

Figure 32.27 *A Guinea worm emerging from an ulcer in the patient's leg.*

the body where they complete their life cycle and the skin symptoms stop.

Hookworm of other animals, e.g. the dog hook-worm after entering the skin of a person cannot get carried away to complete its life cycle. The worm (larva) then travels (migrates) through the skin (cuta), leaving a slow moving inflamed irritated path or line across the skin of the legs or buttocks (where it entered). See Chapter 23 page 359.

Warts (verrucae)

Warts are caused by infection with one of the many human papilloma viruses (HPV).

The virus makes the cells which make the surface layer of the skin grow too much. They make too much skin in that place and cause a lump. In common warts the surface is often rough, or even like cauliflower (see Figure 32.28). Sometimes the surface is flat – plane warts. If warts develop under the feet – plantar warts, they are pressed flat and make a hole in other tissues of the foot. Excess thickened skin can form around them. This can be very painful. In other areas they do not usually cause symptoms. Warts in the mouth in children probably have spread there from their hands. Warts

in the mouth in adults should make you think of HIV infection. Genital warts can be a sexually transmitted disease, can become very many and very large and certain types of these lead to cancers of cervix and penis. If warts suddenly appear in an adult and become very many or very large, think of possible HIV infection.

Most common warts eventually go away without treatment. If you cover warts with sticking plaster for 2–3 weeks they often go away. If you decide that warts need treatment, apply salicylic acid (e.g. 5–20% with lactic acid 5–20% in collodion) to the wart once a day until the wart falls off. It is important that you do not let this treatment get on nearby normal skin because it will cause severe damage to the skin. This can be used for plantar warts covering the area with sticking plaster each night after the liquid has dried. However, just rubbing or cutting off the excess tissue so that under the foot is flat is often all that is needed until it goes away. Genital warts are treated with podophylline but not when pregnant (See Chapter 19 pages 212–213).

Molluscum contagiosum

Molluscum contagiosum is an infectious disease caused by a virus (Figure 32.29).

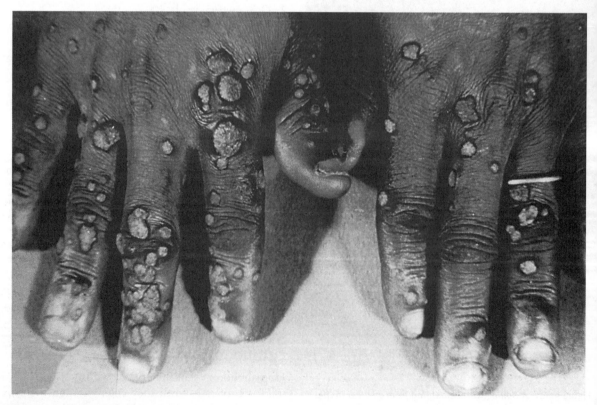

Figure 32.28 *Warts on the hand.*

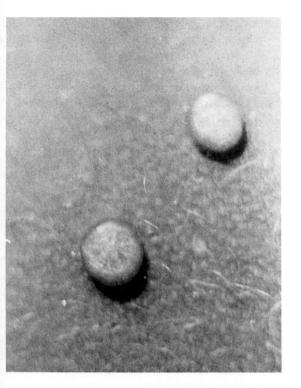

Figure 32.29 *Molluscum contagiosum. (The dark centre is often more obvious than in the photograph.)*

HIV infection; and skin conditions which suggest this may be present

- Herpes zoster (shingles), especially if age less than 50 years (see Chapter 19 page 231)
- Severe chronic seborrhoeic dermatitis (see page 548)
- Molluscum contagiosum in adults (see page 546)
- Pruritis without skin lesions (see Chapter 19 page 230)
- Papular pruritic eruption (or papular folliculitis) (see Chapter 19 page 230)
- Severe candidiasis (see Chapter 19 pages 226–227)
- Herpes simplex (see Chapter 19 page 230)
- Warts, especially anal, genital, oral or very many (see page 546)
- Severe bacterial infections of the skin (e.g. impetigo furunculous) (see page 532)
- Severe mycobacterial infections of the skin (see page 537)
- Severe fungal skin infections (see pages 527–531)
- Severe scabies (see pages 538–540)
- Angular cheilitis (see Chapter 19 page 227)
- Apthous ulcers (see Chapter 19 page 226)
- Severe gingivitis/dental abscesses (see Chapter 19 page 227)
- Severe psoriasis (see page 549)
- More adverse drug reactions than expected
- Kaposi's sarcoma (see Chapter 19 page 232)

Pellagra

Pellagra is a condition caused if there is not enough group B vitamin (niacin) in the food. It is only common in places where maize (corn) or sorghum is the main food, and little else is eaten (e.g. some parts of Africa) or in times of famine or war.

Pellagra causes these conditions:

1. dermatitis – the most common condition;
2. diarrhoea – often with a sore tongue and other gastrointestinal symptoms; and
3. dementia – more often only anxiety and depression; though dementia and even coma can occur; and then
4. death.

The dermatitis of pellagra occurs in areas exposed to sunlight – usually the face and arms. At first there is redness, swelling and discomfort (like sunburn). In acute cases the skin cracks, crusts and ulcerates, and may become infected. In chronic cases the skin becomes dark, thick, dry, rough and scaling. By this stage dermatitis of the vulva, perineum and perianal area is usually also present. (See Figure 32.30.)

It is passed from a patient to another person by close contact or sexual intercourse. It is common in children but not in healthy adults. It is now common in patients with decreased immunity from HIV infection.

The lesions may occur anywhere on the body. There are almost always many of them. They may vary in size from 2 mm up to 2 cm, although large ones are uncommon. They are usually small white tumours of the skin tissue, but the centre is sunken in and is darker. If you press the larger lesions, a white discharge comes out of the centre.

Treatment is not usually necessary as the lesions go away in time. If the lesions are covered with sticking plaster and this is left on and not taken off for a couple of weeks, the lesions are often gone when the plaster is taken off. If treatment is necessary make a small incision in the centre of the nodule. Then squeeze out the white contents. Then put on tincture of iodine 2.5% solution. Use gloves and mask and goggles if the patient may have HIV infection.

Prevention is by avoiding contact with infected persons.

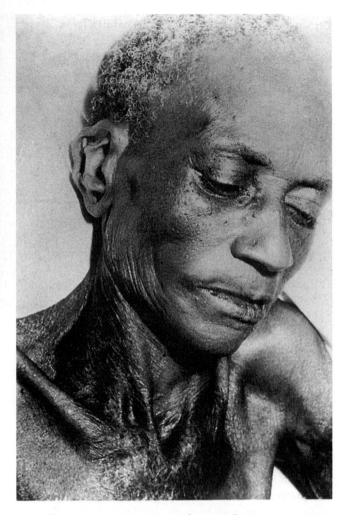

Figurea 32.30 *A severe case of acute pellagra.*

In *treatment*, give nicotinamide tablets 50–100 mg three times a day; but also if possible vitamin B compound tablets three times a day (as other vitamins are probably low); but more importantly, improve the diet by including as many animal products and legumes (peas, etc.) as the patient can afford.

Eczema or eczematous dermatitis

The patient usually complains of an itch or rash. Examination shows an acute or chronic eczematous reaction (see page 523).

You must then find the *cause* of the eczematous reaction. *Always* think of these four things:

1. Contact with things to which the patient's skin has developed a reaction, especially
   - chemicals,
   - metal jewellery,
   - clothing,
   - soap or detergent used to wash the body or to wash the clothes,
   - vaseline or mineral oil or cosmetics or perfume put on to the skin, etc.
2. Infections or infestations, e.g. scabies and lice,
3. Drugs taken for other conditions, and
4. Scratching.
5. Skin on which sun shines after certain drugs taken.

There are also two special types of dermatitis for which the cause is not known:

1. *Atopic dermatitis.* The likelihood to get this is inherited. The patient and the patient's family are likely to have had, or to develop also allergic rhinitis (hay fever), asthma and urticaria. The condition may be brought on by dryness of the skin, heat, infections, irritation or anxiety. Usually, this dermatitis affects areas behind the knees and in front of the elbows, but can be on the face and trunk (like infants).
2. *Seborrhoeic dermatitis.* This affects the scalp, eyebrows and eyelids, the sides of the nose and the front of the chest. There are usually thick greasy scales on the affected area.

   Note that seborrhoeic dermatitis can get worse with HIV infection.

Treatment

1. Treat any underlying cause – look for and treat at least the four conditions above. This is essential.
2. Explain to the patient the likely cause of the condition; and the treatment; and that if the cause is not removed or comes back again, the dermatitis will come back again.
3. Stop the use of any irritants on the skin such as vaseline, mineral oil, cosmetics, perfume, soap or detergent.
4. Use aqueous cream (not soap) when bathing. Do not use hot water. Use cold or warm water.
5. If the condition is acute, use potassium permanganate solution in a dish or bucket for bathing. Put aqueous cream on the skin after bathing. If the condition does not settle 1% hydrocortisone cream could be added.
6. If the condition is chronic and the skin thick and dry: Put urea 5–10% cream or preferably ointment on the skin after bathing If the condition does not settle, coal tar ointment could be used at night (washed off in the morning) and betamethasone (cream or) ointment 0.1% put on in the morning (but do not use this steroid

cream on the face or genitalia or on babies; use instead hydrocortisone).

7. Stop scratching.
Use an antihistamine, e.g. promethazine 25 mg nocte or amitriptyline 10–25 mg nocte to help.

8. If seborrhoeic dermatitis add an imidazole cream (see page 528) twice daily.
See also pages 523-526.

Urticaria

Urticaria are areas of swelling and redness (though often with a pale central part) and at times very irregular edges which may quickly come and change in size and shape and go; but involving only the surface layers of the skin; and are due to oedema from fluid coming out of dilated (widened) capillaries in that area. It is called angio-oedema if tissues under the skin are affected and can be serious if the lips, eyes and mouth are affected and breathing is blocked. The cause of the oedema is the release of histamine and other chemicals in that area.

Causes of the histamine, etc. release include:

- allergens in things breathed in, touched, swallowed or injected (including by insect stings);
- drugs, especially acetylsalicylic acid, NSAIDs, ACE inhibitors, but any drug;
- contact dermatitis;
- heat, cold, pressure;
- infections;
- unknown causes in many cases.

Treatment includes the following.

1. Try to find the cause (especially allergy or acetylsalicylic acid or NSAID) and stop it.
2. Topical preparations. Try calamine lotion. If not effective try betamethasone 0.1% cream, but if on face only hydrocortisone 1% cream.
3. Antihistamines (see Chapter 10 pages 44–45).
4. Epinephrine/adrenalin injection if the condition is severe; especially if swelling on the face or neck threatens to block breathing (see Chapter 10 page 44).

Psoriasis

In psoriasis, patches of redness and inflammation of the skin covered by silvery scales appear. The lesions do not itch or cause pain. The edges of the patches, where they join the normal skin, are very definite (see Figure 32.31). The finger and toenails are often pitted, thickened and the nail is not attached properly to the nailbed under it towards the end of the nail, which often becomes white, then brown. The scalp, elbows,

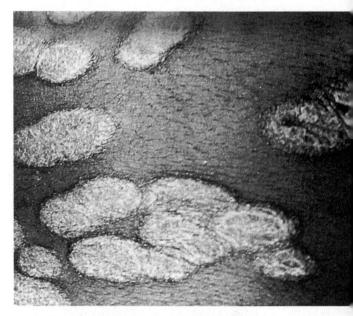

Figure 32.31 *Typical skin lesions of psoriasis. Note the definite edge. These patches are covered by scales.*

knees and also buttocks and around the umbilicus are often affected.

If the patient has HIV infection psoriasis may be severe.

Treatment

1. Explain there is no cure, but treatment may help the lesions when they are worrying the patient.
2. Keep the skin moist. Urea cream, but more likely ointment, twice daily should help.
3. Some exposure to sunlight often helps.
4. Salicylic acid 5–10% twice daily, *or*
Coal tar 5–10% at night, *or*
Sulfur 5–10% at night may help.
Try to get ointments containing these or make up the ointment yourself using 10% urea ointment to which you add the other chemicals.
5. Discuss the patient with the Medical Officer and ask about other treatment including dithranol, corticosteroids and others.

Acne vulgaris

In acne, blackheads and pimples form in the skin. Some may become infected and cause boils. Scars and keloids may occur. (See Figures 32.32 and 32.33.)

Treatment includes:

1. stopping the use of vaseline or mineral oil or greasy cosmetics, etc. which block the pores of the skin;
2. washing the area with a little soap and water;

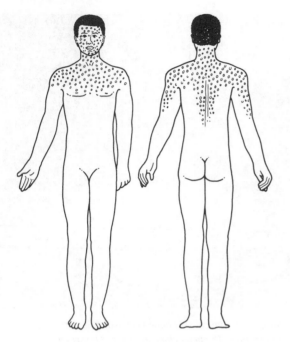

Figure 32.32 *Diagram to show the parts of the body where lesions of acne vulgaris most commonly occur.*

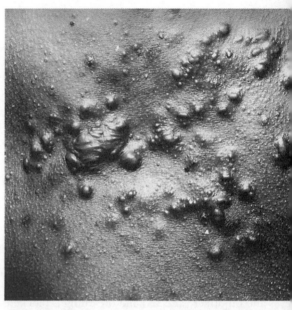

Figure 32.33 *Photograph showing a close up view of skin affected by acne. You can usually see 'blackheads' on the patient more easily than in this photograph.*

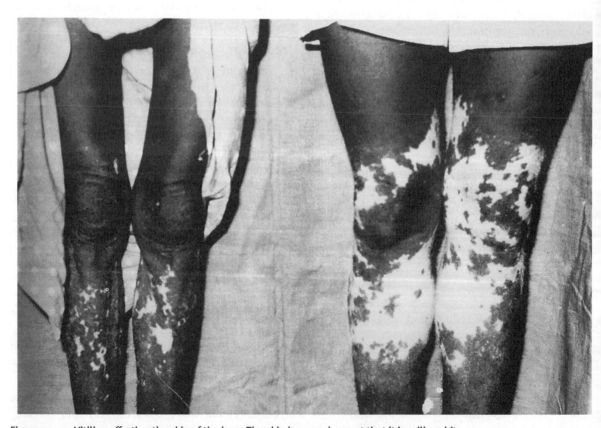

Figure 32.34 *Vitiligo affecting the skin of the legs. The skin is normal except that it is milky white.*

3. getting the surface layer of the skin to 'peel' off using salicylic acid 5% in spirit or benzyl peroxide 5% cream or lotion once daily;

4. if not pregnant, oral doxycycline 100 mg daily or tetracycline 250 mg four times a day for several months;

5. special treatment, which is expensive and which the patient may buy, is a lotion or cream of retinic acid or tretinoin 0.05% but which if female must never be used if is or could get pregnant;

6. a very special, very expensive (and dangerous if pregnant) oral drug, isotretinoin, which could be ordered by the Medical Officer if the patient is willing to buy it, if the above are not effective.

Vitiligo or leucoderma

In vitiligo, patches of normal skin lose their pigment and become white (see Figure 32.34). The skin is otherwise perfectly normal. There is no loss of sensation over the patches.

Do not mistake leprosy, late yaws, late onchocerciasis, etc. for vitiligo.

No treatment for vitiligo is necessary or possible at the health centre, except very importantly, to protect the skin from sunburn (see Albinism). Vitiligo is not dangerous and is not infectious.

At the time of writing even the latest treatment, which is very expensive, helps (and does not cure) at the most only 20% of patients. It is important to encourage patients to accept the problem and not waste a lot of money on treatment that is of little use.

Albinism

Albinism is a hereditary condition in which there is not enough pigment formation in the body (Figure 32.35).

The irises of the eyes are pink or red, and the hair and the skin are white. The skin does not become darker in the sun.

The main complication is skin cancer caused by the sun continually burning the skin, which is not protected by pigment.

There is no cure for this condition.

Treatment includes wearing clothes to keep the sun off the skin – hat, long sleeved shirt and long trousers or dress, etc. all the time during the day. The person should keep away from the sun as much as possible. He should put on a sunscreen with an SPF factor of 15 or more (e.g. 5% para aminobenzoic acid in ethanol) twice daily or more often, before going in the sun. These things are essential.

If the patient develops any sores that do not heal, *refer* or *transfer* him non-urgently for biopsy and probable excision of lesion, in case it is a skin cancer.

Common skin symptoms and signs

Itch (with or without rash)

Do a full history and examination (see Chapter 6 pages 21–26).

Test the urine for protein, sugar and bile.

Note especially:

1. where the itch is, and

2. the details of any skin lesions (rash) present.

Diagnosis depends on where the itch and rash is.

Treat as in this book (see Index) or see a specialist medical reference book.

Rash between fingers or on wrists or on elbows or on genitalia; but not on face, then

• scabies – see pages 538–540.

Rash in hair or around waist or in eyelashes or in pubic area, then

• lice – see page 540.

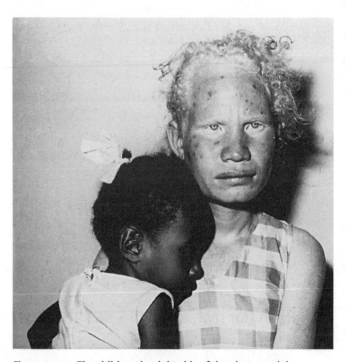

Figure 32.35 *The child on the right side of the photograph is an albino. Note the sun-damaged white skin. She looks older than her age because the sun damage to her skin is the same as for a much older person with normal skin.*

Rash only on uncovered areas (arms, legs, face), then

- insect bites, or
- contact with irritants (contact dermatitis), or
- sunshine and a drug taken or put on skin (e.g. tetracycline) (photosensitive dermatitis).
- HIV infection – itch usually in other places also and small lumps usually develop which become dark.

Itch around anus, then

- candidiasis – see pages 529–530, or
- enterobius (threadworm) – see Chapter 23 page 357, or *Strongyloides* – see pages 357–358, or
- haemorrhoids or anal fissure, or
- diabetes mellitus (glucose in urine) – see Chapter 30 pages 499–504.

Itch of vulva, then

- all conditions as for anus, or
- *Candida* (thrush) or *Trichomonas* infection, or
- after menopause – oestrogen hormone deficiency needing treatment with oestrogen cream twice weekly

Itch all over, then

- onchocerciasis if there are skin nodules over bony areas and especially if there is trouble with the eyes – see pages 542–544, or
- HIV infection – see Chapter 19 page 230, or
- drugs and other causes of allergy – see page 549 and Chapter 10 pages 44–45, or
- jaundice – see Chapter 24 pages 392, 402, or
- chronic kidney failure – see Chapter 26 page 449.

Itch where there is a rash of round patches which are worse at the edges, anywhere on the body, then

- tinea – see pages 527–531.

Itch where there is a rash on face or behind knees and in front of elbows and is either

1. *lesions which are thick and very dry or*
2. *small blisters which burst leaving moist red areas*, then
- atopic dermatitis – see page 548.

Itch where there are the signs of an eczematous dermatitis (see above and page 548).

- eczematous dermatitis – see causes page 548.

Rash (for rash and itch – see also itch)

Do a full history and examination (see Chapter 6 pages 21–26).

Test the urine for protein, bile and sugar.

Note:

1. where the lesions are, and
2. the type of lesions they are.

Diagnosis depends on the features below.

Treat as in this book (see Index) or see a specialist reference book.

Acute start; fever; general rash (face, trunk and limbs) then

- chickenpox – see Chapter 16 pages 152–153, or
- measles – see Chapter 16 pages 151–152, or
- other viral diseases – see Chapter 16 pages 153–154.

Vesicles, pustules, yellow crusts, then

- impetigo – see pages 532–533.

Dry skin patches:

1. *no loss of sensation; itching, healing in centre*, then
   - tinea – see pages 527–531.
2. loss of sensation and thick nerves, then
   - leprosy – see Chapter 15 pages 130–133.

Nodules

1. *severe itchy dermatitis and eye trouble*, then
   - onchocerciasis – see pages 542–544.
2. *other signs of leprosy*, then
   - leprosy – see Chapter 15 pages 138, 130–133.
3. drugs given recently or other causes of allergy, then
   - allergic reaction – see page 549 and Chapter 10 pages 44–45.
4. other signs of leprosy and patient is sick or has tender nerves or iritis, then
   - leprosy reaction – see Chapter 15 page 138.

Eczematous reaction (small blisters which burst leaving moist red areas with itch or thick dry areas). Then

- eczematous dermatitis – see page 548.

Skin ulcer

Do a full history and examination (see Chapter 6 pages 21–26).

Test the urine for protein, sugar and bile.

Note especially where the ulcer is – there are three common places:

1. genitalia,
2. breast, and
3. leg.

But ulcers can occur anywhere.

Diagnosis depends on the features of the ulcer (see below).

Ulcer on genitalia

Then most likely syphilis or other STD – see Chapter 19 pages 198 and 204.

Ulcer on breast

Acute start in young woman, then

- most likely breast abscess see Chapter 36 pages 592–593 and a surgery book. Transfer if needed.

Chronic start in older woman, then
- most likely cancer. See a surgery or gynaecology book. Refer to Medical Officer.

Ulcer on leg or foot but also anywhere

Ulcer started acutely and spread very quickly and was itchy and painful and smelly. Ulcer becomes chronic, if untreated, then
- tropical ulcer – see pages 533–534.

Ulcer started after injury or infection.
Ulcer is like an ulcer anywhere but is slow to heal, then
- bacterial infection (treat as for tropical ulcer).

Ulcer started as nodule which ulcerated.
Ulcer has undermined edges.
Ulcer spread quickly and surrounding ulcers may have developed.
AFB in smear from edge of ulcer or positive biopsy, then
- *Mycobacterium ulcerans* ulcer – see Chapter 32 page 537.

Painful ulcer or ulcers on feet.
Papillomas or ulcers in other areas also.
In area where yaws occurs.
Serological tests for syphilis positive.
- yaws – see pages 535–536.

Ulcer started as a vesicle which ruptured and quickly became 2–3 cm across.
Edges are inverted and slightly undermined.
The ulcer is deep and covered with gray exudate or a dark crust. Surrounding skin is erythematous or blue.
May be paralysis of limb or food swallowed comes back through nose, then
- diphtheritic ulcer (see also Chapter 20 page 284).

Treat with penicillin and dressings as for tropical ulcer (see pages 533–534).
If paralysis transfer urgently for anti-toxin.

Ulcer started as a blister with general allergic reaction, fever and often vomiting. Blister burst and itchy ulcer developed, relieved by cold water.
Outline of worm under skin or end of worm seen in ulcer, then
- guinea worm – page 545.

Ulcer after chronic anaemia, often jaundice, no bile in urine, infarction crises and especially attacks of bone pain, then
- sickle-cell anaemia ulcer (treat as for tropical ulcer; but Eusol and antibiotics are not necessary if there is no infection).

Ulcer most often under foot.
Loss of sensation under foot.
Enlarged nerves or patches with loss of sensation, then
- leprosy – see Chapter 15 pages 135–136, 146–148.

Ulcer most often under foot.
Loss of sensation under foot.
No enlarged nerves or patches with loss of sensation.
Sugar in urine, then
- diabetes mellitus – Chapter 30 pages 499–504.

Ulcer under foot.
Loss of sensation under foot.
Painless.
Not due to leprosy or diabetes.
Serological test for syphilis positive.
- syphilis (see Chapter 19 pages 208–210).

Ulcer anywhere (see leg or foot also).
Ulcer anywhere and keeps on getting larger despite treatment.
- possibly cancer – biopsy or transfer to Medical Officer.

Punched out looking ulcer.
No pain.
No inflammation.
Not healed despite treatment.
Serological test for syphilis positive.
- gumma (from syphilis or yaws) (see Chapter 19 pages 208–210 and page 535).

Ulcer anywhere

Ulcer anywhere, you can see pus and bone, then
- chronic osteomyelitis – see Chapter 28 page 477.

Ulcer anywhere, in an area where dermal leishmaniasis occurs, then
- dermal leishmaniasis (oriental sore) – see Chapter 18 pages 175–181.

Ulcer on face, especially if near nose or mouth or on neck, especially if near a sinus or enlarged lymph nodes.
Chronic cough.
Enlarged lymph nodes.
Weight loss.
Smear from edge positive for AFB, then
- tuberculosis – see Chapter 14 page 537.

If on face and diagnosis not certain, send urgently to Medical Officer before a lot of the face is destroyed.

33 Bites and Stings

Find out in your area:

1. What venomous animals exist.
2. What the effects of their venoms are.
3. What is the best first aid and then treatment for them.
4. What antivenoms are available and when to give them, as these may be different in your area from the usual ones which follow in this chapter.

Snakebite

When a snake bites a person, in only about half of the cases does the snake inject enough venom (its poison) to cause any significant harm (envenomation). However, sometimes enough venom is injected to cause death, even when the place where the snake bit cannot be seen. If a patient claims to have been bitten by a snake, always believe him and give proper first aid. Admit him to the health centre for 24 hours for observation to see if symptoms and signs of injection of the venom develop and if he needs treatment or not.

If a snake injects its venom when it bites, the effects of the injected venom may include any or some or all of the following groups of conditions.

1. Damage to body cells at the site of the bite.
   - Pain where the bite occurred may appear almost immediately. Pain may occur not long after in nearby lymph glands and later also in the abdomen, as the venom travels through the lymph vessels.
   - Acute inflammation of the conjunctivae and cornea may occur if the snake spat the venom into the eye.
   - Inflammation where the bite occurred. Swelling may start in 2–3 hours and become very large by about 2–3 days, and may eventually involve half or more of a limb; blisters may appear on the surface, cellulitis may develop and eventually there may be large ulcers.
2. Poisoning of the cardiovascular system.
   - Shock or heart failure from fluid leaking out of damaged blood vessels or from the heart not pumping well because of damage to its muscle may occur.
3. Poisoning of the nervous system.
   Drowsiness and even unconsciousness may occur. Paralysis of the motor part of the nervous system so

that muscles become weak or paralysed.
   - If the throat muscles become paralysed, the patient's airway may become blocked. The patient cannot breathe and dies.
   - If the swallowing muscles become paralysed, the patient cannot swallow his saliva and aspirates it into his lungs (breathes it in). He 'drowns in his own saliva' or gets pneumonia.
   - If the breathing muscles become paralysed, the patient cannot breathe and suffocates.
4. The clotting proteins in the blood may be 'activated' and all used up; then the blood will not clot and the patient can bleed to death.
5. Damage to muscle cells may occur, with aching, stiffness and weakness of the muscles. Also muscle cells die and the myoglobin from inside the muscle cells makes the urine dark and can damage the kidneys.
6. Damage may occur to the red blood cells with haemolysis (breaking open of red blood cells) in the blood vessels with dark urine from haemoglobinuria and kidney damage.
7. Acute kidney failure (see Chapter 26 page 453) may occur due either to 5 and 6 above or direct poisoning of the kidney cells.

The most serious problems caused by snakebite:

1. Paralysis – not being able to breathe.
2. Blood not clotting – bleeding to death.

If early signs of any of these conditions develop (called 'envenomation') *give antivenom*. Antivenom is made from the blood of a large animal, e.g. horse or sheep. The animal is first injected with very small and safe doses of venom, to which it will make antibodies. Then increasing and eventually very large doses of venom, from which it is protected by the previous antibodies, are given. These large doses make the animal produce even more antibodies. Blood is then taken from the animal and antibodies taken out of the blood; this is what we call 'antivenom'. Some antivenoms can now be made in the laboratory. Antivenom, then, contains antibodies which, if given to a patient with envenomation from a snake, will destroy the venom in the patient and stop more symptoms and signs of envenomation and death occurring.

If signs of envenomation do not occur, *do not give antivenom*. Often when snakes bite people, they do not inject enough venom to cause envenomation, and the patient does not need antivenom.

The type of antivenom you give depends on which type of snake bit the patient.

You must find out for your area:

1. What types of snake are present.
2. What the effects of their bites are.
3. What antivenoms are available.
4. When you should give these antivenoms.
5. What doses of these antivenoms you should give.

If kits are available to determine what kind of venom is on/in the patients, use these kits to tell you what kind of antivenom to use; but only if the patient develops signs of envenomation. Tests are done on venom left on the skin at the site of the bite (or in urine). These tests do NOT tell you whether to give an antivenom or not. A negative test does NOT mean the patient was not bitten. The test tells you only what kind of antivenom to give IF antivenom is needed.

First aid

1. Make sure no further bites occur.
2. Stop any panic. Comfort the patient. The patient should not move. Tell the patient to lie down, keep still and rest. The patient must not walk. Take transport to the patient, or carry the patient to transport or the health centre. Do not move the bitten part to take off clothes.
3. If no kits for testing for the type of venom are available, quickly wash the wound (but only if there is water available immediately) or gently wipe away venom on the skin. If the venom was spat into the eye, wash out the eye with a lot of water. If a venom testing kit is available, do not wash the wound until after venom for the test is taken.
4. Do not cut the wound or treat the wound in any other way.
5. Do not tie anything around the limb (tourniquet).
6. Bandage and splint the limb. Bandage around the area of the bite and then from the end of the limb across the bite area and as far up the whole limb as possible (tightly as for a sprained ankle). Use a bandage or torn up clothing. Remove any other thing (tourniquet) tied around the limb by others when you are about to bandage across it. Then put all the limb in a splint. If the limb cannot be bandaged, put it in a sling or splint. If you are in an area where snakebites may cause swelling of the bite area, check the colour and temperature and pulse of the limb, below the bandage, every half hour.

If the limb becomes cold or white or blue, or if the pulse becomes weak or is not present, or if there is a lot of swelling of the bitten area, and the bandages become too tight, remove the bandages. Bandaging the limb stops the venom being absorbed through the lymph vessels and then being taken to the rest of the body until antivenom is available.

> The patient must not move the bitten limb or walk. Bandage the bite area and then all the limb firmly. Then put all the limb in a splint.

7. Do not give anything to eat or drink.
8. If there is any problem with unconsciousness, paralysis, difficulty in breathing, or vomiting, lay the patient on his side and give routine care for an unconscious patient, and if needed, artificial ventilation (see Chapters 25 page 422, and 37 page 607).

Management

> Management includes:
>
> Admit all patients who say they have been bitten.
>
> 1. Comfort the patient.
> 2. Make the patient rest.
> 3. Set up an IV drip.
> 4. Take blood. Test it for the time it takes to clot.
> 5. Examine to see if there are signs of envenomation. Repeat the examination every hour. Look for:
>   - paralysis,
>   - abnormal bleeding, and
>   - other signs of envenomation.
> 6. Give antimalarial drug if needed.
> 7. Give antivenom carefully, but ONLY if signs of envenomation are present or develop. Look carefully for reactions. Treat any reactions quickly.
> 8. Treat any complications in the usual way. Do not give any IM injections.
> 9. Do not give acetylsalicylic acid, morphine or pethidine.
> 10. Give tetanus prophylaxis later.
>
> Transfer to Medical Officer, if envenomation is probable or present and if there is no antivenom available; or you cannot give antivenom because a reaction occurred; or if another complication occurs.

Admit all patients who say they have been bitten by a snake (for observation and treatment if treatment becomes necessary).

You cannot always tell if envenomation is probable by looking at the bite area.

1. Comfort the patient. Tell him that you can save him.
2. Make the patient keep still, rest in bed and not move the bitten limb.
3. Set up an intravenous drip of 0.9% sodium chloride (1 litre every 12 hours).
4. Put 5 ml of venous blood in a clean glass (not plastic) test tube or bottle and let it stand still. Note the time. Tilt the tube after 10 minutes and after 20 minutes to see if the blood has clotted or not (it should have). If the blood has not clotted by 20 minutes, the patient has had enough venom to need antivenom. Repeat the test on newly collected blood 4 hours after the bandages are taken off.
5. Examine for any clinical signs of envenomation (see below). Repeat and write down these observations:
   • hourly for 12 hours if suspected snakebite,
   • hourly for 24 hours if a definite snakebite,
   • $\frac{1}{4}$ hourly if signs of envenomation are present or develop.

Write the headings on the observation chart so that your staff know what observations to take.

Observations include:
(a) Symptoms and signs of *paralysis*, which are:
   • ptosis (drooping of eyelids),
   • double vision or paralysis of movements of the eyes,
   • speech 'thick', or like a drunken man,
   • jaw hanging open, by more than 2 cm,
   • cannot swallow properly, or saliva collects in the throat, and
   • cannot take a deep breath and cough.
(b) Symptoms and signs of *abnormal bleeding*, which are:
   • venous blood put in a test tube does not clot in 20 minutes (do this once only on admission; but repeat it later if you suspect abnormal bleeding and 4 hours after the compression bandages are taken off),
   • bleeding from the place of the snakebite,
   • blood in the sputum, vomit, urine, stool, nose, etc., and
   • bleeding into the skin.
(c) Symptoms and signs of envenomation in other parts of the body, which are:
   • pulse fast or irregular,
   • blood pressure low,
   • shock or heart failure,

   • respiratory rate fast,
   • level of consciousness below normal,
   • severe swelling and tenderness of lymph glands,
   • abdominal pain and vomiting,
   • swelling and blisters at the place of the bite, and up to the knee or elbow (if the bite was on the foot or hand), or swelling of more than half of the limb, and
   • urine is pink or brown or black from haemolysis or muscle damage (examine urine every time it is passed).

6. Give an oral antimalarial drug if you are in a malarious area (see Chapter 13 pages 79, 80). If a rigor occurs later, then it will probably not be caused by malaria.
7. Give antivenom only if needed.
   Once a drip is running and antivenom is available, if the patient still has no signs of envenomation take the bandages off the limb.
   Give antivenom only if:
   (a) any signs of envenomation are already present when you first see the patient – usually twice the standard dose of the type indicated (give this before taking off the bandages and splint);
   (b) signs of envenomation develop while you are observing – give one full standard dose of the type indicated;
   (c) signs of envenomation are the same (including the blood taken on admission still not clotted) or are getting worse 4 hours after you gave antivenom – give two standard doses of polyvalent antivenom.
   You must find out the *type of antivenom* indicated for your area and their doses.

Dose of antivenom
You must find this out for your area. The dose of antivenom in one ampoule is usually the dose to neutralise the amount of venom injected by one usual snakebite. The size of the dose in ampoules in your area may be different.
(a) One usual bite – give one standard dose.
(b) If more than the usual amount of venom was injected and there was more than one bite – give more than the standard dose (usually two; but more than two may be necessary).
(c) Children – dose the same as for adults.

How to give antivenom
(a) Make sure the antivenom is clear. If it is cloudy it is probably not active, and may be dangerous.

(b) Give antivenom by IV drip.

(c) Put the antivenom into a side drip in a drip that is running.

(d) First inject an antihistamine, e.g. promethazine 25 mg IV *(but only if the antivenom you are using needs it)*.

Keep the syringe at the bedside with a (or another) dose of antihistamine.

(e) Then inject epinephrine/adrenaline tart. 1:1000 solution one half ($\frac{1}{2}$) of the usual dose given for asthma (i.e. 0.25 ml ($\frac{1}{4}$ ml) for an adult) subcutaneously (but only if the antivenom you are using needs it). Draw up into a syringe 0.5 ml ($\frac{1}{2}$ ml) of epinephrine/adrenaline tart. 1:1000 solution and keep this syringe at the bedside with another full ampoule of epinephrine/adrenaline available.

(f) Draw up the antivenom, and inject it into another 500 ml bag of IV fluid, (e.g. normal saline or 5% dextrose) and run this, as a side drip, into the original IV drip and commence at 1 ml/minute for 5 minutes.

(g) Wait 5 minutes. Take PR and BP, look for skin rash or itch, look for swelling of the face or neck and listen for cough and wheezes.

(h) If there is no reaction after 5 minutes, inject the rest of the antivenom, slowly over 30 minutes (never in less than 10 minutes).

(i) Observe as in (g) every 15 minutes for 1 hour.

(j) Remove the bandage and splint from the bite area when you have given the antivenom if envenomation present.

If a reaction to the antivenom occurs:
(a) stop giving the antivenom,

(b) give the epinephrine/adrenaline tart. 1:1000 solution 0.5 ml ($\frac{1}{2}$ ml) SCI immediately, and

(c) give the antihistamine, e.g. promethazine 25 mg (1 ml) IVI immediately.

If a severe reaction to the antivenom occurs and especially if the patient looks as if he may die:
(a) give epinephrine/adrenaline tart. 1:1000 solution 0.5 ml ($\frac{1}{2}$ ml) diluted to 5 ml IV slowly over 5 minutes, i.e. 1 ml/minute immediately,

(b) give antihistamine, e.g. promethazine 50 mg (2 ml) IV with another syringe immediately,

(c) give hydrocortisone 100–300 mg intravenously if it is available, and

(d) repeat the epinephrine/adrenaline after 5 minutes if necessary.

Then see the instruction paper with the antivenom and a specialist reference book for further

management. In most cases the antivenom can be started again but given much more slowly with, if needed, further epinephrine/adrenaline.

8. Treat any complications in the usual way.

If paralysis occurs after you have given a repeat double dose of antivenom, or if you cannot give antivenom because of a reaction, transfer and
(a) nurse the patient on his side (head down if necessary),

(b) suck out the airway every hour (or more often if necessary – noisy breathing or snoring means a blocked airway), and

(c) give artificial ventilation if necessary.

If bleeding occurs, give fresh, whole blood (but only if you have safe (HIV and HBV negative) cross-matched blood); *but first give* a repeat double dose of polyvalent antivenom. Arrange urgent (emergency) transfer to hospital while you do all this.

If shock occurs, if it is soon after the bite, give an antihistamine and epinephrine/adrenaline as for anaphylactic shock, although if it is when the bitten area is very swollen, give fluids as for dehydration. If in any doubt, treat both ways. (See Chapter 27 pages 468–470.)

If a lot of swelling or inflammation of the bitten area occurs, treat it as you would treat a burned area and give antibiotics.

If vomiting occurs repeatedly, give metoclopramide 10 mg IVI and repeat if needed.

If the eye shows corneal ulcers or iritis, treat in the usual way. (See Chapter 31 pages 514 and 515.)

9. Do not give acetylsalicylic acid (which may make bleeding worse) or morphine or pethidine (which could reduce breathing). If the patient is frightened, restless or in pain, give explanation and comfort and intranasal oxygen. If a drug is really necessary, give rectal or oral diazepam and/or paracetamol. If there is no paralysis after 24 hours and pain is severe, morphine could then be used.

10. Give tetanus toxoid 0.5 ml ($\frac{1}{2}$ ml) SCI, and finish the course later if the patient is not immunised. If someone has cut the wound, and it may be infected (and the patient is not immunised), then give also tetanus immunoglobulin 250–500 units IMI.

Transfer to Medical Officer care
Urgently (emergency) if:

• there is a definite bite of a known poisonous snake; *or*

- there are symptoms or signs of envenomation (weakness or bleeding, etc.);

and if also

- there is no antivenom available; *or*
- you cannot give antivenom because the patient is allergic to antivenom (more than just an itchy swelling of the skin which you can treat with epinephrine/ adrenaline and antihistamines); *or*
- the patient is not cured by a repeat dose of 2 ampoules of polyvalent antivenom.

Non-urgent transfer is necessary if other complications which you cannot manage at the health centre occur.

Prevention

Teach people to be careful in areas where snakes are common. Never disturb snakes, even *apparently* dead snakes, unless people are ready and skilled to kill them. Children must not collect or play with *any* snakes. Discourage young men from climbing trees after snakes. Encourage people to wear shoes and long legged clothing and tap the ground to warn snakes someone is coming. As well as this, when walking at night, carry a light.

Seasnake bite

The effects of a bite by a seasnake are as for landsnakes; but cell poisoning of muscle is more common. Pain and stiffness of the muscles; then severe pain if the muscles are moved; and then paralysis can occur. The urine becomes red or brown or black from myoglobin (like haemoglobin but from inside a damaged muscle).

If there are real signs of envenomation (especially if there is red or brown or black urine or paralysis), give seasnake antivenom. If there is no seasnake antivenom available, give polyvalent landsnake antivenom and other treatment, as for landsnakes (see pages 555–558), and transfer to a Medical Officer urgently.

Venomous fish

Stings from such fish can cause:

1. Severe cell poisoning in the stung limb, with very severe pain; oedema; weakness; sometimes necrosis; and later, abscesses.
2. Nausea and vomiting, excessive saliva, diarrhoea; irregular pulse and shock; difficulty breathing; nervous system stimulation with muscle spasms or even convulsions or nervous system depression with sometimes, paralysis of all the muscles, including those used for breathing.

Treatment includes:

1. Put and keep the affected limb into very hot water (45°C). The heat, for many fish venoms, destroys the venom and helps the pain. This is very effective treatment. Make sure you do not burn the patient (test with your own hand and also put the patient's unbitten limb into the water). The heat treatment may be needed for up to a couple of hours.
2. If hot water is not available, apply a firm bandage and splint (see page 555) immediately.
3. Infiltrate the sting area with local anaesthetic lidocaine (lignocaine) 5 ml 2% or 10 ml in solution. This is very important if hot water treatment is not immediately available.
4. Put up an intravenous drip.
5. If the sting was from a stonefish give stonefish antivenom (with precautions as for snake antivenom – see pages 556–557) if there is still severe pain or if general signs are present *after* the above treatment. (Antivenom is not available for most other fish stings.)
6. Treat any other complications in the usual way.
7. Remove any remaining barb or foreign body from the wound.
8. Give tetanus prophylaxis (see page 557).
9. Treat any secondary bacterial infection with antibiotics (e.g. doxycycline).

Prevention is by wearing shoes and shuffling (not walking with steps) when walking in water to avoid stepping onto venomous fish.

Stings from jellyfish (and similar sea stings)

Box jellyfish cause the most severe types of stings:

1. very severe pain,
2. severe skin inflammation, like third degree burns,
3. sometimes paralysis of breathing, shock and stopping of the heart.

Other jellyfish and other marine stingers, e.g. Irukanji syndrome, cause less severe similar conditions; but some after some minutes severe body pains and sometimes high blood pressure, fast and irregular pulse, rapid breathing, severe anxiety and later sometimes shock or heart failure.

Treatment includes:

1. Immediately get the patient out of the water. The rescuer must take care not to be stung (as the tentacles may trail 3 metres behind the jellyfish).
2. If the patient's breathing is not enough, or if it stops, give artificial ventilation (see Chapter 37 page 607).

If shock develops, treat as for shock caused by acute allergic reaction (see Chapter 27 pages 468–470). If the heart stops, give external cardiac massage (see Chapter 37 page 609).

3. If box jellyfish (*or any sting which leaves tentacles on the patient*), immediately 'disarm' the tentacles on the patient (i.e. stop them injecting more venom). Pour 2–10% acetic acid in water, e.g. household vinegar over the affected parts and the tentacles. Pour more on as it runs off. Leave the area covered with vinegar for at least 30 seconds. (In parts of the Atlantic a mixture of sodium bicarbonate (baking soda) and water in equal amounts is said to be effective. Ask about your area.)
   If no acetic acid is available, dry the tentacles by throwing dirt or sand or other dry powder on them before removing them.
   Do not put spirit or alcohol (of any sort) onto the affected area (as used to be recommended). *Do not put any water onto the affected area for 2 hours.*
4. Pull (or shave with a razor blade) the tentacles off the affected area as soon as possible. Do not rub the stung area. If not box jellyfish or no tentacles on skin, wash area with seawater.
5. If a box jellyfish, apply cold (ice) packs as quickly as possible once the tentacles have been either disarmed by vinegar or pulled off. See 7 below.
6. Give analgesics. Try lidocaine/lignocaine 2 or 4% or other local anaesthetic jelly or cream. Usually repeated small doses of IV morphine are necessary, because of the severe pain. If a nitrous oxide–oxygen mixture (often used at childbirth) is available, give the patient this to breathe. A general anaesthetic with ketamine may be better for the pain than large doses of morphine (which may stop breathing).
7. For stings from other than box jellyfish, it has recently been shown that the best relief from pain is heat treatment – not cold packs. As soon as possible, put the affected area all under hot water at 45° (make sure the patient is not burned) for at least 20 minutes.
8. Give antivenom, if available, if there are problems with breathing, shock or cardiac arrest or if there are still significant symptoms and signs after the above (see pages 556–557).
9. Treat the skin as for burns.

Octopus stings

Stings can cause complete paralysis and stop breathing, but usually they cause no pain. Treat with artificial ventilation (see Chapter 37 page 607) until the patient starts to breathe again.

Coneshell stings

Coneshell stings can cause:

1. pain,
2. strange sensations in the body, and
3. paralysis which can stop breathing.

   Treatment:

1. Wash the wound and put on a firm bandage and splint (see page 555).
2. Infiltrate the sting area with local anaesthetic lidocaine (lignocaine) 2% to relieve the pain.
3. Give artificial ventilation (see Chapter 37 page 607) if the patient stops breathing, until he starts to breathe again.

Scorpion stings and centipede stings

The effects of scorpion stings can be different from place to place. The effects are usually much more severe in children than in adults.

1. Most stings cause severe pain, often with swelling, and sometimes bleeding, at the place of the sting.
2. Some stings cause many types of severe unusual symptoms and signs due to stimulation of the parasympathetic and then sympathetic nervous systems. There may be increased temperature, sweating, increased production of saliva, diarrhoea, vomiting, incontinence, penile erection and abnormalities of blood glucose and slow pulse, high blood pressure, heart failure, etc.
3. Some stings cause unusual signs in the nervous system – fitting, paralysis and death by stopping breathing.
4. Some stings can cause fast pulse, very high blood pressure, 'goose bumps' and severe heart failure and pulmonary oedema.
5. Some stings cause heart failure and shock.

   Treatment will depend on what type of scorpion is present in your area. For pain, local anaesthetic injections are often very helpful. Morphine, however, may be needed. In shock, besides giving the usual treatment, if the pulse is slow, give atropine 0.6 mg repeated as necessary until the pulse is over 60 and if peripheral blood vessels are contracted. If the skin is cold, try the effect of sublingual glyceryl trinitrate 0.6 mg repeated if necessary, but not if the blood pressure is less than 100. Prazosin, if available, is particularly helpful for treating high blood pressure and fast pulse and heart failure. If the patient fits, give paraldehyde or diazepam. (See Chapter 25 page 425.) If the patient stops breathing, give artificial ventilation. (See Chapter 37 page 607.)

If antivenom is available, give this as soon as possible if there are serious signs of envenomation, as well as the above. See page 556 for method and precautions.

Spider bites

Only a few spiders cause severe or fatal bites. *Effects* may include:

1. There may be severe pain at the place of the bite with swelling and redness developing quickly. Later on, an ulcer may form.
2. The pain may soon spread all over the body and cause muscle spasm (muscles contract and are then tight all the time) and pain. Shaking and fits can occur.
3. Many different types of general symptoms and signs can occur.
4. Shock may occur.

Treatment includes:

1. Wash or clean the bite.
2. Bandage and splint as for snakebite (see page 555).
3. Give analgesics as necessary for the pain (see Chapter 7 pages 33–34).
4. Give diazepam for severe muscle pain and spasm or for fitting (see Chapter 25 page 425). Calcium gluconate 10 ml of a 10% solution given slowly over 10 minutes intravenously is said to be helpful for muscle spasm.
5. Give atropine 0.6 mg (1 ml) if the pulse is very slow and repeat as often as needed.
6. Treat shock if it occurs (see Chapter 27 page 468).
7. Give spider antivenom if indicated and if available (see pages 556–557).

Insect stings

Insect stings can cause:

1. Severe pain at the bite area.
2. General symptoms and signs of cell poisoning, but usually only if there are many stings.
3. Allergic reactions, which are usually much more common and dangerous than either of the above two. These reactions may cause death from swelling of the bitten area, especially if it is the face, tongue or neck which could block the airway; asthma; shock; etc.

Treatment includes:

1. Give analgesics.
2. Comfort the patient.
3. Remove sting with the point of a needle, if it is from a bee, and take care not to squeeze the sting sac as this will force more venom into the tissues.
4. Wash the affected area.
5. If there is an allergic reaction, give epinephrine/adrenaline SC or IM or IV if necessary and antihistamine orally or IM or IV if necessary and, if available, hydrocortisone IV (see Chapter 10 pages 44–45).

Tick paralysis

The bites of some ticks can cause paralysis and stop breathing, if the tick stays in the body for a few days.

Remove the tick with a needle. Do not squeeze it and inject more venom into the patient. Give artificial ventilation (see Chapter 37 page 607) if necessary and transfer the patient urgently to a hospital.

The patient will get better if ventilated until the paralysis goes. Tick antivenom may be available.

Bats

Bites or scratches from bats (and possibly even breathing in dust from their excretions) may lead to serious diseases. These may include Ebola, Marburg, SARS, Hendra (like rabies) and Nipah (pneumonia and encephalitis) and other virus infections. These viruses infect bats but do not cause disease in bats most of the time (i.e. bats are carriers). It is safest to avoid bites or scratches from bats or breathing in dust from where they live (although in many places many people are not harmed by them). If unusual brain, liver or lung illness occurs, find out if the patient was exposed to bats.

Animal and human bites

If a person has been bitten think of
1. bacterial infection at the site,
2. tetanus,
3. special diseases carried by the animal (rabies from all but especially dogs, fever and arthritis from rats, fever and enlarged lymph nodes from cats, HIV from humans, etc.).

Treatment includes:

1. (a) careful cleaning of the wound; but do not suture it closed; and transfer to Medical Officer if severe or a joint is involved.
   (b) antibiotic usually; amoxicillin and clavulanic acid is the most effective for all; otherwise penicillin and clindamycin (or metronidazole); doxycycline only if the above not available.
2. tetanus prophylaxis (see Chapter 25 pages 419–420).
3. special prophylaxis if needed (e.g. HIV, rabies).

34 Poisoning and Drug Abuse

Acute poisoning is almost always caused by a poison that a person swallows and absorbs through the gastro-intestinal tract. Sometimes acute poisoning is caused by a poison that a person breathes in and absorbs through the lungs; or caused by a poison that a person gets on the skin and absorbs through the skin; or caused by a poison that a person has injected.

The commonest chemicals that cause poisoning are drugs, petroleum products such as kerosene, herbicides (weedkillers) and insecticides (insect killers).

The poisoned person often takes the poison accidentally, e.g. children find and eat coloured tablets or a person drinks kerosene or weedkiller from a bottle which normally has a drink in it.

The poisoned person sometimes takes the poison to commit suicide (kill himself). People often take poisons not to really commit suicide, but to influence another person (to make him feel sorry or guilty, or to make him behave in a different way). This is called 'self-poisoning', (and *not* 'attempted suicide') and is a form of neurotic mental abnormality or acting out (see Chapter 35 pages 569–570).

Overdoses of drugs of abuse and other chemicals which are dangerous to health and life are often taken by drug addicts either accidentally (as the strength of the drug taken is not known) or purposely (to get a stronger effect).

When a person says they have been poisoned, you *must always* admit and treat the patient, even if you do not know if it is true; or even if you think it is not true.

The treatment of poisoning is an emergency. *Treat the patient immediately.* If he has to wait for treatment to start, the patient is more likely to die.

You cannot usually treat acute poisoning by giving an antidote, because there are no antidotes for most poisons. (An antidote is a chemical that will work against a poison and stop the effects of the poison.)

But you can treat most patients who have been poisoned. You must always do two things when a patient is poisoned. If you do these two things quickly, most poisoned patients get better.

1. Stop the patient absorbing any more poison into his body.
   If the patient swallowed the poison, get the poison out of the patient's gastrointestinal tract by making him vomit and giving him diarrhoea and stopping the poison being absorbed (see page 562).
   You *must not make the patient vomit*, however, if:
   (a) it is more than 1 hour after the patient has swallowed the poison (it is too late),
   (b) the patient is not fully conscious,
   (c) the patient has swallowed a petroleum product (e.g. kerosene),
   (d) the patient has swallowed acid or alkali,
   (e) the patient does not agree.
   You must not try to cause diarrhoea, however, if:
   you do not have polyethylene glycol or other colonoscopy preparation fluid to cause diarrhoea without causing problems with salt and potassium in the blood.
   If available, give activated charcoal after vomiting or gastric lavage has finished, as it may join or bind with poisons still in the gastrointestinal tract and stop any more of the poison being absorbed.
   If the patient absorbed the poison through his skin, remove all his clothes and wash him all over with soap and water. Wear gloves when doing this.
   If the patient breathed in the poison, immediately take the patient into fresh air; and give artificial ventilation and oxygen if necessary. Do not breathe in the poison yourself.
   If the poison was injected, put a firm bandage and a splint on the limb that was injected similar to that used for snakebite. The patient must not move the injected limb or walk around (see Chapter 33 page 555).

2. Keep the patient alive by treating any symptoms and signs that develop, until his liver and kidney and other parts of his body remove the poison already absorbed.
   If the patient becomes unconscious, give care for unconscious patient (see Chapter 25 page 422).
   If the patient stops breathing, give artificial ventilation (see Chapter 37 page 607).
   If the patient develops fitting, give diazepam or paraldehyde (see Chapter 25 page 425).
   If the patient develops shock, treat shock (see page 468).
   You may need to transfer the patient to Medical Officer care for the treatment of some symptoms and signs.

> If you do these two things:
>
> 1. stop the patient absorbing any more poison, and
> 2. keep the patient alive, by treating any symptoms and signs which develop,
>
> then you can keep most poisoned patients alive.

There are two other things which you must do:

1. Give antidotes if there are any.

   The only antidotes you probably have in a health centre are naloxone (or nalorphine), which you give for an overdose of morphine, pethidine or codeine, or atropine which you give for organophosphate/carbamate poisoning. The Medical Officer has only a few other antidotes.

2. Stop the poisoning occurring again.

   If the patient poisoned himself then you must give social or psychiatric help.

   If the patient was poisoned accidentally, then you must give health education about the storage of drugs and poisons. The most common kind of poisoning is a patient who has swallowed a poison.

Poisons (and drug overdoses) swallowed

Admit for inpatient treatment all cases of suspected poisoning. Find out:

1. what the patient has swallowed (ask a relative to bring a sample and the original container);
2. how much he swallowed; and
3. when he swallowed it.

Treatment of swallowed poisons

For *petroleum products* (e.g. kerosene), see page 564.

For *strong acids or alkalis,* see page 564.

If the patient is not fully conscious, see page 565.

If it is more than an hour since the patient swallowed the poison, it may be too late for 1, 2 and 3.

For the few other cases treat as follows:

1. Immediately make the patient vomit (to remove the poison from the stomach), *but not if he is not fully conscious or has swallowed a petroleum product (e.g. kerosene) or a strong acid or it is more than an hour since he took the poison.* Rub the back of the tongue and pharynx with several wooden tongue depressors held together.
2. Make the patient drink 200 ml (1–2 cups) of milk or water, *but not if not fully conscious.*

Then make the patient vomit again. *But not if the patient has swallowed a petroleum product (e.g. kerosene) or a strong acid.*

Do this many times until he vomits only water or milk and no food or poison. (The milk or water also dilutes the poison and slows its absorption.)

> For chloroquine, amodioquine or quinine poisoning, the most important part of the treatment is to make the patient vomit *immediately* and then again many times (or wash the stomach out – see 3 below). Then give a large dose of laxative to quickly cause severe diarrhoea.

3. Wash out the stomach if patient will not vomit; *but not if more than an hour since the poison was swallowed.* Lay the patient on his (preferably left) side with his head lower than the rest of his body. Put a large diameter (1.5 cm or $\frac{3}{4}$ inch) tube into the stomach. Then siphon out (by putting the end of the tube lower than the end of the tube in the patient's stomach) or aspirate (suck out with a large syringe on the end of the tube) the stomach contents. Then wash out the stomach, by putting 200 ml (1 cup) of milk or water down the tube and then aspirating it again. Do this at least 20 times, until the aspirated fluid is clear and contains no food or drugs. (It may need, e.g. 100 times.)

4. Give activated charcoal (if available) 50 g immediately and then 25–50 g 4 hourly. Mix with a cup of water. Make the patient drink this after vomiting is finished, or put it down the tube if the stomach is washed out.

5. The only safe laxatives are sorbitol 1–2 g/kg, polyethylene glycol or colonoscopy preparation fluid of any type which you probably will not have. Other laxatives may cause upset of the salt and potassium in the body. However, for very dangerous poisoning, especially quinine, chloroquine and amodiaquine, it is worth that risk; and give magnesium sulfate (Epsom salts) 30 g (30 ml of crystals in a measuring glass or 1 tablespoonful) in two cups of water. Make the patient drink this when the vomiting is finished, or put it down the tube after the stomach is washed out. (This should cause diarrhoea and removes the poison from the intestines.) Repeat the dose in half an hour if there is no diarrhoea.

6. Give an antidote, if there is one and if available (usually neither is), but if paraquat or if organophosphate or carbamate poisoning see page 564 or if isoniazid overdose see page 564.

7. Observe the patient every hour for level of consciousness, breathing rate and depth of respiration, PR, BP, and any other complications which the poison may cause. Note any complications that are developing before they become severe (especially loss of consciousness, not breathing properly and shock).

8. Treat any complication in the usual way, e.g.
   • fitting – anticonvulsants (see Chapter 25 page 425);
   • unconsciousness – routine care of unconscious patient (see Chapter 25 page 422);
   • cyanosis – intranasal oxygen 2–4 litres/minute;
   • not breathing – artificial ventilation after clearing the airway (see Chapter 37 page 607);
   • shock – elevate the legs and give IV 0.9% saline (see Chapter 27 page 468);
   • pain – use *small* preferably IV doses of morphine if there is a risk of depression of breathing (usually give for only swallowed acid).

9. Transfer the patient to Medical Officer care if complications which you cannot treat at the health centre occur (see page below).

10. Use any case of poisoning to give health education on the proper storage and use of drugs and poisons (see below).

11. Check the patient's mental state. Treat any psychiatric condition. Help to solve any problem (see Chapter 35 pages 579–583).

Transfer
Transfer a patient who has swallowed poison or drug overdose (but only after previous treatment) if:

1. You think the dose of the poison he has swallowed is more than:
   • acetylsalicylic acid – 300 mg/kg (more than 15 g in adult),
   • chloroquine, amodiaquine and quinine – twice the normal treatment dose (*but* contact the Medical Officer first) (see below),
   • corrosive acid (e.g. battery acid) – anything more than a little,
   • ferrous sulfate (iron) – 100 tablets (but small doses, e.g. 10 tablets are very poisonous to children),
   • methanol (methyl alcohol) – 10 ml, or methylated spirits – 200 ml,
   • paracetamol – 150 mg/kg (or 15 or more tablets in an adult) after giving (if available) N-acetyl cysteine injection, or
   • phenobarbital – 20 mg/kg or more.
2. If poisoned with
   • phenolic weed killers (e.g. dinitro-ortho-cresol (DNOC), dinitrophenol (dinoseb)), after give chlorpromazine 100 mg IMI and cool the patient,
   • paraquat weed killer (e.g. Gramoxone, Gramixel, Priglone, Weedol),
   • arsenical poisons,
   • organophosphorous insect killers (e.g. parathion, TEPP, malathion), after give oxygen and atropine 2 mg IMI.
3. The patient has a dangerous level of consciousness, or breathing, or pulse or BP.
4. The patient's level of consciousness, breathing *or* BP gets worse every hour for 4 hours.
   Transfer the patient then, before the levels of consciousness, breathing and BP, etc. become dangerous.
5. Complications occur that you cannot treat properly in the health centre (especially unconsciousness that continues for more than 24 hours).
6. If you think the patient may try to commit suicide again and that you cannot stop him in the health centre.

> Always check the patient's mental state if he tried to commit suicide.

Treat with chlorpromazine and transfer the patient if he has severe psychotic depression, or you have another good reason to think that he may try to commit suicide again.

If not, try to solve the patient's problems and treat in the usual way. Do *not* supply phenobarbital or antidepressants to take home as the patient may take it as another overdose.

Prevention of poisoning
Use any case of poisoning to teach people:

1. Always store all poisons and drugs away from children.
2. Never put poisons, especially kerosene, in drink bottles (soft drink or beer or wine bottles, etc.).
3. Always put a label on all bottles that contain drugs and poisons.
4. Always throw away (into the toilet) any old medicines, tablets or the contents of any bottle that has no label.

Notes on specific poisons and drug overdoses

Swallowed chloroquine, amodiaquine and quinine overdose
More than the proper treatment dose is dangerous. More than twice the proper treatment dose will probably cause death.

These drugs are absorbed very quickly and cause death usually within 1–6 hours.

The most important part of the treatment is to empty the stomach and intestines *as quickly as possible. Immediately* make the patient vomit many times or wash out the stomach. For other treatment see 5 on page 562.

If the dangerous dose of these drugs has already been absorbed, there is not much the Medical Officer can do, unless he has special equipment and drugs. Urgently contact the Medical Officer and ask if you should transfer the patient urgently (emergency).

Swallowed petroleum product (e.g. kerosene)

1. Do *not* make the patient vomit.
2. Give 1–2 cups of milk or water to drink.
3. Do *not* wash out the stomach.
4. Give safe laxative if available.
5. There is no antidote.
6. Make routine observations (see page 563).
7. Treat pneumonia when it occurs. Give oxygen if it is severe.
8. Transfer if severe pneumonia develops, especially if you do not have oxygen.
9. Use the case to give health education that kerosene should never be stored in drink bottles and should always be stored away from children.
10. Treat any mental disturbance in the usual way.

Swallowed strong acids or strong alkalis

1. Do *not* make the patient vomit.
2. Give 1–2 cups of milk or water to drink.
3. Do *not* wash the stomach out.
4. Do *not* give a laxative.
5. Do *not* try to give an antidote (e.g. do not give alkali if acid swallowed).
6. Make routine observations (see page 563).
7. Treat any complication in the usual way.
8. Transfer all patients who have swallowed any strong acid or alkali to Medical Officer care (urgent). Meanwhile, the patient must not eat at all or drink large volumes of fluid.
9. Use the case to give health education that no poison should be stored in a drink bottle, and that all poison should be stored away from children.
10. Treat any mental disturbance in the usual way.

Swallowed paracetamol overdose

More than twice to four times the normal daily dose (i.e. > 8 g) may cause liver failure and death after some days (especially if the patient has poor nutrition or drinks a lot of alcohol).

Treat the patient even if he looks well.

1. Give all the usual treatment for swallowed poisons (see pages 562–563).
2. Give the specific antidote if available while organising transfer of the patient to Medical Officer care:
   - (N-)acetyl cysteine 150 mg/kg in 200 ml 5% dextrose over 15 minutes, then
     50 mg/kg in 500 ml 5% dextrose over 4 hours, then
     100 mg/kg in 1 litre 5% dextrose over 16 hours (but what to give after this needs blood tests to work out),
   or if N-acetyl cysteine not available
   - 2.5 g methionine orally each 4 hours for 4 doses only, i.e. 10 g in all.

Swallowed organophosphate or carbamate

Any poisoning is likely to lead to death, but special care from the Medical Officer may help.

1. Give all the usual treatment for swallowed poisons.
2. While waiting for transfer,
   if pulse slow, diarrhoea, vomiting, frequently passing urine, sweating, excessive saliva, wheezing, small pupils, muscle twitches,
   give if available:
   (a) atropine 1.2–2.4 mg IVI repeated each $\frac{1}{4}$–1 hourly if needed to control these symptoms and
   (b) pradidoxime 30 mg/kg by slow IVI (or obidoxime).

Swallowed isoniazid overdose

1. Give all the usual treatment for swallowed poisons.
2. If nervous system side effects give pyridoxine 100–200 mg if can safely swallow.

Swallowed or injected opioid overdose

- Morphine or codeine from health centre drugs.
- These and heroin, methadone, pethidine, dihydrocodeine and dextroprophoxyphene if drug addict.
- Often also needle marks in skin over veins.
- Consciousness level decreases, breathing slows, pupils are small, blood pressure falls and death from stopping breathing follows.

1. Treat as any other patient who is not fully conscious.
2. Give a specific antidote if available:
   Naloxone 0.5–1 mg (or nalorphine 5–10 mg) IVI. This dose may need repeating each 2 minutes until the patient, especially breathing, becomes near normal.

As the naloxone does not last as long as the drug causing poisoning, about two-thirds of this dose *may* be needed each hour for up to 24 hours.

3. If no noloxone or nalorphine is available, IV aminophylline in dose as given IV for severe acute asthma (see Chapter 20 page 296) may be effective.

Treatment if the patient is not fully conscious

1. Do *not* make the patient vomit.
2. Do *not* give fluids to drink.
3. Do *not* wash out the stomach.
4. Do *not* give laxatives.
5. Give naloxone 0.5–1 mg or nalorphine 5–10 mg for pethidine, morphine or codeine or other opiate overdose. If these specific antidotes are not present and breathing is less than needed, IV aminophylline may be effective. (See Chapter 20 page 296.)
   Do not give other antidotes or stimulants.
6. Make routine observations (level of consciousness, size of pupils, breathing rate and depth of breathing, PR, BP).
7. Treat complications in the usual way.
   (a) Give special nursing care for an unconscious patient (see Chapter 25 page 422).
   (b) Check that there is a good urine output (125 ml/hour). Give IV fluids if necessary.
   (c) Treat shock if it occurs (raise legs, give IV 0.9% saline and see 'Shock', Chapter 27 page 468).
   (d) Give artificial ventilation and arrange urgent (emergency) transfer if the patient is not breathing enough, or stops breathing (see Chapter 37 page 607).
8. Transfer any patient whose level of consciousness or whose respiration or BP becomes dangerous. Also transfer any patient who is getting continually worse, before the levels become dangerous.
9. Use the case to give health education that no drugs and poisons should be stored in drink bottles and that all drugs and poisons should be stored away from children.
10. Treat any mental disturbance in the usual way.

Poisoning from seafoods

Fish or shellfish can cause poisoning, even though the food looks good and tastes normal. Symptoms and signs include:

1. gastroenteritis,
2. strange sensations in the body,

3. weakness which can develop into complete paralysis and death from paralysis of breathing, and
4. other symptoms and signs.

Treatment is as in the 10 principles for other types of poisoning above.

If weakness of the respiratory muscles develops, treat with artificial ventilation (Chapter 37 page 607) and *transfer* urgently to Medical Officer care.

Drug or substance abuse

Drugs and chemicals can be taken to try to change the way a person feels, thinks and acts. They are usually taken to try to change the mood and make the person feel good, not tired, full of new exciting thoughts, etc., i.e. 'high'; but sometimes to cause the feeling of relaxation or intoxication (drunkenness). The person then thinks and acts like he feels.

This, however, is dangerous as the drugs have also other effects.

1. The person may injure himself or others while under the influence of the drug.
2. A high dose of the drug may have severe or fatal acute effects on other parts of the body, e.g. high blood pressure, fast irregular pulse, cardiac arrest; shortness of breath, stopping breathing; fitting, unconsciousness, cerebral haemorrhage; high body temperature, etc.
3. The person may develop paranoid ideas or become very frightened (for no other real reason) or be aggressive or become psychotic.
4. Other parts of the body may be damaged. Lung disease (especially if the drug is smoked), cardiovascular disease, gastrointestinal disease, hormonal and sexual disorders (especially men having difficulty having sexual intercourse or women getting pregnant), etc. are all common.
5. HIV infection is more likely when a person is under the influence of such drugs from sharing needles to inject the drugs and from having unprotected sex.
6. The person's time becomes so taken up with how to get the drug and use the drug that there is not enough time left for his normal family, social and work life.

Numerous stimulant drugs and chemicals can be abused and are considered below. They include:

1. Cocaine orally or inhaled or injected IV or smoked 'crack'.
2. Marijuana and cannabis usually smoked.
3. Amphetamines orally including 'Ecstasy' or IV.

4. Lysergic acid diethylamide (LSD) usually orally.

5. Antihistamines usually orally.

6. Many others.

Depressant drugs include:

1. Alcohol.

2. Benzodiazepines, e.g. temazepam, diazepam, etc.

3. Barbiturates.

4. Opiates, e.g. codeine, morphine, heroin.

5. Organic solvents, e.g. petroleum, glue, plants, etc. inhaled ('sniffed').

These are considered in Chapter 23 page 382 and Chapter 35 page 575.

It is very difficult in the health centre without a laboratory to do tests to tell what a patient may have been taking to cause the problem which has led him to being seen; and many of the problems are difficult to treat in a health centre even if the chemical is known; but especially if the patient has taken more than one drug (which is common).

If a patient is seen with acute side effects, treat as for any other poisoning – keep the patient alive by treating any symptoms or signs he has or later develops, until his liver or kidney or other parts of the body remove the drug. See page 561 for details. It is, however, common for the drugs to cause high blood pressure or a fast or irregular heart rate. If you knew that these cardiovascular events were due to cocaine, give a beta blocker such as propranolol or atenolol, whereas if they were due to an amphetamine then give an alpha adrenergic drug such as prazosin; but these would probably not be available.

Psychosis would be treated in the usual way (see Chapter 35 page 580); but if the patient stops the drugs of abuse the psychosis may go away without many days of treatment (but it does not always do this).

Chronic diseases of other body systems caused by the drugs would be treated in the usual way.

Counselling and the help of family and community leaders; keeping the patient in the health centre for a week to do this and treat any health problems that have developed; getting the patient to stay away from the situations where he is likely to use drugs, as well as providing alternative worthwhile activities and work to try to stop the patient wanting to continue to use these drugs, are all essential.

Take all opportunities for health education to stop young people and others trying these drugs.

35 Psychiatric Conditions

Mental disorders and mental diseases

A person in good mental health can think, feel and act in a way his own community expects and understands. He accepts himself, is comfortable with other people and is satisfied carrying out the normal duties of life.

> A mental disorder or disease is present when a person cannot think, feel and act in the way his own society expects or understands.

Remember that:

1. What may be abnormal in one society may be normal in another society.
2. A criminal can behave in a way society expects; but he chooses not to.

There are two groups of psychiatric conditions:

1. conditions with an organic cause, i.e. an alteration in the structure or function of part of the body which causes the psychiatric condition (see page 568); and
2. conditions without an organic cause, i.e. there is no diagnosable alteration in the structure or function

of any part of the body (which has so far been found) that causes the psychiatric condition (see page 569).

There is also an important difference between:

1. psychotic conditions or diseases (psychoses) (see page 570); and
2. non-psychotic conditions or disorders (see page 570).

The above two classifications of mental disorder and disease were the basis of a previously fairly simple classification of all mental conditions, which is still used by many (see Table 35.1).

The new ICD-10 (International Classification of Diseases 10th edition) classifies mental disorders and diseases, however, as shown in Table 35.2 (greatly simplified). We do not have to learn this classification or know all the conditions in it, but it will help us in understanding mental diseases and disorders.

Mental disorders and diseases are very common. Up to 2% of the population may have psychotic disorders, up to 15% have less severe mental disorders and up to 25% of patients in outpatient clinics may be there because of mental problems. Increasing use of alcohol and drugs by the population increases these numbers.

Table 35.1 A simple classification of mental conditions.

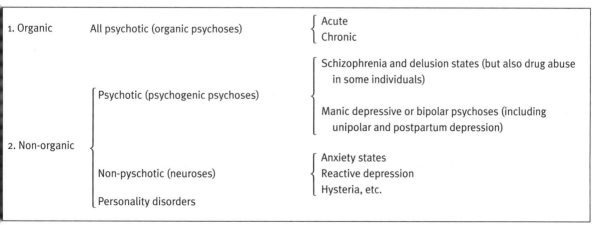

1. Organic	All psychotic (organic psychoses)	{ Acute { Chronic
2. Non-organic	Psychotic (psychogenic psychoses)	{ Schizophrenia and delusion states (but also drug abuse in some individuals) { Manic depressive or bipolar psychoses (including unipolar and postpartum depression)
	Non-pyschotic (neuroses)	{ Anxiety states { Reactive depression { Hysteria, etc.
	Personality disorders	

Table 35.2 Classification of mental disorders according to the 10th edition of the *International Classification of Diseases* (ICD-10). (Adapted and reproduced from WHO ICD-10 *International Classification of Diseases*, 10th ed, by permission of the WHO.)

F0	**Organic**
	Acute, e.g. delirium
	Chronic, e.g. dementia
F1	**Substance misuse**
F2	**Schizophrenia and delusional disorders**
F3	**Mood (affective) disorders**
	Depression
	Mania
	Recurrent affective disorders
F4	**Neurotic, stress-related and somatoform disorders**
	Anxiety disorders:
	Generalised anxiety
	Phobic anxiety
	Panic disorder
	Obsessive compulsive disorder
	Reaction to severe stress:
	Acute stress disorder
	Post-traumatic stress disorder
	Adjustment disorder
	Dissociative (conversion) disorder
	Somatoform disorder
	Neurasthenia
F5	**Behavioural syndromes associated with physiological disturbance**
	Eating disorders
	Sleep disorders
	Sexual dysfunction
	Puerperal mental disorders
F6	**Personality disorders**
F7	**Mental retardation and others**

Adapted from: World Health Organization *ICD-10. International Classification of Diseases,* 10th edn. Geneva, WHO.

Causes of psychiatric conditions

Organic causes of psychotic diseases

1. *Any disease of the brain[1] especially*
   - head injury
   - high fever of any cause, especially hyperpyrexia

---

1 *Note* that these two lists of causes of organic psychoses are almost the same as the two lists of causes of unconsciousness or of convulsions, etc. (see Chapter 25 page 422). An organic psychosis is only another way the brain does not work properly when there is a disease of the brain or abnormality of the blood going to the brain.

- meningitis (all types)
- cerebral malaria
- HIV infection
- viral encephalitis of other types
- African trypanosomiasis
- syphilis
- encephalitis of other types
- cerebral tumour of any type, including cancers, schistosomiasis, TB, cysticercosis
- cerebrovascular disease/stroke
- malnutrition and in particular:
  - vitamin B_1 or thiamine deficiency (Wernicke's encephalopathy)
  - niacin deficiency (pellagra)
  - vitamin B_{12} and/or folic acid deficiency
- epilepsy and the postepileptic state
- damage to the brain at birth (mental subnormality)
- wearing out of the brain in old age (senile dementia)
- Alzheimer's disease
- and others (see a specialist reference book).

2. *Abnormalities in the blood going to the brain[1]*
   - alcohol, drugs and poisons (including some local traditional ones) – both intoxication with or withdrawal from
   - low oxygen from any cause, e.g. shock, heart failure, severe anaemia, etc.
   - dehydration from any cause
   - toxins from severe infections in the body, especially malaria, septicaemia, pneumonia, typhoid, typhus, etc.
   - toxins from the body when organ failure – liver failure, kidney failure
   - blood glucose too high (diabetic ketoacidosis) or too low (diabetic hypoglycaemia from insulin but also from some other illnesses and drugs).

Organic psychoses caused by a disease of the brain or an abnormality of the blood going to the brain can be of two types:

1. an acute organic psychosis, or
2. a chronic organic psychosis.

1. *An acute organic psychosis*
   (a) Has started recently – hours or days and not over a month ago.
   (b) Patient on examination:
   - not fully conscious;
   - memory poor for recent events;
   - not orientated in time and place;
   - intelligence usually cannot be tested, i.e. confused or delirious.

Has a lot of other abnormalities too, including features of a psychosis but the above four features are diagnostic of his illness being 'organic'.

(c) Usually, this type of psychosis can be treated successfully if cause found and correct treatment for cause given.

(d) Often patient will die if cause not found and correct treatment for cause not given.

2. *A chronic organic psychosis*

(a) Has been present for a long time (at least one month).

(b) Patient on examination:
- may or may not be fully conscious;
- memory poor for recent events;
- not fully orientated in time or place;
- intelligence not as it should be for the person's education and previous position in society, i.e. he is demented (loss of previous intelligence when fully conscious) and confused.

Has a lot of other abnormalities too, including features of psychosis but the above four are diagnostic of it being 'organic'.

(c) Often this type of psychosis does not have a cause that can be easily found and successfully treated even if found.

(d) Patient not likely to die quickly so urgent diagnosis and treatment not essential.

To discover the cause of organic psychoses, always:

1. Take a full history from the patient and his family or friends.
2. Do a full physical examination.
3. Take a malaria smear and give antimalarial drugs if malaria possible.
4. Do a lumbar puncture and treat for meningitis if present.
5. Look carefully for evidence of any infection. Treat if infection possible with antibiotics or other drugs.
6. Do blood sugar. Give glucose orally or intravenously if blood sugar low or cannot be done.
7. Look carefully for head injury. Transfer urgently to Medical Officer if significant injury possible.
8. Smell the breath. Ask if there is any possibility of alcohol or drug overdose or withdrawal; or the taking of poisons. Treat if needed.
9. Look for evidence of malnutrition. Give thiamine 50 mg IVI and multivitamin B tablets or injection if malnutrition possible.
10. Test the urine.
11. Send blood for serological test for syphilis and if needed for HIV infection and any other special tests needed.

Always think of an *organic* cause first in every patient who has *any* mental disturbance.

Especially always think of an acute *organic* cause first in any patient with an *acute* mental disturbance who was not mentally abnormal before.

Always consider first that the *cause is organic if*:

1. level of consciousness decreased;
2. recent memory poor;
3. not orientated in time and place;
4. intelligence not normal or not able to be tested.

Non-organic causes of psychiatric conditions

Non-organic causes include the experiences the patient has had. Most important are the relationships he has had with his family (especially as a child), friends, girlfriends, wife, etc. Also important are events at home, school, work, etc.

These *relationships and events can cause stress*. Two things especially cause stress. (1) Separation from people important to him. (2) A decision which the person should but cannot or does not make.

Stress causes anxiety. In anxiety, the brain stimulates certain nerves and the adrenaline producing adrenal gland. This causes dry mouth; sinking feeling in the abdomen; nausea and diarrhoea; palpitations; sighing or deep breathing; urinary frequency; sweating, cold hands and feet; a feeling of weakness; tightening of muscle groups (tension which can cause headache or backache if it remains for some time), etc. Anxiety is unpleasant but normal. The best way to remove the anxiety is to solve the problem causing the stress; or if this is not possible, to cope with it in a healthy mature way. If anxiety continues for a long time or if the anxiety is very great, then the stress and anxiety can cause mental disorders and diseases.

Stress and anxiety can cause non-organic non-psychotic conditions. These are called *neurotic stress-related and body-related disorders* (or by many people just 'neurotic disorders').

Specific neurotic disorders are:

1. Anxiety disorders
- Generalised anxiety
- Phobic anxiety
- Panic disorder

2. Obsessive compulsive disorder
3. Reaction to severe stress
   • Acute stress disorder
   • Post-traumatic stress disorder
   • Adjustment disorder
4. Dissociative or conversion disorder of 'acting out'
5. Somatoform disorder
6. Neurasthaenia or chronic fatigue syndrome

Stress and anxiety can also start some other, very serious psychotic diseases.

1. An *acute psychotic reaction* occurs when a person's anxiety and fearful thoughts completely take over his normal thoughts.
2. *Schizophrenia and manic depressive psychoses* may occur in people who have an inherited likelihood to get them. But they may not develop the disorder until they reach a stressful time in their lives, e.g. schizophrenia starting at a time of great stress – young person going to school or getting married, etc.

Experiences help to form a person's personality. The personality is the characteristic or normal way in which a person thinks, feels, acts. Personality depends on what the person has inherited from his parents; anything that has happened to his brain; and the experiences that he has had, especially as a child. Some people have *abnormal personalities*, such as antisocial personalities, sexual deviations, and alcoholism or drug abuse. The experiences a person has are non-organic causes of the psychiatric condition of abnormal personality. A person's life experiences are the cause of the following disorders.

1. Behavioural syndromes associated with physiological disturbance
   • Eating disorder
   • Sleep disorders
   • Sexual function disorders
   • Puerperal mental disorders
2. Personality disorders

Psychotic or non-psychotic disorder?

Psychotic diseases (or psychoses)

Psychoses have some important typical features. In a psychosis there is a *severe disturbance of the patient's personality*.

The patient's *personality* is the way he thinks, feels and acts. (His acts include his appearance, his behaviour and his speech or talk.) A normal person feels and acts in a way that other people expect him to and that they understand. In a normal person, thinking, feeling and acting are all co-ordinated.

In a psychosis, there is a change in the way the patient thinks, feels and acts. The person is now different. He does not think and feel and act as normal. Also thinking, feeling and acting may not be co-ordinated, e.g. a person may act in a happy way but feel sad.

1. Most commonly in a psychosis there is a *disorder of thought*. The patient *cannot organise his thoughts* or get them 'straight'. His thoughts may suddenly stop or jump from one thing to another. He may have *hallucinations* (see, hear, feel, smell and taste things which are not there). He may have *delusions* (false beliefs which cannot be corrected by logical argument). These delusions are often that a person or something is trying to hurt or kill him; and he may react violently. This delusion of persecution is called a 'paranoid delusion'.
   In organic psychoses (when the patient may not be fully conscious and cannot completely understand or remember what is happening) he may have *illusions* (wrongly understand and interpret real events and physical sensations) and may become *confused* and *delirious*.
2. There may be a *disorder of mood* (the usual 'feelings' of the person).
   He may be *manic* (too happy) or *depressed* (too sad) or seem to have *no feelings*, or the *mood may not be the usual one for the circumstances* (e.g. happy when very bad things are happening).
3. Because of the disturbance of thought and mood the *actions* (appearance, behaviour and speech) may be very *abnormal*.
4. Because of one or more of these things, the patient *loses contact with reality* (does not live in the real world; but lives in his own private world of unreal and strange thoughts and feelings).
5. The patient loses *insight* (to a small or large degree), i.e. he does not know what is really happening. The patient may not know he is sick. You may not be able to convince him he is sick. The patient may think he is normal and everyone else is abnormal. However, there is not always loss of insight (or at least this complete loss of insight) in psychotic illnesses.

Non-psychotic disorders

Non-psychotic disorders are different from psychoses. There is *no change in the patient's personality* (or the way he thinks, feels and acts). The person's anxiety causes feelings that are stronger or continue longer than in a mentally healthy person. This results in an exaggeration or lengthening of thoughts and actions. This can also occur in mentally healthy people but they can control it.

1. The patient does not have a thought disorder. He *does not have hallucinations or delusions*. He is *not confused*. His thoughts are often not normal; but you can understand them and they 'make sense' if you know about his stresses and anxiety.

2. The patient's *mood* is appropriate to his thoughts and circumstances. The mood is often not normal; but you can understand it, and it 'makes sense' if you know about his stresses and anxiety and thoughts.

3. The patient's *actions* may not be normal and they may be very disturbed; but you can understand them and they 'make sense' if you know about his stresses and anxiety and his mood and thoughts.

4. The patient *does not lose contact with the real world*.

5. The patient *does not lose insight* and he knows that he is sick. However, he may deny this; but you can usually eventually convince him by logical explanation. In some non-psychotic patients, however, there is some or at least temporary loss of insight.

When you see a patient with a psychiatric disorder, you must find out:

1. Is there an organic cause or not? (pages 568–569)
2. Is this a psychosis or not? (pages 570–571)
3. Is there a cause for stress and anxiety? (pages 569–570)

You must do a routine history and examination of *both* physical *and* mental states to find the answers to the three questions:

1. Is there an organic cause or not?
2. Is this a psychosis or not?
3. Is there a cause for stress and anxiety or not?

Psychiatric history and examination

Psychiatric history

When you take a normal history, also take this special psychiatric history *from the patient and other witnesses*.

1. *Admission note*
   (a) Reason for admission. (If the police bring the patient, they must give a signed statement saying why they brought the patient.)
   (b) Names and addresses of those who referred the patient.
   (c) Names and addresses of patient's relatives *and*

the people who were with the patient when the illness started.

2. *Complaints and duration*

3. *History of present illness*
   (a) What does the patient say has happened? What does the patient say is the cause?
   (b) What do other people say has happened? What do other people say is the cause?
   (c) What do *you* think really happened? What do *you* think the cause really is?

4. *Specific interrogation*
   Usual questions (see Chapter 6).

5. *Past history*
   Any previous psychiatric disorder?
   • When did it occur?
   • How long did it continue?
   • What form did it take?
   • Did the patient get completely better?
   • Has the patient been taking any treatment?
   Note especially head injury, drugs, alcohol and the usual questions (see Chapter 6).

6. *Family and contact history*
   Any mental illness and the usual questions (see Chapter 6).

Psychiatric examination

When you do a normal examination of the patient, make these eight observations instead of just the level of consciousness.

1. Check if the patient can *communicate* physically (find out if he can hear, see, talk, move, etc.).

2. Check the *level of consciousness*.

3. *Memory*
   (a) recent events – e.g. What did you eat today?
   (b) long past events – e.g. Ask a fact of local importance,

4. *Orientation*
   (a) person – e.g. Who are you? What are you?
   (b) time – e.g. Is it morning or afternoon? What day is it?
   (c) place – e.g. What is this building? Where is the toilet?

5. *Intelligence* – Ask a problem suitable to the patient's education.

6. *Thoughts* by
   (a) speech,
   (b) appearance and
   (c) behaviour.
   Especially:
   (a) clear logical thinking or muddled up thinking?
   (b) delusions, e.g. Do people treat you normally or

in some special way?
(c) hallucinations, e.g.
   • Are any strange things happening?
   • Do you hear voices when you can see no one there?
   • Do you see people when no one else can?
(d) any special thing the patient thinks about all the time.

7. *Mood* by
   (a) speech,
   (b) appearance,
   (c) behaviour.
   Especially:
   (a) manic (too happy) ⎫ e.g. How do you
   (b) depressed (too sad) ⎭ feel in yourself?
   (c) co-ordinated with the patient's thoughts and actions or not?

8. *Insight*
   (a) does he think he is sick?
   (b) does he know the *real* cause of the illness?

In examination of the appearance, behaviour and speech, note the points listed below.

1. *Appearance*
   • facial expression – happy, sad, or worried
   • posture
   • clothing
   • hygiene
   • anything odd or unusual
2. *Behaviour*
   • overactivity
   • underactivity
   • aggression
   • odd or unusual
   • sensible under the circumstances
   • care of bodily needs – does he eat and drink? does he rest and sleep?
3. *Speech*
   • fast
   • slow
   • none
   (shows what thoughts are and what stream of thoughts is like)

Important psychiatric conditions

Acute organic psychoses

In an acute organic psychosis the brain does not work properly as there is an *acute* (i.e. started recently) *under-lying disease of the brain or abnormality of the blood coming to the brain* (see page 568).

This causes a disturbance in level of consciousness.

The typical features of an organic psychosis are therefore:

1. Disturbance of level of consciousness, which causes:
2. Poor memory (especially for ⎫ These are
   recent events), and   ⎬ called
3. Loss of orientation, and ⎭ 'Confusion'.
4. Loss of normal level of intelligence, also
5. The patient cannot understand ⎫ This may
   things that are happening and has ⎬ be called
   illusions and hallucinations.   ⎭ 'Delirium'.

> A patient who has recently become confused or who is delirious has an acute organic psychosis.

Disturbance of the level of consciousness can be from just a little less alert than normal to drowsy to coma. This means the patient cannot pay the usual attention to what is happening. He therefore cannot remember what has happened, how he came to be where he is, or what time it is.

Also, as the brain does not work properly, he sees things but thinks they are different things from what they really are, e.g. illusions, where a shadow on a wall may be thought to be a rat or spider. He also has delusions where he may see or hear things that do not exist. His thoughts by then are all mixed up and he has difficulty in thinking. He is usually quiet. If he is frightened, however, from delusions or hallucinations, he may become violent. (Visual hallucinations are common during drug intoxication or withdrawal.)

The mood is usually in keeping with what he is thinking. His appearance will get worse as he does not remember to take care of his bodily needs.

Typical features of an acute organic psychosis are therefore:	
• Level of consciousness decreased • Memory poor • Orientation in time and place decreased	'Organic'

• Thinking mixed up
  — illusions
  — hallucinations
  — delusions
• Mood variable
• Speech rambling
• Appearance not cared for
• Behaviour quiet, but can be aggressive
	'Psychotic'

You can treat most causes of acute organic psychosis, and often you can cure them. But, if you do not give proper treatment quickly, then these conditions either cause death or permanent damage to the brain. A good example is acute bacterial meningitis causing acute organic psychosis. See pages 568 for common causes of acute organic psychoses and page 569 for diagnostic procedures you must do on all patients with acute organic psychosis. 'Rule' treatments may apply in some areas because some conditions may be very common there, e.g. in areas where alcohol excess or vitamin deficiencies are common such a rule may be 'give all patients with acute organic psychoses injections of vitamin B group vitamins'. Find out if any such 'rules' apply in your area.

> If a patient has an acute organic psychosis you must quickly find the cause and give effective treatment.

Chronic organic psychoses

In chronic organic psychosis there is a *chronic* (i.e. did not start recently) underlying *disease of the brain*. So the brain does not work properly.

This causes the typical features of chronic organic psychosis:

1. Level of consciousness in psychoses that develop after acute attacks may be abnormal. However, in those that develop very slowly and are usually called 'dementia', the level of consciousness is at first normal.
2. Poor memory, especially for recent events, is the earliest and most typical feature. Recent things are not remembered but far past things are. Family members may notice these things first. The patient forgets where he puts things and what he is doing or talking about.
3. Some loss of orientation follows as the patient does not remember what has brought him to the present time and place.
4. Loss of previously good intelligence and not being able to learn new things are typical. The patient is no longer able to do what he previously was able to do or to hold his previous position in society or the family.
5. Thinking gets less and less and the patient does not seem to think of the results of his actions. He may be rude when previously he was polite. He may steal things. He may use bad language. He may be incontinent without being worried about this. He does not think about new things. He does not take an interest in what is going on.

6. Mood changes are common. Often the patient is irritable but may suddenly change from one mood to another. Eventually, he does not seem to be affected by anything that goes on.
7. Insight is to a smaller or greater extent lost so that the patient does not really understand what is happening.

The patient has 'dementia'. There is a long history of the condition. Most of the causes cannot be treated or cured. See page 568 for a list of the causes of chronic (and acute) organic psychoses and page 569 for the diagnosic procedures you must do.

Patients with organic causes for their mental disorder do have disorders of thought and mood and insight and therefore have a psychosis, either acute or chronic organic psychosis.

> In every case of a mental disorder always first look for an organic cause (disease in brain or abnormality in blood going to the brain). This is especially important if
>
> 1. The level of consciousness is not normal.
> 2. Orientation is not normal.
> 3. Memory for recent events is not normal.
> 4. Intelligence is not normal.
> 5. There are sudden changes in mood.
>
> i.e. Delirium or Confusion or Dementia
>
> These signs do not occur in non-organic mental disease. If these signs occur the patient has an organic psychosis. You must find and treat the cause of the organic psychosis if possible. If the condition started recently urgent diagnosis and treatment are essential.

Non-organic psychoses

If the patient does not have:
- decreased level of consciousness, and
- recent memory loss, and
- loss of orientation in time and place, and
- abnormality of intelligence;

but does have:
- disorder of thought,
- disorder of feeling or mood,
- loss of insight,

then that patient has *a* so-called non-organic

psychosis of which there are only two important groups:

1. Schizophrenia – a disorder of thinking
2. Depression or bipolar mood disorder – a disorder of feeling or mood.

It is important to remember:

1. A schizophrenic-like state can be brought about by the misuse of certain drugs or substances (see page 575).
2. A depressive state (also others) can be brought on by childbirth and the few months after it.

There is some evidence now that patients with the so-called non-organic psychoses may in fact have very specific or particular types of organic change in parts of their brain which do not affect the whole of their brain (as the conditions which cause organic psychosis do). Although these cannot be found by normal tests now, some abnormalities in the brain activity (shown on brain scan) and chemistry, which in fact have been shown to be present, may be the cause. The fact that schizophrenic-like states can be temporarily caused by misuse of drugs and other substances would fit with this idea too. However, we do have to wait to find out if these non-organic psychotic patients do have a particular localised or specific type of organic lesion or not.

A patient with:

- level of consciousness decreased,
- memory for recent things decreased,
- orientation and time and place decreased,
- intelligence decreased,

must be assumed to have an organic condition and will be psychotic.

A person who has:

- level of consciousness normal,
- memory normal,
- orientation normal,
- intelligence normal,
- thought disorder or
- mood disorder, and possibly
- loss of contact with reality, and possibly
- loss of insight,

has a psychosis which is not organic and is probably either:

- schizophrenia – a disorder of thinking, or
- substance or drug misuse, or
- unipolar depression or bipolar disorder of mood.

Schizophrenia

Schizophrenia is a non-organic psychosis. You will not find an underlying disease of the brain or abnormality of the blood going to the brain.

There are *abnormal thoughts often with delusions and hallucinations* even though *the patient is fully conscious and orientated*. Mood is also often disturbed and feelings may not be co-ordinated with thoughts and actions, or the patient may appear to have no feelings. So appearance, behaviour and speech, etc. may be very abnormal. The patient may have little or no insight and often says he is not sick at all.

In the acute stage the thought disorders may be very severe with strange hallucinations and delusions. Especially important are paranoid delusions (thoughts that someone is trying to hurt the patient when this is not true).

The main problem seems to be that the patient cannot tell the difference between experiences coming from the world outside him and those coming from inside his body and his mind.

The following disorders of thought are common in people with schizophrenia all over the world. There are changes in mood which may follow. The patient may tell you, or you will find out on questioning, that he has some of the following:

1. His thoughts have been put into his mind by another person; or he is thinking someone else's thoughts (thought insertion).
2. His own thoughts are just suddenly taken away from him (thought withdrawal).
3. His thoughts are known to other people – he may be broadcasting them like a radio transmitter or sending them some other way (thought broadcasting).
4. His body movements and feelings are being controlled by another person or thing, not himself (passivity feelings).
5. He can hear voices talking about him, sometimes just saying all he is doing but at other times making critical remarks about him. The voices may also be talking all of his thoughts out loud (auditory hallucinations).
6. He can tell the significance of certain actions, although others do not agree on what they mean, e.g. he saw a child with a dog and this meant that the world would come to an end today.

Other less common disorders of thought include:

1. Thoughts become mixed up and one thought does not follow on from the previous one.
2. Newly made up words are used.

3. Delusions become marked and of special kinds, e.g. paranoid (someone or something is trying to kill him (and the patient may attack that person to protect himself)), grandiose (that he is an important person), sexual (that he is capable of extraordinary sexual feats), religious (that he is a religious person or God).

4. Hallucinations of tasting, smelling, feeling, touching things that are not there.

The patient may also have:

• mood changes where he appears not to understand what is happening to him, or

• mood changes which are inappropriate to his thoughts, e.g. laughing at terrible things.

Some patients adopt very strange positions or postures and remain in these for hours or longer. Others at times become aggressive and wild.

Eventually, if the disease proceeds, the patients seem to have:

• few thoughts and just tend to sit there,

• no feelings,

• hardly any speech.

Proper treatment helps especially in acute cases. It seems about 20% of patients make a full recovery and never have any more attacks. About 35% recover completely, but they do have further attacks with full recovery between attacks. About 35% have repeated attacks but after each attack are not quite as well as before that attack and therefore gradually get worse. About 10% quickly get worse without getting better at any time.

In *acute schizophrenia*, the patient is fully conscious, fully orientated, but has abnormal thoughts (especially delusions and hallucinations) and possibly abnormal feelings.

In *chronic schizophrenia* (after many years) the patient may appear to have few thoughts, very little feeling about anything, and may behave like a child.

If a patient:

1. is fully conscious and orientated with a good memory and reasonable intelligence, but

2. has abnormal thoughts especially hallucinations or delusions, and

3. possibly has inappropriate or no feelings,

then the patient probably has schizophrenia or a drug or substance misuse.

Check, however, that the patient does not have an acute organic psychosis.

Drug and other substance misuse including withdrawal (including alcohol)

The most commonly abused drug is alcohol. Any more than 2(–3) standard drinks for a male and 1(–2) for a female in 24 hours (or 14–21 for a male and 7–14 for a female in a week), can have significant effects on health. (A standard drink contains 9–10 g alcohol and is contained in 1 glass (425 ml) of beer or 1 wine glass of wine or 30 ml of spirits.) Many patients who drink excessive alcohol do not eat a good diet and all the vitamin B deficiency disorders can occur and contribute to the brain not working properly.

Other sedative drugs (besides alcohol) are benzodiazepines such as temazepam and diazepam; barbiturates; opiates including morphine, codeine and heroin; and organic solvents such as found in glues.

If the above sedative drugs including alcohol are taken regularly, they not only have a bad effect on a person's health and behaviour but the nervous system gets used to being depressed by them and has to, as it were, be more stimulated to keep the person going. If these drugs are suddenly stopped, this excess stimulation, which is no longer needed, can cause a psychotic state ('withdrawal symptoms') something like schizophrenia, but usually with frightening visual hallucinations and also shaking and shivering and sometimes even fitting. (See alcohol withdrawal syndrome, Chapter 23 pages 382–383.)

There are other drugs which are not sedatives but stimulants. These include cannabis (marijuana or hashish), amphetamines such as dexamphetamine and a drug made from it called 'Ecstasy'; cocaine and another drug made from it called 'Crack'; and hallucinogenic drugs such as lysergic acid diethylamide (LSD) and psilocybin ('magic mushrooms'), which themselves stimulate the nervous system and can produce psychotic states like schizophrenia. See Chapter 34 pages 565–566.

Manic depressive psychosis

Depression and mania or bipolar mood disorders are non-organic psychoses. You will not find an underlying disease of the brain or abnormality of the blood going to the brain. (However, a specific chemical or other abnormality of part of the brain controlling only mood may yet be found.)

There is a *disturbance of the mood*. (Another word for 'mood' is 'affect'.) The patient has a definite feeling which he thinks will not stop. It may be of great happiness (mania). It may be of great unhappiness (depression). There is no real cause for this feeling in what is happening to the patient. The patient appears fully conscious and orientated with a normal memory, but he thinks and acts in co-ordination with the feelings he has; so there may be some delusions, usually of being a very important person or God, in mania; or of being a very bad person or of having a terrible disease, in depression. Sometimes there are vague hallucinations. So appearance, behaviour and speech may be very abnormal. The patient has little insight and often says he is not mentally abnormal.

The abnormal mood of the patient often goes after some weeks or months. Sometimes the patient can change from one mood to the other, i.e. from being too happy for no reason to being too sad for no reason. (This change does not usually happen quickly.)

Depression is much more common than mania and often occurs by itself. Mania tends to occur in younger people and become less common as they get older, but it is almost always associated with periods of depression.

Occasionally, a patient has symptoms and signs of both depression and mania. This is called a 'mixed affective state'.

Depression (unipolar depressive mood disorder)

The characteristic features of depression are (at least three of the following, including two of the first three; as long as these are different from what the patient usually is; and are not due to an illness; and are present for most days for at least 2 weeks).

- feeling depressed, sad or empty
- feeling unable to enjoy things which are normally enjoyed
- feeling no energy or fatigued or tired
- problems sleeping; usually less sleep and especially waking in the early hours of the morning and not being able to go back to sleep (and feeling depressed); but occasionally sleeping too much
- feeling guilty and blaming himself for things he is not to blame for
- feeling unworthy or worthless
- feeling that does not want to eat and loses weight (more than 5%); but occasionally feeling hungry and gaining weight
- feeling cannot think or concentrate or make up his mind
- feeling hopeless and being negative or bad thoughts about the future

- feeling nervous and anxious
- feeling no interest in sexual intercourse
- feels would be better off dead and planning about suicide (or has already tried it).

Sometimes patients who feel very depressed not only try to commit suicide themselves, but sometimes also try to kill their families as they feel they also would be better off dead.

About 15% of people have significant depression at least once. It is more common in women. It occurs more often in some families. It often starts in early adult life. An attack may last for weeks to a year. Every time the patient gets another attack, the more likely it is that they will have further attacks.

If a patient has only depressive episodes, the condition is called unipolar (depressive mood disorder) because it is like being at one end of the pole of the earth (i.e. North Pole or South Pole) (as 'uni' means only one). Mania is like being at the other pole of the earth (as far away as it is possible to get from depression) and though it occurs rarely it almost always at times changes to the other pole of depression, and the person is said to have bipolar mood disorder (as 'bi' means two). Most normal people live between these two poles – depressed, but not abnormally depressed at times; and happy, but not abnormally happy (manic) at other times; but most of the time between these two extremes of mood.

As well as this kind of depression for no known cause (psychotic or endogenous depression) (endogenous means coming from within the patient), depression can come from obvious causes in the environment (non-psychotic or reactive or exogenous) (exogenous means things from outside the patient). This depression is different.

Many people are depressed because of illness, side effects of drugs needed for treatment of another illness or life situations which would make any normal person depressed, e.g. death of a loved one or loss of possessions in an earthquake or fire or tsunami. There are reasons for these other sorts of depression and we all can understand why the patient is depressed. The patient feels like we would expect him to feel in the patient's condition. This is reactive or exogenous depression and is normal. It is not the same as endogenous psychotic depression.

Bipolar mood disorder

Bipolar mood disorder is said to exist if as well as an episode of depression the patient has had an episode of mania (bipolar I) or hypomania (but not mania) (bipolar II).

The characteristic features of mania (or manic episode) are two or more of the following for at least a week; and of hypomania, are two or more of the following for at least 2 days but for less than a week.

- increase in mental and physical energy, i.e. thoughts keep racing from one thing to another
- more talkative than usual or seems as if pressure to keep talking
- can't settle or be still for long
- gets little sleep (as feels rested after a few hours sleep)
- feels happier (than should be)
- does things on impulses without thinking
- ideas he is of more importance than he is or has special skill or power
- says things seem more real than usual – colours are brighter, smells are stronger, etc.
- excessive involvement in pleasurable activities which are likely to cause painful results, e.g. buying things he does not need and cannot afford; inappropriate sexual behaviour; gambling, thinking he is winning or will win when he is not and cannot; driving cars at high speed; etc.
- irritability (especially if stopped from doing what he wants).

In severe acute manic delusions, almost all the above things may be similar to those of schizophrenia. Stimulant drugs, thyrotoxicosis, neurological diseases including HIV infection and stroke, etc. may also cause appearances which are very similar.

Manic symptoms will not be recognised by the patient as being abnormal. It is often the history from relatives or friends which makes it clear the behaviour is not normal for the patient.

If a patient:

1. is fully conscious and orientated with a good memory and reasonable intelligence
2. has abnormal feelings (he is too happy or too sad) for which there is no real cause
3. possibly has abnormal thoughts co-ordinated with the abnormal feelings

then the patient probably has depression or bipolar mood disorder.

Check that the patient does not have acute organic psychosis.

In the non-organic psychoses there is a disturbance in thoughts or mood. The patient *does not have*;

1. disturbance in level of consciousness,
2. disturbance of recent memory,
3. disturbance of orientation,
4. disturbance of intelligence, or
5. sudden swings in mood.

i.e. Delirium or Confusion or Dementia

It the patient has any of these things, look for a disease of the brain or an abnormality of the blood going to the brain.

Neurotic, stress-related and somatoform disorders

All neurotic stress-related disorders

If a patient diagnosed with a neurotic stress-related disorder:

- is not fully conscious,
- has poor memory for recent events,
- is not fully orientated,
- does not have normal intelligence for him,
- has disorder of thought especially
  - abnormal thoughts,
  - hallucinations,
  - delusions,
- has disturbance of mood not in keeping with his circumstances,
- has lost contact with reality,
- has no insight into what is going on;

then

- the diagnosis is incorrect and the patient does not have a neurotic stress-related disorder;
- look for organic causes if not fully conscious or not fully orientated or poor memory or intelligence not normal (especially if confused or delirious or demented);
- look for disorders of thought or mood or substance misuse if none of the features of organic disease present.

Anxiety disorders
Generalised anxiety
The cause of anxiety is stress (see page 569). The symptoms of anxiety are the physiological results of stimulation of parts of the patient's body by the nerv-

ous system and epinephrine/adrenaline which are normal for everyone at the time of stress. They include both physical and mental effects.

The effects of generalised anxiety are some, not usually all, of the following:

1. Physical:
   - shaking
   - sweating
   - heart beating fast
   - chest pain
   - shortness of breath
   - headache
   - dizziness
   - diarrhoea
   - urinary frequency
   - not able to go to sleep when go to bed
   - not able to concentrate
2. Mental:
   - feeling that something terrible is about to happen
   - worry about everything
   - irritable
   - feeling as if not in their own body

If the patient has excessive or continuing stress, then some or all of these symptoms will continue. Sometimes only one symptom will continue when the others are no longer noticed by the patient. The patient may then be particularly aware of this symptom and not remember how it started. He will then start to worry that he has a disease problem, i.e. he then has another cause of stress and anxiety. The anxiety can then keep itself going. Of course, if the patient does not solve the cause of the original anxiety, this can also keep the anxiety state going.

Phobic anxiety

When anxiety occurs only in certain situations, it is called a phobia. Agoraphobia occurs when there are anxiety symptoms which come on only when people go out into open spaces and see people. A social phobia occurs when people have to meet other people. Animal phobias are when a patient has a particular fear of a particular animal such as a spider. Other specific phobias include fears of flying, heights, etc.

Panic disorder

When all of the anxiety symptoms happen suddenly in a certain situation, the patient is said to have a panic attack.

Obsessive compulsive disorder

This is said to exist when a special thought or impulse to do something repeatedly pushes itself into the patient's mind despite their trying to stop it. For instance, a patient may know that they have washed their hands and that they are clean, but they have to get up and wash their hands again and then the tap in case their hands got dirty from the tap when they turned it off, and then the door handle in case their hands got dirty from this, etc. Eventually, they may have to spend hours washing their hands, taps, handles, etc. Other such rituals can also develop.

Reactions to severe stress

1. *Acute stress disorder* at the time of an event can cause confusion, anxiety, anger, depression and extreme over-activity or extreme withdrawal.
2. *Post-traumatic stress disorder* occurs weeks or months after a severe stress such as occurs in wars, murders, torture, etc. The patient may suddenly get memories they do not want of the event (flashbacks), not be able to sleep, get episodes of acute anxiety, have nightmares, avoid any situation which reminds them of the traumatic event, tend to use alcohol, drugs, etc.
3. *Adjustment disorders* occur as a reaction to a normal stressful life event and are the processes whereby people get over death by grief reactions, etc.

Dissociative or conversion disorder

It is thought that if a patient has stress and anxiety that they cannot solve, they may unconsciously (without realising it) develop symptoms in their body which mean that their cause of stress and anxiety is solved. However, there is nothing really wrong with the part of their body that has the symptoms. For instance, a student who has not studied enough to pass an examination may develop paralysis of his writing hand and thus solve the problem of possibly failing an exam. Patients may appear to develop disturbance of walking, loss of function of a limb, loss of voice, epilepsy, loss of sensation, blindness and even loss of memory. For the diagnosis to be made, there must be a symptom that usually does not fit with anatomical or physiological organic disease, but rather with non-medical ideas of function and disease; there must be no evidence of organic disease; and there must be a cause for the stress and anxiety which development of this problem solves.

One problem about this diagnosis is that it can be incorrectly made and the patient can then go on to develop severe disability or die because they have had the mistaken diagnosis of 'hysteria' (the old name for dissociative or conversion disorder) made when in fact they have an organic disease. Always be very unwilling to make this diagnosis until the patient is cured.

Somatoform disorders

Patients are said to have these disorders when they come for repeated consultations for physical symptoms for which no cause can be found. In many cases, history will show that there has been a close relationship with some stressful life event in the past or the start of a continuing conflict when these physical symptoms started. They include pains, nausea, vomiting, diarrhoea, headache, dizziness, urinary symptoms, sexual difficulties, etc. At times, there may be a collection of symptoms; at other times it may relate to just one thing (such as heart beating faster than usual, having to take deep breaths or having diarrhoea). The characteristic thing about these patients is that they remain well for years despite having serious symptoms and that tests never show any significant change. However, the symptoms are characteristic if care is taken to find out about them.

Chronic fatigue syndrome or neurasthenia

Numerous causes for this condition probably exist. Some may follow viral infections. Some may be a form of mild depression. Some, however, may be due to anxiety from stress.

Acute psychotic reaction (with no organic cause)

This is any type of severe mental disturbance when these things occur:

1. The patient (who is usually young) has a problem which he cannot solve and which causes great anxiety.
2. Fear replaces clear thinking and controls the thoughts, feelings and actions of the patient. Any type of psychotic (or non-psychotic) behaviour may result. The patient may appear to have schizophrenia or mania (i.e. a non-organic psychosis). Singing, shouting and other disturbing behaviour are common. Irritable answers to all questions are common. But hallucinations and delusions are not common.
3. Once the problem is found and solved the patient becomes normal again within days or weeks.
4. There may be repeated attacks with repeated problems; but after each attack the patient gets completely better. But the patient may never cope well with problems.
5. The behaviour may be, in that particular society, a socially acceptable and understood way of behaving if a person is under excessive stress.

An acute psychotic reaction is different from a non-organic psychosis (schizophrenia or manic depressive psychoses). In most cases of non-organic psychoses:

1. the patient does not become completely normal even when his problems are found and solved, and/or
2. if the patient had a previous attack he was not completely normal before this attack.

This acute psychotic reaction is presumably a form of the neurotic stress-related disorders 'acute stress disorder' or 'dissociative or conversion or hysterical reaction'.

> In every patient who has very disturbed behaviour, you must try to find out if the patient has a big problem. If he does, you should try to solve it. Until you do this, you cannot know if the patient's mental disorder is caused by an acute reaction to anxiety or caused by a non-organic psychosis.

You cannot make a diagnosis of acute reaction when you first see the patient. You can only make it when the patient gets better. If the patient does not get completely better, he probably has schizophrenia or another condition.

Management of patients with psychiatric conditions

Principles of management with psychiatric conditions

1. Treat symptoms and signs (i.e. give symptomatic treatment).
   Control the patient, if necessary (see page 580).
   Look after the patient's bodily needs.
2. Change the patient himself by:
   (a) treatment of any organic cause,
   (b) 'counselling' (talking to the patient),
     • first try to find out any cause of stress and anxiety,
     • then try to solve this cause of stress and anxiety,
     • teach the patient to talk to others about his needs and worries,
   (c) drugs, especially chlorpromazine, but also antidepressants and others, and
   (d) electroconvulsive therapy.
3. Change the patient's environment by:
   (a) 'counselling' (talking to the patient's family, friends and the people he lives and works with),
     • first try to find out any cause of stress and anxiety,

• then try to solve this cause of stress and anxiety,
• show the people how they can help the patient,

(b) sometimes change the patient's school, work, etc.,

(c) sometimes send the patient back to his home area, if he is away from it,

(d) sometimes send the patient to a rehabilitation village if a suitable one is available.

4. Follow up the patient to see if he needs further treatment or help.

Management of a psychotic patient

This includes patients with schizophrenia, schizophrenic state due to drug or substance misuse, mania, depression, acute reaction, organic psychosis.

Management includes four things:

1. *Treat the cause* (see this page)
   (a) Treat any organic cause in the usual way.
   (b) Try to solve any cause of stress and anxiety.
   (c) Give chlorpromazine for thought, mood and behaviour disorders, diazepam for drug withdrawal psychosis and amitriptyline or fluoxetine for depressive psychosis.

2. *Treat the psychotic behaviour* (see this page)
   (a) Admit with a helpful friend or relative. Educate the friend (see below).
   (b) Check that the patient cannot hurt himself or others (see below).
   (c) Give chlorpromazine; or amitriptyline or fluoxetine; or diazepam (see below and Appendix 1 page 583). Reduce the dose of chlorpromazine when the patient improves. But, if it is a non-organic psychosis continue a maintenance dose (see below).
   (d) Give benztropine or promethazine or diazepam if muscle side effects of chlorpromazine develop (see below).

3. *Transfer some patients* (see page 582)
   Most patients are best treated in the health centre.
   A few patients need transfer (see below).
   Before transfer, make special arrangements (see below), and give special treatment (see below).

4. *Change the patient's environment if necessary*
   See 'Principles' No. 3 pages 579–580.
   Follow up the patient regularly to check that he takes any chlorpromazine or other drugs necessary; and to find out if he needs more treatment before the condition becomes severe again.

Treat the cause

1. *If organic psychosis* – treat the underlying disease affecting the brain, or the condition affecting the blood going to the brain (including substance abuse).

2. *If acute reaction* (to stress and anxiety) – try to solve the problem causing stress and anxiety.

3. *If non-organic psychosis* – treat with
   • chlorpromazine, etc. for schizophrenia and manic depressive psychosis, especially manic phase and substance misuse,
   • diazepam for drug withdrawal psychoses,
   • amitriptyline, etc. for depressive psychoses.

Treat the psychotic behaviour (the main treatment of non-organic psychoses too)

1. *Always admit the patient with a responsible friend or relative.*
   Tell the friend how to care for and comfort the patient. Check that the staff and other patients do not tease the patient.

2. *Check that the patient cannot hurt himself or anyone else.*
   • Nurse the patient on the floor if he is throwing himself around.
   • Do not leave articles which the patient could use as a weapon (e.g. knife, piece of wood, etc.).
   • If necessary, get four men to put the patient into a chair. Two strong men can then hold him until the drugs make the patient quiet or he goes to sleep.

3. *Give chlorpromazine* (25 mg *or* 100 mg tablets) and solution for injection 25 mg/ml (50 mg in 2 ml amps) *to produce the neuroleptisation syndrome.*

Choose a suitable oral dose chlorpromazine (see below).

• Give this dose regularly 6 hourly and hourly if necessary.
• Give twice this dose immediately and last dose at night.

Choose a suitable IM dose chlorpromazine if the patient refuses to take any of these oral doses. (Give the oral dose too when the IM dose settles the patient, see below.)
Increase the dose if necessary (see below).

(a) *Give chlorpromazine tablets regularly every 6 hours.*
   • Choose the dose that will probably be necessary (from 50 mg to 200 mg).
   • Try 50 mg for a small, old or sick patient, and for a patient who is quiet and is not very disturbed by hallucinations or delusions.
   • Try 200 mg for a large or young patient, and for a patient who is violent or very active.

and for a patient who is very disturbed by frightening hallucinations or delusions.

- Most patients need between 50 and 200 mg.

(b) *Give an extra dose of chlorpromazine tablets (use the same dose as above)*:
- when you first see the patient,
- with the last regular dose at night,
- every hour *if necessary* for violent behaviour or very disturbed speech and thoughts that are not controlled by the regular doses.

(c) *Give chlorpromazine by injection every time the patient refuses to swallow ANY ONE of the regular 6-hourly or the hourly 'if necessary' doses*
- Choose the dose that will probably be effective (50–100 mg (2–4 ml)).
- Give the oral dose that was refused *also*, when the patient starts to settle after the IM dose.

(d) *Every day, note the total amount of oral and IM chlorpromazine given the day before, and divide this by 4 to give the new 6-hourly regular dose (which is also the 'as necessary' and the night dose).*

(e) *If the patient has schizophrenia or bipolar disorder with mania*
- Leave him on the dose which settled him for 1 week (after he has settled well).
- Then slowly reduce the dose by 100–200 mg every week to 100–200 mg every night.
- Discharge the patient on 100–200 mg each night.
- It may be possible to stop the chlorpromazine after 3 months but usually it is given for 1 year.
- Follow up the patient every month.
- If the disease comes back soon or often after the treatment stops, then continue the treatment all the time.
- Follow up the patient and give him a supply of chlorpromazine every month (or at the least each 3 months).

(f) *You can stop chlorpromazine quickly if*:
- the psychosis is a reaction to a problem that has been solved, or
- the psychosis is caused by an organic disease that has been cured, or
- the psychosis was due to substance misuse that has stopped.

(g) *If the patient is not reliable in taking chlorpromazine himself,* chlorpromazine-like drugs are now available in long-acting injections, e.g. fluphenazine decanoate or enantate 25 mg/ml, the dose being 12.5–25 mg each 5–14 days depending on effect

and side effects. This is very useful if the patient has stopped chlorpromazine himself and had a relapse.

4. *Treat any side effects of chlorpromazine.*
   If the patient has shaking, muscle spasms, tongue or face spasms, eyes turned up, head bent back, limbs held in unusual positions, etc. *then* biperiden 4 mg or benztropine 4 mg or benzhexol 5 mg or procyclidine 5 mg (or if these are not available, promethazine 25 mg) IMI or IVI; then biperiden 2–4 mg 2–4 times daily or if not available promethazine 25 mg twice daily. If none of the above is available, try diazepam 5 mg IVI slowly over 5 minutes, then 5 mg orally twice daily
   and continue the chlorpromazine.
   Other side effects include low blood pressure, especially if chlorpromazine is given by injection. (Do not give larger first doses than recommended and do not give by IMI if blood pressure already low for other reasons.) Excessive sedation with increased appetite and weight gain can occur. Encourage friends and relatives to make the patient physically active. Some problems with dry mouth, blurred vision, constipation, urinary difficulty and impotence can occur, but usually can be accepted until the dose is decreased. Some allergic type reactions with hepatitis or skin rash occasionally occur. Stop chlorpromazine if allergic reactions occur.

5. *If the patient is psychotic because of the effect of alcohol or drugs being stopped,* the most helpful other treatment would be diazepam 5–20 mg orally regularly (up to 4(–12) hourly), this dose being slowly reduced every day to zero by 5–7 days. Much less chlorpromazine would then be needed.

6. *If the patient has depression,* amitriptyline or fluoxetine, specific antidepressant drugs, would be better than chlorpromazine. Chlorpromazine might be needed as well for other symptoms. Give only one antidepressant drug. Combinations of antidepressant drugs are no better than one alone and have more side effects. Amitriptyline is most widely available but has more side effects. It may be better, however, for patients who are agitated and cannot sleep. Give 25–50 mg three times a day when started, but at home the whole dose of 150 mg would be taken at night. It may take up to 3 weeks to improve the depression and the drug should be continued for several months before being stopped. If the patient is not very depressed and is started on treatment as an outpatient with amitriptyline, start with 25 mg at night and slowly increase the dose each 3–4 days.

If the patient is an inpatient, warn about side effects and start 25 mg three times a day and increase to 50 mg three times a day in a couple of days. Side effects include dry mouth, dizziness, difficulty passing urine (in an old man with the urethra partly blocked by the prostate or a stricture). Do not use amitriptyline if the patient has glaucoma. Fluoxetine is given as one 20 mg tablet in the morning. Occasionally, the dose will later need to be 40 mg. This drug is as effective as amitriptyline, but is much safer if an overdose is taken and has fewer cardiovascular and other side effects. It can, however, cause nausea and diarrhoea or constipation; nervousness, headache, insomnia and even agitation; and difficulty in having intercourse. Diazepam may be needed at night to help the patient to sleep. If available, it is the better drug to use if the patient has any cardiovascular problem or may take an overdose of the drug or has had side effects or no help from amitriptyline.

If the patient has repeated attacks of depression or bipolar disorder, the usual drug used for these, lithium, cannot be used for treatment at a health centre because regular blood levels are needed but cannot be measured. Ask your Medical Officer if a trial of carbamazepine (or other 'mood stabilising' drug) taken all the time would be worthwhile.

Transfer

Transfer only these patients to Medical Officer care:

1. an organic psychosis; but you cannot find or treat the cause (urgent);
2. a patient who is not better after 200–800 mg chlorpromazine every day for 3 weeks (non-urgent);
3. a patient who is very depressed and wants to kill himself and does not quickly improve on drug treatment (urgent);
4. side effects of chlorpromazine are not controlled by drugs as on page 581 or some side effects of other drugs;
5. a patient who has committed a serious crime (the police are responsible for transfer);
6. if a patient with schizophrenia, who has not settled back into normal life even with treatment, can be accepted into a special psychiatric rehabilitation village (which is often very successful in improving people enough to get them home again).

When transferring a psychiatric patient, discuss with Medical Officer first and make the following special arrangements:

1. Always send a letter to the Medical Officer with details about the patient and the reasons for his transfer.

2. Always send a reliable friend or relative who can speak the patient's language and whom the patient trusts.
3. For medico-legal reasons, send a letter from the patient's nearest relative requesting the patient's transfer, admission and treatment.
4. Control the patient's behaviour with drugs before transfer (see page 580 and below).
5. Send also a health worker, who can physically manage (control) and treat the patient.

Before transferring a psychotic or disturbed psychiatric patient by air:

1. Make sure the patient's behaviour has been controlled by chlorpromazine.
   - Give another *extra* dose of chlorpromazine 150 mg orally $1\frac{1}{2}$ hours before departure.
   - Fifteen minutes before departure, check the patient again.
   - If the patient is not *very* quiet, give chlorpromazine 50 mg (2 ml) IMI.
2. If you are worried the patient may still not be controlled, also give paraldehyde 0.2 ml/kg (usually 10 ml) IMI or diazepam 5 mg IMI.
3. *Never* transfer the patient alone. There must be a health worker (and, if necessary, another person) with the patient, who can physically control the patient, if he behaves abnormally, and who has chlorpromazine and paraldehyde injections and can give them.
4. Always explain all the details to the pilot.

Management of a non-organic non-psychotic disturbance

This includes patients with anxiety state, acting out, reactive depression, etc.

1. Do a full history and examination (see Chapter 6) and any tests necessary. Check that you look for all the causes of the patient's symptoms. If you find no cause for the patient's symptoms, think of a mental disorder and do these things;
2. Find out if the patient has a cause for stress and anxiety. See the patient often to find out. Also see relations, friends, etc. You can only diagnose mental disorder as the cause of the patient's symptoms, if you find a cause for stress and anxiety (as well as no organic cause).
3. Try to *solve the cause of the stress and anxiety*. This is the most important part of the treatment.
   You may need the help of a social worker, policeman, religious worker, employer, teacher, family, etc. to do this.

4. Then explain to the patient how the stress and anxiety can cause the symptoms he has (e.g. if a headache, explain how the tightening of the forehead and neck muscles for a long time causes pain in the head, just as exercising the arm or leg muscles for a long time causes pain in them).

5. If necessary, give sedative drugs to help reduce the anxiety. Use diazepam 5 mg, which is much better and safer than phenobarbital 15–30 mg three times a day for 1–2 weeks. If diazepam is not successful, try chlorpromazine 25–50 mg (1–2 × 25 mg tabs) three times a day for 1–2 weeks.

Do not keep the patient on drugs. Only give the drugs for a few weeks and then stop. The patient must solve his problem to stop the anxiety. The patient must not depend on drugs (or alcohol) to control the symptoms of his anxiety.

6. Show the patient how to relax and encourage him to do this.

Tell the patient how exercise and sport will help. Encourage him to do these.

7. If the problems cannot be solved, the patient may improve just by talking to you about how he is.

8. Refer or non-urgently transfer a patient to the Medical Officer when all this does not help the patient, or you cannot be certain that there is no organic cause for the symptoms. There are special psychiatric and psychological types of treatment which may be very helpful and which the Medical Officer may be able to organise.

Prevention of psychiatric conditions

1. You can:
- help to improve family life in the community;
- help to educate parents and community leaders in good ways of bringing up children;
- help to improve the environment in which the families live; and
- help to meet the other real needs of families.

These things will help children to grow up with normal ways of thinking, feeling and acting and to reduce the possibility of developing psychiatric conditions.

You need to co-operate with others in doing things to improve family life.

2. Give help to people at times of stress and anxiety. Important times of stress and anxiety include:
- leaving home – going to school,
- getting a job,
- tertiary education,
- getting married,
- having children, and
- sickness or death in the family.

If a person's problems can be solved or helped at such times, then the mental disease which may be caused by these will not develop.

You can co-operate with others in giving this help.

3. Early diagnosis and early effective treatment of psychiatric conditions will stop mild cases from becoming severe cases.

4. Effective rehabilitation of patients into the family and the community after treatment will reduce the effect of the condition on the patients, the families and the whole community.

Appendix 1

'Antipsychotic' drugs

Chlorpromazine was the first specific antipsychotic drug developed. A large number of similar drugs were later developed. These are called 'typical' or 'conventional' antipsychotics.

Recently, new unrelated antipsychotic drugs have been developed. These include risperidone, olanzapine, quetiapine, amisulpride, aripiprazole and others. These new drugs are called 'novel' (i.e. new) or 'atypical' (i.e. not like the others) antipsychotics.

Both typical and atypical antipsychotic drugs can give good control of psychoses.

The atypical drugs, however, are better tolerated, i.e. have fewer side effects (in particular fewer muscle spasms) and may help the 'negative' symptoms (not wanting to do anything much, not talking much, etc.), and the ability to think clearly. They may help to prevent the chance of recurrences more than the 'typical' antipsychotics. However, (1) they are much more expensive, (2) some new side effects have been found, and (3) none at the time of writing are on the WHO Model List of Essential Medicines. It may be that in the future some become available and you may be told to use them in place of chlorpromazine.

Antidepressant drugs

Amitriptyline was one of the first effective antidepressant drugs developed. A number of other similar drugs were made and together are called 'tricyclic antidepressants' (TCAs) and are 'non-selective monoamine re-uptake inhibitors'.

After this, a number of different groups of antidepressants were developed with different advantages and different side effects. One important group is the 'selective serotonin re-uptake inhibitors' (SSRIs).

The SSRIs are effective and have fewer cardiovascular and sedative side effects than amitriptyline and are safer if an overdose is taken. But they are more expensive. At the time of writing, fluoxetine, an SSRI, is the only one of the newer antidepressants on the WHO Model List of Essential Medicines.

It may be that in the future further ones from different groups will become available and that you will be told to use particular antidepressants for particular types of patients with depression.

36 Some Common Symptoms and Signs

Pyrexia of unknown origin (PUO) (fever of unknown cause)

There are many causes of a fever. But there are usually other symptoms or signs, or positive results of tests, in the patient with the fever. These other things usually show you the diagnosis for the patient. You (and the patient) then accept the fever as part of the disease and do not worry about the fever. You treat the cause of the disease and the fever goes away with the rest of the illness.

Sometimes when you first see a patient with a fever you can find no other symptoms and signs or abnormal tests to show you the diagnosis. If you ask the patient every day about his symptoms, and if you carefully examine the patient every day, you can usually find the cause of the fever and make a diagnosis when new symptoms or signs or tests come.

Sometimes you can only find the cause of a fever after all these things:

• history repeated many times,
• examination repeated many times,
• blood tests at a hospital,
• urine tests at a hospital,
• X-rays at a hospital
• biopsies at a hospital,
• laparotomy at a hospital,
• therapeutic trials of drugs, etc. at a hospital

but this is *very* unusual (see page 587).

Causes of fever include:

1. infections of all types in all organs – these are the most common and important causes of a fever;
2. non-infective inflammatory diseases including:
   • rheumatoid disease and other similar or auto-immune diseases,
   • trauma, and
   • allergic reactions of certain types;
3. neoplasm;
4. drugs and chemicals;
5. inherited diseases; and
6. many other causes.

Infections that cause fever

There are three groups of infections that cause fever:

1. Infection of *a particular part of the body which is caused by one of many different organisms*. The disease is often named after the part of the body infected (e.g. pneumonia when the lung (pneuma) is infected; hepatitis when the liver (hepar) is infected: meningitis when the meninges are infected). There is no one specific organism that infects these places. The organisms may be viruses or bacteria or worms, etc. *These infections occur in all parts of the world*. See Chapters 19–32, and septicaemia in Chapter 12.

2. *A specific organism that causes a specific disease which often affects more than one part of the body*. The disease is often named after the specific organism (e.g. measles, chickenpox). No other organism causes the same disease as this specific organism does. *These types of disease occur all over the world*. See specific viral diseases in Chapter 16, malaria in Chapter 13, TB in Chapter 14, leprosy in Chapter 15, HIV and some of the diseases in Chapter 19.

3. Another group of diseases is similar to group 2. *One particular organism causes disease*, which may affect *more than one part of the body*. But *these diseases occur only in certain parts of the world*. Diseases in this group which cause a short fever (a fever present for a week or less, although it may return) are in Chapter 17. Diseases in this group that cause longer fevers are in Chapter 18. If some of the diseases in Chapter 17 and Chapter 18 do not occur in your country, or where the patient has travelled, do not think of them. Think only of the diseases that the patient can possibly have.

Always include these infections in the differential diagnosis of a patient with a fever.

1. A non-specific infection of a part of the body which can occur anywhere in the world:
   • meningitis
   • septicaemia
   • upper respiratory tract infection, especially otitis media and sinusitis
   • influenza
   • pneumonia (especially in an upper lobe, where it is more difficult to find on examination)
   • gastroenteritis (see the many possible causes)
   • intra-abdominal abscess, especially pelvic inflammatory diseases, appendix abscess and liver abscess
   • urinary tract infection
   • osteomyelitis
   • acute bacterial ('septic') arthritis
   • abscess in another place, especially pyomyositis and injection abscess

2. A specific infection which can occur anywhere in the world:
   - malaria (the most important one to never forget)
   - tuberculosis
   - leprosy with reaction
   - measles
   - mumps
   - chickenpox
   - HIV infection
   - glandular fever
   - typhoid fever
   - brucellosis
   - leptospirosis
   - Q fever
3. A specific infection which occurs in your area. If any of these occur in your area, they are likely to be the cause of your patient's fever:
   - relapsing fever
   - typhus fever
   - plague
   - bartonellosis
   - arbovirus infections which do not cause haemorrhagic fever (can include dengue)
   - yellow fever, dengue and other arbovirus infections which do cause haemorrhagic fevers
   - haemorrhagic fevers caused by other virus infections which are spread man-to-man or rat-to-man or monkey-to-man
   - leishmaniasis
   - trypanosomiasis
   - allergic reactions to schistosomes and other worms or parasites in the body

The management of a patient with a fever of unknown cause

1. Do a full medical history.
2. Do a full clinical examination.
3. Do routine tests.
   - haemoglobin estimation,
   - urine in *all* cases for protein, pus, sugar and bile,
   - rapid diagnostic test for malaria if slide not possible,
   - others as indicated.

   Take tests to send to the laboratory, depending on which diseases occur in your area:
   - blood slide, for malaria and relapsing fever in all cases,
   - blood for HIV serology,
   - blood or lymph gland or other aspirate for leishmania and trypanosomes if these occur in your area,
   - others as indicated.

4. Write down a differential diagnosis of all possible causes. See list on this page for common infectious diseases.
5. Look for symptoms and signs to check for these diseases in 4.
6. Do tests to check for these diseases in 4, e.g.
   - tuberculin test (but positive test does not mean the patient has fever due to TB),
   - lumbar puncture (if any signs of meningitis).

   Take tests to send to the laboratory to check for these diseases in 4, e.g.
   - sputum for AFB,
   - blood for HIV (if not already done),
   - others as indicated.
7. Treat any cause you find.

   Also give *all* patients antimalarial drugs as indicated (see Chapter 13 pages 79, 80) if the patient is in or from an area where malaria occurs.
8. See the patient daily.
   - Ask for new symptoms daily until the patient is cured. Examine for new signs daily until he is cured. Remember to examine the ears and do a pelvic examination at least once more.
   - Test the urine again.
   - If not cured in 2 days, treat as in 9 or 10.
9. *If you find no other abnormalities and the patient looks 'sick' and does not improve after 2 days (antimalarials for 2 days):*
   - Transfer to Medical Officer care.

   If transfer is not possible, and the patient gets worse:
   - Give IV artesunate 2.4 mg/kg IVI or IMI or artemether 3.2 mg/kg IMI or quinine 20 mg/kg slow IV infusion or IMI and a companion drug and see Malaria Chapter 13 pages 80–81 if the patient is from or in an area where malaria occurs (see Chapter 13).
   - Give IVI fluids.
   - Give chloramphenicol 2 g IVI or IMI and see antibiotics as for septicaemia (see Chapter 12 page 64).
   - If patient is not greatly improved in 2 days, transfer.
   - If transfer is still not possible, and patient may die before transfer is possible, start anti-TB treatment (see Chapter 14 pages 114–122). (Transfer is essential later, even if the patient improves, unless positive sputum proves the diagnosis of TB.) If treatment for TB is started, the patient must complete the full course.
10. *If you find no other abnormalities, and the patient does not look 'sick' but does not improve after 3 days (antimalarials for 3 days):*

- Repeat a course of antimalarials. Give an artemisinin drug or quinine and companion drug (see Chapter 13 pages 80–81). Observe carefully to check that the drug is swallowed and absorbed (no vomiting or diarrhoea) or give by injection.
- Give also SMX 800 mg and TMP 160 mg twice daily for 7 days.
- If the patient still has fever after the above give chloramphenicol 1 g four times a day for 7–10 days.

11. If the patient still has a fever after the above, transfer is essential.
    - If transfer is really impossible and the fever continues for 4 weeks start anti-TB treatment (see Chapter 14). (Transfer is essential later, even if the patient improves, unless positive sputum proves the diagnosis of TB.) If treatment for TB is started, the patient must complete the full course.

Hospital management of PUO

1. Full history
2. Full examination especially for:
   - malaria,
   - respiratory infections including pneumonia and otitis media and sinusitis,
   - urinary tract infections,
   - HIV,
   - STD, PID,
   - abscesses in all places including abdomen and musculoskeletal system,
   - meningitis (especially chronic).
3. Basic tests for:
   - infections,
   - non-infective inflammatory diseases,
   - cancers,
   - intestinal diseases,
   - drug caused fever.

   AND usually
   - Malaria smears and/or rapid diagnostic test.
   - HIV serology.
   - Full blood count.
   - Sputum microscopy for Gram stain, AFB, fungi, pneumocystis at times, ova, etc. and culture for bacteria, *M. tuberculosis*, fungi, etc.
   - Electrolytes and liver function tests and protein.
   - Urine microscopy, including for parasite eggs and AFB and culture including for *M. tuberculosis*.
   - Stool microscopy, including for parasites and eggs and AFB and cultures including for *M. tuberculosis*.
   - Blood cultures including for *M. tuberculosis*.

- Chest X-ray for pneumonia, including atypical pneumonia and TB including atypical TB, etc.

AND often
- Trial off any drugs being taken in case this drug the cause of the fever (with appropriate replacement if for TB, HIV, etc.).
- LP and CSF examination, including for *M. tuberculosis*, fungi, protozoa, etc. causing chronic meningitis.
- Blood tests including serology (if appropriate) for:
  Relapsing fever
  Typhus fever of various types
  Typhoid
  Brucellosis
  Leptospirosis
  Q fever
  Cryptococcus and other fungal infections in some areas
  Toxoplasma and other protozoal infections
  Viral and other opportunistic infections if the patient has HIV
  Bartonellosis
  Hepatitis
  Dengue and other arbovirus infections
  Other virus infections in area
  Leishmaniasis
  Trypanosomiasis.
- Blood tests for autoimmune diseases, cancers, inherited and blood diseases.
- Aspiration/biopsies for:
  AFB/*M. tuberculosis* culture
  Leishmania
  Trypanosomiasis
- X-rays or scans for abscesses, cancers, others.
- Bronchoscopy, endoscopy, colonoscopy, nasendoscopy, cystoscopy, etc. for infections, cancers, others.

AND sometimes
- Trial of NSAID to determine if inflammation or neoplasia the cause.
- Trial of specific anti-infection treatment if a particular non-diagnosed infection seems likely.
- Biopsy of possibly affected organs.
- Others.

> Careful history and examination, repeated if necessary, and simple tests and continued observation as long as the diseases likely in that area and in that particular patient are always thought of each time the patient is seen, will usually diagnose the cause of the fever without most of the above tests or even sending the patient to hospital.

Malaise (patient feels unwell)

1. Do a full medical history.
2. Do a full clinical examination
3. Do routine tests: (a) Hb if pale, (b) urine test in *all* cases.

   Take tests to send to the laboratory for the common infectious diseases in your area (see pyrexia or fever, page 585).
4. Write down a differential diagnosis of all the possible causes.
5. Look for symptoms and signs to check for these diseases in 4.
6. Do or send tests to check for these diseases in 4. Especially remember
   - blood slide for malaria and relapsing fever,
   - tuberculin test,
   - sputum for AFB,
   - blood test for HIV infection.
   - lumbar puncture,
   - blood or lymph gland or other aspirated material for examination for leishmaniasis or trypanosomiasis,
7. Treat any cause you find *and* give *all* patients anti-malarial drugs as indicated, if the patient is in or from an area where malaria occurs (see Chapter 13 pages 78, 80).
8. See the patient daily.
   - Ask about new symptoms daily until he is cured. Examine for new signs daily until he is cured. Remember to examine the ears and do a pelvic examination at least once.
   - Test the urine again.
   - Manage as in 9, 10 or 11 below.
9. *If it is an acute illness and you find no abnormalities and the patient looks 'sick':*
   - If it is an acute illness and does not improve after 3 days (and antimalarials for 3 days), treat as for 9 (page 586) in pyrexia of unknown cause page 585.
10. *If it is a chronic illness and you find no abnormalities and the patient does not improve after 2 weeks:*
    - Treat as in 10, pages 586–587 (pyrexia of unknown cause).
    - If does not improve and transfer is not possible, send blood for Hb, white cell count (total and differential), liver function tests, urea and serology tests for HIV infection. Send sputum for AFB. Send urine for full examination. Do a tuberculin test. Send the appropriate tests for any other diseases common in your area.

- Ask the Medical Officer to send you a *report on what the tests mean.*
- See 11 below also.

11. *If you find no abnormalities and the patient does not look 'sick':*

    Think of a mental disturbance. Find out if the patient has a problem or a cause for stress and anxiety. But diagnose a psychiatric cause only if:
    - you find *no* organic cause (see Chapter 35 page 568) and the patient does not look 'sick' *and*
    - a *real* cause for stress and anxiety *is* present, *or*
    - positive signs of a non-organic psychosis (see Chapter 35 pages 570, 573) are present.
12. If the patient is not diagnosed and treated by the above, ask the Medical Officer to see him non-urgently.

Generalised oedema (swelling of the whole body)

Do a full history and examination (see Chapter 6). Test urine for protein, sugar, bile, blood and pus.

1. Check that the *whole* body (legs *and* back and sometimes face) has oedema.

   Lymphoedema or elephantiasis usually affect only the limbs (usually legs) and the lymph glands are usually enlarged.

   If oedema only in some parts, see page 590.
2. If the urine contains protein, look for:
   (a) nephrotic syndrome (*much protein (>$\frac{1}{8}$ or +) and much oedema*),
   (b) pre-eclamptic toxaemia (*female, pregnant 20 or more weeks, BP higher than 120/80, protein in urine; or just BP 140/90 or above*),
   (c) chronic kidney failure (*nausea, wasted, anaemic, BP high*),
   (d) acute nephritic syndrome or acute glomerulo-nephritis (*blood in the urine, BP high, fever*),
   (e) heart failure (*see below*).
3. Look for heart failure
   (a) The signs of heart failure are:
   - *raised jugular venous pressure* ⎫ almost
   - *enlarged liver* ⎬ always
   - *oedema*
   - *fast pulse* – usually
   - *cyanosis* – often
   - *crackles in lower lungs* – sometimes
   (b) You can usually find the cause of the heart failure, e.g.
   - *chronic obstructive lung disease*
   - *pneumonia*

- *severe anaemia*
- *IV fluids given too quickly*
- *other,* see Chapter 27 pages 462–464.

4. Look for severe anaemia.

5. Look for malnutrition (unusual in an adult) or chronic disease of the gastrointestinal tract (especially chronic vomiting or chronic diarrhoea or dysentery).

6. Look for cirrhosis (chronic liver disease):
   (a) *you can find no other cause and*
   (b) *ascites that is worse than the oedema*
   (c) *very thin arms and shoulders, very swollen abdomen, moderately swollen legs* } the typical appearance of cirrhosis see Figure 24.5

Management

Give diuretics

Do not give diuretics if it is toxaemia of pregnancy or malnutrition.

Give hydrochlorothiazide 25–50 mg daily. Increase the dose to 100 mg daily if necessary.

Also give furosemide/frusemide 40 mg daily if necessary. Increase the dose slowly to 160 mg daily if necessary.

Give potassium if necessary

1. If the patient is not eating a tuber diet (i.e. sweet potatoes, etc.), *or*
2. he is taking digoxin and diuretics, *or*
3. he is taking furosemide/frusemide and hydrochlorothiazide, then give potassium chloride slow release tablets 1200 mg three times a day.

Treat the cause if possible and transfer to Medical Officer care if necessary

Nephrotic syndrome

- Give prophylactic antimalarials (see Chapter 13 pages 88–89).
- Give treatment for intestinal worms (see Chapter 23 page 355).
- Refer to Medical Officer if the patient is not cured in 6 weeks (some cases can be helped by other drugs).

Pre-eclamptic toxaemia

The patient must rest in bed.

If the patient not cured in 2 days or if she gets worse at any time or if she has fitting, treat (see an obstetrics book) and transfer urgently.

If fitting, give 5 g (10 ml of a 500 mg/ml solution) of magnesium sulfate IMI each buttock then 4 g (8 ml of 500 mg/ml solution) IV slowly over 10 minutes. Give a maintenance dose of 5 g IMI 6 hourly. Give further doses of IV magnesium sulfate and also rectal

or IV diazepam if further fitting. See obstetrics book and transfer as emergency.

If she is cured after 2 days rest in bed, keep her in the health centre on observation or tell her to return every week for examination, until delivery.

Chronic kidney failure

The patient must drink 3 litres of fluid daily. Give chlorpromazine 25 mg every 6 hours if necessary IMI if there is vomiting or orally if there is nausea.

The patient must take as much salt as possible without causing oedema or heart failure – if these develop, reduce salt until these go.

No high protein foods.

See Chapter 26 pages 449–450.

Acute glomerulonephritis

See Chapter 26 page 446 and a medical reference book.

Heart failure

Diuretics are the most important treatment in most cases (see Chapter 27 pages 464–466). If there is acute, severe heart failure give furosemide 40 mg IV.

Give oxygen if there is acute shortness of breath or cyanosis.

If there is chronic obstructive lung disease, see Chapter 20 page 298.

If there is pneumonia, see Chapter 20 pages 289–291 and give digoxin (see Chapter 27 page 465).

If there is anaemia, see Chapter 21 pages 316–319 and transfer for blood transfusion.

If IV fluids were given too quickly, stop or slow the drip.

If there is no cause obvious, give thiamine 50 mg immediately and daily for 2 weeks (the first dose IMI if available).

If other treatment is necessary (e.g. enalapril, digoxin, etc.) see Chapter 27 pages 464–466.

Transfer to Medical Officer care *if*

1. you have not diagnosed a cause which you can treat, especially if the pulse is irregular, *or*
2. you have diagnosed a cause that you can treat but proper treatment is not available or does not cure it.

Severe anaemia

See Chapter 21 pages 316–319 and transfer for blood transfusion.

Malnutrition or chronic gastrointestinal disease

Check that the patient has a good mixed diet of enough food, at least six times a day.

Give drugs for intestinal worms (see Chapter 23 pages 354–359).

Treat any cause of vomiting or diarrhoea (see Chapter 23 pages 384–386, 387–388).

Diuretics should not be given.

Transfer the patient if he does not improve.

Cirrhosis

Check the patient has a good mixed diet with high protein but no salt (tinned meat and fish usually have too much salt).

Give treatment for intestinal worms.

Diuretics are often necessary for the rest of the patient's life (usually a smaller dose after the ascites goes). See Chapter 24 pages 397–398.

Transfer if the diagnosis is not certain, especially if there are masses or tenderness in the abdomen.

Localised oedema (swelling of one part of the body)

1. *Check for swelling of the rest of the body*. If generalised oedema, see page 588.
2. *Check that the swelling is oedema* and not a lump from another cause.

   Types of lumps include
   (a) Congenital (the patient was born with it)
   (b) Traumatic (caused by injury)
   (c) Inflammatory
   - infection
   - trauma
   - allergy
   - bites, stings, toxins
   (d) Neoplastic (cancer)
   (e) Degenerative. Remember especially:
   - hernia
   - prolapse
   - thrombosis (clotting) in a blood vessel
   - calcification
   - swelling caused by a blocked duct
3. *Look for causes of localised oedema*, especially:
   (a) Injury. *History. Type of lesion. Haematoma often present (bruise).*
   (b) Infection. *If acute* – red or shiny; swollen; tender; hot; the part cannot work properly.
   (c) Lymph vessel and lymph gland disease (see Chapter 22 pages 333–343) especially:
   - acute bacterial infection
   - acute filarial inflammation
   - chronic bacterial infection including some STDs
   - chronic filarial inflammation
   - tuberculosis

- cancer
- chronic chemical (silica) inflammation (podoconiosis) (usually farmers who work without shoes on red rocky soil)
   (d) Snakebite. *History*.
   (e) Allergic reaction. *Swelling and often redness and itch but little tenderness.*
   (f) Varicose veins
   (g) Clots in main deep veins. *History of little recent leg movement (e.g. operation, illness, long trip) or of injury to limb or of IV injection or of infection; you can find no other cause. Note risk of pulmonary embolus.*
4. *Treat any cause you find.*
   (a) Injury. See a surgery book.
   (b) Infection. See Chapter 11 pages 56–61.
   (c) Lymphatic disease. See Chapter 22 page 333.
   (d) Snakebite. See Chapter 33 pages 554–558.
   (e) Allergic reaction. Give promethazine 25 mg 1–3 times daily and, if necessary, adrenaline tart. 1:1000 0.5 or $\frac{1}{2}$ ml each 6 hours.
   (f) Clots in the main deep veins. If it is in the leg, transfer urgently to Medical Officer care as risk of pulmonary embolus. In other cases treat with sling, acetylsalicylic acid, heat and antibiotics.
5. *Treat the affected part.*
   (a) Keep it higher than the rest of the body if possible, e.g. blocks under the foot of bed; arm in sling.
   (b) protect from further injury, especially if chronic, e.g. wear shoes if the leg or the foot is affected.

Generalised wasting

Do a full history and examination (see Chapter 6). Test the urine for protein and sugar.

Send sputum for AFB if there is a cough. Look for signs of these conditions:

1. Malnutrition. History of eating – what and how much and how often? (see Chapter 23 page 374).
2. Chronic disease of the gastrointestinal tract, especially if there is chronic vomiting (usually transfer) or chronic diarrhoea (possibly treat with albendazole and metronidazole and tetracycline (Chapter 23 pages 387–388) and transfer if this does not cure it).
3. Chronic infections, especially:
   (a) tuberculosis (*chronic cough or enlarged lymph glands*), see Chapter 14.
   (b) HIV infection usually with diarrhoea, see Chapter 19.
   (c) malaria (attacks of fever, anaemia, large spleen), see Chapter 13.

(d) hyperreactive malarious splenomegaly or tropical splenomegaly syndrome (*anaemia, very large spleen*) see Chapter 21 pages 319–321.

(e) visceral leishmaniasis (*fever, very enlarged spleen, enlarged lymph nodes, anaemia, diarrhoea, skin infiltrations sometimes*) see Chapter 18 pages 175–181.

(f) trypanosomiasis (*history of skin lesions at first, fever, enlarged lymph glands, enlarged spleen, enlarged liver, anaemia, fast pulse, nervous system disease*), see Chapter 18 pages 181–186.

4. Repeated attacks of ordinary infections.
5. Chronic, non-infectious diseases, especially:

(a) chronic obstructive lung disease (*chronic cough, sputum AFB negative*) see Chapter 20 pages 297–298.

(b) chronic kidney failure (*protein in urine, anaemia, nausea, BP high*), see Chapter 26 pages 449–450.

(c) cirrhosis (*thin shoulders, some swelling of legs and back, severe swelling of abdomen, no protein in urine*), see Chapter 24 pages 397–398.

(d) thyrotoxicosis (*eating much, staring eyes, shaking hands, fast pulse*), see Chapter 30 pages 498–499.

(e) diabetes (*eating and drinking much, passing much urine, sugar in urine*), see Chapter 30 page 499.

6. Cancer of any organ (*often enlarged organ or lumps or bleeding*).
7. Others (see a specialist medical reference book). Transer non-urgently if no cause found.

Dehydration

Dehydration is present when there is not enough salt and/or water in the body.

The body normally contains 60% water.

If 0–5% of the body weight is lost (3 kg in 60 kg person, i.e. 3 litres) there is mild dehydration.

If 5–10% of the body weight is lost (6 kg in 60 kg person, i.e. 6 litres) there is moderate dehydration.

If 10–15% of the body weight is lost (9 kg in 60 kg person, i.e. 9 litres) there is severe dehydration which will probably soon cause shock and death.

Causes include:
1. Too much fluid lost from
   • intestines (vomiting, diarrhoea)
   • skin (sweating)
   • urine (diabetes, chronic kidney diseases)
   • lungs (fast breathing in high fever).
2. Not enough fluid taken in
   • too sick to drink
   • unconsciousness

• woman in labour
• no water to drink.

The most important *signs* in adults are:
• fast pulse,
• low BP,
• inelastic skin,
• little urine passed and urine dark colour,
• sunken eyes, and
• dry mouth.

Do not mistake inelastic skin from weight loss (wasting) or old age, for the inelastic skin of dehydration.

For *management* of patient with dehydration, see Chapter 23 pages 363–366.

Loss of weight

Find out *how long* the condition has taken to develop.

1. In a few hours
   • loss of fluid (dehydration), from any cause (see above).
2. In a few days
   • loss of fluid (dehydration), from any cause (see above).
   • not taking in fluid (dehydration), from any cause (see above).
   • not eating.
3. In a few weeks or months
   • wasting condition, from any cause (see page 590).
   • malnutrition (see Chapter 23 pages 375–381).

Note only loss of fluid or not taking in fluid can cause rapid (in a few hours or days) loss of weight.

Lumps (masses)

Examination of lump

Note especially:
• Site
  – in what tissue or organ?
  – where in that tissue or organ?
• Size
• Shape
• Surface
• Consistency
• Fluctuancy
• Tenderness and other signs of inflammation
• Fixed to surrounding tissue or not
• Function of the affected tissue or organ
• Regional (or nearby) lymph nodes

Types of lumps

1. Congenital
2. Traumatic
3. Inflammatory
   • infection
   • trauma
   • allergy
   • bites, stings, toxins
4. Neoplastic
5. Degenerative – remember
   • hernia
   • prolapse
   • thrombosis (clotting) in a blood vessel
   • calcification
   • swelling caused by a blocked duct

If a lump is neoplastic, these signs will usually help you to find out what type of neoplasm it is:

If it is a simple or benign lump, it –	If it is a malignant lump, it –
has clear regular edges	has irregular edges
is not hard	is hard
can be moved	is fixed to other tissues
grows slowly (years)	grows fast (weeks or months)
does not grow into surrounding tissues	grows into surrounding tissues
does not spread to lymph nodes	spreads to lymph nodes
does not spread to other organs	spreads to other organs
rarely forms ulcers	often forms ulcers

Abscess

An abscess is a collection of pus in one part of the body.

Diagnosis of an abscess

1. There are usually general symptoms and signs of infection.
2. There are local symptoms and signs of inflammation.
3. There are signs of fluctuation in *two directions* at right angles; but only if the abscess is near the surface of the body. Place the index and middle fingers of one hand on the swelling. Then press down quickly between the two fingers with a finger of the other hand. If fluctuation is present, you will feel the 2 fingers being lifted. Then put the 2 fingers at right angles (or 90°) to the first position and do the test again. If fluctuation is *again* present, then there is fluid (e.g. pus) under the 2 fingers. Note that fluctuation in one direction only does *not* mean there is fluid under the fingers (normally muscle 'fluctuates' in one direction).

Treatment of an abscess

1. Give *antibiotics* only if:
   (a) There are severe general symptoms and signs of infection (fever, fast pulse, etc.).
   (b) The infection is spreading into the surrounding tissue (cellulitis) or lymph vessels (lymphangitis) or lymph glands (lymphadenitis).
   (c) The bone may be infected (osteomyelitis) (continue for at least 4 weeks).
   (d) The muscle is infected (i.e. it is a pyomyositis).
   (e) It is a breast abscess.
   (f) It is a hand or finger abscess.
   See Chapter 11 pages 56–61 for choice of antibiotic.
2. *Incise and drain* the abscess (but only if you have been trained how to do so) if:
   (a) Pus is definitely present (i.e. if fluctuant in two directions at right angles; or soft); and also:
   (b) A breast abscess has not improved after 2 days of antibiotics or has already been present for 4 days when you first see it, or
   (c) It is a hand abscess and patient cannot sleep for 1 night after you start antibiotics (transfer to Medical Officer is best), or
   (d) It is pyomyositis or osteomyelitis. Incise immediately if it is very swollen; or after 2 days if it is not almost cured by antibiotics.

• Use anaesthetic topical spray if it is a small superficial abscess (except hand).
• Use general anaesthetic (ketamine) or lytic cocktail or regional block if it is a large or deep abscess or in the hand.

> Use these anaesthetics only if you have had special training and have all the necessary resuscitation equipment available.

• Do not cut or damage other structures.
• Cut the skin and subcutaneous tissues with a scalpel.
• Push a closed pair of artery forceps into the abscess, and then open the forceps.
• Make a hole big enough to insert your finger (except hand abscess).
• Destroy all walls inside the abscess with your finger (inside a sterile glove). Feel if the bone is affected.

- Leave a rubber drain in the abscess, that comes out through the skin.
- Pack the wound with gauze soaked in Eusol or strong 3% saline if it bleeds much.
- Apply a Eusol dressing.

3. Give *drugs for pain* if necessary See Chapter 7 pages 32–34.
4. *Dress after incision.*

Dress when necessary (at least daily, but more often if necessary).

- Use either a little acriflavine emulsion smeared on an absorbant pad soaked in strong (3%) saline or an absorbant pad soaked in Eusol.
- Remove any pack in 1 day.
- Remove the drain when there is only a little discharge (2–3 days).
- When the sore is clean and there is no more pus and slough, dress with a weak (1%) saline dressing or a vaseline gauze dressing.

Transfer to the Medical Officer any case where the abscess is deep, or near important structures in the neck, chest, abdomen, or in the hand.

Abdominal pain

1. *Take a full history* (see Chapter 6). Ask about the pain, especially
   - is it a colic? (if colic, see below)

   or
   - is it a constant pain? (if constant pain, see page 594)
   - where exactly is the pain?

   Remember to ask about
   - recent trauma to abdomen,
   - the date of last normal menstrual period.
2. *Do a full examination* (see Chapter 6). Remember to check carefully for:
   (a) temperature (? infection)
   (b) PR; BP; skin elasticity; hands and feet warm or cold (? dehydration, ? shock)
   (c) colour (? anaemia, ? bleeding)
   (d) abdominal
      - distension
      - movement on breathing
      - hernia and scars
      - tenderness – guarding – rigidity
      - masses
      - enlargement of organs
      - intestinal bowel sounds
      - pelvic examination 'PR' or 'PV' for tenderness, masses or enlarged organs

   (e) chest disease (pain referred to abdomen)
   (f) spinal disease (pain referred to abdomen)
3. *Test urine for protein, pus, bile, sugar.*
4. *Look at any vomit or abnormal stools or vaginal discharge to see what it contains.*

The pain is a colic
(if pain is constant, see below and page 594)

Colic is caused by obstruction or inflammation of:

- the gastrointestinal tract (stomach or small intestine or large intestine), *or*
- the female reproductive tract (tubes or uterus), *or*
- urinary tract (ureters) (often more a constant pain with times when it is worse), *or*
- biliary tract (bile ducts) (less often) (see page 399).

See Figure 36.1.

Causes of colic in these organs include:

1. Gastrointestinal tract (see Chapter 23 page 348)
   (a) Gastroenteritis (*diarrhoea, central abdominal colic, sometimes vomiting; no definite abdominal tenderness; often dehydration and fever*).

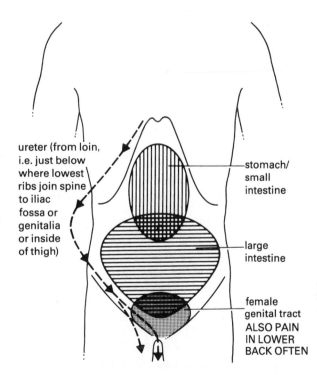

ureter (from loin, i.e. just below where lowest ribs join spine to iliac fossa or genitalia or inside of thigh)

stomach/small intestine

large intestine

female genital tract ALSO PAIN IN LOWER BACK OFTEN

Figure 36.1 *Diagram to show the place in the abdomen where the patient feels colic from the various organs that can cause colic.*

(b) Intestinal obstruction (*constipation; central abdominal colic; vomiting; abdomen distended, not tender*).

(c) Enteritis necroticans ('pigbel') (*signs of obstruction and peritonitis*) (see Chapter 23 page 370).

(d) Others, including gall bladder (page 399).

2. Genital

(a) Labour (*large, non-tender uterus; no fever or shock*).

(b) Antepartum 'accidental' haemorrhage (*large, tender uterus; often anaemia and shock*).

(c) Miscarriage (*PV bleeding; uterus enlarged; no abdominal or pelvic masses or tenderness*).

(d) Ectopic pregnancy (*1–2 periods late or missed; some dark red PV bleeding; usually also constant lower abdominal or general abdominal pain and tenderness; often fainting; often pale or shocked*) (see an obstetrics book).

(e) period pains (dysmenorrhoea) (*history of similar pain with periods; on examination NAD*).

3. Ureters

Stones (*pain in typical place* (see Figure 36.1); *kidney sometimes tender; often blood in the urine*).

If the pain is a colic

1. Where is the pain? What organ is probably causing it? (See Figures 36.1 and 36.2.)

2. What condition is probably affecting this organ? (See above.)

3. What is the management of this condition?

The pain is constant

(If the pain is a colic, see above.)

Constant pain is caused by:

• inflammation or swelling or stretching,
• of the organ or of the peritoneum,
• at the place of the pain (see Figure 36.2 for position of organs; the peritoneum is around the whole abdomen).

Tenderness in one area means:

• inflammation or swelling or stretching,
• of the organ or of the peritoneum,
• under the place of the tenderness (see Figure 36.2 for position of organs; the peritoneum is around the whole abdomen).

Tenderness all over the abdomen (generalised), often with guarding and rigidity means:

• inflammation or irritation of the whole peritoneum by,
• pus (peritonitis), or
• blood from trauma or ectopic pregnancy.

Note. Tenderness over an area is more accurate than pain over that area for diagnosing inflammation or swelling or stretching of the organ or peritoneum under that area.

See Figures 36.2 and 36.3 and below under 'Transfer' for causes of constant abdominal pain.

Note *also* these four causes of constant abdominal pain.

1. All over
   • pus in peritoneum (peritonitis)
   • blood in peritoneum (trauma or ectopic pregnancy)

2. Any part – spinal disease (fracture or bacterial or tuberculous infection) with referred pain.

3. Upper abdomen – chest disease (pneumonia or pleurisy) with referred pain.

4. From where lower rib joins spine to genitalia or upper, inner thigh – ureteric colic (stones).

If the pain is constant

1. Where is the pain?
   What is the organ that is probably causing it? (See Figure 36.2.) (If the pain is all over, the peritoneum is affected.)

2. What condition is probably affecting this organ? (See Figure 36.3.)

3. What is the management of this condition?

Transfer

Transfer urgently to Medical Officer if (but, first start treatment, see next page):

1. Generalised peritonitis or blood in the peritoneal cavity. In both
   • *constant generalised pain*
   • *often vomiting and constipation*
   • *the abdomen is distended and does not move well on breathing*
   • *the abdomen is tender all over, often with guarding and rigidity*
   • *intestinal sounds are not present.*
   If peritonitis
   • *pulse fast, temperature raised, BP normal (later BP low and shock).*
   If bleeding
   • *pale, pulse fast, BP low (sometimes shock), usually no fever.*

2. Localised peritonitis (e.g. appendicitis)
   • *constant pain in one part of the abdomen*
   • *abdomen does not move well over affected area and is tender over affected area, often with rebound tenderness and guarding*

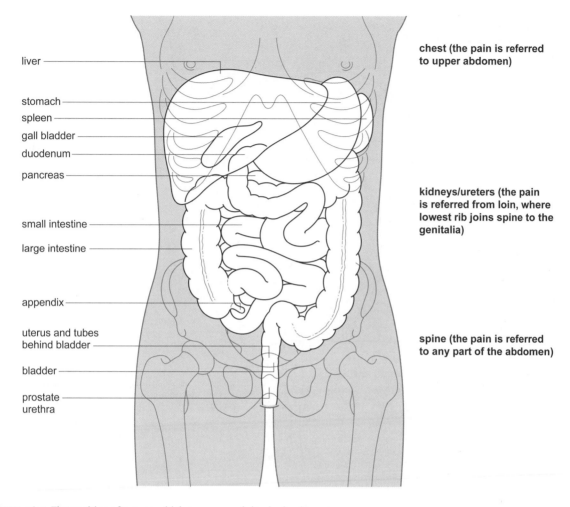

liver

stomach
spleen
gall bladder
duodenum

pancreas

small intestine

large intestine

appendix

**uterus and tubes
behind bladder**

bladder

**prostate
urethra**

**chest (the pain is referred
to upper abdomen)**

**kidneys/ureters (the pain
is referred from loin, where
lowest rib joins spine to the
genitalia)**

**spine (the pain is referred
to any part of the abdomen)**

Figure 36.2 *The position of organs which can cause abdominal pain.*

• *pulse fast*
• *temperature raised.*
But you can treat liver abscess and hepatitis, or pelvic inflammatory disease, or splenic inflammation (not trauma), at the health centre.
3. Obstruction of intestine
(a) *colicky abdominal pain*
(b) *vomiting*
(c) *constipation*
(d) *abdomen*
   • *distended*
   • *no tenderness unless strangulation when tender over one area or over a hernia*
   • *intestinal (bowel) sounds increase when the pain comes.*
4. Ectopic pregnancy or
severe 'Pelvic inflammatory disease'

(a) *missed or late or irregular or heavy periods,* and
(b) *lower abdominal pain,* and
(c) *vaginal bleeding or discharge* and
(d) *uterus enlarged and also tender* or
   • *a mass or tenderness next to the uterus* or
   • *tenderness of all the abdomen often with guarding and rigidity and no intestinal sounds* and
(e) • *pulse fast, BP low, pallor, normal temperature*
      − *if there is bleeding (ectopic, miscarriage, antepartum haemorrhage)* or
   • *pulse fast and temperature raised − if there is infection (septic abortion, pelvic inflammatory disease and sometimes ectopic pregnancy).*
5. Antepartum haemorrhage.
   • *large tender uterus*
   • *anaemia often*

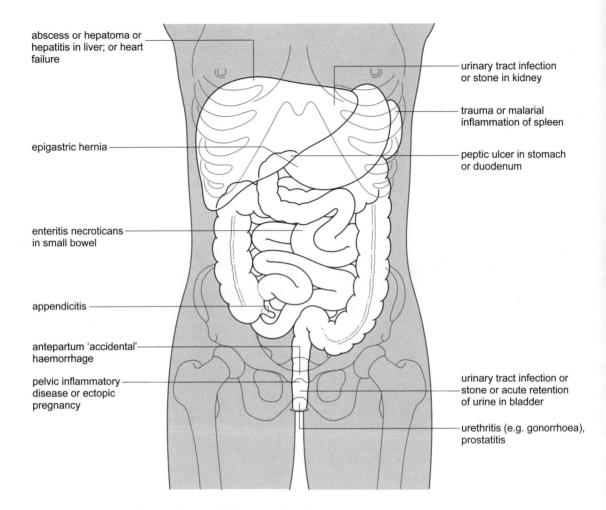

abscess or hepatoma or hepatitis in liver; or heart failure

urinary tract infection or stone in kidney

trauma or malarial inflammation of spleen

epigastric hernia

peptic ulcer in stomach or duodenum

enteritis necroticans in small bowel

appendicitis

antepartum 'accidental' haemorrhage

pelvic inflammatory disease or ectopic pregnancy

urinary tract infection or stone or acute retention of urine in bladder

urethritis (e.g. gonorrhoea), prostatitis

Figure 36.3 *Common conditions of organs which cause abdominal pain.*

• *shock often*.
See an obstetrics book.

6. Acute retention of urine that you cannot cure with catheterisation of bladder and treatment of urinary infection.

7. Ureteric colic (non-urgent).

Acute 'surgical' abdomen

(Peritonitis, bleeding into peritoneum, obstruction of the intestine)

1. The patient must not eat or drink.

2. Start an IV drip.

• Give IV fluids as necessary.

• If there is shock – see Chapter 27 pages 468–470.

• If bleeding into the peritoneum is probable (you suspect it from the history, examination, progressive pallor, rising pulse, etc. in absence of evidence of severe infection) – see Chapter 27 page 469 and arrange emergency transfer for urgent blood transfusion.

• If there is dehydration – see Chapter 23 pages 364–366.

• If only maintenance fluids are needed 0.18% sodium chloride in 4% dextrose 1 litre each 8–12 hours.

- If you do not know if the patient is taking enough fluid and patient cannot pass urine, insert an indwelling urethral catheter and measure the urine passed every hour (it should be > 30 ml/hour). Increase the IV fluids until the urine passed is > 30 ml/hour.

3. Give chloramphenicol, unless infection is not probable.
   - Give chloramphenicol 2 g immediately and then 1 g every 6 hours.
   - Give by IVI if there is shock or a drip running; and by IMI to other cases.

4. Give an antimalarial drug by injection as indicated (see Chapter 13 pages 80–81).

5. Do nasogastric suction if there is evidence of intestinal obstruction (repeated vomiting and distension and colic) or ileus (paralysis) (repeated vomiting and distension).
   - Put a tube through the nose into the stomach.
   - Aspirate (suck out) all the fluid and gas possible, immediately and every hour.
   - Leave the end of the tube open, and hang it over the side of the bed, lower than the patient. Fluid will drain from it.
   - Check the volume of all the fluid which comes out of the tube, and is vomited each hour.

6. Treat the underlying condition.
   - Abdominal surgery will almost always be necessary. Transfer to the Medical Officer urgently for the necessary surgery.
   - In enteritis necroticans (pigbel) and a few other conditions, the above treatment may be enough.

7. Treat any other conditions present, or any complications that develop, in the usual ways.

8. Transfer the patient urgently (emergency) to the Medical Officer at a hospital. First get the patient's written permission for any tests, treatment or surgery which may be necessary.

9. Give analgesics unless the Medical Officer can see the patient almost immediately. (If so, do not give analgesics because they may make the tenderness and signs in the abdomen less.)
   Give IM morphine
   - 7.5–10 mg to a small adult (< 50 kg)
   - 10–15 mg to a large adult (> 50 kg)

Abdominal tenderness – guarding – rigidity

You discover abdominal tenderness, guarding and rigidity during palpation of the abdomen.

Palpate the abdomen to discover three things.

1. Tenderness. If it is present, where is it? Also, are rebound tenderness and guarding and rigidity present?
2. Are normal organs enlarged? – liver, spleen, uterus and bladder.
3. Are there masses or lumps in other places including hernia and lymph glands.

Do palpation only *after* inspection.

Palpate first for tenderness – guarding – rigidity like this:

1. Be gentle. If you hurt the patient with your first palpation, the patient may not relax again. The examination will then be difficult.
2. First move the *palm* of your hand gently over the whole abdomen. This helps the patient to relax. Also, you can often find an area of tenderness by feeling the patient's abdominal wall muscles contract (and seeing his eye or face muscles also contract) when your hand moves over the tender area.
3. Then palpate with the *palm* of your hand held flat and not the tips of the fingers (Figures 36.4, 36.5 and 36.6). Again, look at the patient's face and feel the abdominal muscles contract to find tender parts.
   Palpate carefully all over the abdomen. Do not forget the loins (kidney area at the back), or any other part.
   Start in a place which is probably normal. Palpate a place you suspect is abnormal last.
4. If you do not find any tenderness with 2 and 3, then palpate more deeply. Again, palpate all areas of the abdomen.
5. If it is difficult to decide exactly where the most tender place is, you can do a gentle 'one finger palpation' in the place where you found the tenderness. If you look at the patient's face, feel the abdominal muscles contract and ask the patient where it hurts most, you can usually decide which is the most tender place with 'one finger palpation' (Figure 36.7).

Causes of abdominal tenderness – guarding – rigidity

Inflammation, swelling or stretching of an organ or of the peritoneum causes *tenderness* on palpation over the organ or peritoneum. If the condition is mild, tenderness may be the only sign that you find.

You can find *rebound tenderness* if you quickly remove the palpating hand (which is pressing firmly on the abdomen) from the abdomen. The release of the pressure on the contents of the abdomen causes movement and, therefore, pain over the inflamed or stretched organ or peritoneum (e.g. in appendicitis, if you suddenly lift your hand off the abdomen during palpation of the left iliac fossa, the patient will feel pain in the right iliac fossa, where the inflamed appendix is).

If the inflammation or swelling or stretching of the organ or peritoneum is more severe and acute, then *involuntary guarding* may occur. When you do the palpation, the overlying muscles contract. This stops the palpation putting more pressure on the affected organ or peritoneum and causing more pain. The patient cannot completely stop this muscle contraction, even if you help him to relax (e.g. by talking to him) or he tries himself. (This is different from voluntary guarding, which is often caused by worry and goes if the patient does not think about his abdomen when you palpate it.)

Rigidity occurs if the inflammation, swelling or stretching of the organ or the peritoneum is even

more severe and acute. The muscles do not relax at any time.

Localised tenderness – guarding – rigidity occur over the affected organ or peritoneum. The exact place of this tenderness usually shows which organ is affected, see Figure 36.8 (e.g. right iliac fossa, appendix, appendicitis; epigastrium, stomach/duodenum, peptic ulcer).

Abdominal mass

To find out what an abdominal mass is, you must decide:

1. Where is the mass? *or*
   In which organ or structure is the mass?
2. What type is the mass? *or*
   Is this mass congenital or traumatic or inflammatory or neoplastic or degenerative, etc. (see pages 591–592)?

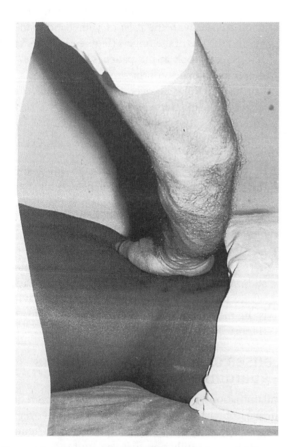 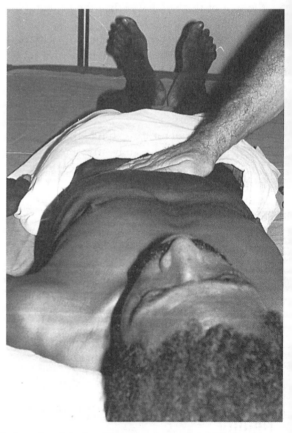

Figure 36.4 and 36.5 *The proper way to palpate an abdomen, with the palm of the hand held flat. Do not bend the fingers, or use the tips of the fingers.*

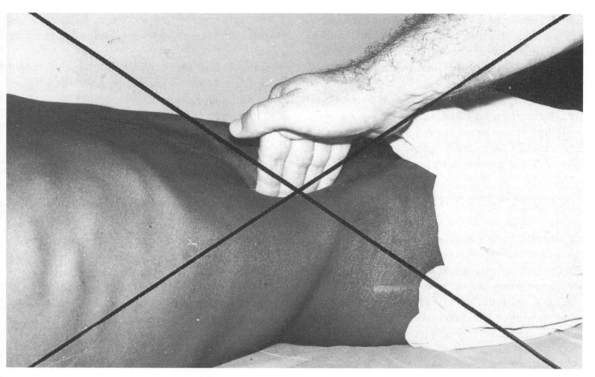

Figure 36.6 *The wrong way to palpate an abdomen.* Use the palm of the hand. *DO NOT USE THE TIPS OF THE FINGERS LIKE THIS.*

A full history and examination is necessary. A pelvic examination 'PR' and/or 'PV' is often also necessary.

It is also usually necessary to:

- test the urine – protein, pus, blood, sugar, bile,
- look at the stools,
- look at any vomit, and
- look at any vaginal discharge.

Where is the mass?

Think of all the structures and organs in the area which could be affected and could contain the mass.

Start at the skin on the anterior (front) of the abdominal wall, and think of all of the organs under it to the skin on the posterior (back) abdominal wall. See Figure 36.8.

Remember that if the patient contracts his anterior abdominal muscles (e.g. by lifting his head when he is lying on his back), any mass that you can still feel must be anterior to (in front of) the muscles. You cannot

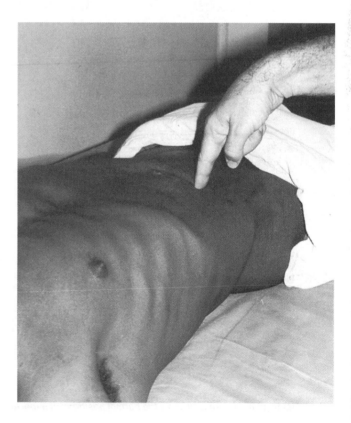

Figure 36.7 *One finger palpation. Only do this when you have found a tender place with normal palpation, but you cannot decide which is the most tender place. Press the point of one finger gently onto different parts of the tender place like this, until you find the most tender area.*

easily feel masses behind the hard contracted muscles.

If you think that a certain organ probably contains the mass, then look for other signs in history, examination and tests to show if the organ has abnormal function and disease, or not: e.g. if you think the mass is in the pelvic colon, then ask carefully about bowel colic, constipation or diarrhoea, blood in the stool, weight loss, etc.; examine for weight loss; do a careful rectal examination to try to feel if the mass is in the bowel wall; and carefully look at the stool for blood.

What type is the mass?

The mass may be congenital or traumatic or inflammatory or neoplastic or degenerative, etc. in any of the organs or structures in that area.

Some types of mass are more probable in some organs than in others (e.g. the spleen is probably enlarged by malarial inflammation or leishmaniasis or lymphomatous cancers or blood disease – other types of mass such as congenital or degenerative are not probable).

For inflammatory masses, see in Chapter 3 page 14. For neoplastic masses, see Chapter 3 page 15 and below.

You can find other signs of the type of mass in history, examination and tests, e.g. fever, fast pulse, etc. if it is an inflammatory mass; or weight loss, enlarged hard fixed lymph nodes, etc. if it is a neoplastic mass.

Common causes of abdominal masses

You can find the causes of most masses if you answer these questions:

1. Where is the mass or in which organ or structure is the mass? and

2. What type is the mass? and then look for

3. other signs of disease in the suspected organ, and

4. other signs of the nature of the pathological process suspected.

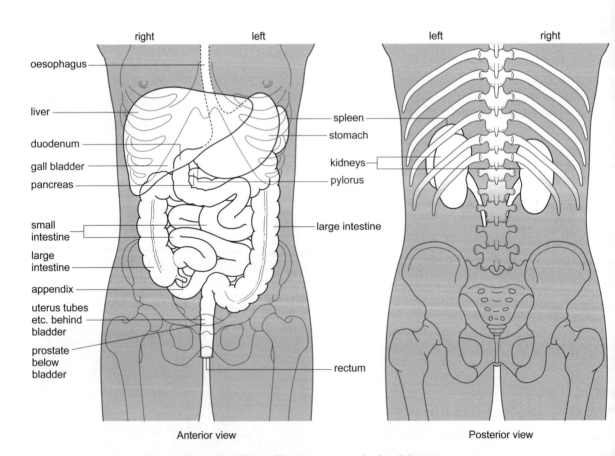

Anterior view

Posterior view

Figure 36.8 *Diagrams to show the normal positions of important organs in the abdomen.*

Common causes of abdominal masses include:

1. *Generalised enlargement* of:
   • liver
   • spleen
   • uterus
   • bladder
   • kidney
   • lymph glands on posterior abdominal wall
2. *Inflammatory masses* (e.g. abscesses) of:
   • any of the organs in 1 (above)
   • part of the gastrointestinal tract, or
   • the peritoneum
3. *Neoplastic masses* of:
   • any of the organs in 1 (above)
   • part of the gastrointestinal tract, or
   • the peritoneum

Especially common causes of masses in the abdomen include:

1. *In the right iliac fossa*
   • appendicitis/appendix abscess
   • amoeboma of the intestine
   • cancer of the intestine
   • tuberculosis of the intestine
2. *In the left iliac fossa*
   • amoeboma of the intestine
   • schistosomiasis of the intestine
   • cancer of the intestine
   • diverticulitis/diverticular abscess
3. *In the lower abdomen*
   • distended bladder
   • pregnant uterus
   • ectopic pregnancy
   • pelvic abscess
   • cancer of the ovary or uterus
4. *In the left upper abdomen*
   • spleen (malaria, hyperreactive splenomegaly syndrome, visceral leishmaniasis, trypanosomiasis,

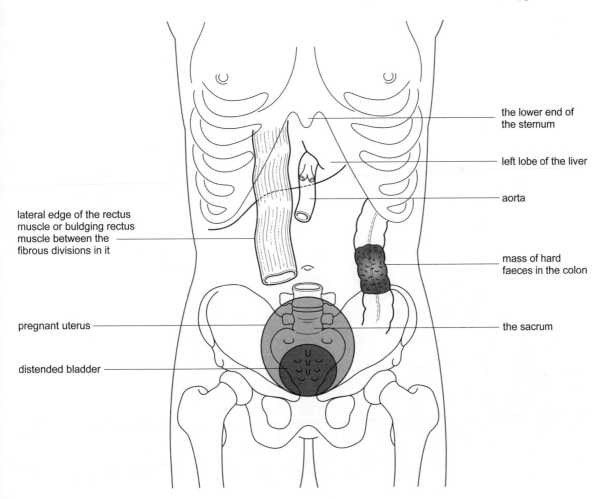

Figure 36.9 *Normal structures which you may mistake for pathological masses.*

schistosomiasis, lymphoma, thalassaemia, sickle cell anaemia and other blood disorders, subcapsular rupture of the spleen)
- kidney tumour or infection (e.g. TB) or swelling caused by a blocked ureter

5. *In the right upper abdomen*
- liver, gall bladder (amoebic abscess, hepatoma, secondary cancer, heart failure, leishmaniasis, trypanosomiasis, TB occasionally, obstructed bile duct)
- kidney tumour or infection (e.g. TB; or swelling caused by a blocked ureter)

6. *In the epigastrium*
- cancer of the stomach
- liver (amoebic abscess, hepatoma, secondary cancer, leishmaniasis, trypanosomiasis; TB occasionally; but also sometimes a normal large left lobe of the liver)

Do not mistake normal structures for pathological masses (see Figure 36.9).

Generalised abdominal swelling

Causes of swelling of the whole abdomen include five groups of conditions:

1. A solid mass inside the abdomen
   (a) *Generalised enlargement of any organ*, especially:
   - the liver
   - the spleen
   - the uterus (or ovary or tubes)
   - the bladder
   - the kidney, or
   - the lymph glands on the posterior abdominal wall
   (b) *Any large inflammatory mass* of:
   - any of the above organs, or
   - part of the gastrointestinal tract, or
   - the peritoneum
   (c) *Any large neoplastic mass* of:
   - any of the above organs, or
   - part of the gastrointestinal tract, or
   - the peritoneum
2. Fluid inside the abdomen
   (a) *Fluid (ascites, blood or pus) in the peritoneal cavity usually shown by 'shifting dullness'* (see below)
   Ascites (clear fluid)
   - cirrhosis of liver
   - schistosomiasis
   - heart failure

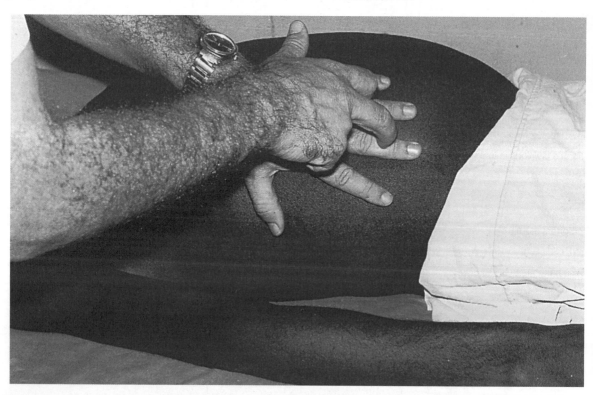

Figure 36.10 *The method of percussion of the abdomen for fluid. Note that the finger on the abdomen is kept parallel to the patient's bed. See also Figure 36.11A and B.*

- nephrotic syndrome
- kwashiorkor
- tuberculous peritonitis
- cancer of peritoneum

Blood
- bleeding ectopic pregnancy
- ruptured spleen, liver or other organ
- tuberculous peritonitis
- cancer of the peritoneum

Pus
- peritonitis
  (b) *Fluid in an ovarian cyst* (see Figure 36.12)
3. Gas (flatus) and fluid in the intestines
   - Obstruction of the intestines
   - Paralytic ileus
   - Enteritis necroticans ('pigbel')
   - Peritonitis
4. Fat

5. Abdominal wall swellings
   - Hernia
   - Lipoma
   - Cellulitis

Inguinal swellings

Causes of inguinal swellings include:

- hernia (see a surgery book),
- lymph gland enlargement (see Chapter 22 pages 340–341),
- inflammation – cellulitis, abscess, etc., and
- traumatic swelling.

'Shifting dullness'

Shifting dullness is a sign which shows that *fluid (ascites or blood or pus)* is *in the peritoneal cavity*.

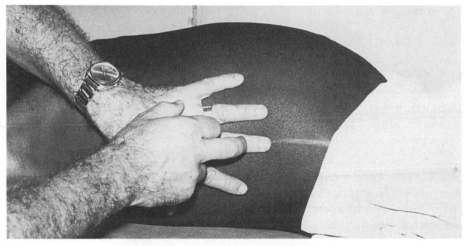

A

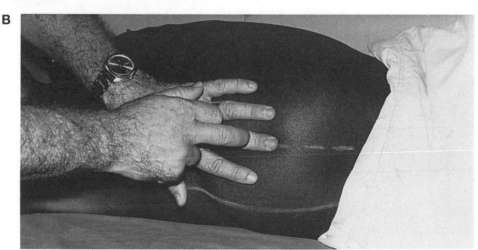

B

Figure 36.11 A and B *These figures show how to find if there is fluid in the abdomen (see text for details).*

For *causes* of fluid (ascites, blood and pus) in the peritoneal cavity, see causes of 'Generalised abdominal swelling' (see page 602).

Test for shifting dullness in all cases when the *abdomen is distended* or when *ascites or blood or pus* in the peritoneal cavity is possible.

The patient lies on his back, facing up. Percuss the abdomen as in Figure 36.10. The abdomen is resonant (hollow) on top and dull on both sides, as the gas in the intestine floats that part of the intestine to the top and the fluid runs down on both sides.

Find the place where resonance changes to dullness and mark it with a pen or chalk (see Figure 36.11A).

In Figure 36.11A the patient is lying on his back facing up. The place where dullness changed to resonance is marked with an unbroken chalk line. In Figure 36.11B the patient is lying on his side. Fluid from the other side of the abdomen has run down to join fluid on this side of the abdomen. The new place where dullness changed to resonance is marked with a dotted chalk line. The 'dullness' has 'shifted' (moved) up. The patient has fluid in the abdomen.

The patient then rolls on to the other side. The dullness will then move to the other side of the abdomen. The places where dullness was marked will now be resonant. The dullness will now be in the area posterior (behind) the line on the other side of the patient, and will also shift closer to the umbilicus.

> Note that shifting dullness means only that fluid is present in the peritoneal cavity. It does not diagnose what type of fluid is present in the peritoneal cavity. Use other symptoms and signs and tests to find out what type of fluid is causing the shifting dullness.

The main differential diagnosis is a very large ovarian cyst (Figure 36.12).

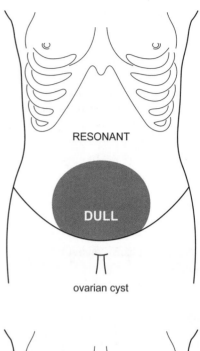

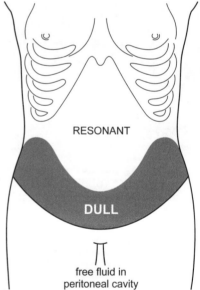

Figure 36.12 *Diagrams to show one way of diagnosing an ovarian cyst or fluid in the peritoneal cavity. The patient is lying on her back facing up. A cyst can become so large that it seems to fill the whole abdomen.*

Bowel sounds

Intestinal or bowel sounds may be:

• normal, or
• increased, or
• decreased or absent.

Intestinal sounds are increased when the patient feels colic, when there is:

• obstruction of the intestine or
• gastroenteritis.

Intestinal sounds are decreased or absent if there is:

1. pus in the peritoneal cavity (peritonitis from any cause), or
2. blood in the peritoneal cavity (e.g. bleeding ectopic pregnancy or ruptured spleen or other organ), or
3. paralytic ileus.

Listen for at least 2 minutes (10 minutes if possible), before you decide that bowel sounds are reduced or absent.

37 Emergency Resuscitation

Inhaled foreign body

If the foreign body is in the larynx or trachea, it will cause obstruction of the airway which may be complete or not complete.

If the obstruction is complete, the patient usually clutches his neck, cannot talk, makes no noise if he tries to cough and makes violent breathing movements, with indrawing of the ribs. If you ask 'Are you choking?' he will nod. Cyanosis and death quickly occur without treatment. Sometimes complete obstruction causes only sudden unexpected unconsciousness and no breathing and then death.

If the obstruction is not complete, there is severe shortness of breath, stridor and indrawing of the ribs on breathing in; but the patient can answer, cough and breathe.

Obstruction of the larynx or trachea may occur when the patient is eating ('food choking'). Suspect it in every case of respiratory distress or loss of consciousness which occurs during eating. It is also common if the patient was holding a foreign body in his mouth or if he was drunk. It is more common in patients with chronic bronchitis.

> If you suspect obstruction, act immediately.

If the patient cannot get the foreign body out by coughing, but is still conscious and standing or sitting, then you should try to get it out by up to five back blows.

- Stand to the side and slightly behind the patient.
- Lean the patient forward, holding him with one hand in front of his chest (so that anything that comes out of the airway into the mouth will fall out and not be sucked back in again with the next breath in).
- Hit the patient hard between the shoulder blades with the heel of your other hand.

This will force some air out of the lungs and should expel (push out) the foreign body.

Only if hitting on the back does not work, try the *abdominal thrust* method as follows. However, do not try this if
1. the patient is too obese for you to get your arms around them, or

2. the patient is in the late stages of pregnancy.
In these cases, see next step.
For the abdominal thrust:
- The patient is standing or sitting.
- Stand behind the patient and put your arms round his upper abdomen.
- Make a fist of one of your hands and hold this fist with the other hand. Put the fist on the patient's anterior abdominal wall between the umbilicus and the ribs.
- Then pull up and in with the arms quickly and strongly towards the back and chest of the patient (see Figure 37.1).
Repeat up to five times, if needed.

This is not just squeezing the patient – it is like a punch; but with the fist starting on the abdominal wall and helped by the other hand. This should force air out

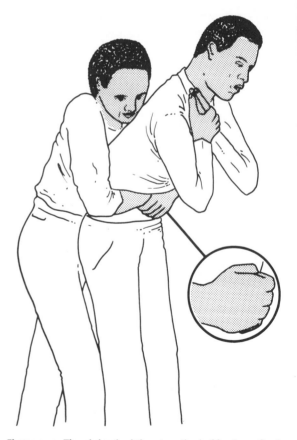

Figure 37.1 *The abdominal thrust method of forcing a foreign body out of the trachea or larynx.*

of the lungs through the trachea and the larynx and expel (push out) the foreign body (see Figure 37.1).

If the patient is or becomes unconscious:

- Lower him carefully to the floor and turn him onto his back.
- Make sure the airway is open.
- Start the chest compression of CPR, which may well force the foreign body out of the airway.

If these methods do not work, you can sometimes get the foreign body out of the throat, if you push your fingers down deep into the back of the patient's throat and pull out what is there or suck with powerful electrical or mechanical suction apparatus.

Artificial ventilation (artificial 'respiration'), heart stimulation and external heart (cardiac) massage

Artificial ventilation is necessary if the patient cannot breathe enough.

This is done only when the patient:

- is not breathing (even if breathing occasionally and even if this occasional breathing is deep).

Causes include:

- near drowning,
- paralysis from snakebite,
- an unconscious patient whose airway becomes blocked,
- very deep unconsciousness (especially after a drug overdose),
- sometimes after anaesthetics or operations,
- cardiac arrest (stopping of heart), and
- others.

Chest compression (external cardiac massage) is necessary if the heart has stopped. This is diagnosed if the patient:

1. stops breathing properly – even if occasional deep breaths.
2. is not responsive (is unconscious) – shake the patient's shoulder and ask loudly 'Are you all right?' If there is no answer the patient is unconscious. Start cardiopulmonary resuscitation (CPR). Do not try to feel if there is a pulse. This cannot be done reliably when done quickly. Harm will be done if the heart has stopped and CPR is not started immediately. No harm will be done if the heart is still beating and CPR is started.

This is done when not only has breathing stopped but the patient is also unconscious.

Causes include:

- electrocution,
- reaction to drugs,
- shock that is not treated,
- low oxygen from any cause,
- breathing stops and no one gives artificial ventilation,
- myocardial infarction (heart attack),
- pulmonary embolus, and
- others.

Do artificial ventilation and chest compression only if the patient may recover and return to normal life. The underlying condition must be treatable. The patient must have suddenly or unexpectedly collapsed. Do not do these things if the patient is slowly getting worse with a fatal disease or even with all possible treatment.

If the patient is unconscious and not breathing or is breathing with only a few breaths,

then immediate emergency cardiopulmonary resuscitation is necessary.

If you do not do this immediately, the patient will die or have severe brain damage from which he cannot recover.

Artificial ventilation of the lungs

It is unusual that this alone is needed. However, it may be needed if breathing is reduced due to a drug or anaesthetic overdose or snakebite, etc. but the heart is still going and the circulation is still good. Give artificial ventilation while waiting for the effect of drugs or anaesthetic to wear off or for antivenom to work. Normally, it will also be done with chest compression.

Clear the airway

Extend the head (or move the head back on the top of the neck). Hold the back of the neck with one hand and push the top of the head back with the other hand. This will bend the head back on the top of the neck as far as possible.

Push the angle of the jaw forward from behind *or* pull the jaw forward from under the front of the jaw. This jaw positioning will stop the tongue from blocking the airway (see Figure 37.2).

Extract (get out) anything from the mouth or throat which could block an airway. Use your fingers (and, if necessary, a cloth).

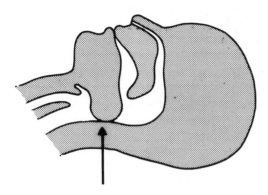

A The tongue is blocking the
throat of an unconscious
patient. Compare the
tongue in B

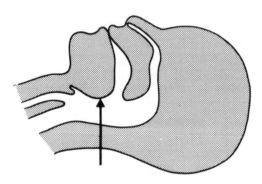

B Normal airway in a
conscious patient

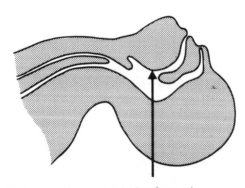

C The head extended and the jaw forward.
In this position the tongue does not block
the throat; the air passages are not
obstructed, even in an unconscious patient

Figure 37.2 A, B and C. *Diagrams to show how to stop the
tongue blocking the airway of an unconscious person.*

Suck out the airway if you have a sucker (but do
not leave the patient unattended while you find one).

Mouth-to-mouth ventilation

See pages 611–612 about 'barrier methods' to protect
the health worker from infection from the patient.

• Separate the patient's lips.
• Put the face shield over the patient's face and into
  his mouth.
• Hold the patient's nostrils together.
• Take a deep breath.
• Open your mouth widely (Figure 37.3).
• Seal your lips around the patient's mouth.
• Blow your breath into the patient's lungs.
• Look to see if the patient's chest rises as you blow air
  into the patient's lungs.
• Then remove your mouth from the patient's mouth.
• Look to see if the patient's chest falls when you stop
  blowing air into the patient's chest (Figure 37.4).

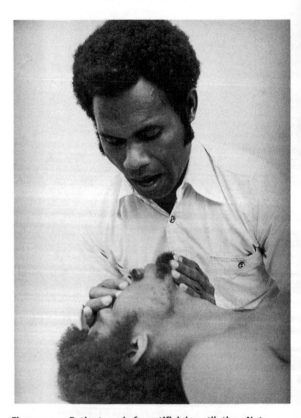

Figure 37.3 *Patient ready for artificial ventilation. Note
(1) airway cleared, (2) head extended, (3) jaw held forward,
(4) nostrils held, (5) mouth open. It is essential now to also
use a face shield. See Figures 37.7 and 37.8.*

Continue artificial ventilation

Repeat the artificial ventilation about 20 times every minute, i.e. about 1 second to blow the air in and 2 seconds for it to come out until the patient can breathe enough for himself.

Check for cardiac arrest

After each minute check if the patient has a cardiac arrest or not, i.e. not unconscious and the pulse is present and at a reasonable rate (60–120/minute). If not so, start CPR.

Cardiopulmonary resuscitation (CPR) or basic life support (BLS)

UNRESPONSIVE?

- Shout for help.
- Open airway.

NOT BREATHING NORMALLY?

- Send for another health worker to help.
- 30 chest compressions, then
- 2 rescue breaths, then
- 30 compressions.

Basic life support consists of the following sequence of actions:

1. *Make sure the patient, any bystanders and you are safe.*
   - Be particularly careful of live electric wires, poison gases or vehicles which may come past.
2. *Check the patient for a response.*
   - Shake his shoulders and ask loudly, 'Are you all right?'
3. (a) *If he responds:*
   - Leave him in the position in which you find him as long as there is no further danger.
   - Try to find out what is wrong with him and get help if needed.
   - Reassess him regularly.
   (b) *If he does **not** respond:*
   - Shout for help.
   - Turn the patient onto his back and then open the airway using head tilt and chin lift.
     Place your hand on his forehead and gently tilt his head back.
     With your fingertips under the point of the patient's chin, lift the chin to open the airway.
4. *Keeping the airway open, look, listen, and feel for normal breathing.*
   - Look for chest movement.
   - Listen at the patient's mouth for breath sounds.

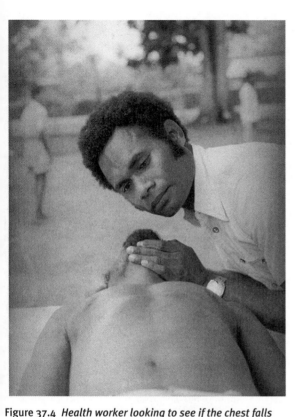

Figure 37.4 *Health worker looking to see if the chest falls after he stopped blowing his breath into the patient.*

If the chest does not rise and fall check that
- the head is extended,
- the jaw is well forward, and
- the airway is not blocked by foreign bodies, and
- then try the mouth-to-mouth ventilation again.

If the chest still does not rise and fall, start chest compression. This will force air in the lungs through the airway and often expel (push out) any foreign bodies in the lower airway, which are blocking the air going into the lungs. (See Figure 37.1 page 606 for another method.)
Then repeat the mouth-to-mouth ventilation again.

Mouth-to-nose ventilation is as effective as mouth-to-mouth ventilation. It would be used if
1. the patient's mouth is seriously injured,
2. the patient's mouth cannot be opened,
3. artificial ventilation if being done while getting a drowning patient out of water as a mouth-to-mouth seal is then often difficult to get.
Hold the patient's jaw up (Figure 37.4) but also hold the lips together if needed.
Make a seal with the mouth around the nose and blow the air in through the nose.

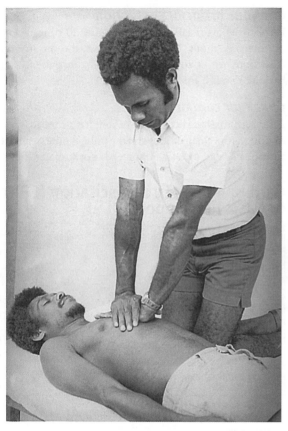

Figure 37.5 *A health worker giving external cardiac massage.*
Note that he has placed his hands in the centre of the chest.
Note that the elbows are straight and that he uses the
weight of his body to push down the sternum as he moves
backwards and forwards. (He is not pushing the sternum
down by bending and straightening his elbows.)

- Feel for air on your cheek.
- In the first few minutes after cardiac arrest, the patient may be breathing a little, or taking infrequent noisy gasps. This is not normal breathing.
- Look, listen, and feel for **no more** than **10 seconds** to find out if the patient is breathing normally.
- If you have any doubt whether breathing is normal, act as if it is **not** normal.

5. (a) *If he is breathing normally*:
   - Turn him into the recovery position (see Chapter 25 page 424).
   - Send or go for help.
   - Check for continued breathing.
   (b) *If he is **not** breathing normally*:
   Ask someone to call for help or, if you are on your own, do this yourself; you may need to leave the patient. Start chest compression as follows:

- Kneel by the side of the patient.
- Place the heel of one hand in the centre of the patient's chest.
- Place the heel of your other hand on top of the first hand.
- Interlock the fingers of your hands and ensure that pressure is not applied over the patient's ribs.
- Do not apply any pressure over the upper abdomen or the bottom end of the sternum.
- Position yourself vertically above the patient's chest and, with your arms straight, press the sternum down about one third the depth of the chest. In most adults, this will be 4–5 cm (2–2½ inches). The pressure needed is about 20–30 kg.
- After each compression, release all the pressure on the chest without taking your hands off the sternum. Repeat at a rate of about 100 times a minute (a little less than 2 compressions a second).
- Compression and release should take an equal amount of time.

6. (a) *Combine chest compression with artificial ventilation (rescue breaths).*
   - After 30 compressions open the airway again using head tilt and chin lift.
   - Pinch the soft part of the patient's nose closed, using the index finger and thumb of your hand on his forehead.
   - Allow his mouth to open, but maintain chin lift.
   - Put the protective face shield over the patient's face and into his mouth.
   - Take a normal breath and place your lips around his mouth, making sure that you have a good seal.
   - Blow steadily into his mouth whilst watching for his chest to rise; take about 1 second to make his chest rise as in normal breathing; this is an effective breath.
   - Keep the head tilted and chin lifted. Take your mouth away from the patient and watch for his chest to fall as air comes out.
   - Take another normal breath and within 2 seconds blow into the patient's mouth once more to give a total of two effective breaths. Then return your hands immediately to the correct position on the sternum and give a further 30 chest compressions.
   - Continue with chest compressions and rescue breaths in a ratio of 30:2.

• Stop to recheck the patient only if he starts breathing *normally; otherwise do not interrupt resuscitation.*

If your artificial ventilation does not make the chest rise as in normal breathing, then before your next attempt:

• Check the patient's mouth and remove any visible obstruction.

• Recheck that there is adequate head tilt and chin lift.

• Do not attempt more than two breaths each time before returning to chest compressions.

If there is more than one rescuer present, another should take over CPR about every 2 minutes to stop the rescuer getting tired and not doing CPR properly. Make sure there is no delay in chest compression during the changeover.

If a mask and self-inflating bag is available for ventilation and a health worker is able to use this efficiently, then this would be used for giving 8–10 breaths each minute (only 1 second for each breath in). The chest compression should continue at 100/minute and then not stop for this ventilation.

(b) *Chest compression only CPR.*

• If you are not able, or are unwilling, to give rescue breaths, give chest compressions only.

• If chest compressions only are given, these should be continuous at a rate of 100 a minute.

• Stop to recheck the patient only if he starts breathing *normally; otherwise do not interrupt resuscitation.*

7. *Continue cardiopulmonary resuscitation.*

Continue cardiopulmonary resuscitation until the patient

1. is breathing normally himself,

2. has good pulse and BP himself, *or*

3. has been transferred to the Medical Officer, *or*

4. after 30 minutes:

• is still not breathing normally himself,

• is still unresponsive (unconscious),

• has had no pulse without ECM, and

• has widely dilated pupils, and

• is obviously dead.

Barrier methods to try to prevent cross-infection during mouth-to-mouth ventilation

Special devices have been produced to try to reduce the risk of infection of the health worker by HIV and HBV and TB and other organisms from infected patients.

The risk of infection is very small unless the patient has blood on his face or in his mouth and the health worker has a cut or sore on his lips or mouth. There is also as yet no published scientific evidence that these devices do protect the health worker. Laboratory tests have shown that they do stop organisms from the patient's mouth getting into the health worker's mouth. These devices therefore do give some protection and if possible should be used.

It is important that you find out from your Health Department what the risks are in your country, what special precautions should be taken and what are you to do about a device for mouth-to-mouth ventilation. If you are to use a device, then you must make sure you are trained how to use it correctly and *always have one with you, e.g. in your pocket,* so that you can use it in an emergency.

Face masks (Figure 37.6) are probably the safest for the health worker; but they are expensive, difficult to carry and difficult to use correctly.

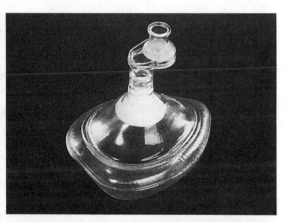
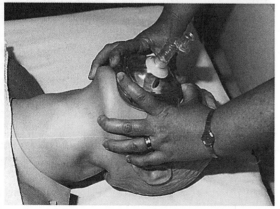

Figure 37.6 A and B. *A typical face mask with valve (Laerdal Pocket Mask).*

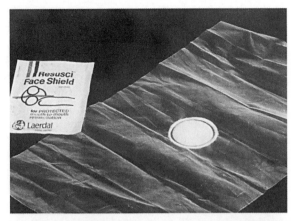

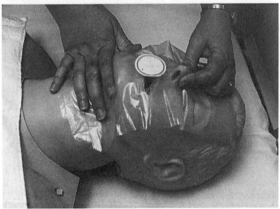

Figure 37.7 A and B. *A typical face shield with filter (Laerdal Face Shield).*

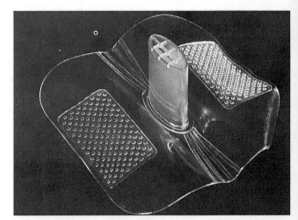

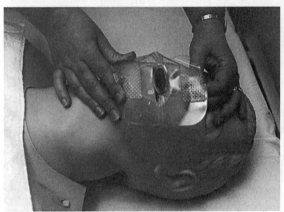

Figure 37.8 A and B. *A typical face shield with valve (CPR Microshield).*

A face shield (Figures 37.7 and 37.8) has a plastic sheet, which covers the patient's nose and mouth, and has a central filter or valve, which goes over the patient's mouth, through which the health worker blows.

Near drowning

Start resuscitation immediately you see the patient, even before he is brought out of the water.

Resuscitation includes:

1. Clear the airway (see page 607).
2. Give mouth-to-mouth or mouth-to-nose ventilation, if the patient is not breathing properly (see page 608).
3. Start chest compressions if the patient is unconscious as soon as he is out of the water (see page 609).
4. Change from mouth-to-mouth ventilation to ventilation with a self-inflatable bag and oxygen as soon as possible.

5. When possible, put down a nasogastric tube to get air and fluid out of the stomach (which may be stopping good ventilation by pushing the diaphragm up).
6. Make sure the patient's temperature is not low. If rectal temperature is 35°C or less, warm the patient with heated blankets or by other means. Keep all near-drowned patients warm with a temperature of about 37°C.
7. If all this does not cause return of normal breathing and heart beat, and if the patient is still alive, and if you can continue resuscitation while you transfer the patient to a hospital or Medical Officer care; then continue resuscitation and arrange urgent (emergency) transfer.
8. If these things are not successful, and if the patient is not starting to recover within 1 hour, then stop the treatment.
9. If the patient's breathing and circulation do improve, treat like this:
   (a) Give intranasal oxygen 2 litres/minute for some hours.

(b) If the patient nearly drowned in salt water and becomes shocked, treat with IV fluids as in shock (see Chapter 27 pages 468–470).

(c) Check the urine output carefully. If there is no urine output or only a little red or brown urine with protein in it, start treatment for acute kidney failure (see Chapter 26 page 453) and arrange urgent (emergency) transfer to hospital.

(d) Give antibiotics as if the patient had pneumonia (see Chapter 20 pages 289–291).

(e) Do not discharge the patient for at least 24 hours. Sometimes complications and death occur hours after the patient seems to have recovered.

Emergency laryngostomy

Complete block of the upper airway can occur from infection, e.g. acute epiglottitis or diphtheria or oedema (angio-oedema from insect bite or acute anaphylactic reaction) or inhaled foreign body – which cannot be got out by back blows then abdominal thrusts then chest thrusts of CPR – or other cause. There may be increasing stridor, insuction and rib retraction, the pulse gets faster, the patient develops cyanosis and is extremely distressed and breathing can stop, the heart stop and the patient become unconscious. Immediately do the following, as the patient will otherwise soon die.

Push large-bore cannulas or needles through the cricothyroid membrane into the trachea. If this does not allow the patient to breathe well enough, do an emergency laryngostomy. See below for method of doing both.

The patient is laid on his back facing straight upwards. The patient's *head is extended* (head tipped right back) and *held in the midline* (i.e. facing straight up if the body is facing straight up) by an assistant. *These two things are **very** important.* Do not start the operation until these two things are done.

Feel for the bottom part of the thyroid cartilage. The thyroid cartilage is the large hard lump, often somewhat pointed at the top, in the middle of the front of the neck, which can be seen to move up then down during swallowing (Adam's apple). Below this, at the top of the trachea, the cricoid cartilage can be felt. The cricoid cartilage is the next hard piece of tissue felt going across the neck straight under the thyroid cartilage. Between the thyroid and cricoid cartilages is a hollow – the cricothyroid membrane (see Figure 37.9).

Push one or two 13-gauge needles, otherwise four or more of the largest available needles, through the membrane, pointing them backwards and downwards. If air can go through all, then oxygen may be run in through *one* of the needles. Artificial ventilation may be able to be given by blocking the other needles with the fingers until the oxygen going in fills the lungs, and then taking the fingers off the needles to allow expiration.

If the patient is still not able to breathe or is not ventilated enough, do an emergency laryngostomy as follows. However, laryngostomy is:

1. used only in cases of desperate emergency (patient stopped breathing or about to stop breathing),
2. only temporary,
3. suitable for use in adults only.

Put on glasses or goggles and a waterproof mask as blood will be sprayed into the air and sucked into the lungs with each breath.

If there is time, make a transverse incision about 2 cm (1 inch) long across the neck in this area. If there is time, use local anaesthetic and clamp any bleeding points with artery forceps.

Then, with or without the above incision, either a pair of closed pointed scissors or the cutting end of a scalpel is pushed downwards and backwards as close to the upper border of the cricoid cartilage as possible. Either will easily go through the cricothyroid membrane into the lower larynx and upper trachea.

Then turn the instrument (and open the blades if it is a pair of scissors). Turning the instrument will open a hole between the larynx and trachea and the air outside. The patient will then be able to breathe through this hole.

If possible, push a short stiff wide-bore tube through the hole. Use the cut-off end of a 20 or 10 ml disposable syringe barrel; or test-tube with the bottom end broken off (put the top end with the flange or widened part into the hole); or a piece of pipe, tube, or hard plastic or rubber hose. Have the tube as short as possible, e.g. 3–5 cm (1–2 inches). Pull out the scissors or the knife when the tube is in place. The membrane will close on the tube and will keep a lot of the blood out of the trachea as the blood comes mostly from outside the membrane.

An oxygen tube can be put through the tube into the trachea. The trachea can be sucked out with a soft catheter on a sucker.

If the patient does not immediately start to breathe, artificial ventilation can be given by blowing into the tube.

The bleeding vessels can then be clamped with artery forceps and tied off.

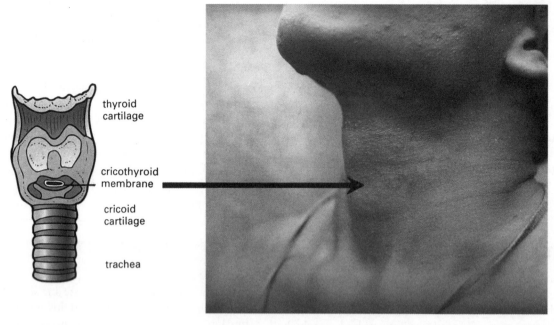

thyroid
cartilage

cricothyroid
membrane

cricoid
cartilage

trachea

Figure 37.9 *Diagram and photograph showing the place for putting needles or doing laryngostomy incision (arrow) through the cricothyroid membrane.*

Stick the tube firmly with plaster so that it cannot fall into the trachea or out of the hole in the larynx.

The patient is then transferred urgently (emergency) to Medical Officer care for further treatment and probably proper tracheostomy.

Emergency treatment of an anaphylactic reaction

Think of this if the patient has:

- recently been stung by an insect or been given a drug by injection or by mouth,
- difficulty breathing, especially if wheezing or asthma,
- low blood pressure or shock,
- urticaria or angio-oedema,
- past history of allergy especially.

Immediately treat as follows:

1. Give oxygen 4–6 litres by mask or nasal cannula if available.
2. Give epinephrine/adrenaline (1–1000 solution, i.e. 1 mg/ml) 0.5 mg (0.5 ml) IMI. Repeat in 5 minutes if not improved.
3. Put in IV needle or cannula.
4. Give antihistamine, e.g. chlorphenamine 10–20 mg IV (or IMI) or promethazine 25–50 mg IV (or IMI).
5. Give hydrocortisone 300 mg IVI if available, or if not available and patient can swallow, prednisolone 50 mg immediately and daily.
6. If wheezing or dyspnoea, give salbutamol 5 mg nebulised or one puff from a 100 mcg per puff metered aerosol through a large volume spacer, then repeat this dose 10 times. Repeat these doses if needed in 10 minutes, 1 hour and 2–4 hourly.
7. If the patient is in shock and does not immediately improve on the above, start 0.9% saline 1 litre as fast as it will go, and then if needed another litre so that 2 litres are given quickly.
8. If severe shock or is not improving, give epinephrine/adrenaline 1 in 10,000 solution (i.e. 1 ml of 1–1000 solution or 1 mg in 1 ml ampoule diluted with 9 ml of saline to 10 ml) at 1 ml/minute; but stop if improves.
9. Cardiopulmonary resuscitation if needed.

Appendix: Incubation Periods

Incubation periods can be misleading in areas where diseases are endemic. In practice, in such areas it is probably sufficient to remember whether the incubation period is of long, medium or short duration.

Amoebiasis	Medium–long	14 days to many months
Anthrax	Short	2–5 days
Bacillary dysentery	Short	1–7 days
Brucellosis	Long	Days to months
Chancroid	Short	2–5 days
Chickenpox	Medium	14–21 days
Cholera	Short	Hours–5 days
Dengue	Short	2–7 days
Diphtheria	Short	2–5 days
Filariasis	Long	3 months–years
Gonorrhoea	Short	2–5 days
Hepatitis A	Medium–long	2–6 weeks
Hepatitis B	Long	6 weeks–6 months
HIV	Long	1–3 months but can be shorter or much longer
Lassa fever	Medium	7–14 days
Leishmaniasis cutaneous	Medium–long	1 week–months
Leishmaniasis visceral	Medium–long	2 weeks–2 years
Leprosy	Long	2–5 years but can be shorter or much longer
Leptospirosis	Medium	1–3 weeks
Malaria	Medium–long	2 weeks–months but cannot be shorter than 8 days
Measles	Medium	7–14 days
Meningococcal meningitis	Short–medium	2–10 days
Mumps	Medium	12–21 days
Plague	Short	3–6 days but less if pneumonic
Poliomyelitis	Short–medium	3–21 days
Rabies	Medium–long	Usually 4–8 weeks, minimum 9 days, can be many months
Rubella (German measles)	Medium	14–21 days
Schistosomiasis	Long	Weeks–years
Syphilis	Medium–long	10–90 days
Trypanosoma gambiense	Long	Weeks–years
Trypanosoma rhodesiense	Medium	14–21 days
Tetanus	Medium	2 weeks but can be as short as 2 days or longer
Typhoid fever	Medium	7–21 days
Typhus fever	Medium	7–14 days
Tuberculosis	Long	Months–years
Whooping cough (pertussis)	Short	7–10 days

Useful Publications

Publications of particular value for health workers include the following:

Crofton, J., Horne, N. and Miller, F. (2nd edition, 2002) *Clinical Tuberculosis*. London, Macmillan Education.

Boon, N. *et al.* (2006 or latest edition) *Davidson's Principles and Practice of Medicine*, 20th edn. Edinburgh, Churchill Livingstone, 1203 pp. (low-priced edition available).

Douglas, S. (ed.) (2005 or latest edition) *MacLeod's Clinical Examination*, 11th edn. Edinburgh, Churchill Livingstone (low-priced edition available).

Evian, C. (2005) *Primary HIV/AIDS Care*. Macmillan Education.

Fountain, D. (2008) *Primary Diagnosis and Treatment*. Macmillan Education.

Huband, S. *et al.* (2006) *Nursing and Midwifery: A Practical Approach*. Macmillan Education.

Lawrence, D.R., Bennett, P.N. and Brown, M.Y. (1997 or latest edition) *Clinical Pharmacology*, 8th edn. Edinburgh, Churchill Livingstone (low-priced edition available).

Malaria Consortium (2007) *Malaria: A Handbook for Health Professionals*. Macmillan Education.

von Massow, Fr., Ndele, J.K. and Korte, K. (1997) *Guidelines to Rational Drug Use*. London, Macmillan Education.

Publications of particular value for Medical Officers in adult internal medicine in the tropics include:

Cook, G.C. (ed.) (2008 or latest edition) *Manson's Tropical Diseases*, 22nd (or latest) edition. London, W.B. Saunders.

Eddleston *et al.* (2008 or latest edition) *Oxford Handbook of Tropical Medicine*, 3rd (or latest) edition. Oxford, Oxford University Press.

Gill G. and Beeching, N. (eds) (2004 or latest edition) *Lecture Notes on Tropical Medicine*, 5th (or latest) edition. Oxford, Blackwell Science.

Hayman, D. (ed.) (2008 or latest edition) *Control of Communicable Diseases Manual*, 19th (or latest) edition. Washington DC, American Public Health Association.

Teaching Aids at Low Cost in the United Kingdom has numerous low-priced books, CD ROMs, downloads, DVDs, videos, slide sets, featured publications, accessories, etc. Catalogues are available (www.talcuk.org and PO Box 49, St Albans, Herts AL1 5TX, UK).

The World Health Organization has all kinds of information online, including policy guidelines, statistics, training manuals, disease updates, journal articles, etc. which can be downloaded. It also has books for sale (www.who.int and World Health Organization, CH-1211, Geneva, 21, Switzerland).

Index

Numbers in **bold** refer to major references.

abacavir (ABC) 241, 243, **249**
abbreviations 10–12
abdominal
  examination 24, 593–605
    gastrointestinal 348–9
    if pain 593–8
    liver 393
    spleen 343
  mass 598–602
  pain 348, **593–8**
  rigidity 597
  shifting dullness 602–4
  swelling 602–4
  tenderness/guarding 597
  transfer indications 594
  see also pelvic inflammatory disease
abscess 592–3
  brain 421–2
  breast 592–3
  liver 398
  lymph nodes (bubo) 332
  muscle 478–9
ACE inhibitor 440, 471–2
acetaminophen (paracetamol) 32, 33
  overdose 564
acetylsalicylic acid 32–3
  not in malaria 81
  overdose 562
acid, swallowed 564
acne vulgaris 549
acute, defined 9
acute diarrhoeal disease 360–6; *see also*
  gastroenteritis
acute necrotising ulcerative gingivitis/
  periodontitis 227
acute psychotic reaction 579
acute surgical abdomen 596–7
addiction 32, **382–3**, **565–6**, **575**
adjustment disorder 578
admission notes 21, 571
adrenal gland 504
adrenal insufficiency 504
adrenaline
  in allergy/anaphylaxis 44, 614
  in asthma 294–7
  in bleeding nose 283
aetiology 7, 16, 37
AFB (acid fast bacilli)
  in leprosy 127, 141
  in TB 101, 108
  in *Mycobacterium ulcerans* ulcer 537
African trypanosomiasis 181–4
AIDS
  definition 236
  see HIV infection 216–61

airborne spread 53, **124**
airway block 285, 606
albendazole 338, **355**
albinism 551
albuminuria: *see* proteinuria 455
alcohol and alcoholism 382–3
alcohol, standard measure 397
algid malaria (shock) 73, 82
alkali, swallowed 564
allergic reaction 44–5, 614
  causing shock 466–70
  treatment 44–5, 614
allergic rhinitis 284
aluminium acetate 524–6
alveoli 267
American trypanosomiasis 184–7
amlodipine 472
aminoglycosides 60
amitriptyline 581, 583
amodiaquine 85, 93
amoebiasis 371–2
amoebic liver abscess 398
amoebic ulceration, genital 215
amoxicillin/amoxycillin 57, 58, 61
amphotericin B 180
ampicillin 57, 58, 61
amyloid disease 17
anaemia 314–24
anaesthesia in leprosy 130–5, 146–7
analgesic choice 32–4
anaphylaxis 44–5, **614**
anaplastic nasopharyngeal carcinoma
  339
anatomy, defined 7
Ancylostoma duodenale 355
angina pectoris 472–3
angular cheilitis 227
antacids 353
anthrax 536–7
antibacterial drug 55, 56–61
  choice 61
  listed 56–61
  skin preparations 524
antibiotic antagonism 61
antibiotic for eye infections 508
antibiotics with antimalarial activity 100
antibodies 41, 42–5
anticoagulants
  for tests 27
  for treatment 301–2
anti-convulsants 425–6
anti-retroviral drugs (ARD)/therapy
  (ART) 240–55
antidote 562, 564–5
antifolate drugs 97

antigens 41
antihistamine 44–5
anti-inflammatory drugs 146
antivenom 554, 556–7
anuria 453
anxiety disorders 577–9
anxiety management 582–3
aphthous ulcers in HIV 226
appendicitis 375
arbovirus infections 166–72
  arthritis 492
  dengue fever 167
  encephalitis 169
  haemorrhagic fever 170–2
  hepatitis 169–70
  symptoms and signs 166
  yellow fever 169
aromatic diamidine injections 180
artemisinin drugs
  artemether 79–80, 99
    and lumefantrine 79–80, 98, **99**
  artemisinin 99
  artemisinin combination therapy
    (ACT) 77–9, **98–9**
  artesunate 79–80, 98, **99**
    and amodiaquine 79–80, 98, **99**
    with mefloquine 79–80, 98, **99**
arteries 456, 457, 460
arthritis
  acute bacterial 485
  acute in many joints 492
  acute in one or few joints 493
  allergic 492
  aspiration 481–4
  brucellosis 174–5
  chronic in one or few joints 493
  physiotherapy 485, 489, 491–2
  reactive/Reiter's 488
  rheumatic fever 475, 486
  rheumatoid 486
  septic 485
  spine 490–2
  spondyloarthritis 487
  symptoms and signs 481
  traumatic 482
  tropical 488
  tuberculous 489–90
  virus 492
artificial ventilation 607–9
  barrier methods 611–12
Ascaris lumbricoides 354
ascites 602–4
aspiration of joints 481–4
aspirin (acetylsalicylic acid) 32, 33
  overdose 56

asthma 294–7
  from worms 299
astigmatism 519
atheroma 472
atopic dermatitis 548
atovaquone 78, 96
atropine 474, 564
auriscope examination
  ear 267
  eye 507, 509
  nasal 268
autoimmune disease 45
avian influenza 36, 279
azithromycin 60
  for trachoma 513

bacillary index (BI) 141
backache 494
back stiffness 428
bacteria 40, 42
  antibacterial drugs 55–61
bacterial endocarditis 475
bacteriology specimens 29
balanitis 214
barrier methods in artificial ventilation
      611–12
barrier nursing 30, 35
bartonellosis 161–2
Basic Life Support (BLS) 609–11
basic observations 23
bats 560
BCG
  and leprosy 150
  immunisation for TB 124–6
bed nets, insecticidal 87, 100
beef tapeworm 358–9
bejel (endemic syphilis) 536
Benedict's test 455
benign cancer 15, 16
benznidazole 186
benzoic acid and salicylic acid, ointment
      and cream 524–6, 527–9
benzoin lotion or cream 524–6, 549,
      551
benztropine 581
benzyl benzoate 524–6, 538–40
benzylpenicillin 57, 58
betamethasone ointment or cream
      524–6, 548
beriberi 380
beta (β) blockers 471–2
bile 390–1
  test for in urine 445
bile duct 390–1, 399–400
bilharziasis: see schistosomiasis 187–91
biliary colic 399–400
bilirubin 390, 392
biochemistry specimens 29
bipolar mood disorder 576–7
bites and stings 554–60
  animal 560

bats 560
  human 560
Bitot's spots 515
blackwater fever 73, 82
bladder 437
bleeding
  causes in blood 312–13
  causing shock 466–70
  from acetylsalicylic acid 32–3
  from malaria 74, 83
  from septicaemia 64
  in bartonellosis 161–2
  in bowel motions (dysentery)
      melaena 387–9
  in haemorrhagic fever 173–4
  in leptospirosis 156
  in liver disease 396
  in schistosomiasis 187–91
  in snakebite 554–8
  in sputum (haemoptysis) 304–5
  in TB (haemoptysis) 102
  in typhoid fever 173–4
  in typhus fever 164
  in urine (haematuria) 454–5
  in vomit (haematemesis) 386
  into eye 519
  into joint (traumatic arthritis) 482
  into peritoneum/haemoperitoneum
      350, 603
  nose 283
blindness 520
blood clots
  in veins and lung 301–2
  in arteries 472–4
blood: see also bleeding
  anatomy 312
  circulation 456–9
  disorders 314–23
  history and examination of 313
  HIV transmission in 217, 257
  pathological changes 313
  physiology 312
  production organs 313
  tests 26–9, 325–7, 328
blood film 26–9, 312
  examination 312, 328
  malaria 90
  relapsing fever 160, 170
  sickle cell anaemia 321
blood pressure 461
blood pressure, high 470–2
blood sample taking 26–9
blood specimens, laboratory despatch
      291
blood sugar/glucose 499–504
  in diabetes 502–3
  in fitting 426
  in malaria 73, 82
  in unconsciousness 423
blood transfusion 328
  for anaemia 316

hepatitis 394
  and HIV 257
  malarial patients 82
blood vessel damage
  atherosclerosis 472–3
  coronary heart disease 473–4
  diabetes mellitus 500
  hypertension 470–2
  stroke 418–19
blood vessel disease 17, 301–2, 418–19,
      472–5
blood volume, and shock 466–70
Body Mass Index (BMI) 377
body, water content 591
  weight 376–7
boil (furuncle) 532
bone marrow 312
bone diseases 476–9
  destruction by yaws 535
  in leprosy 138
  neoplasm 478
  osteomalacia 477–8
  osteomyelitis 476–9
  sickle cell anaemia 321–3
bowel: see intestine
  sounds 605
box jellyfish 558–9
brain tumour 421–2
breast abscess or ulcer 592–3
breastfeeding, and HIV 217, 258
breath sounds 271–2
breathing 262–5
  rate and type 270
  shortness of breath 305–6
  see also respiratory disease
bronchi 262
  cancer 300
bronchial breathing 272
bronchial narrowing
  asthmatic 294
  in COLD 297
  treatment 294–7
bronchial obstruction 273
bronchiectasis 299
bronchitis
  acute 268
  chronic: see COLD 297–8
bronchodilators 294–7, 308–9
bronchopneumonia 286–7
brucellosis 174–5
bubonic plague 162
Burkitt's lymphoma 338–9

Calabar swellings 544
calamine lotion 524–6
calipers for leg paralysis 418
calcium antagonists 471–2
calcium channel blockers 471–2
cancer (neoplasm) 15, 16
  anaplastic nasopharyngeal carcinoma
      339

benign 15, 16
Burkitt's lymphoma 338–9
malignant 15, 16
  of bone 478
  of brain 421–2
  of breast 552–3
  of conjunctiva 519
  of intestine 375
  of kidney 455
  of liver (hepatoma) **399**, 402
  of lymph node 339
  of oesophagus 384
  of pancreas 401
  of stomach 354
pathology 15
venereal warts 212–13
Candida albicans 529–31
  in HIV 226–7
  vaginal discharge 198, 203
capillaries 456–7
cardiac failure 461–6
cardiac massage 609–11
cardiopulmonary resuscitation (CPR)
  609–11
cardiovascular system: *see* heart and
  blood vessels 456–75
carriers 52
cataract 517
catheterisation and urinary tract
  infection 444, 446
  and septicaemia 64
CATT test 183
CD4 lymphocytes 41
  in HIV 219–20, 223, 250
ceftriaxone 58
cellular immunity 41
cellulitis 538
centipede stings 559
cephalosporins 58
cephalothin 58
cerebral embolism/haemorrhage/
  thrombosis 418–19
cerebral malaria 72, **82**, 413
cerebral tumour in HIV 229
cerebrospinal fluid (CSF) 406
  laboratory examination 435–6
  naked eye examination 408
  rapid diagnostic tests 408–9
cerebrovascular disease 418–19
Chagas' disease 184–7
chancre, syphilis 209
chancroid 210–11
chemicals
  disease from 17, 301, 561–6
  in eye 511
chemotherapy: *see* drug treatment 32,
  55–61
chest
  compression (CPR/BLS) 609–11
  examination of 270–5
  pain 307–8

chickenpox 152
chigoe (tungiasis) 540
Chlamydia pneumoniae and *psittaci*
  causing atypical pneumonia 287–91
Chlamydia trachomatis
  lymphogranuloma venereum 212
  trachoma – eye 512–13
  urethritis 198, 204, 208
  urinary tract infection 443–6
  vaginitis 198, 204, 208
  with gonorrhoea 198
chloramphenicol 55, 58–9, 61
chloramphenicol resistant organisms
  66–7
chloroquine 84–5, 92, 93
  leprosy reaction treatment 146
  malaria prophylactic 93
  malaria resistance to 77–9
  poisoning from 563
chlorpromazine 580–2, 583
  side effects 581
choking 606
cholecystitis 399
cholera 36, 367–70
chronic, defined 10
chronic bronchitis: *see* COLD 297–8
chronic fatigue syndrome 579
chronic liver disease 395
chronic obstructive lung disease COLD
  COAD COPD 297–8
chyluria 336
CIATT test 183
ciprofloxacin 60
circulatory system: *see* heart and blood
  vessels 456–75
cirrhosis of liver 395
classification of disease 16–18
clavulanic acid 58
clawing 135–7
clindamycin 60
clinical staging in HIV 221–3
Clonorchis sinensis 400
clofazimine 143, 145
cloxacillin 58
clubbing of nails 274–5
coal tar solution 524–6, 548
codeine 32, 33
cold (viral infection) 278
cold chain 49–51
colic 593–4
  biliary 399
  genital 594
  intestinal 348
  renal or ureteric **450**
coma 422–4
communicable diseases 52–5
community diagnosis 19
complaints 21; *see also* symptoms
complications 8
concentration (chemical) 12
condoms 259–61

condyloma acuminatum (venereal
  warts) 212–13
condylomata lata (syphilis) 209–10
coneshell stings 559
confusion 572
congenital disease 16
conjunctiva 505–7
conjunctival foreign bodies 511
conjunctivitis 510, 511–13
constipation 389
consultation 9, **31**
contact dermatitis 548
contact history 7, **22**
contagious diseases 52–5
conversion disorder 578
convulsions (fits) 424–6
cornea 505–7
corneal foreign body 513
corneal ulcer 514
coronary arteries 458, 460, 473
coroner 9, 36
cortisone 504
co-trimoxazole 56–61
  in HIV infection 239
cough 303–4
  airborne and droplet spread 124
  in HIV 225
  tuberculosis spread 101
counselling
  in HIV 236–9
  in psychiatric disorders 579, 582–3
counterfeit drugs 34
course 8
crackles 272–3
cretinism, endemic 497
Crimean congo haemorrhagic fever
  170
crust 522–3
Cryptococcus 414–15
  in HIV 224, 229
crystal violet (methylrosanilinium) 524
cutaneous larva migrans 359, 545–6
cutaneous leishmaniasis 176, 178
cyanosis 274
cysticercosis 358
cystitis 443–6
Cytomegalovirus (CMV) 154

dapsone 55, 196, 143, 145
Darrow's solution 364, 369
deafness 302
death notification 36
deep venous thrombosis (DVT) 301
degenerative diseases 17
dehydration **362–6**, **591**
  cholera 367
  diagnosis 362
  infarction crisis 322
  intestinal obstruction 351
  shock from 466
  signs 362, 369

dehydration *continued*
  treatment 364, 366; *see also*
    rehydration
delirium 572
delusion 570
  paranoid 574–5
dementia 568–9, 573
  in HIV 229
dengue fever 167
depression 576–7
  antidepressants drugs 583–4
  in HIV 236
  management 579–83
dermatitis 523, **548**
desert sore 284
dexamethasone 504
diabetes mellitus 499–504
diagnosis 8, 21
diarrhoea
  acute (gastroenteritis) 360–6
  causes and diagnosis 387
  from cholera 367–9
  drugs for 365
  giardia 373
  in HIV 227
  from pellagra 380
  from schistosomiasis 189
  treatment 363–6
dicloxacillin 58
didanosine (ddl) 241, 248, 254
diethylcarbamazine 504
differential diagnosis 8, **25**
digestive system: *see* gastrointestinal
    system 346–89
digoxin 465
dihydroartemisinin 99
diloxanide 372
diphtheria 284
  vaccine 44, 46
direct contact 52
discharge patient procedure 31
disease
  causes of 16–18
  control and prevention 37–9
  notifiable 36
  under surveillance 36
  see also infectious disease
diseases under surveillance 36
disinfection 62–3
dissociative disorder 578
dithranol 524–6, 549
diuretics 397, 448, 465
dizziness 424
dogs 176, 416–17
Donovanosis 211–12
DOTS: *see* tuberculosis, treatment 113
doxycycline 59, 61
dressings 525–6
drinks, standard measures 397
droplet spread 53, **124**
dropsy, epidemic 464

drowning, resuscitation method 612–13
drugs
  abuse 382, 565–6, 575
  cost 35
  counterfeit 34
  definition 31
  disease from 17, 31, 561–6
  fake 34
  non-compliance 35
  routes of administration 31
  traditional 2–3, 35
  treatment 31–5
duodenal ulcer 352
dysentery 387–9
dysphagia 384
dysuria 451–2
dystonic reactions 581

ear
  deafness 302
  discharge from 302
  drum 264, 280
  examination 267–8
  external ear inflammation 282
  foreign body in 282
  middle ear inflammation 281
  pain 302
  signs of disease 266
  symptoms of disease 265
  toilet 282
Ebola fever 170
Echinococcus granulosus 359
ectopic pregnancy and STD 199, 206
  and abdominal pain 594
  and haemoperitoneum **350**
eczema 523, 548
efavirenz (EFV/EFZ) 241, 243, 250
eflornithine 183
elephantiasis 336, 338
emergency resuscitation: *see*
    resuscitation 606–14
emphysema: *see* COLD 297–8
emtricitabine (FTC) 241, 243, 248
enalapril 472, 474
encephalitis 229, 415–16; *see also*
    cerebral malaria 72–3, 82
endemic 52
endemic goitre 496
endocarditis (bacterial or infective) 475
endocrine glands 495–504
Entamoeba histolytica 215, 371
enteric fever: *see* typhoid 173
enteritis necroticans 370–1
Enterobius vermicularis 357
entropion 513
envenomation 554–60
EPI 43, 44
epidemic 52
epidemiology 7, 19–20, 37
epididymitis 196, 199
epigastric pain 348, 352

epilepsy 425–6
epistaxis 283
Epstein–Barr virus (EBV) 154
erythema nodosum leprosum (ENL)
    138, 146
erythromycin 59–60, 61, 100
eschar 165–6
espundia 179
ethambutol 113–20
etiology 7, 16, 37
Eusol solution 524, 525
evidence-based medicine 1
examination 8, **23–5**, 571
exophthalmos 498, 520
'expatriate syndrome' 336
Extensively Drug Resistant TB (EDR-
    TB) 123
external ear inflammation 282
eye, disorders of
  anaesthesia for 507
  anatomy 505–6
  cataract 517
  chemicals in 511
  cloudy anterior chamber 516
  conditions in patients with HIV
    519–20
  conjunctivitis 511, 512
  corneal ulcer 514
  diabetic retinopathy 578
  foreign bodies, conjunctiva 511,
    cornea or sclera 513
  history and examination 506–7
  iritis, acute 515–16
  glaucoma 517
  injuries to 579
  long sight (hypermetropia) 518–19
  macular degeneration 578
  onchocerciasis 516–17
  painful or 'red eye' 520
  retinal detachment 518
  short sight (myopia) 518–19
  strabismus (squint) 518
  stye 509
  trachoma 512
  treatment of 507–9
  visual loss/blindness 520
  vitamin A deficiency 514–15
  xerophthalmia 515
  see also blindness
eyelashes
  infected (stye) 509
  turned-in (entropion) 513

face, tumour (Burkitt's) 238–9
face mask or shield for CPR 611–12
fainting (syncope) 424
fake drugs 34
family history 7, 22
Fasciola hepatica 400
fat, digestion 347, 390, 391
fear 569–70, **579**

febrile fit 72
feet, anaesthetic 135–6, 146–8, 500–1
fever 585–7
    hyperpyrexia 72, 81–2
    in HIV 227, 231
    malarial 59–60, 65–6
    management 71–5, 81–2
    unknown cause 585–7
fibrous tissue, and scar formation 14–15
filarial worms: see filariasis, loiasis,
        onchocerciasis
filariasis 334–8
fish poisoning 565
fit: see convulsions 424–6
flea control 165
flea, jigger (tungiasis) 540
flea vectors 162, 165
flucloxacillin 58
fluid, IV, and heart failure 463, 466
flukes, liver 400
fluoquinolones 60
fluorescein stain 507, 509
fluoxetine 582, 584
fly larvae infestation (tungiasis) 540
fly vectors: see under vectors
folic acid 316, 318, **381**
food, digestion 346–7
food poisoning 282, 283, 360, 373
    Salmonella 373
    toxin type 373
foreign body, cornea 513
formaldehyde gel test for leishmaniasis
        180
formalin for histology specimens 29
frequency of disease 19
fungi 40
    antifungal drugs 55
        Candida 227, 531
        Cryptococcus 224–5, 414–15
        Penicilliosis 225
furosemide/frusemide 397, 448, 465
furuncle 532

gall bladder 391, 399–400
gangrene **17**, 500–1
gastric ulcer 352
gastroenteritis 360–6
    causes 360
    complications 363
    control and prevention 366
    dehydration treatment 364
    diagnosis 362
    epidemiology 360–1
    symptoms and signs 362
    treatment 363–6
gastrointestinal system
    anatomy, physiology 346–7
    history and examination 348–9
    disorders of 349–89
gastro-oesophageal reflux 351
genital lumps, sores, ulcers 198, 204

gentamicin 60
gentian violet (methylrosanilinium)
        524
German measles (rubella) 151, 615
    immunisation 46–9
Giardia lamblia 373
gibbus 105, 106
glands: see endocrine glands; lymphatic
        node
glandular fever 154
glaucoma 517
glibenclamide 502
glomerulonephritis 446–7
glucose-6-phosphate dehydrogenase
    deficiency (G6PD) 84, 96–7,
    324
glucosuria 455
glyceryl trinitrate 473, 474
goitre 496–9
gonorrhoea 198, 203, 205–8
    incubation period 615
    urinary tract infection 443–6
grain toxins 396, 399
granuloma inguinale: see Donovanosis
        211–12
Graves' disease 498–9
griseofulvin 529
groundnuts 396, 399
guarding, abdominal 597–8
Guinea worm 545
gumma 209, 535
gut obstruction 363, 385

haematemesis 386
haematology specimens 29
haematuria 454–5
haemoglobin, HbS 321
haemoglobin estimation 324–7
haemoglobin level 314
    and anaemia treatment 318
haemoglobin physiology 312, 392
haemoglobinuria 73, 82, 454
haemolysis
    and anaemia 315
    caused by primaquine 96–7
    in glucose-6-phosphate
        dehydrogenase deficiency
        (G6PD) 324
    in hyperreactive splenomegaly
        319–21
    in malaria 73, 82
    jaundice from 401–2
    in sickle cell anaemia 321–3
    snakebite 554
haemoperitoneum 350
haemoptysis 305
haemorrhage: see bleeding
haemorrhagic fever 166, 167, 170
haemotology specimens 29
hallucination 570
halofantrine 95

hands
    anaesthetic 135, 146–7
    trembling/shaking/tremor 498
Hanta virus 170
Hartmann's solution 364, 368–9; note
        1, 364
hay fever 284
HBV: see hepatitis viral
headache 427–8
    in HIV 229
health education 1, 2, 5, 30, **37–9**
hearing tests 268
heart and blood vessels
    anatomy and physiology 456–8
    atherosclerosis 472
    coronary heart disease 473
    failure 461–6
    pathology 458–9
    rheumatic fever 475
    symptoms and signs 459–61
    systemic vascular hypertension 470–2
    shock 466–70
heart attack 473–5
heart massage 609–12
height, weight, measurement 376–7
Helicobacter pylori 352
helminths 41
    anti-helminthic drugs 55, **355**
hepatitis
    acute viral 393–4
    differential diagnosis 394
    from drugs 402
    in acute severe infections 401–2
    in haemorrhagic fever 170
    jaundice from 401–2
    urine examination 445
hepatoma 399
Herpes simplex infections **226, 230**
    genital 213–14
    in HIV 226, 230
Herpes zoster 153
    in HIV 231
histology specimens 29
history of present illness 7, **21**–2, 591
HIV infection/AIDS 216–59
    AIDS definition 236
    Anti-retroviral drugs (ARD)/anti-
        retroviral treatment (ART)
        240–55
        after possible HIV infection 253–4
        choice of drugs 242–7
        dose 248–51
        failure to control HIV 253–4
        if infant born to HIV infected
            woman 246
        if patient has hepatitis 247
        if patient has TB 244
        if patient in child-bearing age 245
        if patient pregnant 245
        indications 241–2
        interactions with other drugs 244

HIV infection/AIDS   *continued*
    monitoring efficiency of treatment 247
      side effects of treatment 248–53
    condoms 259–61
    control and prevention 255–8
    counselling 236–9
    differential diagnosis 236
    epidemiology 216–18
    eye conditions 519–20
    management 236
    opportunistic infections 223–33
    prophylactic drugs to stop infections 239, 258
    publications about 216
    symptoms and signs 218–36
    tests 233, 235
    see also AIDS
Hodgkin's lymphoma 339
homicide
    if paranoid delusions 570
    in depression 576
honey skin dressing 526
hookworm 355–7
    treatment 356
hormones 495
hydatid disease 359
hydration assessment 362
hydrochlorothiazide: *see* diuretics
hydrocoele 336
hydrocortisone 504
    ointment or cream 524–6, 548
hyperglycaemia
    in diabetes 501–2
    in psychiatric conditions 568
    in unconsciousness 422–3
hypermetropia 518–19
hyperpyrexia 72, 81–2
hyperreactive malarious splenomegaly 319–21
hypersensitivity: *see* allergy 44–5
hypertension: *see* blood pressure, high 470–2
hyperthyroidism 464, 498–9
hypoglycaemia
    in diabetes 501–2
    in fitting 426
    in malaria 73, 82
    in psychiatric conditions 568
    in unconsciousness 422–3
hypolactasia 374
hypopyon 515–16
hypothyroidism 499
hypoxia 34
    in anaemia 315, 316
    malaria 73, 82
    treatment with oxygen 34
hysteria 578

ibuprofen 33
ileus, paralytic 363, 385

illusions 570
imidazole drugs 528
Immune Reconstitution Inflammatory Syndrome (IRIS) 248, 252
immune system 42–9
immunisation 42–9
    WHO programme (EPI) 44
immunity
    antibodies 41
    cellular 41
    classified 41–9
    humoral 41
    and leprosy type 128–30
    and septicaemia 65–6
immunodeficiency disorder 45; *see also* HIV
immunological reaction
    encephalitis 416
    iritis 515–16
    diabetes mellitus 499
    glomerulonephritis 440, 446–7
    nephrotic syndrome 447
    peripheral neuritis 420–1
    rheumatic fever 475
    rheumatoid disease 486
    thyrotoxicosis 498
    see also allergy 41–5
impetigo 532
incidence of disease 7, 19
incontinence of urine 452–3
incubation periods 54, 615
indinavir (IDV) 241, 251
industrial lung disease 501
infarction crisis in sickle cell anaemia 322
    myocardial 473–5
infection 40–2
    bacterial, drug choice 56–63
    control 54–5
    and cortisone 504
    defence against 41–4
    and lymph node enlargement 42, 333
    and nutrition 376
    opportunistic (HIV) 223–33
    spread 52–4
infectious diseases 52–5
    chemotherapy 55–61
    drug choice 61
    sera/vaccines 42–4, 46–9
infectious mononucleosis 154
infectious period, defined 52
infective endocarditis 475
inflammation **14–15, 16, 42**
    anti-inflammatory drugs
      acetylsalicyclic acid 32, 146
      chloroquine 146
      clofazimine 146
      non-steroidal 33
      prednisolone 504
influenza 278–9
    avian 36, 279

inguinal lymphadenitis 199, 204
    bubo 212
inguinal swelling 603
inhaled foreign body 606–7
injection 31
injury of eye 519
insects 41
insect stings 560
insecticides for
    fleas 164
    lice 165, 540
    mosquitoes 87, 100
    reduvid bug 186
    sandfly 176–7
    ticks 160
insecticide-treated nets (ITNs) 87, 100
insight 570, 571
insulin 392, 499–504
insulin (soluble, clear, unmodified, short acting) 501, 502, 503
insulin depot 501
Intermittent Prophylactic Treatment (IPT) for malaria 88–9
Intermittent Prophylactic Treatment (IPTP) for malaria in Pregnancy 88–9
International Health Regulations (IHR) 36
intestinal
    bowel sounds 605
    cancer 375
    obstruction 351
    paralytic ileus 363, 385
    worms 354–9, 374
intestine 347
    gastroenteritis and intestinal infections 360–73
intracranial mass 421–2
investigations 8, **25**, 26–9
iodine and thyroid 496–8
iodine for skin disinfection 524–5
iridocyclitis 515
IRIS 248, 252
iritis 515–16
iron treatment 317–18
    IMI 318, 327
    IV drip 318, 327
    thalassaemia 324
irukanji syndrome 558
isoniazid 113–20, 126
    poisoning 564
isosorbide dinitrate 474
itch
    anti-itch preparations 524–5
    diagnosis 551–2
ivermectin 337, 540, 543, 544

Japanese encephalitis 169
jaundice 390, 392, **401–2**
jaw
    Burkitt's 338–9
    tetanus 419–20

jellyfish stings 558–9
jigger flea (tungiasis) 540
joint disorders 480–93
 aspiration 482–4, 485
 symptoms and signs 481
 types 480
jugular venous pressure (JVP) 461–3
Junin virus 170

kala azar: *see* leishmaniasis, visceral
  179–81
Kaposi's sarcoma 232
Kernig's sign 428
ketamine 32, 34
ketoacidosis 503
kidney: *see* urinary system
kidney diseases 443–50
kidney failure
 acute 439, 453
 chronic 449
kwashiorkor 17

lactose intolerance 374
lamivudine (3TC) 241, 243, 248
large intestine (colon) 347
large volume spacer 310–11
larva migrans 359
laryngeal infection 286
laryngeal obstruction 285, 606, 613
laryngostomy (emergency) 613
Lassa fever 170
leishmaniasis 175–81
 classification 176
 control and prevention 176–7
 diagnosis
  skin 178
  visceral 179
 in HIV 179, 180, **231**
 skin and mucous membrane 179
 treatment
  skin 178
  skin and mucous membrane 179
  visceral 179–81
 visceral (kala azar) 179–81
length, defined 12
leprosy 127–50
 biopsy 141–2
 cause 127
 classification of types 138–40
  multibacillary 138–40
  paucibacillary 138–40
 control and prevention 149–50
 course and complications 142
 definition 127
 drug side effects 144–5
 epidemiology 127–30
 management 145–50
 multidrug therapy (MDT) 142–3
 nerve changes 133–8
 pathology 127
 skin changes 130–3

skin smears 141
 surgery 148
 symptoms and signs 130–40
 transfer to Medical Officer 149
 treatment 142–8
leptospirosis 156, 170
lesion 10
leucoderma (vitiligo) 551
leukaemia 313, 345
leukoplakia 225
levamisole 355
lice
 control 165
 pediculosis **540**
 relapsing fever 161
 typhus 165
 vectors 161, 165
lidocaine/lignocaine 34
light reflex 268, 280
lignocaine/lidocaine 34
lime, in eye 511
liver
 abscess 398
 anatomy 590
 cancer 399
 cirrhosis 395
 diseases 393–400
 enlarged 401
 examination 392–3
 flukes 400
 functions 390–2
 tender, diagnosis 401
Loa loa/loiasis 544–5
lobar pneumonia 287–91
local anaesthetic, eye 507, **509**
lobes of lung 265–6
Long Lasting Insecticidal Nets (LLINs)
  87, 100
long sight/hypermetropia 518–19
lopinavir/ritonavir (LPV/r) 241, **250**,
  254
louse: *see also* lice above
louse-borne relapsing fever 161
louse-borne typhus 165
lumbar puncture 429–35
lumefantrine 79–80, 98, **99**
lumps 591–2
 genital 192, **198**
 in abdomen 598–602
lungs
 anatomy 262–5
 consolidation 287
 cancer 300
 diseases of 286–302
 disease symptoms and signs 268–75
 flukes in 300
 postural drainage 299
 schistosomiasis damage 189
 tuberculosis 102, 104
lymph node (glands) 331, 332–3
 cancer 338–9

enlarged 340–2
 examination 332–3
 infections and infestations 333–8
 in HIV 223
 plague 162–4
 vessel obstruction 333–8
lymphadenitis
 acute 333
 all causes 340–2
lymphadenitis
 chronic 333
 filarial 334–8
 tuberculous 334
lymphadenopathy 340–2
lymphangitis 333
 filariasis 334–8
lymphatic system 330–45
lymphocytes 41, 219–20, 223, 254
lymphoedema 333–8
lymphogranuloma venereum: *see*
  inguinal bubo 212
lymphoma 339
 in HIV 333
 of orbit/eye 520

macrolides 59
macular degeneration 518
macule 521–2
Madura foot 531
maggot infestation 540
malabsorption, post-infective 374
malaise, diagnosis 588
malaria
 acute attacks 71–4
 blood smear 90
 Burkitt's lymphoma 75, 338
 chronic malaria 74–5
 definition, frequency, cause 68, 69
 diagnosis
  clinical diagnosis 75
  parasitological diagnoses 75
  Rapid Diagnostic Test 91
 differential diagnosis 170
  arbovirus infections 166
  pyrexia of unknown origin (PUO)
   585
  septicaemia Chapter 12
 epidemics 76
 epidemiology 68–71
 hyperreactive splenomegaly 75, 319
 late complications of malaria 75
 nephritic syndrome 75, 447
 prevention and control 87–9
 semi-immunity to malaria 68, 75
 severe/complicated malaria 72–4
  abnormal bleeding 74
  acidosis 74
  acute anaemia/hypoxia 73, 82
  cerebral malaria 72, 82, 413
  complicating bacterial infections
   74

severe/complicated malaria *continued*
  gastrointestinal malaria 73, 82
  hyperparasitaemia 74
  hyperpyrexia 72, 81
  hypoglycaemia 73, 82
  kidney failure 73, 82
  malarial haemoglobinuria
      ('blackwater fever') 73, 82
  pulmonary oedema 73, 82
  shock ('algid malaria') 73,
      82
  stable malaria 76
  symptoms, signs, course and
      complications 71–6
  tests for 75
  unstable malaria 76
malignant, cancer 15, 16
malnutrition 17, 375–83
management, defined 8, 39
mania 577
manic depressive psychosis 575–6
Mantoux test 109–10
marasmus 17
Marburg disease 170
marine stingers 558–9
mass in abdomen 598–601
mass or lump 591–2
mass, unit of measurement 12
measles (morbilli) 151, 615
  vaccine 44, 46–9
mebendazole 355
medical examination 23–5
medical history 7, **21–2**, 591
mefloquine 95
Meibonian cyst 509
melarsoprol 183
melaena 352, 389
melioidosis 161
  in HIV 224
memory loss 573, 578
meningeal tuberculosis 106, **414**
meninges 406
meningism 428–9
meningitis
  acute bacterial 409–13
  cerebral malaria 413
  CSF examination for 408–9,
      435–6
  cryptococcal 414
  in HIV 228–9
  neck stiffness 428
  signs 23, 428
  tuberculous 414
  viral 415
meningococcal vaccine 412–13
mental disorders: *see* psychiatric
      disorders 567–84
mental health 567, 583
metformin 502
methylrosanilinium 524–6
metriphonate 190

methyldopa 471
miconazole ointment or cream
      524–6, 529–31, 548
microbicides 256
microfilaria 334–7, 542–4
mid-arm circumference 377, 379
middle ear inflammation 280–2
milk, lactose intolerance 374
miltefasine 180
minocycline 59, 143
mites 166
mitochondrial dysfunction 253
Mochipo virus 170
molluscum contagiosum 546
  in HIV 231
Monilia 529–31
  in HIV 226–7
  vaginal discharge 198, 203
mononucleosis 154
mood disorder 575–7
morbilli (measles) 151
morphine 32, 34
morphological index (MI) 141
mosquito
  arbovirus infections 166–72
  control 87–9
  filariasis 334
  malaria 68, 71
mosquito nets 87, 100
motor system 405–6
mouth 278, 284–5, 346, 349
  Burkitt's lymphoma 338–9
mouth-to-mouth ventilation 607–9
  barrier methods 611–12
mucocutaneous leishmaniasis 179
multibacillary leprosy 139
Multi Drug Resistant TB (MDR-TB)
      123
Multi Drug Therapy (MDT) for leprosy
      142–5
mumps 155; *see also* 349, 615
murder
  in depression 576
  if paranoid delusions 570
murine typhus 165
muscle
  arthritic symptoms and signs 481
  contracture 481
  examination 24
  infected (pyomyositis) 478–9
mustard oil 464
mycetoma (Madura foot) 531
Mycobacterium ulcerans ulcer 537
  tuberculosis 101–3
Mycobacterium leprae 127–30
myiasis 540–1
myocardial infarction: *see* heart attack
      473–5
myopia 518–19
myositis, tropical 478–9
myxoedema: *see* hypothyroidism 499

nails, tinea 528
narcotics 32–4
  poisoning 564
nausea 384–6
near drowning 612–13
Necator americanus 355
neck muscle strain/torticollis 429
neck retraction 410
neck stiffness 428
nelfinavir (NFV) 241, 251
neomycin and bacitracin ointment
      524–6, 532
neoplasm: *see also* cancer 15, **16**
nephritic syndrome, acute 446–7
nephrotic syndrome 447–9
nerve cells 403–6
nerve damage
  internal nerves
      from Chagas' disease 186
      from diabetes mellitus 500
  peripheral nerves 420–1
      HIV 186, 230
      leprosy 133–8
nervous system 403–36
  anatomy and physiology 403–7
  cerebrospinal fluid (CSF)
      examination 408–9, 435–6
  diagnosis and management of
      common symptoms and signs
      422–8
  diseases affecting 409–22
  symptoms and signs 422–8
nets 87–8, 100
neural leprosy 139
neurasthenia 579
neuritis (neuropathy): *see* nerve damage
      above
neuroleptisation syndrome 580–1
neurotic disorders 570, 577–8
nevirapine (NVP) 241, 243, 249
niclosamide 191, 358
nifedipine 472
nifurtimox 186
night blindness 515
nits (head lice) 540
Nocardia
  in lungs 290
  in CNS 422
  in HIV 224
nodule 521–2
nodule
  in leprosy 132, 138
  in onchocerciasis 542
non-gonococcal urethritis/cervicitis
      208
non-Hodgkin's lymphoma 339
non-steroidal anti-inflammatory drug
      (NSAID) 33
non-typhoid *Salmonella* (NTS) 322, 373
  in HIV 65–7, 227–8
  osteomyelitis 477

nose
  anatomy 263
  bleed 283
  discharge from 302–3
  disease symptoms 265–7
  examination 268
  foreign body 283
  leprosy damage 138
  mucocutaneous leishmaniasis
    (espundia) damage 179
  washing out 393
  yaws 535
notifiable diseases 9, **36**
  influenza (avian) 279
  poliomyelitis 417–18
  SARS 280
  smallpox 36
nutrition and infection 376
nutritional disorders 375, 383

obesity 381
obsessive compulsive disorder 578
obstruction
  laryngeal/tracheal 285, 606, 613
  intestinal 351
obstructive sleep apnoea syndrome
    (OSAS) 285
octopus stings 559
oedema
  generalised (of whole body) 588–90
  localised (of one part of body) 590
oesophagus 346, 351, **384**
ofloxacin 60, 143, 145
oliguria 453
onchocerciasis (river blindness) **542–4**
  eye disease 516–17
opiates 32–4
  poisoning from 564
opportunistic infections in HIV 223–4
oral drug administration 31
oral hairy leukoplakia 226
orchitis 155, 199
organ failure cause of disease 17
oriental sore: *see* skin *under* leishmaniasis
    178
orientation loss 568–9, 572–3
osmotic pressure 12
osteoarthrosis (osteoarthritis) 491
  of spine 492
osteomalacia 477–8
osteomyelitis 476–7, 491
otitis externa 282
otitis media 280–1
ovarian cyst 604
overdoses 561–6
oxamniquine 190
oxygen treatment 34

pain 32–4
painful or red eye 520
pain in abdomen 593–8

pallor 313, 317
palpitations 469, 498
pancreas 391, 400
pancreatic cancer 401
pancreatic juice 347, 400
pancreatitis 400–1, 500
panic disorder 578
pannus formation 512
papule 521–2
paracetamol 32–3
  overdose 564
paraldehyde 420, **424–6**
paralysis 426–7
paralytic ileus 363, 385
paranoia 570, 575
paraplegia 427
parasite: *see specific parasite or disease*
parasite rate in malaria 74–6
paratyphoid fever 173
paromomycin 180
parotitis 155, 161, **349**
past history 7, **22**
pathogenicity 41
pathology 7, 14
paucibacillary leprosy 139
peak expiratory flow meter 310–11
pediculosis 540
pellagra 380, 547–8
pelvic inflammatory disease 199, 204
pelvis
  anatomy 442, 443
  examination 24, 200, 442–5
penicillin 55, 57, 58
penis
  cancer 215
  lumps, sores, ulcers 198, 204,
    208–14
  other important conditions 214–16
  urethral discharge 198, 203
pentamidine 183
pentavalent antimony 180
peptic ulcer 352
pericarditis pain 460
pericardium 460 (Figure 27.7)
peripheral neuritis/peripheral
    neuropathy 420–1
  in HIV 230
peritoneum 348
  shifting dullness (fluid) 603–4
  haemoperitoneum 350
peritonitis 349–50, 596–7
permethrin, cream/lotion 524–6,
    538–40
  as insect repellent/insecticide 87
  treated bed nets 87, 100
persistent generalised lymphadenopathy
    (PGL) 223
personality 570
pertussis: *see* whooping cough 155
pethidine 32, 34
petroleum poisoning 564

phenobarbital 424–6
phenytoin 424–6
phobia 578
photophobia 409
photo-sensitive dermatitis 548
  quinolones 60
  tetracycline 59, other drugs
physical examination 8, **23–5**, 571,
    585–605
physical signs 8, **23–5**, 572–4,
    585–605
physiology 7
physiotherapy
  for chest (including postural
    drainage) 299
  for joint diseases 482–94
  for leprosy 146–8
pigbel (enteritis necroticans) 370–1
pimple 549, 532
pinta 536
piperaquine 100
placebo effect 4
plague 36, 162–4
plantar ulcers 146–8
plasma 312
plasma volume expander 468
Plasmodium: *see* malaria 66
platelets 312–13, 314
pleura 262–3, **266**
  haemothorax 292
pleural aspiration 291–2
pleural fluid 291–3
pleural rub 273
pleuritic pain 307
Pneumocystis jeroveci (carinii) pneumonia
    224
pneumonia
  atypical 288
  broncho- 286–7
  and HIV 224–6
  and influenza 278–9
  jaundice 401
  lobar 287–91
  not resolving (getting better) 291
  opportunistic 224–6
  pneumocystis 224–6, 287–91
  tuberculosis 102, 104
  from worms 298–9, 300
pneumonic plague 162
pneumothorax 293
podophyllum 524–6, 546, 212–13
pointing sign (peptic ulcer) 352
poisons 17, 561–6
  acetylsalicyclic acid 563
  antidotes 562
  corrosive acid 563
  inhaled 561
  injected 561
  isoniazid 564
  opiates 564
  organophosphates or carbamates 564

poisons *continued*
  paracetamol 564
  petroleum 564
  skin absorption 561
poisoning: *see* poisons
  dangerous dosages 563
  seafoods 565
  swallowed poisons 561, 562–4
  unconscious patient 565
poliomyelitis 36, 417–18
pork tapeworm 358–9
portal system 391–2
Post-Traumatic Stress Disorder (PTSD) 578
postural drainage (chest) 299
potassium
  loss causing paralytic ileus 363
  raised in acute kidney failure 453
  needed in cholera 367
  needed in gastroenteritis with paralytic ileus 365
potassium chloride orally 397, 448, 465
potassium chloride IV 503
potassium permanganate 524–6
Pott's disease 106
PR examination 200, 442, 444
praziquantel 190, 422
prazosin 472
pre-eclamptic toxaemia 588–9
prednisolone/prednisone 504
prefixes 10
pregnancy
  backache 494
  chloramphenicol not given 58
  co-trimoxazole not given 57, 61
  ectopic pregnancy and STD 199, 206
    haemoperitoneum 350
  goitre 496
  gonorrheal infection 207
  herpes infection needing caesarian section 213
  HIV 245
  and malaria prevention 89
  and malaria treatment 80, 86
  medical examination 24
  medical history 22
  pelvic examination 24
  rubella 151–2
  syphilis 210
  tetanus, and birth 420
  tetracyclines contraindicated 59
  urinary frequency 451
  vomiting 385
presbyopia 518–19
pressure, defined 13
prevalence 7, 19
prevention 9, 37–9
primaquine 84, 96–7
prions 40
prognosis 9, 26
proguanil 96

propranolol 472, 474
prostatitis 440, 443, 451–2
protein production 392
proteinuria 455
proton pump inhibitors 353
protozoa 40
  antiprotozoal drug 55
provisional diagnosis 8, **25**
psoriasis 549
psychiatric disorders 567–84
  acute organic psychoses 572
  acute psychotic reaction 579
  antidepressant drugs 583
  antipsychotic drugs 583
  anxiety disorders 577
  causes 568–70
  chronic organic psychoses 572
  classification 567–8
  conversion disorder 578
  depression, unipolar mood disorder 576
  depression, bipolar mood disorder 576
  drug and substance misuse 575
  history and examination 571–2
  management of non organic
    psychotic disturbance 582
    psychiatric conditions 57
    psychoses 580
  manic depressive (bipolar) mood disorder 575
  mental health 567
  neurotic stress related disorders 577
  non-psychotic disorder 570–1
  obsessive compulsive disorder 578
  prevention 583
  psychotic disorders 570
  reactions to severe stress 578
  schizophrenia 574
  somatoform disorder 579
  transfer of patient 582
psychological causes of disease 17, 569
psychoses 570, 572–7
pulmonary
  embolism (PE) 301–2
  malaria 73, 82–3
  oedema 461–2
  tuberculosis 102, 104
pulse rate, regularity and volume 460–1
pulse rate slow 170, 474
pupil 507, 515–16, 517
purified protein derivative (PPD) for tuberculin test 109
pus 42
pustule 521–2
PV examination 200, 443
pyelonephritis 443–6
pyloric stenosis 352, 354
pyomyositis 478–9
pyrantel 355
pyrazinamide 113–20

pyrexia: *see* fever
pyrexia of unknown origin 585–7
pyridoxine 114
pyrimethamine 77, 89, 97
pyuria 455

Q fever 156
qinghaosu 98
quadriplegia 427
quinine 79–83, 93–5
  poisoning by 563
quinolones 60

rabies 416–17
ranitidine 353
rash 552
reaction: *see* immunological reaction
rebound tenderness 597
rectal examination 444
reduvid bug 184, 186
referral 9, **31**
reflex action 405
reflux (GOR) 351
rehydration 364, 366
  cholera 368
  dengue haemorrhagic fever 167
  oral solution 366
Reiter's syndrome 208, 488
relapsing fever 158–61, 170
renal diseases 443–455
  failure, acute 439, **453**
  failure chronic 439, 449
  ureteric colic 450
reproductive system 193, 194
  HIV infection 216–59
  other conditions of genitalia 214–16
  pain 196–9, 594
  sexually transmitted diseases 192–214
reserpine 471
reservoirs of infections 52
respiratory disease
  anatomy and physiology 262–5
  diseases of 278–302
  prevention of disease 277–8
  symptoms and signs 265–75, 302–8
  treatment methods 276–8
respiratory system 262–311
resuscitation 606–14
  anaphylactic reaction 614
  artificial ventilation of lungs 607–9
  barrier method to prevent cross-infection 611–12
  cardiopulmonary resuscitation (CPR) 609–11
  emergency laryngostomy 613–14
  inhaled foreign body 606
  near drowning 612–13
retinal detachment 518
retinol treatment 380, 515
retinopathy, diabetic 518
rheumatic fever 468, **475**

rheumatoid disease 486
rhinitis 278, 282, 284
ribavirin 170, 172
rickettsiae 40, 164–6
rifampicin 113–20, 144
Rift Valley Fever 170
Ringer's lactate 364, 368–9
ritonavir 241, 251
river blindness: see onchocerciasis
    516–17, 542–4
roundworm 354
roxithromycin 60
rubella: see German measles 46–9, 151
rule treatment 30

saline solution for skin treatment 526
salivary glands 155–6, 346, 349
Salmonella
    food poisoning 373
    non-typhoid *Salmonella* (NTS) 373
        in HIV 65–7, 227–8
    osteomyelitis 322–3, 447
    septicaemia 66–7
Salmonella typhi 173
salicyclic acid solution and ointment
    524–6
sandfly 176–7
saquinavir (SQV) 241, **251**
SARS 36, 280
scabies 538–40
scales 522–3
scarring 14
schistosomiasis 187–91
    control and prevention 190–1
    differential diagnosis 190
    distribution 187–8
    symptoms and signs 189
    tests 189–90
    treatment 190
schizophrenia 574–5
sclera, foreign bodies 513
scorpion stings 559
scrotal swelling 199
scrub typhus 166
scurvy 381
seafood poisoning 565
seasnake bite 558
seborrhoeic dermatitis 548
sedatives 583
selenium sulfide 524–6, 529
self-poisoning 561
sensory system 404–5
septicaemia 64–7
    differential diagnoses
        infections that cause fever 585–6
    pyrexia of unknown origin 585
    see also
        arbovirus infection 166, Table 17.1
        haemorrhagic fever 170–2
septicaemic plague 162
septic arthritis 485

sera (immunisation) 45–9
seroconversion reaction 219
serology for HIV 233–4
serology specimens 29
serum specimens, laboratory despatch 29
Severe Acute Respiratory Syndrome
    (SARS) 36, 280
severe bacterial infections 64–7
sex, high risk/safe 256–7
sexually transmitted disease (STD)
    192–261
    control and prevention 201–3
    drug treatment 203–4
    symptoms, signs, syndromes 196–200
    tests 200–1
shellfish poisoning 565
shifting dullness 602, 603–4
Shigella 363, **372**
shingles 153
shock 466–70
    malaria 73, 82
    snakebite 554–8
shortness of breath 305–6
short sight (myopia) 518–19
SI units 12
sickle cell anaemia 321–3
sight, loss of 520
sight testing 507
signs 8, **23–5**, 572–4, 585–605
sinuses 263
sinusitis 283
skeleton 476
skin
    anatomy and physiology 521
    biopsy 141–2
    common symptoms and signs 551–3
    diagnosis 523, 551–3
    diseases 526–53
    examination 521–3
    itch 551–2
    lesions 521–2
    pathology 521–3
    rash 552
        in viral diseases 153
    treatment 523–6
    ulcer diagnosis 522–3
skin smear (leprosy) 141
skin snip (onchocerciasis) 543
sleeping sickness: see trypanosomiasis,
    African 181–4
'slim disease' 227–8
smallpox 36
smoking and lung disease 277
snails 187–91
snakebite 554–8
sodium thiosulfate 524–6, 529
somatoform disorders 579
spacer for inhaled drugs 309–10
specific agents of infection 19, **40–1**
specific interrogation 7, **22**
specimens, preparation and despatch 29

spider bites 560
spinal canal 430
spinal cord 403, 427, 430
spinal pain in chest 308, 492, 494
spine
    anatomy 429–32
    and backache 400–1
    deformity 492
    osteoarthrosis 492
    osteomyelitis 477, 491
    tuberculosis 105, 490
spleen 343–5
    blood cell destruction by 343
    disease symptoms and signs 343–4
    enlarged (splenomegaly) 344–5
    hyperreactive malarious 75, 319
    rate in malaria 76
    ruptured 345
spondyloarthritis 487–8
sporadic 52
sprue 374
sputum 304–5
    AFB test 108–9
    removal from lungs 276
squint (strabismus) 497, 507, 519
Staphylococcus aureus 58
sterilisation of instruments 63
Stevens–Johnson Syndrome **117**
stings 558–60
stomach 346, 351–4; see also
    gastrointestinal system
stomach cancer 354
stonefish sting 558
stools, blood in 387–9
strabismus 497, 507, **519**
streptomycin 60, 61, 113–20
stress 569–70, 582–3
stridor 306–7
stroke 418–19
Strongyloides stercoralis 357
Stuart's transport medium 29, 201, 206
stye 509, **511**
subacute 10
subarachnoid haemorrhage 418–19
substance abuse 382, 565, 575
suffixes 10
sugar
    Candida infection 529
    paste – skin dressing 526
    storage, in liver 392, 499
    sugar diabetes 499–504
    in urine 455
sugar (glucose) in blood
    in diabetes 502–3
    in fitting 426
    in malaria 73, 82
    in psychiatric disorders 568
    in unconsciousness 423
suicide 561, 576
sulfadoxine 56, 77, 89, **97**
    and pyrimethamine 56, 97

sulfamethoxazole 56, 57
  and trimethoprim 56, 57
sulfonamides 56, 57, 97
sulfonylureas 502
sunlight
  cancer producing 15
  causing photo-sensitive dermatitis
    548 if also
      quinolones 60
      tetracyclines 59
      coal tar 525
  in albinism 551
  in pellagra 547
  in vitiligo 550–1
sunscreen 551
suramin 183
surgical abdomen 596–7
surveillance, diseases under 36
swallowing difficulty 384
sweet potato 370–1, 589
swelling
  generalised 588–90
  localised 590
  of all skin 132
symptomatic treatment 30, 32–4
symptoms 7, **21–2**, 585–605
syncope 424
syndrome 10
syphilis 198, 204, 208–10
  bejel 536
  congenital 210
  endemic 536
  pinta 536
  tests 210

Taenia saginata/solium 358
tapeworms 358
TB 101–26: *see* tuberculosis
temperature 13
  above normal 585–7
  below normal 612
tenderness of abdomen 597–8
tenofovir (TDF) 241, 243, **249**
terbinafine 528
tests 8, **25**, 26–9
tetanus 419–20
tetrachloroethylene 356–7
tetracycline 59, 61
  eye ointment 313
thalassaemia 324
thioacetazone 113–20
threadworm 357
throat
  examination of 268
  infected 284
  sore 303
  symptoms of disease 266–7
thrush **529–31**
  in HIV 226–7
  vaginal discharge 198, 203
thyroid gland, diseases of 496–9

thrombosis, deep venous (DVT) 301
thyrotoxicosis 498–9
thyroxine 499
tick paralysis 560
ticks 158, 165
time, defined 13
tinea 527–9
tinea imbricata 528
tinea versicolor 529
toilets 38
tonsillitis 284
torsion 155, 197, 199
torticollis 429
toxaemia 42
toxins 17, 360
toxoplasma infection 155, 229
trachea 262
  infection 286
  obstruction 285, 606
  pain 268, 307–8
trachoma 512–13
traditional healers 2
trandolopril 472
transfer procedure 9, **31**
transfer of psychiatric patients 528
trauma 16
traumatic arthritis 482
treatment
  components of 8, 30
  by drugs 31–4
  nursing care 30
  of pain 32–4
  procedure 30–5
  specific 30
  symptomatic 30
treatment supervision: *see* DOTS
trichiasis 513
Trichomonas vaginalis 198, 203
Trichuris trichiura 357
trimethoprim 86, 97
  and sulfamethoxazole 56, 57
tropical arthritis
tropical myositis 478–9
tropical splenomegaly syndrome
  319–21
tropical sprue 374
tropical ulcer 533–4
trypanosomiasis, African 181–4
  distribution 182
trypanosomiasis, American 184–7
tsetse fly 181
tuberculin test 109–10
tuberculosis 101–26
  abdominal 107
  AFB in sputum 108
    in gastric aspiration 109
  arthritis 106, 489
  BCG 124
  chest X-ray 110
  contact tracing 122
  continuation chemotherapy 115, **116**

contraception if taking rifampicin
  114
definition, cause, pathology,
  epidemiology 101–2
Directly Observed Treatment (DOT)
  112
Directly Observed Treatment Short
  Course (DOTS) 113
droplet and droplet nuclei spread
  101, 124
drugs treatment
  Category I regimen (WHO) 116
  Category II regimen (WHO) 116
  Extensively drug resistant TB (EDR-
    TB) 123
  fixed dose combinations 113
  health education 122
  HIV 111, 121–2
    drug treatment if present 115
    infection 107
    testing 110
  initial intensive chemotherapy 115,
    116
  latent 103
  lymph node 105, 334, 340
    aspiration 110
    biopsy 110
  Mantoux test 109
  meningeal 106, 414
  miliary 107
    spine 105, 490
  Multidrug resistant (MDR-TB) 123
  prevention 123–6
  post primary 102, **103**
  primary 102, **103**
  prognosis if untreated 107
  prophylactic 126
  pulmonary 102–5
    in HIV 225
  side effects and management **118–20**
  skin 537
  standard code for TB drugs 113, **114**
  symptoms and signs 102–8
  tests 108–11
  transfer 123
  treatment 112–23
  treatment category selection 116, 117
  Tuberculin test 109
  urinary tract 105, 443
  vertebral 105, 490
tumour: *see* cancer
tungiasis (fleas) 540
typhoid 173
typhus fever 164–6

ulcer 522–3
  anywhere 552–3
  black (eschar) 165–6, 536–7
  breast 552–3
  corneal 514
  foot 552–3

genitalia 198, 204, 552–3
oral and HIV 226–7
peptic 352
skin 552–3
unconsciousness (coma) 42
unipolar depressive mood disorder
576–7
universal precautions 61–3
ureteric (renal) colic 450
urethral discharge 198, 203, 205–8
urinary system
anatomy and physiology 437–8
diseases of 443–50
diagnostic problems 450–5
pathology 438–40
symptoms and signs 440–4
tests 441–5
urinary tract infection 443–6
colour 454
frequency 450–1
incontinence 452–3
pain 451–2
urine test abnormalities 454–5
urine testing 441, 445
urticaria 549
uveitis 515–16

vaccination 44–9
vaginal discharge 198, 203, 205–8
vaginal examination 200, 443
vaginitis 198, 203, 205–8
varicella (chickenpox) 152
varicella zoster (shingles) 153, 231
vascular cause of disease 17, 301–2,
418–19, 472–5
vasodilators 465
vectors 53
fish 400
fleas 162, 165
flies (chrysops) (loiais) 544
flies (simulium) (onchocerciasis)
542–4
flies, gastrointestinal infections 360–1
trachoma 512–13
lice 161, 165
reduvid bug 184, 186
sandfly 176–7
snails 187–91

ticks 158, 165
tsetse fly 181
see also mosquito
vector spread 53
vehicle spread 53
veins 456–8
venous thrombosis (DVT) 301–2
venepuncture 27
venereal disease: see sexually transmitted
disease
venereal warts 212–13
venomous fish 558
venoms 17; see also bites and stings
554–60
ventilation (breathing) 262–7
artificial 607–9
verapamil 472
verrucae: see warts 546–7
vertebra 429–33, 476
bacterial 491
osteomyelitis of 477, 491
tuberculosis 490–1
see also spine
vertigo (dizziness) 424
vesicle 521–2
viral
load in HIV 220, 254
arthritis 166, 492
meningitis 415
visceral larva migrans 359
visceral leishmaniasis 179–81
viruses 40, 55
visual loss: see blindness; sight 520
vital signs 23
vitamin A deficiency – eye 514–15
vitamins 379–81
ascorbic acid (vitamin C) 381
folic acid 381
niacin 380
pyridoxine (B_6) 381
riboflavin (B_2) 380
thiamine (B_1) 380
vitamin A 379
vitamin B_{12} 381
vitamin D 380
vitamin K 83, 171, 380
vitiligo (leucoderma) 551
voice, hoarseness or loss 303

volume, defined 12
vomiting 384–6
blood 386
and dehydration 362, 364–6
gastroenteritis 360–6
vulva
cancer 215
discharge 198, 203
sores or lumps 198, 204

walking difficulty 426
in HIV 229
warfarin 380
warts (verrucae) 546–7
venereal 212–13
wasting 590–1
water
content of body 591
treatment to make safe 39
weight loss 590–1
wheezing (rhonchi) 273
treatment 294–8
whipworm 357
white blood cells 312–14
white spot (tinea versicolor) 529
WHO flow charts, STD 192
whooping cough (pertussis) 155
and bronchopneumonia 286–7
vaccine 44, 46
worms 41
drugs for 55, 355
wounds, check for 25
and tetanus 419–20
bites and stings 554–60
animals 560
bats 560
human 560
in HIV 231
preparations for treatment of 524–62

X-ray, chest 275
xanthochromia 408
xerophthalmia 515

yaws 535
and syphilis semi-immunity 208
yellow fever 36, 169, 170

zidovudine (AZT/ZDV) 241, 243, **248**